Clinical Nutrition

Clinical Nutrition

Marion Bennion, Ph.D.
Formerly Professor of Food and Nutrition at Brigham Young University

Harper & Row, Publishers

New York   Hagerstown   San Francisco   London

Sponsoring Editor: John Woods
Project Editor: Eva Marie Strock
Production Supervisor: Marian Hartsough
Designer: Karen Emerson
Illustrator: John Foster
Compositor: Bi-Comp, Inc.
Printer and Binder: Halliday Lithograph

Clinical Nutrition

Copyright © 1979 by Marion Bennion Stevens

Library of Congress Cataloging in Publication Data
Bennion, Marion, 1925-
   Clinical nutrition.

   Includes index.
   1. Diet therapy.   2. Nutritionally induced
diseases.   I. Title.   [DNLM: 1. Diet therapy.
2. Nutrition.   WB400.3 S845c]
RM216.B463   616.3'9   78-18214
ISBN 0-06-453526-6

Contents

Preface

Great interest has been expressed in human nutrition during recent years, on both a national and an international basis. A variety of books discussing topics in normal and clinical nutrition have been written for the lay population. The medical literature includes books on clinical nutrition written primarily by and for physicians. Other texts have been aimed chiefly at nursing students. This textbook was written with the dietetic student in mind, although the material should also be of interest to the medical student and students in other allied health disciplines. The theoretical background for giving nutritional care is treated, with lesser emphasis on the skills involved in dietetic practice. This book should be particularly useful to students in coordinated undergraduate programs in dietetics, traditional dietetic programs, and dietetic internships.

The book is organized into six units. Unit 1 introduces the student to the process of giving nutritional care and describes tools to use in this process. A short discussion of food and drug interactions is included in this section. Unit 2 addresses problems of over- and undernutrition, including discussions of obesity, malnutrition, anorexia nervosa, and nutritional anemias. Unit 3 focuses on nutritional problems in times of stress, with discussions of the effects of trauma, surgery, fevers, and burns. Parenteral and tube feeding are discussed in this unit, as are some of the nutritional problems associated with cancer. Unit 4 describes gastrointestinal disorders and their associated nutritional problems. It also includes a discussion of food allergies. Unit 5 treats various matabolic abnormalities. Diabetes mellitus, liver disorders and alcohol metabolism, hypoglycemia, and gout are discussed. Unit 6 discusses cardiovascular and renal disorders with associated nutritional problems.

The text is documented with a number of pertinent references; these are listed at the end of each chapter. However, the coverage of topics was not meant to be exhaustive. Chapters 5, 13, 15, 17, 21, and 24 include references that are appropriate for use with clients receiving nutritional care. Study questions are included for each chapter as a guide to the student in organizing the major points discussed.

This book is a result of many years spent in the classroom with dietetic students, in both traditional and coordinated undergraduate programs. I wish to thank these many students for their contributions to this manuscript and for the stimulation and enrichment they have added to my life.

Provo, Utah   Marion Bennion

UNIT 1

Introduction to Nutrition Care

1

Nutritional Assessment and Care

Clinical nutrition has been defined by Butterworth (1975) as "that branch of the health sciences having to do with the diagnosis, treatment, and prevention of human disease caused by deficiency, excess, or metabolic imbalance of dietary nutrients." The wide-ranging character of this definition implies that clinical nutrition is of vital importance to all members of society. Nutritional care is the application of the science of nutrition to the health problems or potential problems of people. These people may be hospitalized with severe and extensive medical problems, or they may be apparently healthy individuals within a community. Nutrition is of importance both in the medical setting and the preventive arena.

Several professionals may be involved, directly or indirectly, with the nutritional care of people. The clinical nutrition research scientist is expanding the frontiers of knowledge and furthering understanding of optimal nutritional care. Some physicians, through special interest and training, have developed specialized expertise in clinical nutrition. Some of these are affiliated with medical schools. There are not enough physicians with this background, however, to touch all medical schools. As Krehl (1976) pointed out, physicians, in general, appear to be inadequately trained to provide in-depth consultation to their patients regarding nutrition and dietary recommendations. All members of the health team—including the physician, nurse, dietitian, social worker, pharmacist, physical therapist, medical technologist, and health educator—are concerned with nutritional care in terms of the nutritional effects on the patient and the interaction of these effects with other medical problems. However, registered dietitians are the only professionally educated group whose primary concern is the application of nutrition science to the health care of people (American Dietetic Association, 1974). Clinical dietitians must recognize this important role and use their expertise in giving nutritional care where appropriate as they work with the physician and other members of the health team for the direct benefit of the client.

The giving of nutritional care by the clinical dietitian involves dietary counseling, which has been defined as "the process of providing individualized professional guidance to assist a person in adjusting his daily food consumption to meet his health needs" (Community Nutrition and Diet Therapy Joint Committee, 1969). It has been suggested that the process of diet counseling involves three activities—interviewing, counseling, and consulting—defined by a committee of the Diet Therapy Section of the American Dietetic Association (1975) as follows:

> *Interviewing* is the gathering of information and/or data. Expert interviewing requires training and experience, since accurate, selective information is basic to effective counseling.
>
> *Counseling* is listening, accepting, clarifying, and helping the client to form his own conclusions and develop his own plan of action. The focus is on the client. An effective diet counselor must be able to guide the client's thinking, focus on objectives, and interpret and evaluate information accurately and effectively. The counselor translates for the patient the regimen prescribed by the physician.
>
> *Consulting* involves developing plans or proposals for a client, based on observations and evaluations. The consultant also has the responsibility to enhance the knowledge and understanding of the person seeking help.

This chapter discusses, from a general point of view, some important parts of the process of giving nutritional care. Chapter 2 includes a discussion of tools that may be used in this process. The remainder of the book focuses on discussions of specific disease conditions or abnormalities for which dietary modification and nutritional adjustments are helpful as part of total treatment and care.

1.1 Role of the Dietitian and the Health Care Team

The roles of dietitians are becoming increasingly varied and complex. The American Dietetic Association (A.D.A.) Position Paper on Education for the Profession of Dietetics (1971a) defined four specialty areas in dietetics as:

1. A *general practitioner of dietetics:* a person who is a specialist in the general application of dietetics. This is a person qualified to assist the extended-care facility or the small hospital, probably either as a part-time dietitian or as a dietetic consultant.
2. An *administrator of dietetic services:* a person competent in the management of complex food service operations using a systems approach and integrating nutrition principles; an executive who participates in defining objectives, formulating policies, and who employs all the tools of business management, automation, creative planning, and delegation.
3. A *clinical nutrition specialist:* a person with expertise in nutritional treatment. One who can evaluate the nutritional status of a person, plan his nutritional care, and direct implementation of the plan. Such a specialist would work with other members of the health care team but would accept responsibility for the diet prescription and the patient's nutritional care.
4. A *nutrition educator:* a person proficient in education, motivation, and counseling techniques whose primary role is the improvement of nutrition care to the general population in the community.

Qualifications shared by each of these specialty roles are:

1. Knowledgeable about the principles of nutrition
2. Highly skilled in communication
3. Devoted to conceptual thinking and adept in the application of its products
4. Oriented to research; participating in research and applying the results to the clinical delivery of nutritional care

In the early years of the profession of dietetics, dietitians usually worked autonomously in relatively isolated areas of the hospital, defining their own functional roles and having little communication with physicians or other health personnel (Schiller, 1973). Hospital administrators commonly viewed dietitians as specialists in the "art of feeding" without recognition by colleagues of competence in the "science of nutrition" (Foster, 1975). The dietitian's role has changed from these early images and is continuing to change in the direction of the A.D.A. definitions. Schiller (1974a and b) studied the role of the clinical dietitian as perceived by both dietitians and physicians. Both groups agreed that the dietitian should ideally be a "full and equal member" of and make a positive contribution to the health team. However, there were some differences in the ways that physicians and dietitians viewed the dietitian's role in decision-making processes. Physicians agreed that the dietitian should provide information for the physician. However, there was not a strong consensus among physicians that the dietitian should assist in such decision-making activities as attending medical rounds, contributing to discussion during rounds, initiating dietary prescriptions, and recommending diets following medical evaluation. The dietitian's conception of his or her own role did include these activities. Both groups perceived incongruity between ideal role and actual performance of the dietitian. Dietitians perceived lack of time as the primary reason for deficiencies in role performance, although lack of education, restrictions of hospital policy, and shortage of trained personnel were more important deterrents to ideal performance than were limitations imposed by physicians. Dietitians, and other professionals as well, should constantly examine their roles and performance and implement appropriate objectives for improvement.

The team concept in health care has been widely discussed in recent years. It implies that professional health personnel—physicians, nurses, dietitians, and other therapists—work together in planning, prescribing, implementing, and evaluating patient care (Robinson, 1974). The patient is also an important member of the team and patient involvement promises to improve the quality and quantity of health care available (Etzwiler, 1972). However, the physician is still ultimately responsible for the medical care and treatment of the patient, both morally and legally, and the very nature of an allied or paramedical profession requires a subordinate relationship to the physician (Schiller, 1973). In practice the health care team seldom functions ideally, but the physician is relying more and more on the expertise of allied health professionals as the knowledge explosion demands more than any one practitioner can retain (Foster, 1975).

It is apparent that when services are provided, many physicians are willing and even anxious to allow dietitians to accept a great deal of responsibility for nutritional care of patients (Schiller, 1973). A 1-year trial of prescribing diets by a dietitian was conducted at Yale-New Haven Hospital in Connecticut (Lawler, 1973). The dietitian assigned to this project in a 30-bed medical division (1) reviewed the medical record of each new admission, (2) interviewed the patient and obtained a brief dietary history before recommending a diet, and (3) counseled the patient regarding any dietary modification needed. She reviewed the medical records daily in order to initiate dietary changes when it seemed appropriate. The concept of dietitians prescribing diets was found to be feasible in this pilot study, although some problems were encountered. The chief difficulties involved the reluctance of some physicians to permit the dietitian to determine the dietary order and the need to provide coverage for the unit when the dietitian was off duty. The major advantages for the patients included less restrictive diets in many instances and an opportunity for nutritional counseling earlier during the hospital stay. This resulted in better preparation for discharge.

A high level of responsibility for nutritional care of patients, including the writing of dietary prescriptions, requires a clinical dietitian who is well prepared professionally. It assumes not only a knowledge of the patient's dietary history and evaluation of his nutritional status, but an understanding of the influences of the pathologic condition and of various therapies on the nutritional status. Dietitians must work within the health team in giving this type of nutritional care. They must be available in the patient areas to make daily rounds and consult with other team members. They must make appropriate notations in the medical record. Dietitians must change the dietary prescription when significant alterations in symptoms or laboratory findings warrant a change. Since this process is very time-consuming, the clinical nutrition specialist must delegate more routine duties to other members of the supportive personnel team, which includes dietetic technicians and assistants. This role of the clinical dietitian is the ideal toward which the profession is moving. Even though full responsibility for prescribing diets is not presently part of the role of most dietitians, they can participate to a marked degree in directing the nutritional care of patients by making recommendations to the physician and effectively communicating to all members of the health care team (Robinson, 1974; American Dietetic Association, 1975). Most dietitians would do well to assume an aggressive role in health care (Etzwiler, 1972).

Dietetic professionals, along with other health professionals, have become increasingly aware of the need to engage in self assessment to ensure quality in the delivery of nutritional care. Federal legislation has mandated peer review for hospital care directed by the physician. There may be occasions where it is desirable for dietetic professionals to evaluate the performance of other dietetic professionals on an objective basis. Guidelines for evaluating dietetic practice have been published by the American Dietetic Association (1976).

1.2   Model for Giving Nutritional Care

The American Dietetic Association's Position Paper on the Nutrition Component of Health Services Delivery System (1971b) states that

> *in its broadest sense, nutritional care is provided to the general population through studies of food consumption and nutritional health, mass education, and food assistance programs. As applied to patient care, it has the same components (assessment of food practices and nutritional status, nutrition education, and food assistance) plus dietary counseling and the service of appropriate food. These nutritional care services must be combined and coordinated to meet individual needs.*

The term *nutritional care* therefore, can be used in reference to both group feeding and individual care. In this chapter the concept is developed primarily in terms of the care of individual clients by the clinical dietitian.

The giving of nutritional care is basically a problem-solving process. Its essential elements are (1) assessment, (2) planning, (3) implementation, and (4) evaluation (Kocher, 1972). A model for the process of giving nutritional care is:

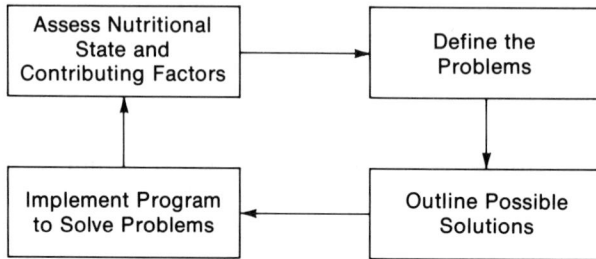

```
┌─────────────────────┐          ┌─────────────────────┐
│ Assess Nutritional  │  ──────▶ │   Define the        │
│ State and           │          │   Problems          │
│ Contributing Factors│          │                     │
└─────────────────────┘          └─────────────────────┘
           ▲                                 │
           │                                 ▼
┌─────────────────────┐          ┌─────────────────────┐
│ Implement Program   │ ◀─────── │ Outline Possible    │
│ to Solve Problems   │          │ Solutions           │
└─────────────────────┘          └─────────────────────┘
```

This is a model of a continuous cycling process. The first step is a data-gathering process in which the nutritional status of the client is assessed. All relevant data are collected. The planning step includes (1) arriving at a clear and concise definition of the nutrition-related problems of the client, after an analysis of the data gathered in the assessment step, and (2) outlining possible solutions to the specific problems. The implementation step involves setting up a program that includes possible solutions to the specific problems. The evaluation step is another assessment of the nutritional state to see if the program has solved or is solving the nutrition-related problems. This begins the cycle again. If nutritional problems are still present, they are reassessed, redefined, other possible solutions outlined and implemented, and the results again evaluated. As long as the client is being followed, this cycling process of giving nutritional care should be continued.

The assessment process includes the collection of all data that are relevant to the nutritional state of the client. Data may be gathered from interviews with the client, the client's family and friends, and other health professionals working with the client; the medical record with reports of medical history, physician's examination, laboratory and other tests, and notes of other health team members; and observation by the clinical dietitian of the physical state of the client. Some physical and clinical signs of good or poor nutrition may be readily observable, whereas others may require more careful testing.

The planning process involves the organization of all data collected in such a way that the real problems can be clearly defined. With experience, this organization process will occur almost automatically, even while data are being gathered. Some problems may be easily defined, but others are more elusive, and several clues may need to be put together to clarify them. The *basic underlying* problem should be sought and possible solutions proposed from this base. A number of alternative solutions should be developed and the most feasible ones selected for implementation. The client should be involved in the process of recognizing problems and selecting possible solutions, as well as in the implementation process, if long-term results are likely to be successful. In the final analysis, the client has the most control over her own nutritional state and is responsible for maintaining it. The clinical dietitian is a counselor who helps the client find her nutritional problems and solve them. Education, directed by the clinical dietitian, is an essential part of this problem-solving process. Both counselor and client are also involved in the continuing evaluation process.

1.3   Assessment of Nutritional Status

A nutritional assessment process has been part of regional or national nutritional surveys of public health programs for many years. A United States Interdepartmental Committee on Nutrition for National Defense (ICNND) was established in 1955 for the purpose of giving assistance to foreign countries on nutrition problems. ICNND assisted with many nutritional appraisal or assessment programs throughout the world (Schaefer and Berry, 1960). Attention was later called to nutrition problems within the United States, and the Ten-State Nutrition Survey was conducted in 1968 to 1970 (Department of Health, Education and Welfare). A plan for ongoing nutrition assessment of the United States population was implemented in the U.S. Health and Nutrition Examination Survey (HANES), and the first nutrition survey under this program was conducted between May 1971 and June 1974 (Department of Health, Education and Welfare, 1974 and 1975; Lowenstein, 1976). The results of a number of limited nutrition surveys are also reported periodically in the scientific literature (Burrill and Schuck, 1962; Driskell and Price, 1974; Sims and Morris, 1974; Armstrong, 1975). More recently, malnutrition has been reported among hospitalized patients and procedures for assessing the nature and extent of nutritional abnormalities in this group have been suggested (Butterworth and Blackburn, 1975; Blackburn et al., 1976).

Methodology

Nutritional assessments or surveys usually include three major parts: (1) dietary studies, (2) biochemical measurements, and (3) clinical and anthropometric evaluation. The results from all three approaches are evaluated together in drawing conclusions from the survey or assessment. Some components of each approach are important to use in the assessment of the nutritional status of either individual clients or population groups.

Dietary Studies.   Dietary studies are used to determine the sources and the amounts of nutrients consumed by individuals or population groups. This information can be used to evaluate present programs or to determine the need for various intervention procedures. On an individual basis where diet counseling will follow, dietary studies will also provide a basis for developing a diet pattern appropriate for the individual's needs and preferences.

The type of dietary information collected may vary from a very rough estimate of food intake to a detailed history, depending upon the purpose of the study. Population surveys often have used a 24-hour recall of food intake as the dietary study, although questions have been raised concerning the validity of this method (Madden et al., 1976). The 24-hour recall is not likely to be useful for a clinical dietitian working with clients, especially in the hospital. If the dietary information collected by a clinical dietitian is to be related to clinical and biochemical measurements and observations, it will need to include an estimate of nutrient intake over a significant period of time. Some type of dietary history, which includes a usual pattern of food intake and estimates of the frequency of consumption for various types of food, is usually taken by the dietitian in interviews with the client and/or family members. From this information, a rough estimate of nutrient intake may be made and used in diet counseling.

When food intake is greatly limited over a period of time, as frequently occurs in the presence of severe or chronic illness, suboptimal nutritional status will be obvious. However, with slight deficiencies in dietary intake and estimated nutrient intakes that are somewhat less than Recommended Dietary Allowances, signs of malnutrition may or may not be apparent. Some reasons for this include (1) differences in nutrient requirements among individuals; (2) additional factors such as concurrent disease or genetic effects that modify an individual's absorption, utilization, requirement, destruction, or excretion of nutrients; (3) the skill of the individual obtaining dietary information and the degree of cooperation and memory of the subject; and (4) the present state of knowledge in the field of nutrition and the ability to detect subclinical deficiencies (Christakis, 1973).

Biochemical Measurements. Laboratory tests allow an objective and reasonably precise method of assessing nutritional status. Blood and urine are the usual biological materials tested for indications of malnutrition. Laboratory measurements may detect marginal nutritional deficiencies in individuals before clinical signs appear, particularly when dietary histories are questionable or unavailable. The medical team, however, should approach the treatment of apparent subclinical nutritional deficiencies in a rational and intelligent way. Factors other than dietary may contribute to low blood or urine levels of a nutrient by interfering with absorption, transport, or utilization in body cells and should be recognized (Pearson, 1962). The reproducibility and reliability of various biochemical tests should also be considered when evaluating results.

The following biochemical indicators of nutritional status may be of value under various conditions (Christakis, 1973; Blackburn et al., 1976):

1. Protein status: serum proteins, particularly albumin, transferrin, and total iron-binding capacity; cellular immune system, indicated by total lymphocyte count and delayed cutaneous hypersen-

sitivity to common recall antigens; urinary urea nitrogen excretion and nitrogen/creatinine ratios; and ratios of specific amino acids in plasma.

2. Minerals: hematocrit, hemoglobin, serum iron; plasma-bound iodine; plasma magnesium, zinc, and possibly other trace elements. Measurement of trace elements in hair samples may be useful in some cases.

3. Water-soluble vitamins: serum ascorbic acid; urinary thiamin excretion and red blood cell transketolase (thiamin-requiring enzyme); urinary riboflavin excretion and possibly red blood cell glutathione reductase (increase in activity due to addition of flavin adenine dinucleotide); urinary N'-methylnicotinamide excretion; plasma or red blood cell folacin; and plasma vitamin B_{12}.

4. Fat-soluble vitamins: serum vitamin A and beta-carotene; and serum vitamin E.

5. Other substances in serum: cholesterol and triglycerides; glucose; hormones, as insulin and glucagon.

Laboratory tests are expensive for a hospitalized patient, and many hospital laboratories are not equipped to routinely determine many of the nutrients. Information on serum and urinary levels of vitamins usually will not be available on a patient. Serum proteins, cholesterol, and hematocrit or hemoglobin appear routinely in medical records. Selected biochemical measurements are included in nutritional assessment of population groups.

Clinical and Anthropometric Evaluations. Physical signs and symptoms can be valuable aids in detecting nutritional deficiencies. In children, stature and weight are among the most important indices of nutritional status and should be accurately determined (Department of Health, Education and Welfare, 1971). Measurement of head and chest circumference is also recommended for infants and preschoolers (Christakis, 1973). Growth curves are commonly used as reference standards for infants and children. New growth charts were published in 1976 by the National Center for Health Statistics and Center for Disease Control, U.S. Department of Health, Education and Welfare. Measurements that fall between the 25th and 75th percentiles on these charts are likely to represent normal growth. Observations of a child's growth over a period of time are important in long-term nutritional assessment. Information about the developmental level of a young child and an evaluation of the level of feeding skill are helpful in assessing his or her nutritional status.

In both adults and children, an indication of body fatness is an important part of nutritional assessment. Standard height/weight tables are often used in estimating overweight or obesity. However, measurement of skinfold thickness gives a better assessment of body-fat content. The thickness of subcutaneous fat over the triceps muscle and at the subscapular site are

Table 1.1   PHYSICAL SIGNS ASSOCIATED WITH MALNUTRITION*

Body Area	Normal Appearance	Signs Associated with Malnutrition
Hair	Glossy; luxuriant; not easily plucked	Lack of natural shine; dull, dry, thin, sparse; color changes; easily plucked
Face	Skin color uniform; smooth, pink, healthy appearance; not swollen	Skin color loss; skin dark over cheeks and under eyes; flakiness of skin on nose and mouth; swollen face
Eyes	Bright, clear, shiny; no sores at corners of eyelids; membranes pink and moist; no prominent blood vessels	Eye membranes pale; Bitot's spots; redness and fissuring of eyelid corners; dry and roughened conjunctivae (xerosis); dull or scarred cornea
Lips	Smooth; not chapped or swollen	Redness and swelling of mouth or lips (cheilosis), especially at corners of mouth (angular fissures and scars)
Tongue	Deep red in appearance; not swollen or smooth	Swelling; scarlet and raw; magenta color; smooth; swollen sores; hyperemic and hypertrophic papillae; atrophic papillae
Teeth	No caries; no pain; bright	May be missing or erupting abnormally; gray or black spots (fluorosis); caries
Gums	Healthy; red; do not bleed; not swollen	"Spongy" and bleed easily; recession of gums
Glands	Face not swollen	Thyroid enlargement; parotid enlargement (cheeks swollen)
Skin	No rashes, swellings, dark or light spots	Dryness (xerosis); follicular hyperkeratosis; flakiness; skin swollen and dark; red swollen pigmentation of exposed areas (pellagrous dermatosis); excessive lightness or darkness of skin; petechiae; lack of fat under skin
Nails	Firm, pink	Spoon-shape (koilonychia); brittle, ridged nails
Muscular and skeletal systems	Good muscle tone; some fat under skin; can walk or run without pain	Muscles have "wasted" appearance; baby's skull bones are thin and soft; round swelling of front and side of head (frontal and parietal bossing); swelling of ends of bones (epiphyseal enlargement); beading of ribs; persistently open anterior fontanelle; knock-knees or bow-legs; bleeding into muscle; person cannot get up and walk properly

* Adapted from Christakis, G. (ed.). 1973. *Nutritional Assessment in Health Programs.* Washington, D.C.: American Public Health Association.

most commonly measured. Assessment of body fatness is discussed more completely in Sec. 4.2.

A simple but accurate method of assessing the skeletal muscle compartment can be made by measuring the mid-upper arm circumference. The calculation of mid-upper-arm-muscle circumference can be made from the arm circumference and the skin-fold measurement of subcutaneous fat. Measurement of urinary creatinine height index also indicates the status of muscle stores (Butterworth and Blackburn, 1975).

Physical signs that may be associated with malnutrition are described in Table 1.1. Few clinical signs of nutritional deficiency are specifically due to the lack of one particular nutrient. Several nutrient deficiencies may contribute to one symptom. Environmental factors (such as excessive heat or sun, wind, or cold), lack of general personal hygiene, and cultural factors can contribute to physical signs that are also associated with malnutrition. Any physical finding that suggests a nutritional abnormality should be considered a clue rather than a diagnosis and pursued further (Christakis, 1973). A study reported by Leevy et al. (1965) of 120 randomly selected low-income patients in a municipal hospital revealed a reduced serum level of two or more vitamins in 59 percent of the subjects and apparent clinical signs of hypovitaminosis in 35 percent. However, no correlation could be established between the presence or degree of hypovitaminemia and clinical signs of vitamin deficiency. Clinical abnormalities were often absent despite marked reduction in serum levels of vitamins. Physical signs, usually attributed to specific vitamin deficiencies, were occasionally observed without significant reduction in serum levels of these vitamins. When clinical methods for detecting nutritional deficiencies are used in a cautious manner along with dietary and biochemical methods, they are valuable in assessing the nutritional status of either individuals or communities (Christakis, 1973).

The Hospitalized Patient

Although there are wide differences among hospitals in the United States, dependent upon size, sponsorship, types of services, and nature of affiliations with educational institutions, they are all basically concerned with the struggle against disease and suffering. Scientific and technological developments have invaded the hospital in recent years and, as in much of modern life, the threat of dehumanization has in many instances become a reality for the hospitalized patient (Knowles, 1973). Thus, the hospital environment has an emotional impact on the patient, with many anxiety-provoking aspects. If a patient does not adapt to the hospital environment, important clinical changes can result, including effects on the cardiovascular and endocrine systems and psychological responses that can influence the course of illness (Kornfeld, 1972). The food served to the patient in the hospital may contribute to a sense of isolation and removal from familiar people and things (Shearman, 1963). The patient may not eat because of loneliness, worries about dependent family members at home or about finances, and fear of disability and pain. Failure to eat, for any reason, may contribute to malnutrition that, in turn, can influence the body's response to disease and injury.

Hospital Malnutrition. In recent years, a condition known as "iatrogenic" or "physician-induced" malnutrition has been described among hospitalized patients, particularly those undergoing major surgery. A number of case studies have been presented documenting nutritional neglect (Bistrian et al., 1974; Butterworth, 1974; Enloe, 1974a and b; Butterworth and Blackburn, 1975). Patients often are not allowed any food by mouth for 3 or more days; they are given 5 percent glucose intravenously and no oral or parenteral vitamin supplements while they receive expensive and elaborate diagnostic studies, complex drug programs, or specialized surgical procedures. The resulting malnutrition, which may develop even in obese subjects, has often gone unrecognized. If recognized, it usually can be effectively treated, if not by oral food consumption, then by appropriate parenteral therapy that supplies a source of nitrogen to control loss of visceral protein and muscle tissue.

The presence of malnutrition in hospitalized patients may delay wound healing, increase susceptibility to infection, and significantly affect the hospital course while having a direct bearing upon morbidity and mortality. Some hospitals are now providing special nutrition support services to ensure proper nutritional care. Before a regimen for nutritional support of a depleted patient can be formulated, however, it is necessary to assess the present nutritional status to determine the nature and extent of the malnutrition. Procedures and suggested standards for nutritional/metabolic assessment have been published by Blackburn et al. (1976) and by Butterworth (1975).

Procedures for Assessment. Assessment is made of (1) lean body mass, (2) fat stores, and (3) visceral protein in the following ways:

1. Lean body mass (body weight minus body fat)
   (*a*) Measurement of mid-upper-arm circumference, which is used, along with measurement of triceps skin-fold, for the calculation of mid-upper-arm-muscle circumference (muscle circumference = mid-upper-arm circumference in cm minus $\pi \times$ skin-fold measurement in cm). The diameter of the humerus is assumed constant. Muscle circumference is decreased in protein-calorie malnutrition.
   (*b*) Measurement of creatinine/height index as an indication of muscle stores and, therefore, a sensitive indicator of degree of protein depletion. The 24-hour urinary excretion of creatinine is generally related to total muscle mass, although it tends to be higher with high dietary intake of lean meat. The creatinine excretion of patients with protein-calorie malnutrition is less than normal persons.
2. Fat stores
   (*a*) Measurement of triceps skin-fold with appropriate calipers gives a reasonable estimate of body fat (see Sec. 4.2).
   (*b*) Measurement of height and weight gives an indirect indication of fat stores unless there is excessive edema present. Rapid weight loss in the hospital usually reflects loss of protein tissue, however, since adipose tissue is lost more slowly.

3. Visceral protein
   (a) Measurement of secretory proteins—serum albumin, transferrin, and total iron-binding capacity (TIBC). Severe depression of these proteins may occur in acute protein malnutrition (kwashiorkor-like state).
   (b) Estimation of cellular immune system by total lymphocyte count and delayed cutaneous hypersensitivity to common recall antigens such as *Candida*. Skin tests are read at 24 and 48 hours. Greater than 5 mm is considered positive, and one positive test indicates intact immunity. Cell-mediated immunity is an important host defense system against infection and is decreased in acute protein malnutrition.
   (c) Measurement of 24-hour urinary urea nitrogen excretion and estimation of nitrogen balance. The following formula may be used to estimate nitrogen balance, assuming a constant nitrogen excretion for skin plus fecal plus urinary nonurea nitrogen as 4* g.

Nitrogen balance = (protein intake in g ÷ 6.25) − (urinary urea N + 4*)

Nitrogen balance will become more negative as the loss of body protein increases.

Two types of malnutrition have been reported to be most common in hospitalized patients undergoing stress, starvation, and physical trauma. (1) Protein malnutrition (adult kwashiorkor) is characterized by loss of visceral protein, with decreased serum albumin, transferrin, and TIBC. It may occur even in obese patients, and no associated weight change may be apparent because of accompanying edema. Depression of cellular immunity is also generally present. (2) Protein-calorie malnutrition (marasmus) describes the obviously malnourished, underweight patient. There is loss of muscle and fat stores with decreased arm-muscle circumference and skinfold thickness. Depression of visceral protein parameters may also occur but is usually less pronounced.

1.4 Nutritional Care Plans

A written plan for the nutritional care of a patient is a management tool to help ensure that appropriate care is given. Since it provides a written record of the care given, the plan improves communication among those who participate in this process. The nutritional care plan is one component of an overall plan of care for the patient and is the component for which the dietitian is primarily responsible. Some dietary departments may use a specific form for recording the development and implementation of a nutritional care plan. An example of this type of form is shown in Fig. 1.1.

In developing a nutritional care plan, the steps outlined in the model

Meals:	AMT	C	P	F		AMT	C	P	F		AMT	C	P	F	
Meat															
Bread															
Fat															
Fruit															
Milk															
Veg. A															
Veg. B															
Sub Total	B					L					D				
Between Meals															
Sub Total	10					2					HS				
TOTAL							MEAL		PATTERN						

Height		Weight	(Ideal)	Patient Diagnosis
Age	Dr.			

Diet PTA

Date	NUTRITION CARE PLAN	Date Achieved

Date	PROGRESS NOTES	Beverage:	LIKES	DISLIKES
		B		
		L		
		D		
		Special Problems:		
		Nourishment:		
		10		
		2		
		8		

Room:	Name:	Selects:	Diet:

Fig. 1.1 A form for recording dietary information and nutrition care plan for hospitalized patients. (Courtesy of Utah Valley Hospital, Provo, Utah.)

for giving nutritional care are followed. Background data are first collected in the assessment process. Pertinent results of the dietary history are recorded on the form being used for the plan. Appropriate nutrition-related notes from the medical record are also recorded. These may in-

DIETARY HISTORY

DIETARY EVALUATION SUMMARY

HISTORY: Social, Med.

FOOD	Daily Serv.	Weekly Serv.
Milk		
Cheese		
Eggs		
Meat, Poultry, Fish		
Legumes, Nuts		
Vegetable—green, yellow		
Citrus Fruit, Tomato		
Other Fruit, Veg.		
Cereal grains, breads—enrich.		
Fats		

Estimated Intake — Compared to RDA

	K Cal	CHO	Pro	Fat	Vit. A	Vit. C	Folic A	Nia.	Ribo.	Thia.	Ca	Fe
RDA												
Intake												

Lab Data:	Hb	Hct	K^+	Na^+	BUN	FBS	Chol	Trigly	Uric A		Enzymes

Medications:

Fig. 1.1 (cont'd.)

clude information from the medical and social history that has a bearing upon the patient's food intake or ability to modify his or her food habits, laboratory data and medications that have nutritional significance, height, weight, and diagnosis or medical problems. An estimate of nutrient adequacy, based upon the diet history, should be recorded on the form. Also, particular food likes and dislikes of the patient should be noted.

The next step is to analyze all the data collected and clearly define the problems. After considering alternative solutions to the problems, specific objectives of the nutrition care plan should be recorded on the form, with the current date. The patient should be included in the process of developing the objectives, as appropriate. An individualized diet pattern may also be developed and recorded.

As nutritional care is given, progress notes will be recorded daily on the form, along with the appropriate dates. As the outlined objectives are achieved, this should be noted on the form. If reassessment and evaluation show a need to change the objectives, the new objectives should be indicated. The nutritional care plan, therefore, is a graphic record of the patient's nutritional care during his or her hospitalization. Notes may also be made on recommendations following discharge from the hospital or other health facility. The nutritional care plan may be used in an outpatient nutrition clinic if the patient is followed there. It may, in some cases, be retained in the dietary department for reference if the patient is readmitted to the facility at a later date.

1.5   Interviewing and Counseling

One factor that contributes to discontent or dissatisfaction among patients with doctors and among doctors with lack of cooperation by their patients is poor communication between doctor and patient. This is an important area of medical care, and clarification of the process is desirable to better prepare medical students. For this reason, doctor-patient communication was studied at the emergency clinic of Childrens Hospital in Los Angeles by Korsch and Negrete (1972). They used audio tape recordings for 800 first-time patient-doctor interactions. After the visit, the patient (usually the mother of the child treated) was questioned concerning what she had expected from the visit and what her reactions were. A final follow-up was then done within 14 days to learn whether she had complied with the physician's instructions. The researchers analyzed the contents of the tapes for communication clues.

Results of this study confirmed that the language used by the physicians was often too technical for their patients. A reference to "incubation period" was taken by one mother to signify the length of time the sick child was to be kept in bed. Another mother, who was told that her child would be "admitted for a work-up," did not realize that he was to be hospitalized. When one mother was told by the physician that he would have to "explore," she had no idea he was talking about surgery. In more than half of the cases studied, the physician resorted to jargon. The most common complaint of mothers who were not satisfied by the visit was that the physicians showed too little interest in the mothers and their great concern for their children. Many mothers felt that they did not have an opportunity or were not encouraged by the physician to reveal important information about their child's illness. In a number of cases, the physician failed to provide a clear diagnostic statement and often offered no prognosis. In some cases, there was a complete breakdown of communication.

From interviews with the mothers, it was found that 40 percent were highly satisfied, 36 percent moderately satisfied, 11 percent moderately dissatisfied, and 13 percent highly dissatisfied with the visit. Their specific reactions, however, were even less favorable. Almost half of them were still wondering when they left the physician what had caused their child's illness. On follow-up it was found that 42 percent of the mothers had carried out all the doctor's medical advice, 38 percent had complied only in part, and 11 percent not at all. The other 8 percent had not received any prescription or advice. There was a substantial correlation between the mothers' expressed satisfaction with the doctor's behavior in the visit and their compliance with the doctor's instructions.

The communication shortcomings found in this study reflect a pattern that is apparently common among many health workers, including dietitians. Attention to effective communication could make a valuable contribution to the quality of health care for the general population. In the area of food and diet, where long established patterns of eating exist, it is essential that the dietitian communicates effectively with the client. Otherwise, desired change in behavior is not likely to occur. In the final analysis, communication is the transfer of meanings from one person to another. According to Brill (1973), meanings are transferred in such a way that a commonness of understanding and participation results; the transferrence occurs through "what we are," through attitudes and feelings as well as ideas, and by both verbal and nonverbal means.

What is counseling? Ohlson (1973) pointed out that the dictionary recognizes both a noun and verb form of the word "counsel." As a verb, *counsel* is defined as "to give or offer counsel or advice, to advise." As a noun, the definition is "interchange of opinions; consultation, deliberation." *Counseling* is defined as "giving or taking of counsel," thus emphasizing the latter meaning involving interchange. The giving of counsel may be a passive process. However, this is of little value where change in behavior is desired. Advice on diet is only effective when the client understands, accepts, and practices it. Therefore, the first precept in dietary counseling, according to Ohlson, must be that the counseling interview should include an active interchange between the counselor and the person being counseled. When the client makes a definite commitment to apply the advice as changed behavior, the interview can be considered successful.

Counseling may be considered a two-part process (Danish, 1975), although these processes overlap. The first part involves the development of rapport, empathy, and a trusting relationship. In the second part, strategies and techniques for bringing about specific behavior change are directed at the client's problems. The particular knowledge and skills about food, food composition, food buying and preparation, recipes, nutritional science, disease pathology, diet modification in disease, and relationships of food to health are learned in various ways by the student of dietetics in the class-room, laboratory, and clinical setting. In the second part of the counseling process, this knowledge is readily organized and applied to an instructional model, adapted for the particular client. The first part of the process is much more difficult to teach and has received less emphasis in dietetic education. It involves the development of a "helping relationship." Danish and Hauer (1973a,b) published a set of manuals, one for the lay leader (a) and one for the trainee (b), as a basic training program that attempts to develop helping skills.

Combs et al. (1971) suggested that the helping relationship is a special one which differs from the usual kinds of relationships people encounter in their daily lives. In most ordinary relationships, both parties are seeking personal enhancement. In the helping relationship, one party decides to set aside her or his own needs temporarily to help another. The helper is not a passive object in the helping relationship. By the way the helper behaves, he "structures" the relationship to help the client discover what the helping encounter is and how to use it most effectively. The helper gives direction to the process of helping. He does this by (1) serving as a model for the client (in the case of the dietitian, a vital, healthy, well-nourished model), (2) reinforcing or rewarding that which is fruitful in the helping dialogue, and (3) suppressing explorations in undesirable directions. According to Brammer (1973), the helping relationship is dynamic; it is constantly chang-ing at verbal and nonverbal levels. The relationship is the chief means for meshing helper problems with helper expertise. Helping in a professional relationship takes place between a person who has a special problem and another person skilled in techniques to decrease or alleviate that problem. The relationship can be established in the first meeting. It is, therefore, important for the health professional who may see a client only once as well as for those who may see a client on a continuing basis. Purtilo (1973) sees a helping relationship, on a professional or therapeutic level, as a personal but not an intimate relationship. It should result in self-dependence on the part of the client.

What makes an effective helper? Combs et al. (1971) suggested that although the professional helper must know her subject, this does not guarantee successful professional work. Neither are there particularly "right methods" of helping others. The effects of stimuli on human behav-ior are not mechanical or chemical responses like a prod with a pin. The professional helper must respond instantaneously and uniquely in the in-terchange with the client and must constantly adjust in this interaction, as appropriate. She must be a thinking, problem-solving person, and the pri-mary tool with which she works is the effective use of self. Thus, according to Combs et al., since the self on each individual is unique, the search for a common knowledge or a common method in the helper is hopeless. The professional helper does respond in a helping relationship, however, ac-cording to a program or pattern. The basis of this program is the helper's values, beliefs, and purposes. The effective professional helper will have (1) specific beliefs about his subject, about what people are like, and why they behave as they do; (2) personal feelings of adequacy; and (3) purposes and approaches oriented toward people and toward aiding or assisting them. Combs et al. look at learning to use the self as an effective instrument in the helping relationship as a matter of personal discovery and a problem in *becoming*—as, *becoming* a dietitian. In the final analysis, it must be a personal thing. However, the *becoming* process may be helped by interaction with the ideas of others, both verbal and written.

Some guidelines for diet counseling to enhance the effectiveness of the "active interchange" were developed by the Diet Therapy Section of the American Dietetic Association (1975). They suggest basing effective methods of counseling on the (1) reason(s) for the session, i.e., therapeutic treatment, general nutritional assessment, nutrition education, and so on; (2) skills and resources of the counselor; and (3) motivation, needs, and interest of the client.

Background knowledge and resources for diet counseling should include:

1. Having an objective—knowing what is expected and why
2. Having certain basic knowledge, including
   (a) Subject matter
   (b) Awareness of self and knowledge of client—physiologically, psychologically, socially, economically
   (c) Familiarity with a variety of methods and techniques for collecting and processing food intake information
   (d) Knowledge and skill in the use of resources and aids, including illustrative or educational tools and community services
   (e) Familiarity with the educational process—how people learn
3. Having appropriate skills, including:
   (a) Competency in diet calculations
   (b) Training and experience in diet history-taking
   (c) Ability to listen actively
   (d) Ability to establish rapport with clients and coworkers
4. Having a plan for accomplishing objectives

The Diet Therapy Committee (1975) also offered some suggestions on the interview itself.

1. Introduce yourself. Be friendly. Talk with the client about the purposes of the visit—hers, the referring agent's, yours. Include family members whenever possible during the initial and follow-up visits.
2. Find our from the client what the physician has discussed with her with regard to her prescribed diet.
3. Describe what you are going to do, and why.
4. Check with the client about usual statistics, such as height, weight, and age, even though this information is available in the medical

record. Find out what the client's occupation is and where she eats her meals. This provides the client an opportunity to become accustomed to the situation and to you; it is also an opportunity for you to begin to know your client and to establish rapport.

5. Obtain a typical day's intake. The purpose of this is to gain some idea of the client's food patterns, amounts eaten, and habits.

6. Ask about specific foods and food groups in terms of frequency of intake and amounts eaten. This may be accomplished through the diet-history technique or any other appropriate method, such as a review of a diet record the client has prepared prior to the counseling session or a self-administered questionnaire. Be thorough. This information is used in evaluating and interpreting the diet, as well as for review in follow-up visits. It is also important in correlating other medical or social information and for writing meaningful notes in medical records and reports.

7. Give the client something to do while you summarize, estimate (or calculate), and evaluate the information on food intake. Have pertinent literature available for her to read, or you might even have her help with the calculations of nutrients.

8. Discuss the results of the evaluation with the client. By this time, she should be an active participant, with some insight into what she will need to do. And, the counselor has had the opportunity to become well acquainted with the client.

1.6   Nutrition Instruction and Education

The dietitian-counselor is in the business of education, specifically nutrition education. An important part of the process of translating the science of nutrition into the skill of furnishing optimal nourishment for people involves teaching. A position paper of the American Dietetic Association on Nutrition Education for the Public (1973) defined nutrition education as the "process by which beliefs, attitudes, environmental influences, and understandings about food lead to practices that are scientifically sound, practical, and consistent with individual needs and available food resources." Leverton (1974) defined nutrition education as "a multidisciplinary process that involves the transfer of information, the development of motivation, and the modification of food habits where needed. It must form the bridge that carries appropriate information from the research and development laboratories to the public, the ultimate user." She further pointed out that the results of nutrition education must be satisfying to the recipient and bring to him returns of discernable value. Nutrition education is a process of producing planned behavioral change in the area of food consumption and eating habits.

The dietitian/nutritionist has a responsibility to participate in nutrition education programs for persons who are healthy as well as those who are ill. There are many opportunities for instruction on normal nutrition as part of preventive medicine in the community. There are also many occasions where hospitalized patients who are not on modified diets may well profit from sound dietary advice and counsel. Effective nutrition education projects, titled "Food for Fun and Thought," were reported in a hospital for children by Rickard and Farnum (1974). A game used as a reinforcing agent for nutrition learning and cooking experiences that used a variety of levels of fine and gross motor skills were most successful in this setting.

The Interagency Committee on Nutrition Education developed four basic concepts for use in nutrition education. These concepts, which may be useful in many different situations, are

1. Nutrition is the food you eat and how the body uses it.
   (a) We eat food to live, to grow, to keep healthy and stay well, and to get energy for work and play.
2. Food is made up of different nutrients needed for growth and health.
   (a) All nutrients needed by the body are available through food.
   (b) Many kinds and combinations of food can lead to a well-balanced diet.
   (c) No food by itself has all the nutrients needed for full growth and health.
   (d) Each nutrient has specific uses in the body.
   (e) Most nutrients do their best work in the body when teamed with other nutrients.
3. Throughout life all persons have need for the same nutrients but in varying amounts.
   (a) The amounts of nutrients needed are influenced by age, sex, size, activity, and state of health.
   (b) Suggestions for the kinds and amounts of food needed are made by trained scientists.
4. The way food is handled influences the amount of nutrients in food, its safety, appearance, and taste.
   (a) Handling means everything that happens to food while it is being grown, processed, stored, and prepared for eating.

In working with a client, it is important to evaluate not only his apparent ability to learn but the manner in which he seems to learn best so that necessary instruction may be adapted for a successful outcome in terms of changing behavior (Slowie, 1971). Ginther (1971) reviewed several categories of learners. One set of categories includes the terms symbolic, ikonic, and enactive. The *symbolic* mode of learning involves learning from symbols and abstractions, which are often given verbally. The *ikonic* mode involves imagery and learning from pictures or illustrations. The *enactive* mode emphasizes acting out or manipulating and handling things in the process of learning. A second set of categories of learners includes: stereopath—one who needs structure in learning situations; non-stereopath—one who is independent of authority and undisciplined;

and rational—one who needs little structure but wants to be left to his or her own devices after knowing the problem and the resources available to solve it. The instructional approach in dietary counseling would be different for each type of learner. It is also important, according to Leverton (1974), to assess how much the client *desires,* as well as needs, to know. Some clients may be very interested in learning detailed information about nutrition, whereas others may not be interested in learning more than they need to know to function adequately.

When instruction is part of the nutrition care plan for a client or a group of clients, the following steps are suggested in the design and implementation of that instruction (Project Continuing Education for Health Manpower, 1974):

1. Determine the purpose of the instruction—what specific outcomes are to be achieved; what are the goals and objectives.

2. Select those strategies most appropriate for achieving the goals that have been set or the outcomes to be achieved.
   (a) Relate the instructional techniques to the expected outcomes.
   (b) Select the type and level of instruction best suited to the client.

3. Conduct the actual instruction.
   (a) Develop interpersonal and communication skills; different skills are demanded by different instructional approaches.

4. Determine the actual effects of the instruction that has been offered; evaluate the information.
   (a) Use continuous evaluative information to make adjustments in the focus, pace, and even style of instruction during the process; make corrections the moment they seem necessary (formative evaluation).
   (b) Use summative evaluation to make valid judgments about the outcome.
   (c) Evaluate in terms of changes effected.

The goals or objectives of an instructional program for a client should come from an analysis of the client's needs. General goals may be formulated and then highly specific instructional objectives written. Objectives should be written in such a way that they can be evaluated upon the basis of clarity, assessability—whether or not their accomplishment can be evaluated—and relevance.

If education is defined in terms of changing behavior, the emphasis in instruction should be on participation by the learner. Teaching sessions should be planned so that the client can actively participate and demonstrate that he can do what is expected of him (Vargas, 1971). This then provides an excellent opportunity for evaluating the effectiveness of the instruction.

REFERENCES

1. American Dietetic Association. 1971a. Position paper on education for the profession of dietetics. *J. Am. Dietet. Assoc.,* **59:** 372.

2. American Dietetic Association. 1971b. Position paper on the nutrition component of health services delivery systems. *J. Am. Dietet. Assoc.,* **58:** 538.

3. American Dietetic Association. 1973. Position paper on nutrition education for the public. *J. Am. Dietet. Assoc.,* **62:** 429.

4. American Dietetic Association. October 1974. Fact sheet, nutritional care-dietary counseling.

5. American Dietetic Association. 1975. Position paper on the dietetic technician and the dietetic assistant. *J. Am. Dietet. Assoc.,* **67:** 246.

6. American Dietetic Association. 1976. Guidelines for evaluating dietetic practice.

7. Armstrong, H. 1975. Nutritional status of black preschool children in Mississippi. *J. Am. Dietet. Assoc.,* **66:** 488.

8. Bistrian, B. R., G. L. Blackburn, E. Hallowell, and R. Heddie. 1974. Protein status of general surgical patients. *J. Am. Med. Assoc.,* **230:** 858.

9. Blackburn, G. L., B. R. Bistrian, B. S. Maini, P. Benotti, A. Bothe, G. Gibbons, M. F. Smith, and H. Schlenn. 1976. Manual for nutritional/metabolic assessment of the hospitalized patient. New England Deaconess Hospital, Boston, Mass. 02215.

10. Brammer, L. M. 1973. *The Helping Relationship: Process and Skills.* Englewood Cliffs, N.J.: Prentice-Hall.

11. Brill, N. I. 1973. *Working with People.* New York: Lippincott.

12. Burrill, L. M. and C. Schuck. 1962. Dietary intakes and nutritional status of 28 South Dakota women in two decades of life. *J. Home Econ.,* **54:** 707.

13. Butterworth, C. E. 1974. The skeleton in the hospital closet. *Nutr. Today,* **9** (No. 2): 4.

14. Butterworth, C. E. 1975. The dimensions of clinical nutrition. *Am. J. Clin. Nutr.,* **28:** 943.

15. Butterworth, C. E. and G. L. Blackburn. 1975. Hospital malnutrition. *Nutr. Today,* **10** (No. 2): 8.

16. Christakis, G. (Ed.). 1973. Nutritional assessment in health programs. Reprinted from *Am. J. Pub. Health,* November 1973, Part Two, Vol. 63, by the American Public Health Association.

17. Combs, A. W., D. L. Avila, and W. W. Purkey. 1971. *Helping Relationships.* Boston: Allyn and Bacon.

18. Community Nutrition and Diet Therapy Joint Committee. 1969. Guidelines for developing dietary counseling services in the community. *J. Am. Dietet. Assoc.* **55:** 343.

19. Danish, S. J. and A. L. Hauer. 1973a. *Helping Skills: A Basic Training Program. Leader's Manual.* New York: Behavioral Publications.

20. Danish, S. J. and A. L. Hauer. 1973b. *Helping Skills: A Basic Training Program. Trainee's Workbook.* New York: Behavioral Publications.

21. Danish, S. J. 1975. Developing helping relationships in dietetic counseling. *J. Am. Dietet. Assoc.,* **67:** 107.

22. Department of Health, Education and Welfare. 1968–1970. Ten-state nutrition survey. DHEW Publication No. (HSM) 72–8134.

23. Department of Health, Education and Welfare. 1971. Screening children for nutritional status: Suggestions for child health programs. PHS, DHEW Publication No. 2158.

24. Department of Health, Education and Welfare. January 1974. Preliminary findings of the first Health and Nutrition Examination Survey, United States, 1971–1972: Dietary intake and biochemical findings. PHS, DHEW Publication No. (HRA) 74–1219–1.

25. Department of Health, Education and Welfare. April 1975. Preliminary findings of the first Health and Nutrition Examination Survey, United States, 1971–1972: Anthropometic and clinical findings. PHS, DHEW Publication No. (HRA) 75–1229.

26. Diet Therapy Committee. 1975. Guidelines for diet counseling. *J. Am. Dietet. Assoc.,* **66:** 571.

27. Driskell, J. A. and C. S. Price. 1974. Nutritional status of preschoolers from low-income Alabama families. *J. Am. Dietet. Assoc.,* **65:** 280.

28. Enloe, C. F., Jr. April 1974a. The view from the catbird's seat, Part 1. *Food and Nutrition News,* National Live Stock and Meat Board, **45** (No. 4): 1.

29. Enloe, C. F., Jr. May–June 1974b. The view from the catbird's seat, Part 2. *Food and Nutrition News,* National Live Stock and Meat Board, **45** (No. 5): 1.

30. Etzwiler, D. D. 1972. The patient is a member of the medical team. *J. Am. Dietet. Assoc.,* **61:** 421.

31. Foster, J. T. 1975. A hospital administrator's view of the shared responsibility. *J. Am. Dietet. Assoc.,* **67:** 539.

32. Ginther, J. R. 1971. Educational diagnosis of patients. *J. Am. Dietet. Assoc.,* **59:** 560.

33. Knowles, J. H. 1973. The hospital. *Sci. Am.,* **229** (No. 3): 128.

34. Kocher, R. E. 1972. New dimensions for dietetics in today's health care. *J. Am. Dietet. Assoc.,* **60:** 17.

35. Kornfeld, D. S. 1972. The hospital environment: Its impact on the patient. *Adv. Psychosom. Med.,* **8:** 252.

36. Korsch, B. M. and V. F. Negrete. 1972. Doctor-patient communication. *Sci. Am.,* **227** (No. 2): 66.

37. Krehl, W. A. 1976. Nutrition: Does the physician know enough? *The Professional Nutritionist,* **8** (No. 2): 3.

38. Lawler, M. R. 1973. One-year trial of prescribing diets by a dietitian. *J. Am. Dietet. Assoc.,* **62:** 280.

39. Leevy, C. M., L. Cardi, O. Frank, R. Gellene, and H. Baker. 1965. Incidence and significance of hypovitaminemia in a randomly selected municipal hospital population. *Am. J. Clin. Nutr.,* **17:** 259.

40. Leverton, R. M. 1974. What is nutrition education? *J. Am. Dietet. Assoc.* **64:** 17.

41. Lowenstein, F. W. 1976. Preliminary clinical and anthropometric findings from the first Health and Nutrition Examination Survey, USA, 1971–1972. *Am. J. Clin. Nutr.,* **29:** 918.

42. Madden, J. P., S. J. Goodman, and H. A. Guthrie. 1976. Validity of the 24-hr. recall. *J. Am. Dietet. Assoc.,* **68:** 143.

43. Ohlson, M. A. 1973. The philosophy of dietary counseling. *J. Am. Dietet. Assoc.,* **63:** 13.

44. Pearson, W. N. 1962. Biochemical appraisal of the vitamin nutritional status in man. *J. Am. Med. Assoc.,* **180:** 49.

45. Project Continuing Education for Health Manpower. 1973. *Fostering the Growing Need to Learn.* Rockville, Md.: Bureau of Health Resources Development.

46. Purtilo, R. 1973. *The Allied Health Professional and the Patient.* Philadelphia: Saunders.

47. Rickard, K. and S. Farnum. 1974. Food for fun and thought: Nutrition education in a children's hospital. *J. Am. Dietet. Assoc.,* **65:** 294.

48. Robinson, C. H. 1974. Basic considerations in prescribing diets. *J. Am. Dietet. Assoc.,* **65:** 161.

49. Schaefer, A. E. and F. B. Berry. 1960. U.S. interest in world nutrition. *Pub. Health Rep.,* **75:** 677.

50. Schiller, R. 1973. The dietitian's changing role. *Hospitals,* **47**: 97.

51. Schiller, M. R. and V. M. Vivian. 1974a. Role of the clinical dietitian. I. Ideal role perceived by dietitians and physicians. *J. Am. Dietet. Assoc.,* **65**: 284.

52. Schiller, M. R. and V. M. Vivian. 1974b. Role of the clinical dietitian. II. Ideal vs. actual role. *J. Am. Dietet. Assoc.,* **65**: 287.

53. Shearman, C. W. 1963. *Diets are for People.* Englewood Cliffs, N.J.: Prentice-Hall.

54. Sims, L. S. and P. M. Morris. 1974. Nutritional status of preschoolers. *J. Am. Dietet. Assoc.,* **64**: 492.

55. Slowie, L. A. 1971. Patient learning—segments from case histories. *J. Am. Dietet. Assoc.,* **59**: 563.

56. Vargas, J. S. 1971. Teaching as changing behavior. *J. Am. Dietet. Assoc.,* **58**: 512.

STUDY GUIDE

The roles of dietitians are becoming varied and complex.

1. Describe several specialty areas in dietetics.

2. What is a health care team, and how might a clinical dietitian participate in this team?

3. What type of professional preparation is necessary for a clinical dietitian who assumes a high level of responsibility for the nutritional care of clients, including the writing of dietary prescriptions?

The primary concern of clinical dietitians is the nutritional care of clients.

4. Describe a model for the giving of nutritional care.

5. Describe three major processes or procedures that are part of most nutritional assessments or surveys, and explain how the information collected by each process may be used in evaluation of nutritional status.

6. What is a diet history, and how might it be effectively used by a clinical dietitian?

7. What biochemical measurements are likely to be of value in assessing the nutritional status of an individual or a population and why?

8. Describe several physical signs and symptoms that may indicate some degree of malnutrition in an individual.

9. What is meant by anthropometric evaluation, and how might it be useful in assessing nutritional status?

10. What is likely to be the nutritional status of many stressed and traumatized hospitalized patients and why? What is the clinical dietitian's responsibility for these patients?

11. Describe a procedure for the nutritional assessment of hospitalized patients that has been suggested by Blackburn and Butterworth. Indicate how the clinical dietitian might be involved in this procedure.

12. Describe major characteristics of kwashiorkor and marasmus as they might occur in hospitalized patients.

13. Describe the essential components of a written nutritional care plan and discuss advantages of having a written record.

Interviewing, counseling, and teaching are important components of the overall process of giving nutritional care.

14. What are some likely purposes of interviews involving the dietitian/nutritionist?

15. Why is it important to consider the physical setting in which an interview takes place? Explain.

16. What is a "helping relationship," and what makes an effective helper? How can a clinical dietitian act as a "helping vehicle" for the client?

17. Describe some things that a clinical dietitian might do to ensure that she or he establishes rapport and a satisfactory relationship in an interview with a client.

18. How can the clinical dietitian stimulate the client to self-motivation in changing undesirable dietary practices?

19. Describe and discuss a satisfactory procedure that might profitably be followed in designing and implementing dietary instruction for a client.

2

Tools for Nutrition Counseling

The dietitian/nutritionist must be well prepared, from an educational and professional standpoint, in order to meet the challenge involved in the delivery of good quality nutritional care. As with all professions, there are particular "tools of the trade" in dietetics that are used in giving professional service. These include a working knowledge of food composition and various techniques for organizing and applying this knowledge in the use of food composition tables, exchange lists, and food group guides. Recommended Dietary Allowances (1974) and U.S. Recommended Daily Allowances (U.S. RDA) are additional tools for use in the delivery of nutritional care. Individual nutrient needs must be translated into specific foods and menus for each client requiring nutrition counseling. For the dietitian/nutritionist working in a medical setting, the medical record provides an important tool that will yield essential information for nutritional care. Some basic tools for nutrition counseling are discussed in this chapter.

2.1 Tables of Food Composition

Reliable tables of data on the nutrient composition of foods are invaluable in many areas of nutrition and food science. They are used in the development of national programs and policies, the nutritional evaluation of food supplies and diets, and the development of guides for food selection. Government agencies, food industries, and research workers in many fields make use of the tables. They are an essential tool for the dietitian/nutritionist in giving nutritional care to clients because they allow the practice of dietetics to be a science as well as an art.

Available Food Composition Data

Several countries have developed composition tables for foods used in their regions. The U.S. Department of Agriculture (USDA) has historically been responsible for the development of basic tables of food composition used in the United States. Dr. W. O. Atwater and his coworkers prepared the first major publication in this area, *The Chemical Composition of American Food Materials,* Bulletin No. 28, which was published in 1896 and revised in 1899 and 1906. Other major publications of the USDA on food composition have included (Watt and Murphy, 1970):

1. *Proximate Composition of American Food Materials,* Circular 549, by Chatfield and Adams (1940)
2. Table 5 of *Food Composition in Terms of Eleven Nutrients,* Miscellaneous Publication 572 (1945)
3. *Composition of Foods . . . Raw, Processed, Prepared,* Handbook No. 8, by Watt and Merrill (1950: rev'd ed., 1963)
4. *Composition of Foods Used in Far Eastern Countries,* Handbook No. 34, by Leung, Pecot, and Watt (1952)
5. *Fatty Acids in Food Fats,* Home Economics Research Report 7, by Goddard and Goodall (1959)
6. *Amino Acid Content of Foods,* Home Economics Research Report No. 4, by Orr and Watt (1957)
7. *Folic Acid Content of Foods,* Handbook No. 29, by Toepfer, Zook, Orr, and Richardson (1951)
8. *Pantothenic Acid, Vitamin B_6, and Vitamin B_{12} in Foods,* Home Economics Research Report 36, by Orr (1969)
9. *Nutritive Value of Foods,* Home and Garden Bulletin No. 72 (1977)
10. *Nutritive Value of American Foods,* in common units, Handbook No. 456, by Adams (1975)
11. *Composition of Foods. Dairy and Egg Products.* Agriculture Handbook No. 8–1 (November 1976)
12. *Composition of Foods. Spices and Herbs.* Agriculture Handbook No. 8–2 (January 1977).

The most recent publications, numbers 11 and 12, begin a new sectional looseleaf format that can be more easily revised as new data become available. They include information on nutrients in 100-g edible portions of food, in common measures, and in edible portions of 1 lb of food as purchased. Data from USDA tables are widely reprinted in textbooks and other reference materials.

In the process of developing food composition tables, USDA staff study both the scientific literature and much unpublished work. They then derive figures for the basic tables that are representative of the products on a year-round, country-wide basis. In this process such factors as variety, breed, stage of maturity, seasonal differences, storage, trimming, manufacturing, and preparation practices are considered (Watt and Murphy, 1970).

The use of "nutrition labeling," as regulated by the Food and Drug Administration (FDA), has stimulated the food industry to analyze many of their products for nutrient content. A wealth of data on food composition is thus accumulating. To handle these data, the USDA created a computerized Nutrient Data Bank to "serve as an international repository for data submitted by industry and experiment stations, from government contracts and grants," and from literature search (Watt et al., 1974). This bank will provide a central place for storing and compiling information on food composition and will facilitate the production of new food composition tables.

Another widely used source of food composition data was originally prepared by Bowes and Church in 1937 and was revised in the 12th edition by Church and Church (1975). These tables include data on eight amino acids and fiber, as well as protein, fat, carbohydrate, and several vitamins and minerals. Information is given in terms of measures and weights of portions commonly used. The Food and Agriculture Organization of the United Nations (FAO) also publishes information on food composition, including *Amino-Acid Content of Foods and Biological Data on Proteins,* by the Food Policy and Food Science Service, Nutrition Division (1970).

The dietitian working with computerized menu planning should find useful the 1975 USDA publication, *Food Yields Summarized by Different Stages of Preparation,* Handbook No. 102. It provides data on percentages of refuse from foods "as purchased."

Food composition data periodically appear in the scientific literature as they are reported by various research laboratories. They provide the practicing dietitian nutrient information on such items as convenience dinners and pot pies (De Ritter et al., 1974), foods sold by fast-food chains (Appledorf, 1974), pizza (Kilgore, 1967), newer brands of margarine (Miljanich and Ostwald, 1970), ready-to-eat foods (Standall et al., 1970), and cholesterol content of foods (Feeley et al., 1972). A series of articles giving information on fatty acids in foods has been published in the Journal of the American Dietetic Association by staff members from USDA (Posati et al., 1975a and b; Anderson et al., 1975; Fristrom et al., 1975; Brignoli et al., 1976; Weihrauch et al., 1976).

Accuracy and Limitations of Food Composition Tables

Although food composition tables are valuable to the dietitian when properly used in giving nutrition care, their reliability and accuracy should be considered and their limitations realized. Food samples vary greatly in composition, and data in food tables are often weighted averages. One cannot assume that the food consumed by a client contains the exact nutrient composition listed in a food table. However, these data can be useful in *estimating* nutrient intake as an aid, along with consideration of clinical and biochemical data, in diagnosing and treating nutritional deficiencies. When using any table of food composition, it is important to read the introductory or explanatory information to understand how the data were collected and derived. What were the sources of data? Are the data averages of a small number of food samples? Have variety and growing conditions been considered in data for agricultural products? Are the data representative values for the nation as a whole?

A number of research reports have been concerned with a comparison of calculated versus determined values for various diets or foods. Groover et al. (1967) tested the accuracy of dietary survey methods by comparing estimates of total kilocalories and kilocalories from fat, as calculated from USDA Handbook No. 8 (Watt and Merrill, 1963), with measurements by the bomb calorimeter. When collection of food samples was unsupervised in the field, the dietary calculations were consistently higher than the calorimeter values. The greatest error on total kilocalories was a calculated value of 189 percent more than the determined value. The errors for fat kilocalories were often greater than this, with only 4 of 15 calculated samples coming within ±20 percent of the calorimeter determination. With supervised field collection of food samples, the correspondence between calculated and measured values was somewhat closer than that achieved with the unsupervised collections, but a significant margin of error still remained. The calculations for duplicate diet samples collected in a hospital were more accurate than those collected in the field. For 50 percent of these samples, calculated values for total kilocalories and kilocalories from fat fell within ±20 percent of the measured values. These authors concluded that data from dietary surveys need to be checked with actual calorimetric determinations if quantitative statements are to be made on the correlation of dietary habits with disease. Errors contributing to the differences could have included inaccuracy in data gathered from subjects or in food samples provided, inaccuracy in estimating weights, or errors in analyses.

In a carefully controlled dietary study to evaluate the effects of low-fat, low-cholesterol diets on the reduction of blood lipids in humans, Marshall et al. (1975) compared calculated and analyzed values for daily diets containing 25 percent and 35 percent of kilocalories from fat. Under laboratory conditions for collection of food samples, they found the analyzed values and those calculated from USDA Handbook No. 8 to be exceptionally close, except for calcium. Total calculated kilocalories were within 7 percent to 8 percent of analyzed values. Differences for total protein were between 3 and 5 percent, and differences for total fat were between 8 and 12 percent. Differences for the various vitamins and minerals were somewhat greater than for the proximate components, but they usually were not greater than ±25 percent.

Walberg and Adams (1965) compared analyzed values with calculated values for nitrogen, calcium, phosphorus, sodium, and potassium in constant diets. In all cases the differences between the determined and calculated values were greater than the experimental variance of the determinations. The greatest differences occurred with phosphorus and sodium.

Variation in composition of food, techniques of food preparation, and laboratory analysis were thought to contribute to the differences found.

Water content of food is one of the most variable figures in analyses. For foods of high water content, such as fruits and vegetables, differences between calculated and analyzed values will be greater than for low-moisture foods, such as dry cereal grains and legumes. Fat content of meats and various mixed dishes often varies widely. The variance with vitamins is usually much greater than with proximate analysis, but calculations can still give useful indications of possible deficiency in clinical practice. Data on minerals, particularly trace elements, are more limited in value than data on other nutrients. There are not only differences in content among foods and some problems with laboratory analyses, but major differences in absorption apparently occur. When limitations of food composition data are recognized, however, they can provide a valuable tool for the dietitian/nutritionist in interpreting dietary histories and diagnosing possible nutritional deficiencies. They are also useful in dietary surveys to assess possible nutritional problems in a population and to evaluate the adequacy of feeding institutionalized groups.

Approximate Assessment of Nutrient Intake

A practicing dietitian is expected to have a good knowledge of food composition. In this area the dietitian is an "expert" and should be relied upon for this expertise as a member of the health care team. Knowledge of food composition that will allow a dietitian to make rapid, approximate estimations of nutrient content of foods and diets is gradually acquired when a conscious effort is made to organize and use this information in dealing with clients. Use of exchange lists, prepared by the American Diabetes Association and the American Dietetic Association (1976), allows rapid estimation of kilocalories, protein, fat, and carbohydrate in foods or meals. For use in clinical practice it is also helpful to develop short lists of significant food sources for major vitamins and minerals with rough quantitative approximations. With use these lists will be automatically memorized and provide an important tool for rapid assessment of gross dietary deficiencies.

Examples of such lists are:

Ascorbic Acid
50 mg in
 ½ cup citrus fruit or juice
 ½ cup strawberries
 ½ cup cooked broccoli or Brussels sprouts
 1 cup cooked cabbage, cauliflower, or greens
10 mg in
 ½ cup pineapple or juice
 ½ cup berries
 1 cup other raw vegetables and fruits

5 mg in
$\frac{1}{2}$ cup other cooked vegetables and fruits

Iron

3 to 4 mg in
1 oz liver

2 mg in
$\frac{1}{2}$ cup cooked dried beans
$\frac{1}{2}$ cup cooked greens

1 mg in
1 oz meat, fish, poultry
1 egg
$\frac{1}{2}$ cup enriched or whole grain cereal
1 oz raisins (2 tbs)

0.5 mg in
1 slice enriched or whole grain bread
$\frac{1}{2}$ cup other vegetables and fruits

Index of Nutritional Quality

A tool for organizing nutrient analysis with computer use, called the Index of Nutritional Quality (INQ), was developed by Sorenson et al. (1976). It is based upon the concept of *nutrient density* and compares the nutritive content of a specified quantity of food with its energy content. Computer generated bar graphs can show at a glance the nutritional quality of a food or dietary intake in relation to its caloric content. U.S. Recommended Daily Allowances have been used as the standard in calculating the INQ. This tool has potential for nutrition education programs at all levels.

2.2 Exchange Lists

Using tables of food composition to calculate nutrient intake from menus, diet histories, or individual diet patterns is a laborious and time-consuming process unless the computer is used. For convenience in working with the special nutritional needs of clients, various groupings of similar foods and averaging of nutrient contributions from these food groups have been done for many years. By the 1940s it became apparent that the great diversity in these groupings and methods of developing diet patterns for therapeutic diets, particularly for patients with diabetes mellitus, was interfering with effective communication among health professionals and education of patients. Therefore, a committee was appointed, with representatives from the American Dietetic Association, the American Diabetes Association, and the Chronic Disease Program of the Public Health Service, U.S. Department of Health, Education and Welfare to study the problems and make recommendations. This committee developed a system of exchange lists (Caso, 1950) for use in meal planning (American Diabetes

Association, 1950). Although the exchange lists were designed for use in the calculation of diabetic diets, they have found widespread use in the calculation of other therapeutic diet patterns, especially low-kilocalorie and low-fat regimens. They also offer an effective tool for the rapid estimation of kilocalories, protein, fat, and carbohydrate in records of dietary intake. Since 1950 many changes have occurred in the types of food available on the market, and in the use of fat-modified diet patterns for treatment and/or prevention of coronary heart disease. The exchange lists therefore recently have been revised by committees from the American Diabetes Association, the American Dietetic Association, the National Institute of Arthritis, Metabolism and Digestive Diseases, and the National Heart and Lung Institute of the U.S. Department of Health, Education and Welfare (1976), to reflect these changes and expand the uses of the exchange lists.

The term *exchange* is used in the sense of "substitute" or "trade." Each exchange list includes a number of measured foods of similar nutritive value that can be substituted interchangeably in meal plans. The following six major exchange lists have been designated:

List 1—milk exchanges: nonfat, low-fat, and whole milk

List 2—vegetable exchanges: all nonstarchy vegetables

List 3—fruit exchanges: all fruits and fruit juices

List 4—bread exchanges: bread, cereal, pasta, starchy vegetables, and prepared foods

List 5—meat exchanges: lean meat, medium-fat meat, high-fat meat, and other protein-rich foods

List 6—fat exchanges: polyunsaturated, saturated, and mono-unsaturated

Table 2.1 summarizes the kilocalorie, protein, fat, and carbohydrate values assigned to each exchange list. These figures are weighted averages for the various foods included in each list. The use of the exchange lists on a national basis has simplified patient education and communication among

Table 2.1 NUTRIENT COMPOSITION OF EXCHANGE LISTS

Exchange List	Protein (g)	Fat (g)	Carbohydrate (g)	Energy (kcal)
List 1—milk exchanges	8	trace	12	80
List 2—vegetable exchanges	2		5	25
List 3—fruit exchanges			10	40
List 4—bread exchanges	2		15	70
List 5—meat exchanges	7	3		55
medium-fat meat		omit $\frac{1}{2}$ fat exchange		
high-fat meat		omit 1 fat exchange		
List 6—fat exchanges		5		45

health professionals as they move from one part of the country to another. The booklet presenting the revised exchange lists (American Diabetes Association, 1976) emphasizes the client's need for a nutrition counselor who is a registered dietitian in order for the client to best utilize the exchange lists. A guide for professionals in using the exchange lists has also been prepared (American Diabetes Association, 1977). Throughout the exchange booklet, nonfat or low-fat food items appear in **bold** type. The meat exchanges are subdivided into three groups on the basis of fat content— lean meat, medium-fat meat, and high-fat meat. The patient adjusts the number of fat exchanges in his meal pattern as he makes choices from the various subgroups that differ in fat content. In the listing of fat exchanges, food items that are high in polyunsaturated fat appear in **bold** type. The revised exchange lists thus may be easily adapted for use with diet patterns requiring modification of type or amount of fat.

Table 2.2 presents the foods included in each exchange list. The amount of each exchange for vegetables is ½ cup, and for meat it is 1 oz. For each of the other exchange lists, the specified amount varies with the food. The usual serving size for meat in menu planning is 3 or 4 oz; thus 3 or 4 meat exchanges may be included in one serving. Starchy vegetables are included in the bread list. Each exchange list should be studied carefully, noting the foods included, the amounts of each, and any adjustments on fat exchanges. The exchange lists have been applied to a wide variety of prepared foods by Cinnamon and Swanson (1976) in the booklet "Everything You Always Wanted to KNOW About Exchange Values for Foods".

If the exchange lists are used in planning a low-kilocalorie diet pattern, foods or food mixtures containing large amounts of fat or sugar must be limited because of the caloric restriction. In diabetic diets of normal calorie levels, sugar-containing food mixtures may be limited because of decreased satiety value after 1 or 2 hours and the resulting tendency to overeat and/or the possible hyperglycemia after intake of large amounts of simple sugars. However, as the patient learns to use the exchange lists in planning a diabetic diet, he may be instructed to calculate the protein, fat, and carbohydrate in a recipe, using food composition tables or exchange lists, and assign appropriate exchange values for a measured serving of the recipe. This will increase the variety in his diet and stimulate enjoyment of eating. Food manufacturers may provide nutrient information on their products that will allow them to be used in a diet pattern based on exchange lists. The patient will need instruction from the dietitian counselor on the use of various manufactured foods.

The exchange lists represent average values for the foods included in them. When different choices are made from the lists, the composition of the menus will not be exactly the same. However, use of these lists in clinical practice has demonstrated that the lists are accurate enough for practical purposes. Over a period of time, diet patterns and menus based upon the exchange lists can bring effective results in weight reduction, diabetic control, and so on.

Table 2.2   EXCHANGE LISTS

LIST 1   Milk Exchanges (includes nonfat, low-fat, and whole milk)—1 exchange of milk contains 12 g carbohydrate, 8 g protein, a trace of fat, and 80 kcal. Those items in **bold** are *nonfat.*

Nonfat Fortified milk

Skim or nonfat milk	1 cup
Powdered (nonfat dry, before adding liquid)	$\frac{1}{3}$ cup
Canned, evaporated—skim milk	$\frac{1}{2}$ cup
Buttermilk made from skim milk	1 cup
Yogurt made from skim milk (plain, unflavored)	1 cup

Low-Fat Fortified Milk

1% fat fortified milk (omit $\frac{1}{2}$ fat exchange)	1 cup
2% fat fortified milk (omit 1 fat exchange)	1 cup
Yogurt made from 2% fortified milk (plain, unflavored) (omit 1 fat exchange)	1 cup

Whole Milk (omit 2 fat exchanges)

Whole milk	1 cup
Canned, evaporated whole milk	$\frac{1}{2}$ cup
Buttermilk made from whole milk	1 cup
Yogurt made from whole milk (plain, unflavored)	1 cup

LIST 2   Vegetable Exchanges—1 exchange of vegetables contains about 5 g carbohydrate, 2 g protein, and 25 kcal. This list shows the kinds of vegetables to use for one vegetable exchange. 1 exchange = $\frac{1}{2}$ cup. (Starchy vegetables are in bread exchange list.)

Asparagus	Greens (cont'd.):
Bean sprouts	Mustard
Beets	Spinach
Broccoli	Turnip
Brussels sprouts	Mushrooms
Cabbage	Okra
Carrots	Onions
Cauliflower	Rhubarb
Celery	Rutabaga
Cucumbers	Sauerkraut
Eggplant	String beans, green or yellow
Green pepper	Summer squash
Greens:	Tomatoes
Beet	Tomato juice
Chards	Turnips
Collards	Vegetable juice cocktail
Dandelion	Zucchini
Kale	

The following raw vegetables may be used as desired:

Chicory	Lettuce
Chinese cabbage	Parsley
Endive	Radishes
Escarole	Watercress

Table 2.2 EXCHANGE LISTS (cont'd.)

LIST 3 Fruit Exchanges—1 exchange of fruit contains 10 g carbohydrate and 40 kcal.

Apple	1 small	Mango	$\frac{1}{2}$ small
Apple juice	$\frac{1}{3}$ cup	Melon	
Applesauce (unsweetened)	$\frac{1}{2}$ cup	Cantaloupe	$\frac{1}{4}$ small
Apricots, fresh	2 medium	Honeydew	$\frac{1}{8}$ medium
Apricots, dried	4 halves	Watermelon	1 cup
Banana	$\frac{1}{2}$ small	Nectarine	1 small
Berries		Orange	1 small
Blackberries	$\frac{1}{2}$ cup	Orange juice	$\frac{1}{2}$ cup
Blueberries	$\frac{1}{2}$ cup	Papaya	$\frac{3}{4}$ cup
Raspberries	$\frac{1}{2}$ cup	Peach	1 medium
Strawberries	$\frac{3}{4}$ cup	Pear	1 small
Cherries	10 large	Persimmon, native	1 medium
Cider	$\frac{1}{3}$ cup	Pineapple	$\frac{1}{2}$ cup
Dates	2	Pineapple juice	$\frac{1}{3}$ cup
Figs, fresh	1	Plums	2 medium
Figs, dried	1	Prunes	2 medium
Grapefruit	$\frac{1}{2}$	Prune juice	$\frac{1}{4}$ cup
Grapefruit juice	$\frac{1}{2}$ cup	Raisins	2 tbs
Grapes	12	Tangerine	1 medium
Grape juice	$\frac{1}{4}$ cup		

Cranberries may be used as desired if no sugar is added.

LIST 4 Bread Exchanges (includes bread, cereal and starchy vegetables)—1 exchange of bread contains 15 g carbohydrate, 2 g protein, and 70 kcal. Those items in **bold** are *low-fat.*

Bread

White (including French and Italian)	1 slice
Whole wheat	1 slice
Rye or pumpernickel	1 slice
Raisin	1 slice
Bagel, small	$\frac{1}{2}$
English muffin, small	$\frac{1}{2}$
Plain roll, bread	1
Frankfurter roll	$\frac{1}{2}$
Hamburger bun	$\frac{1}{2}$
Dried bread crumbs	3 tbs
Tortilla, 6"	1

Cereal

Bran flakes	$\frac{1}{2}$ cup
Other ready-to-eat unsweetened cereal	$\frac{3}{4}$ cup
Puffed cereal (unfrosted)	1 cup
Cereal (cooked)	$\frac{1}{2}$ cup
Grits (cooked)	$\frac{1}{2}$ cup
Rice or barley (cooked)	$\frac{1}{2}$ cup
Pasta (cooked), spaghetti, noodles, macaroni	$\frac{1}{2}$ cup
Popcorn (popped, no fat added)	3 cups
Cornmeal (dry)	2 tbs
Flour	$2\frac{1}{2}$ tbs
Wheat germ	$\frac{1}{4}$ cup

Table 2.2   EXCHANGE LISTS (cont'd.)

LIST 4   Bread Exchanges (cont'd.)

Crackers

Arrowroot	3
Graham, $2\frac{1}{2}''$ sq.	2
Matzoth, $4'' \times 6''$	$\frac{1}{2}$
Oyster	20
Pretzels, $3\frac{1}{8}''$ long $\times \frac{1}{8}''$ diameter	25
Rye wafers, $2'' \times 3\frac{1}{2}''$	3
Saltines	6
Soda, $2\frac{1}{2}''$ square	4

Dried Beans, Peas, and Lentils

Beans, peas, lentils (dried and cooked)	$\frac{1}{2}$ cup
Baked beans, no pork (canned)	$\frac{1}{4}$ cup

Starchy Vegetables

Corn	$\frac{1}{3}$ cup
Corn on cob	1 small
Lima beans	$\frac{1}{2}$ cup
Parsnips	$\frac{2}{3}$ cup
Peas, green (canned or frozen)	$\frac{1}{2}$ cup
Potato, white	1 small
Potato (mashed)	$\frac{1}{2}$ cup
Pumpkin	$\frac{3}{4}$ cup
Winter squash, acorn, or butternut	$\frac{1}{2}$ cup
Yam or sweet potato	$\frac{1}{4}$ cup

Prepared Foods

Biscuit 2" diameter (omit 1 fat exchange)	1
Corn bread, $2'' \times 2'' \times 1''$ (omit 1 fat exchange)	1
Corn muffin, 2" diameter (omit 1 fat exchange)	1
Crackers, round butter type (omit 1 fat exchange)	5
Muffin, plain small (omit 1 fat exchange)	1
Potatoes, french fried, length 2" to $3\frac{1}{2}''$ (omit 1 fat exchange)	8
Potato or corn chips (omit 2 fat exchanges)	15
Pancake, $5'' \times \frac{1}{2}''$ (omit 1 fat exchange)	1
Waffle, $5'' \times \frac{1}{2}''$ (omit 1 fat exchange)	1

LIST 5   Meat Exchanges. Items in **bold** are low-fat.

Lean Meat: 1 exchange of lean meat (1 oz) contains 7 g protein, 3 g fat, and 55 kcal.

Beef:	**Baby beef (very lean), chipped beef, chuck, flank steak, tenderloin, plate ribs, plate skirt steak, round (bottom, top), all cuts rump, spare ribs, tripe**	1 oz
Lamb:	**Leg, rib, sirloin, loin (roast and chops), shank, shoulder**	1 oz
Pork:	**Leg (whole rump, center shank), ham, smoked (center slices)**	1 oz
Veal:	**Leg, loin, rib, shank, shoulder, cutlets**	1 oz
Poultry:	**Meat without skin of chicken, turkey, Cornish hen, guinea hen, pheasant**	1 oz
Fish:	**Any fresh or frozen**	1 oz
	Canned salmon, tuna, mackerel, crab, and lobster	$\frac{1}{4}$ cup
	Clams, oysters, scallops, shrimp	5 or 1 oz
	Sardines, drained	3

Table 2.2   EXCHANGE LISTS (cont'd.)

LIST 5   Meat Exchanges (cont'd.)

Cheeses containing less than 5% butterfat	1 oz
Cottage cheese, dry and 2% butterfat	$\frac{1}{4}$ cup
Dried beans and peas (omit 1 Bread Exchange)	$\frac{1}{2}$ cup

Medium-fat Meat: For each exchange of medium-fat meat omit $\frac{1}{2}$ fat exchange.

Beef:	Ground (15% fat), corned beef (canned), rib eye, round (ground commercial)	1 oz
Pork:	Loin (all cuts tenderloin), shoulder arm (picnic), shoulder blade, Boston butt, Canadian bacon, boiled ham	1 oz
	Liver, heart, kidney, and sweetbreads (these are high in cholesterol)	1 oz
	Cottage cheese, creamed	$\frac{1}{4}$ cup
	Cheese: Mozzarella, ricotta, farmer's cheese, neufchatel, parmesan	1 oz
		3 tbs
	Egg (high in cholesterol)	1
	Peanut butter (omit 2 additional fat exchanges)	2 tbs

High-fat Meat: For each exchange of high-fat meat omit 1 fat exchange.

Beef:	Brisket, corned beef (brisket), ground beef (more than 20% fat), hamburger (commercial), chuck (ground commercial), roasts (rib), steaks (club and rib)	1 oz
Lamb:	Breast	1 oz
Pork:	Spare ribs, loin (back ribs), pork (ground), country style ham, deviled ham	1 oz
Veal:	Breast	1 oz
Poultry:	Capon, duck (domestic), goose	1 oz
Cheese:	Chedder types	1 oz
	Cold cuts	$4\frac{1}{2} \times \frac{1}{8}''$ slice
	Frankfurter	1 small

LIST 6   Fat Exchanges—1 exchange of fat contains 5 g fat and 45 kcal. To plan a diet low in saturated fat, select only those exchanges that appear in **bold** because they are *polyunsaturated.*

---

*Margarine, soft, tub or stick**	1 ts	Butter	1 ts
Avocado (4" in diameter)†	$\frac{1}{8}$	Bacon fat	1 ts
Oil, corn, cottonseed, safflower,		Bacon, crisp	1 strip
soy, sunflower	1 ts	Cream, light	2 tbs
Oil, olive†	1 ts	Cream, sour	2 tbs
Oil, peanut†	1 ts	Cream, heavy	1 tbs
Olives†	5 small	Cream cheese	1 tbs
Almonds†	10 whole	French dressing‡	1 tbs
Pecans†	2 large whole	Italian dressing‡	1 tbs
Peanuts†		Lard	1 tbs
Spanish	20 whole	Mayonnaise‡	1 ts
Virginia	10 whole	Salad dressing, mayonnaise	
Walnuts	6 small	type‡	2 ts
Nuts, other†	6 small	Salt pork	$\frac{3}{4}$-in. cube
Margarine, regular stick	1 ts		

Adapted from Exchange Lists for Meal Planning, American Diabetes Association and American Dietetic Association, 1976.
* Made with corn, cottonseed, safflower, soy, or sunflower oil only.
† Fat content is primarily monounsaturated.
‡ If made with corn, cottonseed, safflower, soy, or sunflower oil can be used on fat-modified diet.

2.3   Food Group Guides

People tend to think of nutrition in terms of food. Lists of required nutrients with quantities specified for optimum health mean little to the average consumer of nutrition services, although this information is vitally important to the nutrition counselor. Nutrient standards, therefore, have often been translated into food groups with recommended amounts to be consumed from each group.

The first national food guide in the United States consisted of five groups and was written in 1916 by Caroline Hunt, a scientific assistant in the USDA Office of Home Economics. The groups were (1) milk, meat, fish, poultry, eggs, and meat substitutes; (2) bread and other cereal foods; (3) butter and wholesome fats; (4) vegetables and fruits; and (5) simple sweets (Hertzler and Anderson, 1974).

The "basic 7" food groups emerged in 1943 and were published in a 1946 postwar version as the "National Food Guide" by the Human Nutrition Research Branch of the Agricultural Research Service, USDA. In 1956 a new plan with only four groups was presented in the USDA publication "Essentials of an Adequate Diet," and the USDA Leaflet No. 424, "Food for Fitness—A Daily Food Guide," was issued in 1958. This leaflet was designed as a nutritionally reliable teaching device for individuals or families with the groups appearing as (1) milk—2 or more cups for adults and 3 to 4 cups for children; (2) meat—2 or more servings; (3) vegetable-fruit—4 or more servings; and (4) bread-cereal—4 or more servings. Although there is only one group of vegetables and fruits in this food guide, the need to select dark green leafy and deep yellow vegetables for vitamin A value and fruits or vegetables that are good sources of ascorbic acid is emphasized. The minimum number of servings from each food group combined should provide a nutritionally balanced diet that approaches the RDAs for protein, calcium, vitamin A, thiamin, riboflavin, niacin, and ascorbic acid. Adjustments in serving sizes can be made to meet the differing nutritional needs of nearly all individuals. Additional kilocalories can be obtained by choosing more than the minimum number of servings from the four food groups. The requirement of women for iron will not be met by the recommended amounts. In fact, it is difficult to meet this requirement by using ordinary foods (Hertzler and Anderson, 1974).

The food group guide is basically a nutrition education tool. It provides a simple plan for teaching consumers how to choose an adequate diet. The four-group Daily Food Guide is adapted to the usual diet patterns in the United States and may not be useful among subgroups that do not follow the usual patterns, such as vegetarians. Although it has limitations, the Daily Food Guide has been widely accepted and is useful in many nutrition education programs sponsored by hospitals and community health agencies.

2.4 Recommended Dietary Allowances (RDAs)

RDAs were first published in 1943 by the Food and Nutrition Board of the National Research Council, National Academy of Sciences. They have been reevaluated and revised periodically. The RDAs are "the levels of intake of essential nutrients considered, in the judgment of the Food and Nutrition Board on the basis of available scientific knowledge, to be adequate to meet the known nutritional needs of practically all healthy persons." They are estimates of "acceptable daily nutrient intakes" or "standards" to serve as a goal for good nutrition on the basis that an individual consuming a diet of usual foods providing RDAs for all nutrients would be unlikely to suffer nutritional deficiencies. However, there may be a small number of individuals with nutrient requirements above the RDA. RDAs can only be used meaningfully within the framework of statistical probability (National Research Council, 1974). RDAs are presented in Table 2.3.

RDAs are useful in estimating the nutrient content of foods available for a population in the planning and procuring process, as guidelines for establishing policy for health and welfare programs, and as standards for assessing the nutritional quality of new food products. Along with clinical and biochemical evidence, RDAs may be used to evaluate information obtained from nutritional surveys. However, the variability of nutrient requirements and intakes within the population surveyed must be considered in interpreting results. When assessing individual dietary records, it is highly unlikely that nutrient intake is deficient when it meets or exceeds the RDA, but the possibility still exists. Also, an intake below the RDA is not, in itself, evidence of nutrient inadequacy. Clinical and biochemical evidence must also be present (National Research Council, 1974).

RDAs have been established for healthy people. They do not take into consideration the needs that result from infections, metabolic disorders, chronic diseases, or other abnormalities. Therapeutic nutritional needs are special problems that must be treated on an individual basis. Routine hospital menus will usually be planned to exceed the RDA for adults, but this does not guarantee that a hospitalized patient, particularly one who is acutely ill, will consume the planned meals. Many must be individually encouraged to eat.

A therapeutic or modified diet is based upon the normal, nutritionally adequate diet. In planning both therapeutic and normal diets, age, sex, size, activity, and environment, as well as individual preferences must be considered. With therapeutic diets, the nature of the disease and condition of the patient also must be considered. The therapeutic diet may be modified in consistency or amount in each feeding. Special foods or nutrients may be increased or decreased. However, essential nutrient requirements of an individual must be adequately supplied in a modified diet, or it must be supplemented. RDAs are often used as general guides in assessing nutrient intake of patients who are ill because other guides are not available. In the

Table 2.3 FOOD AND NUTRITION BOARD, NATIONAL ACADEMY OF SCIENCES— NATIONAL RESEARCH COUNCIL RECOMMENDED DAILY DIETARY ALLOWANCES,[a] REVISED 1974

	Age (years)	Weight (kg)	Weight (lbs)	Height (cm)	Height (in)	Energy (kcal)[b]	Protein (g)	Vitamin A Activity (RE)[c]	Vitamin A (IU)	Vitamin D (IU)	Vitamin E Activity[e] (IU)	Ascorbic Acid (mg)	Folacin[f] (μg)	Niacin[g] (mg)	Riboflavin (mg)	Thiamin (mg)	Vitamin B6 (mg)	Vitamin B12 (μg)	Calcium (mg)	Phosphorus (mg)	Iodine (μg)	Iron (mg)	Magnesium (mg)	Zinc (mg)
Infants	0.0–0.5	6	14	60	24	kg × 117	kg × 2.2	420[d]	1400	400	4	35	50	5	0.4	0.3	0.3	0.3	360	240	35	10	60	3
	0.5–1.0	9	20	71	28	kg × 108	kg × 2.0	400	2000	400	5	35	50	8	0.6	0.5	0.4	0.3	540	400	45	15	70	5
Children	1–3	13	28	86	34	1300	23	400	2000	400	7	40	100	9	0.8	0.7	0.6	1.0	800	800	60	15	150	10
	4–6	20	44	110	44	1800	30	500	2500	400	9	40	200	12	1.1	0.9	0.9	1.5	800	800	80	10	200	10
	7–10	30	66	135	54	2400	36	700	3300	400	10	40	300	16	1.2	1.2	1.2	2.0	800	800	110	10	250	10
Males	11–14	44	97	158	63	2800	44	1000	5000	400	12	45	400	18	1.5	1.4	1.6	3.0	1200	1200	130	18	350	15
	15–18	61	134	172	69	3000	54	1000	5000	400	15	45	400	20	1.8	1.5	2.0	3.0	1200	1200	150	18	400	15
	19–22	67	147	172	69	3000	54	1000	5000	400	15	45	400	20	1.8	1.5	2.0	3.0	800	800	140	10	350	15
	23–50	70	154	172	69	2700	56	1000	5000		15	45	400	18	1.6	1.4	2.0	3.0	800	800	130	10	350	15
	51+	70	154	172	69	2400	56	1000	5000		15	45	400	16	1.5	1.2	2.0	3.0	800	800	110	10	350	15
Females	11–14	44	97	155	62	2400	44	800	4000	400	12	45	400	16	1.3	1.2	1.6	3.0	1200	1200	115	18	300	15
	15–18	54	119	162	65	2100	48	800	4000	400	12	45	400	14	1.4	1.1	2.0	3.0	1200	1200	115	18	300	15
	19–22	58	128	162	65	2100	46	800	4000	400	12	45	400	14	1.4	1.1	2.0	3.0	800	800	100	18	300	15
	23–50	58	128	162	65	2000	46	800	4000		12	45	400	13	1.2	1.0	2.0	3.0	800	800	100	18	300	15
	51+	58	128	162	65	1800	46	800	4000		12	45	400	12	1.1	1.0	2.0	3.0	800	800	80	10	300	15
Pregnant						+300	+30	1000	5000	400	15	60	800	+2	+0.3	+0.3	2.5	4.0	1200	1200	125	18+[h]	450	20
Lactating						+500	+20	1200	6000	400	15	80	600	+4	+0.5	+0.3	2.5	4.0	1200	1200	150	18	450	25

[a] The allowances are intended to provide for individual variations among most normal persons as they live in the United States under usual environmental stresses. Diets should be based on a variety of common foods to provide other nutrients for which human requirements have been less well defined.

[b] Kilojoules (kJ) = 4.2 × kcal.

[c] Retinol equivalents.

[d] Assumed to be all as retinol in milk during the first 6 months of life. All subsequent intakes are assumed to be half as retinol and half as β-carotene when calculated from international units. As retinol equivalents, three-fourths are retinol and one-fourth as β-carotene.

[e] Total vitamin E activity, estimated to be 80 percent as α-tocopherol and 20 percent other tocopherols.

[f] The folacin allowances refer to dietary sources as determined by Lactobacillus casei assay. Pure forms of folacin may be effective in doses less than one-fourth of the recommended dietary allowance.

[g] Although allowances are expressed as niacin, it is recognized that on the average 1 mg of niacin is derived from each 60 mg of dietary tryptophan.

[h] This increased requirement cannot be met by ordinary diets; therefore, the use of supplemental iron is recommended.

final analysis, the individual condition of the patient and the patient's apparent nutrient requirements, evaluated in terms of clinical and biochemical evidence as well as dietary intake, must guide nutritional care. It is helpful for the practicing dietitian to be thoroughly familiar with RDAs, their uses and limitations, as tools in working with clients.

2.5 U.S. Recommended Daily Allowances (U.S. RDAs)

U.S. RDAs have been developed by the Food and Drug Administration (FDA), the U.S. Department of Health, Education and Welfare, and the food industry for use in nutrition labeling. U.S. RDAs have been selected from tables of RDAs published by the National Research Council. They replace the Minimum Daily Requirements (MDRs) previously used by the FDA in labeling. Actually, there are three sets of U.S. RDAs: (1) for adults and children over 4 years of age, (2) for infants and children under 4 years of age, and (3) for pregnant or lactating women. The U.S. RDA for adults are most used on nutrition information panels of packaged foods and vitamin-mineral supplements. The ones for infants and children are used on baby foods and special vitamin-mineral supplements for infants and small children. Table 2.4 lists the U.S. RDAs.

Nutrition information is presented on a food label as in the following illustration for a package of cornflakes (DHEW Publication No. (FDA) 75–2029):

NUTRITION INFORMATION
(Per Serving)
Serving Size = 1 oz ($1\frac{1}{3}$ cup)
Servings per Container = 18

		Cornflakes 1 oz with $\frac{1}{2}$ cup whole milk
Calories	110	190
Protein	2 g	6 g
Carbohydrate	24 g	30 g
Fat	0	4 g

Percentage of U.S. Recommended
Daily Allowances (U.S. RDAs)

Protein	2	10
Vitamin A	25	25
Vitamin C	25	25
Thiamin	25	25
Riboflavin	25	25
Niacin	25	25
Calcium	0	15
Iron	10	10

Table 2.4 U.S. RECOMMENDED DAILY ALLOWANCES (U.S. RDAs)*

Supplement	Adults and Children Over 4 Years	Infants and Children Under 4 Years		Pregnant or Lactating Women
Protein	65 g†	25–28	g†	65 g†
Vitamin A	5000 IU	2500	IU	8000 IU
Vitamin C	60 mg	40	mg	60 mg
Thiamin	1.5 mg	0.7	mg	1.7 mg
Riboflavin	1.7 mg	0.8	mg	2.0 mg
Niacin	20 mg	9.0	mg	20 mg
Calcium	1.0 g	0.8	g	1.3 g
Iron	18 mg	10	mg	18 mg
Vitamin D	400 IU	400	IU	400 IU
Vitamin E	30 IU	10	IU	30 IU
Vitamin B_6	2.0 mg	0.7	mg	2.5 mg
Folacin	0.4 mg	0.2	mg	0.8 mg
Vitamin B_{12}	6.0 mcg	3	mcg	8 mcg
Phosphorus	1.0 g	0.8	g	1.3 g
Iodine	150 mcg	70	mcg	150 mcg
Magnesium	400 mg	200	mg	450 mg
Zinc	15 mg	8	mg	15 mg
Copper	2.0 mg	1	mg	2 mg
Biotin	0.3 mg	0.15	mg	0.3 mg
Pantothenic acid	10 mg	5	mg	10 mg

* For use in nutrition labeling of foods, including foods that also are vitamin and mineral supplements.

† If protein efficiency ratio of protein is equal to or better than that of casein, U.S. RDA is 45 g for adults and pregnant or lactating women, 20 g for children under 4 years of age, and 18 g for infants.

Nutrition labeling is voluntary for most foods, but it is required for foods (1) to which nutrients are added, (2) to which reference is made on the label or in advertising to the caloric value or the nutrient content, other than sodium, and (3) for which any nutritional claim is made on the label or in advertising. When nutrition labeling is used, it must conform to FDA regulations. The percentage of the U.S. RDA in a serving of food must be listed on the label for protein, vitamin A, vitamin C, thiamin, riboflavin, niacin, calcium, and iron. The percentage of the U.S. RDA *may* be listed for vitamin D, vitamin E, vitamin B_6, folacin, vitamin B_{12}, phosphorus, iodine, magnesium, zinc, copper, biotin, and pantothenic acid if these nutrients occur naturally in a food. They *must* be listed, however, if they are added to the food. The percentages of the U.S. RDA are expressed in 2 percent increments up to and including 10 percent, 5 percent increments up to and including 50 percent, and 10 percent increments above the 50 percent level. The fatty acid composition and/or cholesterol content of a food may be listed immediately following the statement of fat content. The nutrient contents stated on a food label cannot be calculated from standard food composition tables but must be determined by laboratory analyses (Ross, 1974).

Nutrition labeling may be an effective nutrition education tool, but many consumers will require considerable motivation to use it. Dietitians should give their clients information and guidance in using nutrition labeling to select more nutritious diets. Labeling will be particulary useful with new food products. Nutrition labeling can be helpful to patients following modified diets, especially when control of kilocalories, fat, or carbohydrate is necessary. If nutrition counseling of clients includes information on nutrition labeling and how it might be effectively used, including relationships with exchange lists, food selection can be more appropriate for the diet the patient is attempting to achieve (Johnson, 1974).

2.5 Medical Records

A record or chart of medical care is kept for each hospitalized patient and is also used in outpatient clinics or treatment centers. There are a number of important purposes for keeping medical records on individual patients. The record serves as a basis for planning and for continuity of patient care; it provides a means of communication among all professionals on the health team as they contribute to the patient's care; it provides an accurate record that could be used in the process of peer review; and it provides data for use in health planning and for research in various morbidity and mortality problems. Medical records have been standardized to contain pertinent information. They usually include:

1. Demographic data obtained on admission—patient's name, address, sex, age, physician, admitting diagnosis, and so on
2. Charts for recording patient's temperature, pulse, respiration, blood pressure, fluid intake and output, weight, and so on
3. Medical history and record of physical examination
4. Physician's progress notes
5. Nursing notes
6. Medication record
7. Intravenous therapy record
8. Reports of radiographic and operative procedures, physical therapy, laboratory tests, and so on
9. Dietary history record (in some cases)

Physician's orders for the patient may also be included in the patient's chart, or they may be kept with orders for other patients in one central place. The medical record is available to authorized hospital or clinic personnel, but it is not available to the patient himself. Information contained in the chart is *confidential* and must not be discussed except in the process of communicating with other health professionals concerning the care of the patient. When the patient has been discharged from the hospital, his chart is stored in the Medical Records Department and may be retrieved on subsequent admissions.

The dietitian has the responsibility to record in the medical record pertinent information concerning the nutritional care of the patient. In some hospitals the chart may contain a page for dietitian's notes, including the dietary history and diet order. In other hospitals the dietitian may record in the Physician's Progress Notes.

The American Hospital Association (1976) has developed guidelines for therapeutic dietitians on recording in patients' medical records. Dietitians should record (1) confirmation of original diet order within 24 hours of admission and all subsequent diet orders; (2) summary of dietary history; (3) pertinent and progressive information on nutritional care therapy, including nutrient intake, patient tolerance and special problems, instruction plans, and requests for referral to community agencies; (4) nutritional care discharge plan; and (5) consultation reports. The method of recording should be compatible with the institution's method for arranging clinical data.

Many health care facilities are using the problem-oriented medical record (P.O.M.R.), which was developed and pioneered by Lawrence L. Weed, M.D. (1968). The P.O.M.R. is not simply a method of writing medical charts that differs from the classical records but an entire philosophy stressing the alignment of the health care team with the patient and her needs (Voytovich, 1973). The medical record is emerging, by this system, as a means of ensuring the recognition of all the patient's problems all the time; it also coordinates the activities of all members of the health team as they focus on the patient. The use of the term *diagnosis* is changed in this system to *problem,* which is anything that the patient presents that requires the health team to (1) obtain more information about, (2) treat, or (3) educate for. A problem appears in the patient's chart because it requires action.

A definitive list of *all* problems pertinent to the patient's care appear in the P.O.M.R. This is followed by a plan for each problem that includes diagnosis, treatment, and patient education. The problem list is maintained at the front of the record and is constantly updated as new information accumulates and as problems are added, dropped, or changed. Progress notes in the chart are related to the problems listed. The SOAP format is used in recording information in the chart, each letter representing one element in the progress note (Voytovich, 1973).

Subjective: What new information is available from talking to the patient?

Objective: What new hard facts (such as laboratory data or the physical examination) are available?

Assessment: What is the impact of this information on understanding the defined problem?

Plan: What are new diagnostic, therapeutic, and patient education ventures?

An example of a progress note written by a dietitian follows (Voytovich, 1973):

PROBLEM: Failure to follow dietary regimen (250 mg sodium).

S̲ubjective: Patient subsists on luncheon meat and skim milk, occasional potato chips, rye bread, canned vegetables.

O̲bjective: Noted peanut butter crackers on night table; in discussion, patient revealed he had no knowledge of low-sodium foods. Social worker says he has no refrigerator in his apartment.

A̲ssessment: Inadequate nutrition education; no refrigerator.

P̲lan: Diagnostic—find out about financial resources. Patient education—visit patient daily at lunchtime to discuss sodium content of foods; stress high sodium content of various prepared foods. Introduce patient to another patient on a low-sodium diet who is willing to discuss common problems and reinforce learning.

s/Jane Doe, Dietitian

The medical record is an indispensable tool for the dietitian in giving quality nutritional care. It provides essential background information, including medical, biochemical, and socioeconomic data, pertinent to an understanding of the patient's nutritional problems. It provides a means of communicating with other health professionals concerning these problems. The P.O.M.R. system, particularly, encourages the dietitian to evaluate the nutritional treatment of every patient with whom he or she works and, when appropriate, points out to the physician and other members of the health care team even more effective measures for nutritional care (Walters and De Marco, 1973). Through use of the medical record and the professional expertise of dietetics, the dietitian may identify nutritional problems of a patient for the physician. Information about normal values for many laboratory tests and the significance of abnormal results is important to the dietitian when using the medical record as a tool for giving nutritional care. Data on laboratory tests appear in the appendix.

REFERENCES

1. American Diabetes Association and American Dietetic Association. 1950. *Meal Planning with Exchange Lists.* Chicago: American Dietetic Association.

2. American Diabetes Association and American Dietetic Association. 1976. EXCHANGE LISTS FOR MEAL PLANNING. Chicago: American Diabetes Association.

3. American Diabetes Association and American Dietetic Association. 1977. *A Guide for Professionals: The Effective Application of "Exchange Lists for Meal Planning."* Chicago: American Diabetes Association.

4. American Hospital Association. 1976. Recording nutritional information in medical records. Chicago: American Hospital Association.

5. Anderson, B. A., J. A. Kinsella, and B. K. Watt. 1975. Comprehensive evaluation of fatty acids in foods. II. Beef products. *J. Am. Dietet. Assoc.*, **67:** 35.

6. Appledorf, H. 1974. Nutritional analysis of foods from fast-food chains. *Food Technol.*, **28** (No. 4): 50.

7. Brignoli, C. A., J. E. Kinsella, and J. L. Weihrauch. 1976. Comprehensive evaluation of fatty acids in foods. V. Unhydrogenated fats and oils. *J. Am. Dietet. Assoc.*, **68:** 224.

8. Caso, E. K. 1950. Calculation of diabetic diets. *J. Am. Dietet. Assoc.*, **26:** 575.

9. Church, C. F. and H. N. Church. 1975. *Food Values of Portions Commonly Used.* Philadelphia: Lippincott.

10. Cinnamon, P. A. and M. A. Swanson. 1976. Everything You Always Wanted to Know About Exchange Values for Foods, rev'd ed. Moscow, Idaho: University Press of Idaho.

11. De Ritter, E., M. Osadca, J. Scheiner, and J. Keating. 1974. Vitamins in frozen convenience dinners and pot pies. *J. Am. Dietet. Assoc.*, **64:** 391.

12. Feeley, R. M., P. E. Criner, and B. K. Watt. 1972. Cholesterol content of foods. *J. Am. Dietet. Assoc.*, **61:** 134.

13. Fristrom, G. A., B. C. Stewart, J. L. Weihrauch, and L. P. Posati. 1975. Comprehensive evaluation of fatty acids in foods. IV. Nuts, peanuts, and soups. *J. Am. Dietet. Assoc.*, **67:** 351.

14. Groover, M. E., L. Boone, P. C. Houk, and S. Wolf. 1967. Problems in the quantitation of dietary surveys. *J. Am. Med. Assoc.*, **201:** 8.

15. Hertzler, A. A. and H. L. Anderson. 1974. Food guides in the United States. *J. Am. Dietet. Assoc.*, **64:** 19.

16. Johnson, O. C. 1974. The Food and Drug Administration and labeling. *J. Am. Dietet. Assoc.*, **64:** 471.

17. Kilgore, L. 1967. Proximate composition and energy value of pizza. *J. Am. Dietet. Assoc.*, **50:** 133.

18. Marshall, M. W., J. M. Iacono, C. W. Young, V. A. Washington, H. T. Slover, and P. M. Leapley. 1975. Composition of diets containing 25 and 35 percent calories from fat. *J. Am. Dietet. Assoc.*, **66:** 470.

19. Miljanich, P. and R. Ostwald. 1970. Fatty acids in newer brands of margarine. *J. Am. Dietet. Assoc.*, **56:** 29.

20. National Research Council. 1974. *Recommended Dietary Allowances.* Washington, D.C.: National Academy of Sciences.

21. Posati, L. P., J. E. Kinsella, and B. K. Watt. 1975a. Comprehensive evaluation of fatty acids in foods. I. Dairy products. *J. Am. Dietet. Assoc.*, **66:** 482.

22. Posati, L. P., J. E. Kinsella, and B. K. Watt. 1975b. Comprehensive evaluation of fatty acids in foods. III. Eggs and egg products. *J. Am. Dietet. Assoc.*, **67:** 111.

23. Ross, M. L. 1974. What's happening to food labeling? *J. Am. Dietet. Assoc.*, **64:** 262.

24. Sorenson, A. W., B. W. Wyse, A. J. Wittwer, and R. G. Hansen. 1976. An index of nutritional quality for a balanced diet. *J. Am. Dietet. Assoc.*, **68:** 236.

25. Standal, B. R., D. R. Bassett, P. B. Policar, and M. Thom. 1970. Fatty acids, cholesterol, and proximate analyses of some ready-to-eat foods. *J. Am. Dietet. Assoc.*, **56:** 392.

26. Voytovich, A. E. 1973. The dietitian/nutritionist and the problem-oriented medical record. I. A physician's viewpoint. *J. Am. Dietet. Assoc.*, **63:** 639.

27. Walberg, S. M. and W. S. Adams. 1965. Calculated and determined values in constant diets. *J. Am. Dietet. Assoc.*, **47**: 37.

28. Walters, F. M. and M. De Marco. 1973. The dietitian/nutritionist and the problem-oriented medical record. II. The role of the dietitian. *J. Am. Dietet. Assoc.*, **63**: 641.

29. Watt, B. K., S. E. Gebhardt, E. W. Murphy, and R. R. Butrum. 1974. Food composition tables for the 70's. *J. Am. Dietet. Assoc.*, **64**: 257.

30. Watt, B. K. and A. L. Merrill. 1963. *Composition of Foods*. U.S. Department of Agriculture.

31. Watt, B. K. and E. W. Murphy. 1970. Tables of food composition: Scope and needed research. *Food Technol.*, **24**: 674.

32. Weed, L. L. 1968. Medical records that guide and teach. *N. Eng. J. Med.*, **278**: 593.

33. Weihrauch, J. L., J. E. Kinsella, and B. K. Watt. 1976. Comprehensive evaluation of fatty acids in foods. VI. Cereal products. *J. Am. Dietet. Assoc.*, **68**: 335.

STUDY GUIDE

As with all professions, there are particular tools that are used by the dietitian/nutritionist in giving nutrition care to clients.

1. Describe several important tools that are widely used by dietitians in giving professional service related to nutrition.

Reliable food composition tables have many important uses in the areas of nutrition and food science.

2. Describe several ways in which food composition tables could be effectively used by professionals.

3. Why should a dietitian/nutritionist be in possession of a comprehensive food composition table?

4. What food composition tables are available and widely used in the United States? How are they usually developed?

5. How accurate are food composition tables? What are their limitations?

Exchange lists have been used for many years in nutrition counseling.

6. How and why were the commonly used exchange lists first developed and later revised?

7. How might the exchange lists be used effectively by the dietitian?

Nutrient requirements are often translated into food group guides for use with lay groups.

8. How might food group guides be used effectively by the dietitian?

Recommended Dietary Allowances (RDAs) and U.S. Recommended Daily Allowances (U.S. RDAs) serve different functions.

9. How are RDAs developed in the United States and by whom? What is the philosophy upon which they are based?

10. What are U.S. RDAs and how do they differ from RDAs? What is the primary purpose of U.S. RDA's?

11. Why is it important for a clinical dietitian who works primarily with modified diets to be thoroughly knowledgeable about RDAs and U.S. RDAs?

A medical record is kept on each hospitalized patient and is available to authorized personnel.

12. Describe several purposes for keeping medical records on individual patients.

13. What types of information are usually included in a patient's medical record, and who usually records this information?

14. What types of information should a dietitian record on a patient's medical record and why?

15. What is the general philosophy and format of the problem-oriented medical record (P.O.M.R.) as developed by Dr. Lawrence L. Weed? Discuss possible advantages of this system over the traditional record.

16. What is the meaning of SOAP in relation to the P.O.M.R.? Give examples of how a dietitian might record relevant information for a patient in a P.O.M.R. system.

3

Drugs and Nutrition

The word "iatrogenic" originally meant "physician-induced," referring to imagined ailments derived from suggestions or attitudes of the physician. It has recently acquired a broader definition that includes side effects of most therapeutic measures (Smuckler, 1977). Many drugs are used by the phsyician in treatment of his or her patients, and adverse drug reactions yearly afflict millions of people. Some drugs may interact with other drugs and with various nutrients, thus influencing the nutritional state of a patient and/or the effectiveness of the drugs. These effects must be considered in giving nutritional care.

Interactions between food substances and drugs may occur in several ways. Drugs may adversely affect nutrient absorption or metabolism, therefore gradually depleting the body of essential substances. Taste and appetite may also be influenced by drugs. On the other hand, foods sometimes affect drug absorption, and a state of malnutrition influences the body's ability to metabolize drugs. In certain cases, foods contain pharmacologically active substances that may interact with drugs to produce unwanted results. This chapter points out some of the more common problems involving food and drugs.

3.1   Drug Metabolism

The majority of reactions involved in metabolism of drugs in the body occur in liver cells within the smooth endoplasmic reticulum (microsomes). The microsomal drug-metabolizing enzymes are membrane-bound and function as a multicomponent electron transport system. They are responsible for the metabolism of a variety of endogenous substances, e.g., steroids, fatty acids, and bile acids, as well as exogenous substrates, such as drugs, insecticides, carcinogens, and many other foreign compounds (Lu, 1976). The metabolism of alcohol by this system is discussed in Sec. 17.5.

The metabolism of drugs usually involves two phases: (1) the processes of oxidation, reduction, and hydrolysis are used to produce intermediate metabolites that are (2) conjugated with substances such as amino acids or glucuronic acid to yield water-soluble compounds which can be excreted in the urine (Drayer, 1974). Many drug interactions are predictable because of known chemical structures, and plans can be made to avoid some of the more common and serious effects (Robinson, 1975).

There is large individual variation in drug absorption, biotransformation, and excretion even for healthy individuals, and disease states add additional variables. Patients with impaired renal function have a high incidence of adverse drug reactions. Metabolism of drugs is altered in liver disease. Since many drugs are bound to albumin or other proteins in the serum, and the amount of bound drug is related to the concentration of the unbound portion, decreased serum protein levels cause higher unbound drug levels and affect intensity of action (Reidenberg, 1974).

3.2 Effect of Drugs on Nutrient Absorption and Metabolism

Drugs can induce malabsorption by exerting their effects in the intestinal lumen or by impairing the integrity of the mucosa. They may also affect motility of the gastrointestinal tract. Some examples of drugs influencing absorption are (Roe, 1976; Hartshorn, 1977; Visconti, 1977):

1. Mineral oil, taken as a laxative, dissolves fat-soluble vitamins and decreases their absorption.
2. Cathartics reduce transit time to less than that for optimal absorption.
3. Neomycin, an antibiotic, and cholestyramine, a hypocholesteremic agent, bind bile acids and thus impair the absorption of fats and fat-soluble vitamins. Absorption of vitamin B_{12} and iron is also affected. In addition, neomycin produces structural changes that cause malabsorption of nitrogen, sodium, potassium, calcium, sucrose, and lactose.
4. Dioctyl sodium sulfosuccinate, a fecal softener, is a surfactant and may increase absorption of cholesterol and vitamin A.
5. Colchicine, an anti-inflammatory agent for gout, creates a structural defect with enzyme damage and decreases absorption of fat, carotene, sodium, potassium, lactose, folic acid, and vitamin B_{12}.

6. The biguanides, metformin and phenformin, used as oral hypoglycemic agents, competitively inhibit absorption of vitamin B_{12}.

7. Estrogens in oral contraceptives may interfere with polyglutamate conjugase resulting in decreased absorption of folic acid.

8. Slow release potassium chloride for potassium repletion lowers ileal pH values and depresses absorption of vitamin B_{12}.

9. Salicylazosulfapyridine (Azulfidine), an anti-inflammatory agent for ulcerative colitis and regional enteritis, causes a mucosal block in folate uptake.

10. Glucocorticoids, used in allergic and collagen diseases, impair calcium transport across the mucosa and lower serum calcium.

11. Aluminum hydroxide, a widely used antacid, combines with phosphates in the intestine and can result in phosphate depletion.

Drugs may affect metabolism of nutrients in various ways. Accelerated catabolism may occur. Hyperexcretion of vitamins and minerals through the urine may cause depletion over a period of time. Antivitamins competitively inhibit the metabolism of vitamins. Some examples of drugs affecting nutrient metabolism are (Roe, 1976; Hartshorn, 1977):

1. The anticonvulsant drugs, diphenylhydantoin, phenobarbital, and primidone, can induce folate deficiency (Haghshenass and Rao, 1973) with resulting macrocytic anemia, and also vitamin D deficiency (Crosley et al., 1975; Lifshitz and Maclaren, 1973) with low serum calcium levels and possibly rickets. Folate deficiency may be a result of hepatic microsomal enzyme induction with increased metabolism of folic acid. The interference with vitamin D metabolism may be at the stage of hepatic conversion from cholecalciferol to 25-hydroxycholecalciferol.

2. Oral contraceptives may cause increased urinary excretion of folate metabolites; decreased levels of serum vitamin B_{12}; increased catabolism of ascorbic acid or change in tissue distribution with lowered levels in serum and in leukocytes; development of a vitamin B_6 deficiency; and riboflavin depletion.

3. Isoniazid, an antituberculous agent, may cause symptoms of vitamin B_6 deficiency from increased urinary excretion of this vitamin, or by inhibition of various vitamin B_6 dependent enzymatic reactions. Pellagra may also occur because vitamin B_6 is a necessary coenzyme in the metabolism of tryptophan to niacin. Adrenal cortical hormones cause a breakdown of glycogen to glucose resulting in hyperglycemia; a breakdown of protein, leading to tissue-wasting; and a peculiar mobility of fat to certain areas of the body, creating the typical "moon face" and "buffalo hump"

commonly seen in patients on high-dose, long-term steroid therapy.

5. Folic acid antagonists, such as aminopterin and methotrexate, used in the treatment of leukemia and other malignant diseases as well as resistant forms of psoriasis, interfere with folate metabolism and thus impair DNA synthesis. Toxic effects include anorexia, abdominal pain, nausea, and ulceration in the mouth and pharynx.

6. Triamterene, a diuretic, has structural similarities to folic acid and apparently inhibits the dihydrofolate reductase enzyme. It may result in megaloblastic anemia, particularly in individuals depleted of folate stores, such as alcoholics and pregnant women.

Certain drugs, such as Parnate or Marplan, frequently are given to depressed patients. These drugs inhibit monoamine oxidase, which maintains the proper levels of a transmitter substance, norepinephrine, in certain nerve endings. This enzyme is also found in the intestinal wall, liver, and kidneys, where it functions to control absorption and circulation of monoamine compounds. Tyramine, a monoamine present in foods such as sharp cheddar cheese, bananas, chianti wine, pickled herring, and broad beans, has the ability to release norepinephrine from inactive intraneuronal storage sites. It is normally inactivated in the intestine by monoamine oxidase but may be absorbed in comparatively large amounts when the inhibiting drugs are being administered. Headache, nose bleed, increased blood pressure, and occasionally a cerebrovascular accident can result from the body's inability to inactivate released norepinephrine under these circumstances (Hartshorn, 1977; Sen, 1969).

March (1976) published a handbook on interaction of selected drugs with nutritional status in human beings.

3.3 Effect of Drugs on Taste and Appetite

Taste acuity may be altered by certain drugs, including griseofulvin (an antifungal agent used to treat certain skin problems), penicillamine (used in Wilson's disease to chelate copper), and lincomycin (used to treat systemic infections). Potassium iodide and bromide-containing medications are excreted by the salivary glands and produce a salty-bitter taste in the mouth. Other drugs, including potassium chloride liquids, chloral hydrate and paraldehyde (hypnotics and sedatives), and vitamin B-complex liquids, are unpleasant tasting. They may cause nausea, anorexia, and gastrointestinal symptoms. Cholinergic agents (given to patients with intestinal distention or urinary retention); expectorants, such as glyceryl guaiacolate, given in large doses; and narcotic analgesics may cause nausea and anorexia. Amphetamines are sometimes given as appetite depressants in weight-reduction programs. Other drugs, including phenothiazine tranquilizers, benzodiazepine antianxiety agents, tricyclic antidepressants, and oral contraceptives have been reported to stimulate appetite (Hartshorn, 1977). Stimulant drugs, dextroamphetamine and methylphenidate, given to hyperactive children have been reported to suppress growth, apparently because of decreased appetite and caloric intake (Lucas and Sells, 1977).

3.4 Effect of Foods in Drug Absorption

Drugs that are particularly irritating to the gastrointestinal tract, such as nitrofurantoin (used in urinary tract infections), phenylbutazone (an analgesic), and aminosalicylic acid (an antitubercular agent), should be given with or immediately after meals to lessen the irritating effect. Other drugs, such as anticholinergic agents, are given shortly before a meal to reduce gastric acid secretion and gut motility. Antibiotics that are destroyed by gastric acidity, such as penicillin G and erythromycin, are best given at least 1 hour before or 2 hours after meals to minimize the acid environment and decrease gastric emptying time. Tetracycline is chelated by calcium or iron present in foods, and thus its absorption is decreased when administered with meals, particularly with milk or iron supplements (Hartshorn, 1977). Griseofulvin is highly lipid-soluble, and its absorption is enhanced by a high-fat meal (Visconti, 1977).

3.5 Malnutrition and Drug Metabolism

A number of animal studies indicate that the hepatic microsomal drug-metabolizing system is markedly influenced by general nutritional status, protein or mineral deficiency, and certain vitamins, as well as by age, sex, stress, and hormones. A reduction in either quantity or quality of dietary protein decreases the activity of the microsomal drug-metabolizing system. This will have an adverse effect if the parent drug is more toxic than the metabolites but may have a beneficial effect if the metabolites are more toxic than the drug itself (Campbell and Hayes, 1976).

The hepatic microsomal enzyme activity decreased in ascorbic acid and in riboflavin-deficient animals (Zannoni and Sato, 1976). Iron-deficient rats showed increased rates of drug metabolism, although this has not been demonstrated in people. Zinc, copper, and calcium deficiencies have been reported to alter the rate of drug metabolism and thus potentially alter the toxicological response (Becking, 1976). Rats fed a diet containing 3 percent corn oil for 3 weeks metabolized several drugs significantly faster than did rats fed a fat-free diet (Wade and Norred, 1976).

Investigations concerning the clinical significance of nutritional deficiency and drug metabolism in humans are desirable. If drug metabolism is markedly altered when nutritional deficiencies are present, whether because of an inadequate diet or the presence of disease, nutritional rehabilitation in people receiving drugs should take into account the special re quirements for drug biotransformation (Roe, 1976).

REFERENCES

1. Becking, G. C. 1976. Hepatic drug metabolism in iron-, magnesium- and potassium-deficient rats. *Fed. Proc.,* **35:** 2480.

2. Campbell, T. C. and J. R. Hayes. 1976. The effect of quantity and quality of dietary protein on drug metabolism. *Fed. Proc.,* **35:** 2470.

3. Crosley, C. J., C. Chee, and P. H. Berman. 1975. Rickets associated with long-term anticonvulsant therapy in a pediatric outpatient population. *Pediatrics,* **56:** 52.

4. Drayer, D. E. 1974. Pathways of drug metabolism in man. *Med. Clin. No. Am.,* **58:** 927.

5. Haghshenass, M. and D. B. Rao. 1973. Serum folate levels during anticonvulsant therapy with diphenylhydantoin. *J. Am. Ger. Soc.,* **21:** 275.

6. Hartshorn, E. A. 1977. Food and drug interactions. *J. Am. Dietet. Assoc.,* **70:** 15.

7. Lifshitz, F. and N. K. Maclaren. 1973. Vitamin D-dependent rickets in institutionalized, mentally retarded children receiving long-term anticonvulsant therapy. I. A survey of 288 patients. *J. Ped.,* **83:** 612.

8. Lu, A. Y. H. 1976. Liver microsomal drug-metabolizing enzyme system: functional components and their properties. *Fed. Proc.,* **35:** 2460.

9. Lucas, B. and C. J. Sells. 1977. Nutrient intake and stimulant drugs in hyperactive children. *J. Am. Dietet. Assoc.,* **70:** 373.

10. March, D. C. 1976. *Handbook: Interactions of Selected Drugs with Nutritional Status in Man.* Chicago: American Dietetic Association.

11. Reidenberg, M. M. 1974. Effect of disease states on plasma protein binding of drugs. *Med. Clin. No. Am.,* **58:** 1103.

12. Robinson, D. S. 1975. Pharmacokinetic mechanisms of drug interactions. *Postgrad. Med.,* **57** (No. 2): 55.

13. Roe, D. A. 1976. *Drug-Induced Nutritional Deficiencies.* Westport, Conn.: Avi Publishing.

14. Sen, N. P. 1969. Analysis and significance of tyramine in foods. *J. Food Sci.,* **34:** 22.

15. Smuckler, E. A. 1977. Iatrogenic disease, drug metabolism, and cell injury: lethal synthesis in man. *Fed. Proc.,* **36:** 1708.

16. Visconti, J. A. May 1977. Drug-food interaction. *Nutrition in Disease* (Ross Laboratories) No. F 412.

17. Wade, A. E. and W. P. Norred. 1976. Effect of dietary lipid on drug-metabolizing enzymes. *Fed. Proc.,* **35:** 2475.

18. Zannoni, V. G. and P. H. Sato. 1976. The effect of certain vitamin deficiencies on hepatic drug metabolism. *Fed. Proc.,* **35:** 2464.

STUDY GUIDE

The metabolism of drugs usually occurs in the smooth endoplasmic reticulum of liver cells.

1. Give examples of endogenous and exogenous substances that are normally metabolized in the microsomal enzyme oxidizing system.

2. Describe two phases or steps that usually occur in drug metabolism.

Drugs may affect nutrient absorption and metabolism.

3. Describe several examples of drugs affecting gut motility and absorption.

4. Describe several examples of drugs affecting nutrient metabolism.

Drugs may affect taste and appetite.

5. Give several examples of drugs that affect taste and/or appetite.

Foods may affect drug absorption.

6. Describe examples of foods affecting drug absorption.

The hepatic microsomal drug metabolizing system is influenced by nutritional status.

7. Discuss possible relationships between drug metabolism and nutrient deficiencies in experimental animals and humans.

UNIT 2

Over- and Undernutrition

4

Obesity - Development and Assessment

Fatness is within reach of most of the population in the United States. Calorie-packed foods in abundance, the automobile, and a great variety of labor-saving devices have made the accumulation of excess adipose tissue not only possible but probable for many people. Obesity has become one of the most common nutritional disorders confronting professional counselors and one of the most difficult to treat successfully. Many factors appear to contribute to the development of obesity, and many forms of treatment have been tried. The problem is multifaceted and continues to be a major challenge for the dietitian. This chapter discusses the varied facets of obesity, with emphasis on development and assessment; treatment is discussed in Chap. 5.

4.1 Definitions

Obesity may be defined as the excessive accumulation of body fat or adipose tissue. It is usually associated, but not synonymous, with the overweight state (Braunstein, 1971). Overweight may be defined as excessive heaviness, which may or may not include an abnormal amount of adipose tissue (Heald, 1972). For example, a professional football player may be considerably overweight when compared with standard height/weight charts, but because of great muscularity rather than fat accumulation. Collection of fluid in the edematous state may also produce an abnormal weight increase without excess adipose tissue. Usually, however, abnormally high body weight reflects accumulation of fatty tissue. On the other hand, excess body fat may occur in a person of relatively normal weight. A diagnosis of true obesity should, therefore, involve some estimation of body fat content rather than measurement of body weight only.

4.2 Assessment

A simple but objective measure of obesity for use in clinical practice is desirable. The appearance of an individual, as evaluated by an experienced clinician, may provide a reliable qualitative guide to diagnosing obesity. Visual assessment has sometimes been called the "eyeball" test. Rauh and Schumsky (1969) used a visual observation scale of body roundness as three trained observers rated 1,130 Cincinnati school children who were clad in indoor clothing. Visual observations showed strong relationships to triceps skin-fold measures and Wetzel grid values for this group of children. The researchers concluded that it is possible to obtain useful and valid differentiation of obesity levels in children with visual ratings made by trained observers. However, they cautioned that further refinements in the procedure for training observers to use their rating scale would be necessary before it could be employed clinically.

Generally, obesity has been assessed in adults by measuring body weights and heights and comparing with arbitrary height/weight standards. The most widely used standard height/weight tables resulted from data collected by the life insurance industry. The original tables were based upon studies of insured persons covering the periods 1885 to 1900 and 1909 to 1927 and listed *average* weights for males and females at specified ages and heights. Newer tables of *average* weights were published from the findings of the Build and Blood Pressure Study of 1959, which covered the experience of several million people insured by 26 large life insurance companies in the United States and Canada during 1935 to 1953. A table of *desirable* weights for men and women was derived from the data, based upon weights associated with lowest mortality, and is given in Table 4.1. It was assumed that no additional weight should be gained after age 25. Some anthropometric data were used in deriving the ranges for small, medium, and large frames, based primarily upon chest breadth and hip width (Metropolitan Life Insurance Company, 1959). In practice no simple, reliable method of estimating body frame is available. The use of desirable weight tables for the assessment of obesity is limited because the data are based upon a special group rather than upon a cross section of the population, there is no indication of the level of excess body weight that should be considered abnormal or obese, and no information on composition of the body weight is available.

An adaptation of the table of the Metropolitan Life Insurance Company was presented by the editorial board of a conference on obesity spon-

Table 4.1 DESIRABLE WEIGHTS FOR MEN AND WOMEN, AGES 25 AND OVER, ACCORDING TO HEIGHT AND FRAME*

Men: Weight in Pounds (indoor clothing)

Height (in shoes)†	Small Frame	Medium Frame	Large Frame
5'2"	112–120	118–129	126–141
5'3"	115–123	121–133	129–144
5'4"	118–126	124–136	132–148
5'5"	121–129	127–139	135–152
5'6"	124–133	130–143	138–156
5'7"	128–137	134–147	142–161
5'8"	132–141	138–152	147–166
5'9"	136–145	142–156	151–170
5'10"	140–150	146–160	155–174
5'11"	144–154	150–165	159–179
6'0"	148–158	154–170	164–184
6'1"	152–162	158–175	168–189
6'2"	156–167	162–180	173–194
6'3"	160–171	167–185	178–199
6'4"	164–175	172–190	182–204

Women: Weight in Pounds (indoor clothing)

Height (in shoes)†	Small Frame	Medium Frame	Large Frame
4'10"	92–98	96–107	104–119
4'11"	94–101	98–110	106–122
5'0"	96–104	101–113	109–125
5'1"	99–107	104–116	112–128
5'2"	102–110	107–119	115–131
5'3"	105–113	110–122	118–134
5'4"	108–116	113–126	121–138
5'5"	111–119	116–130	125–142
5'6"	114–123	120–135	129–146
5'7"	118–127	124–139	133–150
5'8"	122–131	128–143	137–154
5'9"	126–135	132–147	141–158
5'10"	130–140	136–151	145–163
5'11"	134–144	140–155	149–168
6'0"	138–148	144–159	153–173

* Prepared by the Metropolitan Life Insurance Company. Derived primarily from data of the Build and Blood Pressure Study, 1959, Society of Actuaries.
† Allow 1" heels for men's shoes and 2" heels for women's shoes.

sored by the National Institutes of Health in 1973 (Bray, 1975). The adaptation expresses a central weight and a range of acceptable weight (Table 4.2).

Various weight/height ratios have been suggested for use in assessing obesity. Keys et al. (1972) compared the ratios weight/height, weight/height squared, and the ponderal index (cube root of weight divided by height)

Table 4.2   FOGARTY INTERNATIONAL CENTER CONFERENCE ON OBESITY RECOMMENDED WEIGHT IN RELATION TO HEIGHT*†

Height	Men Average	Men Range	Women Average	Women Range
4'10"			102	92–119
4'11"			104	94–122
5'0"			107	96–125
5'1"			110	99–128
5'2"	123	112–141	113	102–131
5'3"	127	115–144	116	105–134
5'4"	130	118–148	120	108–138
5'5"	133	121–152	123	111–142
5'6"	136	124–156	128	114–146
5'7"	140	128–161	132	118–150
5'8"	145	132–166	136	122–154
5'9"	149	136–170	140	126–158
5'10"	153	140–174	144	130–163
5'11"	158	144–179	148	134–168
6'0"	162	148–184	152	138–173
6'1"	166	152–189		
6'2"	171	156–194		
6'3"	176	160–199		
6'4"	181	164–204		

* Height without shoes, weight without clothes. Adapted from the table of the Metropolitan Life Insurance Co. (Courtesy of the Metropolitan Life Insurance Co.).

† G. A. Bray (ed.). 1975. *Obesity in Perspective*, Part 1. DHEW Publication No. (NIH) 75–708.

with height and with subcutaneous fat thickness for 7,424 healthy men. They found the ratio of weight/height squared (termed *body-mass index*) to be best correlated with skin-fold thickness and the ponderal index to be the poorest. Thomas et al. (1976) used the body-mass index (weight/height squared) in a nomograph method for assessing body weight in clinical situations (Fig. 4.1). The scale expresses relative weight as a continuous variable, and the authors encourage the use of clinical judgment in interpreting "overweight" and "underweight." With appropriate caution in interpretation, the body-mass index may offer a reasonable approach to working with patients in a clinical setting.

Since obesity is defined as an excessive accumulation of body fat, a measurement of body fat is usually preferable to the use of height/weight tables in assessing obesity. One of the simplest and most readily available methods of indirectly estimating the amount of adipose tissue in the body is the measurement of skin-fold thickness with the use of calipers. Subcutaneous fat is thought to account for about 50 percent of total body fat, although the constancy of this proportion in extremely obese individuals has not been clearly established (Grande, 1975). It has been suggested that

A Nomograph Method for Assessing Body Weight[1]

Anthony E. Thomas,[2] *Ph.D., David A. McKay,*[3] *M.D., and Michael B. Cutlip,*[4] *Ph.D.*

(*From the American Journal of Clinical Nutrition* **29**: Mar. 1976, pp. 302–304.)

It has long been customary to include measurement of weight in clinical health assessments. Life insurance data have indicated an increased mortality risk for extremes of weight, and the insurance industry's tables showing desirable weights for height have become widely used (1, 2). However, these tables are somewhat cumbersome in practice and require an arbitrary and rather ambiguous classification of the patient by small, medium, or large "body frame."

The ratio of weight to various powers of height is often used in epidemiological studies. Data from diverse populations have indicated the superiority of weight/height^2 as the index of relative weight which is best correlated with other measures of obesity, such as skinfold thickness, and which is least correlated with height independent of weight (3–6). Sometimes designated "Quetelet's index," after an early proponent, this expression is being referred to with increasing frequency simply as the "body mass index" (BMI) (5). The division of weight by the square of height is, however, sufficiently demanding mathematically that this index has received little use in clinical settings. Yet it does offer the advantage of providing a continuous quantitative scale for relative weight which facilitates comparisons of individuals with population norms.

We have therefore developed a nomograph to ease the calculation and use of the body mass index in clinical settings [Fig. 4.1]. It has been derived using the metric system, and the BMI scale units are thus in kilograms/square meter. Conversions to inches and pounds are given on the height and weight scales so that it can be used directly with measurement in those units. As an initial rough guide to BMI interpretation, we have indicated along the scale the approximate range corresponding to the life insurance tables' "desirable weights" and the points that are ±20% of the outside limits of this range. *Horizontal shading* has been used for "medium frame," *upper left to lower right diagonal shading* for "large frame," and *lower left to upper right* for "small frame." However, as no systematic method is available for classing individuals by "frame" (7), these distinctions are more suggestive than categorical and may serve best simply as a reminder to consider the skeletal contribution to relative weight. It is also important to assess clinically the individual proportion of muscle to fat before equating a high BMI with obesty. Indeed, the clinician may prefer to make a preliminary judgment of weight status based on appearance alone before looking at the nomograph data.

Beyond this initial assessment, a photocopy of the nomograph may provide a useful display method for monitoring and encouraging weight control. Based on the index, and taking into account individual motivation and social support as well as body frame and muscularity, one can select an appropriate weight as a goal the individual can aim for in modifying eating and exercise behavior.

It has been suggested that the patient who looks fat usually is but that the diagnosis can be clinched by appropriate pinching (8). Skin-fold calipers have been advocated as a way to quantitate the latter process, but the method has not gained general clinical acceptance. The assessment of relative weight is still widely relied upon and, with appropriate caution in interpretation, seems generally the best guide to nutritional status. While there are limitations implicit both in the body mass index (4) and in the life insurance tables (7), for the present a combination of these methods, as in our nomograph, seems to offer a reasonable approach for working with weight assessment and control.

References

1. Metropolitan Life Insurance Company. New weight standards for men and women. *Statist. Bull.,* **40**: 1, 1959.
2. Build and Blood Pressure Study. Vol. I. Chicago: Society of Actuaries, 1959.
3. Khosla, T. and C. R. Lowe. Indices of obesity derived from body weight and height. *Brit. J. Prev. Soc. Med.,* **21**: 122, 1967.
4. Florey, C. V. The use and interpretation of ponderal index and other weight-height ratios in epidemiological studies. *J. Chronic Diseases,* **23**: 93, 1970.
5. Keys, A., F. Fidanza, M. J. Karvonen, N. Kimura, and H. L. Taylor. Indices of relative weight and obesity. *J. Chronic Diseases,* **25**: 329, 1972.
6. Goldbourt, U. and J. H. Medalie. Weight-height indices. *Brit. J. Prev. Soc. Med.,* **28**: 116, 1974.
7. Brozek, J. A review of build and blood pressure study. *Human Biol.,* **32**: 320, 1960.
8. Mayer, J. Overweight: Causes, Cost, and Control. Englewood Cliffs, N.J.: Prentice-Hall, 1968.

[1] The University of North Carolina, Chapel Hill, North Carolina, and the University of Connecticut, Storrs, Connecticut.
[2] Department of Anthropology, University of North Carolina. [3] Department of Medicine, University of North Carolina.
[4] Department of Chemical Engineering, University of Connecticut.

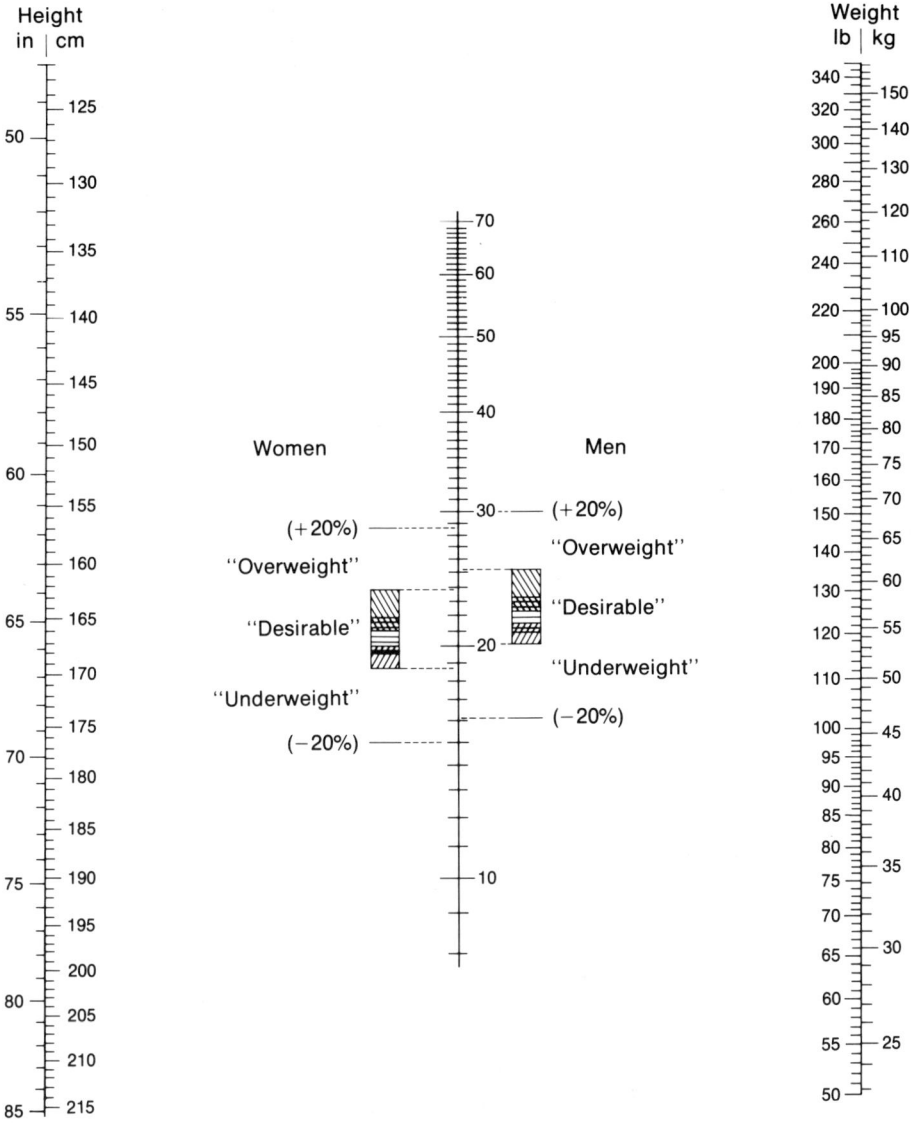

Fig. 4.1 Nomograph for body mass index (kg/m²). The ratio of weight/height² emerges from varied epidemiological studies as the most generally useful index of relative body-mass in adults. The authors present a nomograph to facilitate use of this relationship in clinical situations. While showing the range of weight given as desirable in life insurance studies, the scale expresses relative weight as a continuous variable. This method encourages use of clinical judgment in interpreting "overweight" and "underweight" and in accounting for muscular and skeletal contributions to measured mass. (From A. E. Thomas, D. A. McKay, and M. B. Cutlip, "A Nomograph Method for Assessing Body Weight, *American Journal of Clinical Nutrition,* **29:** 302, 1976; by permission of the authors and publisher.)

calipers used for the measurement of skin-fold thickness should give a relatively constant pressure of about 10 g/mm² over the usual range of measurements, have an optimal face area of approximately 6 × 15 mm, and a scale that reads between 0.5 and 0.1 mm (Edwards et al., 1955). Lange calipers meet these criteria and are manufactured in the United States (Figure 4.2).

When measuring the skin-fold thickness, a full fold of skin and subcutaneous tissue is pinched up with the thumb and forefinger of the left hand at a distance about 1 cm from the site at which the calipers are to be placed. The fold is pulled away from the underlying muscle and held while the measurement is made. The calipers are applied to the fold about 1 cm below the fingers so that the pressure on the fold at the measurement point is exerted by the faces of the caliper and not by the fingers. The handle of the caliper is released and the dial read. Caliper application should be made at least twice for stable readings (Seltzer and Mayer, 1965).

Several sites on the body have been used for the measurement of skin-fold thickness. The Committee on Nutritional Anthropometry suggested the triceps and the subscapular skin-folds as good indices of an individual's overall fatness. The triceps skin-fold measurement is taken on the back of the right upper arm, midway between the acromial process of the scapula and the olecranon process at the tip of the elbow. The midpoint may be measured with a tape. The arm should hang freely during the skin-fold measurement. The subscapular skin-fold measurement is taken

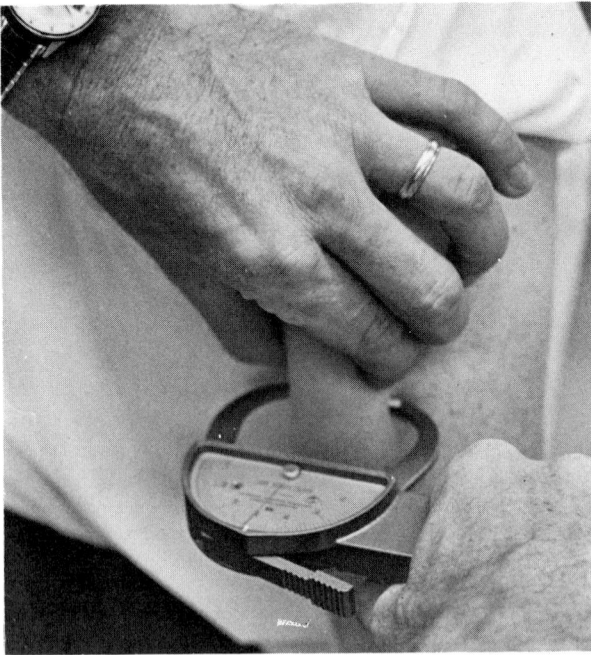

Fig. 4.2   Lange calipers are used for the measurement of skin-fold thickness in the estimation of body fatness. (Courtesy Garth Fisher, Brigham Young University.)

just below the angle of the right scapula with shoulder and arm relaxed. The fold is picked up in a line slightly inclined in the natural cleavage of the skin (Seltzer and Mayer, 1965). The triceps skin-fold is apparently the most representative site for total body fatness and is sometimes used alone in an assessment of obesity.

Data collected on various groups show that skin-fold measurements represent a continuum within certain limits and are independent of height. It is difficult to determine just where on this continuum obesity begins. Seltzer and Mayer (1965) suggested minimum triceps skin-fold thickness that would indicate obesity in Caucasian Americans, based upon the idea that obesity should be reserved for those in whom the triceps skin-fold is greater by more than one standard deviation than the mean (Table 4.3). Butterworth and Blackburn (1975) used a normal standard of 12.5 mm for

Table 4.3 OBESITY STANDARDS IN CAUCASIAN AMERICANS*

Age (years)	Minimum Triceps Skin-fold Thickness Indicating Obesity (mm)	
	Males	Females
5	12	14
6	12	15
7	13	16
8	14	17
9	15	18
10	16	20
11	17	21
12	18	22
13	18	23
14	17	23
15	16	24
16	15	25
17	14	26
18	15	27
19	15	27
20	16	28
21	17	28
22	18	28
23	18	28
24	19	28
25	20	29
26	20	29
27	21	29
28	22	29
29	22	29
30–50	23	30

* C. C. Seltzer and J. Mayer. 1965. A simple criterion of obesity. *Postgrad. Med.* **38**, A–101.

male and 16.5 mm for female triceps skin-fold measurements in assessing malnutrition among hospitalized adult patients.

Several other methods have been used, primarily in research, to study the fat and nonfat compartments of the human body (Grande, 1975). These include measurement of body density or specific gravity, K^{40} analysis, and isotope dilution techniques. Since these methods are usually difficult to administer, they do not find practical use in a clinical setting.

Density of the body can be used to calculate the percentage of body fat since the density of fat is less than that of other body components, and the density of the body thus decreases as body fat increases. Density is equal to weight/volume. The weight of the body is easily measured, and body volume may be obtained by weighing the individual under water, applying Archimedes' principle of water displacement. Correction is made for residual air in the lungs. Equations have been derived to predict both fat and water content of the body from density measurements (Pike and Brown, 1975, pp. 767–769).

The amount of potassium in the body is an indicator of lean body mass. K^{40} constitutes 0.012 percent of naturally occurring potassium and, therefore, from the quantity of K^{40} determined by a low-level, whole-body scintillation counter the quantity of total potassium in the body can be calculated (Anderson and Langham, 1961; Pike and Brown, 1975, pp. 774–776).

Various isotope dilution methods have been used in studying body composition. K^{42} has been given intravenously and allowed to exchange with body potassium. Measurement of K^{42} after equilibrium allows the calculation of total body potassium and, therefore, the estimation of lean body mass and body fat. Total body water may be estimated by injecting a known amount of a substance that penetrates and dissolves in all the water of the body and yet is not rapidly metabolized. After time for equilibration, measurement of the substance in a blood sample will allow calculation of body-water content. Isotopic hydrogen (deuterium or tritium) or antipyrine have been used. Other body compartments may be calculated from the total body-water content (Goodhart and Shils, 1973, p. 16).

4.3   Obesity and Health

Various reports concerning prevalence of overweight in restricted population groups suggest a substantial incidence of obesity in the United States at every age and in both sexes (U.S. Department of Health, Education and Welfare, 1966). However, data have been collected in a number of different ways, the composition of the populations studied has not been the same, and different criteria have been used to define overweight and obesity so that the accuracy of estimates for the general population is limited. Periodic health and nutrition evaluation surveys are now being made in the United

States, and more data are becoming available from the National Center for Health Statistics.

It is important to consider the effects of an obese state on morbidity and mortality. Concern for the health of the overweight person is not new. In 399 B.C. Socrates warned: Beware of those foods that tempt you to eat when you are not hungry and those liquors that tempt you to drink when you are not thirsty (Jordan, 1973). Obesity may be detrimental to health in three different ways: (1) some systems of the body may be affected by the excessive amount of adipose tissue so that they do not function normally; (2) the severity of established diseases may be increased by the presence of obesity; and (3) the risk of developing certain diseases may be increased (U.S. Department of Health, Education and Welfare, 1966).

The respiratory system may be affected by obesity, apparently because of the increased work required to move the thoracic cage, diaphragm, and abdominal wall. Extreme obesity produces a syndrome characterized by plethora, hypoxia, and respiratory acidosis and is labeled the "Pickwickian syndrome" in honor of a Dickens character (Burwell et al., 1956). Lourenco (1969) concluded that an incapacity to increase the activity in the respiratory muscles to levels necessary to overcome the load caused by obesity plays a major role in the genesis of respiratory failure in grossly obese individuals. In less marked obesity, changes in pulmonary function may include, successively, increased work of breathing, reduction of lung volumes, hypoxia, hypercapnia, and pulmonary hypertension. If an individual has chronic pulmonary disease, such as emphysema and asthma, the dysfunction is increased by obesity. Wilson and Wilson (1969) suggested that since obesity is a respiratory stress, it should be vigorously treated—or prevented if it is not present—as soon as obstructive pulmonary disease is diagnosed.

The cardiovascular system is affected by obesity. Heart size, blood volume, cardiac output, stroke volume, and cardiac work are greater in very obese individuals as compared to normal weight subjects. Alexander and Peterson (1972), reporting on the reversibility of these cardiovascular effects for nine obese subjects, concluded that the circulatory effects were largely reversed with weight loss. However, left-ventricular dysfunction persisted for as long as 3 years, suggesting that myocardial hypertrophy had not been reversed. In other studies with grossly obese patients, Alexander (1964) found that cardiac enlargement seemed to increase in rough proportion to the amount of excess body weight.

Evidence for an association between obesity and hypertension has been presented, with more hypertension existing among obese than nonobese individuals. Abnormally elevated blood pressure often decreases as body weight is lost (Salzano et al., 1958; U.S. Department of Health, Education and Welfare, 1966; National Dairy Council, 1975).

Reduction of obesity may have a beneficial effect on some already established diseases, including those with pulmonary dysfunction, congestive heart failure, angina pectoris, intermittent claudication, and varicose. veins. Arthritis, ruptured intervertebral discs, and other types of bone or joint disease may also be somewhat improved with weight reduction in an obese patient. Physical immobility characteristic of many of these diseases may be increased with obesity. Weight reduction is of great benefit to obese diabetic patients. In many cases of maturity-onset diabetes, glucose intolerance may approach normal when weight is decreased to near ideal levels (U.S. Department of Health, Education and Welfare, 1966).

The question of whether or not obesity creates an extra health hazard for otherwise healthy people as it increases their risk of developing certain diseases or decreases life expectancy has not been answered. However, data that are available follow a similar trend in suggesting that obesity is a health hazard. The evidence from life insurance statistics indicates that overweight people are more likely to develop certain diseases (particularly cardiovascular) and to die at a younger age than people of normal weight, although all questions are not answered by the mortality figures available (U.S. Department of Health, Education and Welfare, 1966). Obesity exerted a modest effect on excessive mortality in the Framingham Study, principally from cardiovascular disease. This study did not find a strikingly significant impact of obesity as a risk factor in major manifestations of atherosclerosis. However, relationships were found between the risk of developing angina pectoris and both antecedent weight and weight gain. Obesity was also associated with a higher incidence of sudden death from myocardial infarction, once infarction did occur, although the rate of development of infarction was unrelated to obesity in men. In women no relationship was found between obesity and any of the manifestations of coronary artery disease (Heald, 1972; Kannel et al., 1969). There have been conflicting reports in terms of the effect of obesity as a predictive risk factor in coronary heart disease (Weinsier et al., 1976; National Dairy Council, 1975). Serum triglyceride levels are often elevated in the obese, but serum cholesterol levels are usually no different than those of the nonobese population (Waxler and Craig, 1964; Montoye et al., 1966).

The Framingham Study indicated that overweight subjects developed diabetes three times as often as did lean individuals in the study. Also, adults who gained an excessive amount of weight after completion of growth had two times the risk of developing diabetes as those who did not. Although the diabetic was at greater risk of developing lethal coronary heart disease and stroke than the nondiabetic population, obese diabetics were at even greater risk. The Framingham Study also indicated that obesity was associated with an excessive amount of gout, hyperlipemia, and development of gallstones (Heald, 1972).

A group of 73,532 women in the United States and Canada who were members of TOPS (Take Off Pounds Sensibly), an international weight-control organization, was surveyed by Rimm et al. (1975) for personal health histories. The women reported what they believed they had been told by their physicians concerning illnesses they had experienced. No medical records were consulted. However, crude relative risks, with women who were closest to their ideal weights being used as the base, were calculated for 18 disease conditions from the data collected. Significant risks were found for diabetes, hypertension, gallbladder disease, gout, hypothyroidism, heart disease, arthritis, other thyroid, and jaundice, in descending order of significance.

4.4　Factors Affecting Development and Maintenance of Obesity

Obesity is an enigma in many ways, despite much research aimed at unraveling the puzzle. It invariably results from a greater intake of kilocalories in food than are expended as heat or energy by the body. The law of conservation of energy is obeyed here as elsewhere. Having said this, however, the problems are far from solved. The underlying cause(s) of the energy imbalance must be clarified if a logical approach to treatment of obesity is to be found. Several implicating factors in the development and maintenance of obesity have been suggested, the number and kind varying from one obese individual to another.

Attempts have been made to classify obesities according to primary mechanisms or causes. One such classification divides them into two groups: regulatory, in which there is a defect in the regulatory apparatus governing food intake, and metabolic, which involves some type of primary metabolic abnormality. Van Itallie and Campbell (1972) added a third classification of "constitutional" obesity, under which they categorize obesity characterized by increased numbers of fat cells. This classification is undoubtedly oversimplified. There may be cases, for example, where a basic metabolic abnormality affects the centers that regulate food intake, thus implicating both metabolic and regulatory causes. Conversely, regulatory problems may have direct metabolic consequences.

Genetic Effects

Genetic influences on obesity have been demonstrated in experimental animals. An obese hyperglycemic syndrome with autosomal recessive inheritance has been extensively studied in mice, with the ultimate aim of better understanding human obesity (Mayer, 1965a; Chlouverakis, 1972; Bergen et al., 1975). This syndrome is characterized by extreme adiposity, hypercholesteremia, a marked degree of hyperglycemia in spite of increased circulating insulin, marked hyperplasia of the islets of Langerhans, and several other metabolic and behavioral abnormalities. Presumably the large number of metabolic, anatomic, and behavioral abnormalities stem from one inborn error. The yellow mouse with obesity of autosomal dominant inheritance, the New Zealand obese mouse, which is the result of selective breeding for many generations, the Zucher "fatty" rat that appeared as a spontaneous mutation, and the PBB/Ld mouse that resulted from the inbreeding of a black line of mice have also been studied (Hunt et al., 1976).

It is difficult to demonstrate the hereditary nature of obesity in people. Humans, of course, are different in many ways from other animals, and direct application of results from animal studies to humans is not possible. Also, genetic effects are complex and difficult to study in human populations. Various studies have shown that obesity seems to run in families. A high degree of correlation between overweightness in parents and in their children has been reported (Mayer, 1965a). However, cultural background and family food habits complicate the picture and make it difficult to separate the effects of heredity and environment. Are both parents and children obese because they share a common genetic background or because they eat at the same table and share common food habits?

Body weights of identical twins vary considerably less than weights of fraternal twins or siblings of similar ages. The average percent variation in body weight of identical twins reared and living in dissimilar environments was found to be 3.60 percent compared to 1.39 percent for those reared and living together. In both cases the variation was small, suggesting that although environment plays some role, genetic factors may be of paramount importance in the control of body weight (Mayer, 1965a). Withers (1964) found overweightness of parents to be more highly correlated with overweight in natural children than in adopted ones. However, Garn et al. (1976) found adoptive parent-child pairs to have fatness similarities comparable to those of biological parent-child pairs. Shenker et al. (1974) suggested that overweight foster mothers may have a greater tendency to overfeed their infants than do normal weight foster mothers, based upon a study of weight changes of infants while in foster homes during the first few months of life.

The study of body build or somatotype in groups of obese and nonobese individuals supports genetic and constitutional factors operating in the predisposition to obesity. Somatotyping is a body-type classification system devised by Sheldon in 1940. Three primary components are rated in this system: endomorphy (softness, roundness, and smoothness), mesomorphy (strong bone and muscle development), and ectomorphy (linearity and fragility) (Seltzer and Mayer, 1966). Endomorphy is correlated with amount of body fat, and obesity is synonymous with strength in this type of build. However, Seltzer and Mayer (1964) found that obese adolescent girls differed from nonobese counterparts in other body build features besides those involving endomorphy and the amount of fatty tissue. The obese girls were more endomorphic, of course, but were somewhat more mesomorphic (larger skeleton and muscle structure) and considerably less ectomorphic (less linear, delicate, and fragile) than nonobese girls from a similar population. A group of 94 obese women was also studied with similar results (Seltzer and Mayer, 1969). Apparently obesity rarely occurs in some body build types and is very prevalent in others. Body build is inherited, although the way in which this occurs is not clear.

Several lines of evidence thus lend support to the idea that there· are genetic factors influencing the development of obesity. If children with hereditary tendencies toward obesity are identified early in life, preventive measures can be adopted.

Metabolic Effects

Metabolic obesity implies some type of biochemical lesion or abnormality, including possible enzymatic or hormonal defects. An unequivocal primary biochemical lesion in obesity has not, as yet, been clearly demonstrated. However, this does not mean that such lesions do not exist since unanswered questions remain in the area of bioenergetics. Researchers are attempting to clarify both the input and output sides of the energy equation in humans, although available techniques for measuring the various factors involved in body weight regulation are imprecise (Goldman et al., 1975). A recent revival of interest in overeating experiments in people has resulted from the awareness that there are metabolic differences between the lean and the obese (Miller, 1975). Normal humans and animals can adapt, within limits, to an increase in caloric intake without gaining weight. For many years, farm animals have been cultivated for their metabolic efficiency in converting feed to edible meat. Metabolic abnormalities accompany obesity in certain strains of animals that are genetically predisposed to develop obesity. It is also apparent, even from casual observation, that there is wide variation in the number of kilocalories required by various individuals to maintain body weight within normal range.

Several metabolic abnormalities have been reported to be more prevalent among obese human subjects than among normal weight controls, including:

1. Elevated fasting level of plasma free fatty acids (FFA) (Rath et al., 1970; Goldberg and Gordon, 1964). Although the levels are high after an overnight fast, in some patients with longstanding obesity FFA fail to increase markedly above this level with longer periods of fasting when compared to nonobese subjects (Gordon, 1960).
2. Elevated fasting level of plasma ketones (Rath et al., 1970). The elevation appears to be related to the amount of body fat. However, less marked ketosis has been observed in the obese during a 5-day fast than in nonobese controls, particularly for subjects in a "stabilized" as compared with a dynamic stage of obesity.
3. Increased fasting levels of plasma glucose (Kalkhoff et al., 1971).
4. Increased fasting levels of plasma insulin (Kalkhoff et al.; Schultz, 1973). This abnormality has been reported also for many maturity-onset diabetics. It has been suggested that insulin antagonism is present in obesity but the site is not clear (Davidson, 1972).
5. Abnormal oral glucose tolerance test (Kalkhoff et al.; Knittle and Ginsberg-Fellner, 1972; Jourdan et al., 1974). The higher plasma

glucose and longer time of elevation after a glucose load are similar to the responses of mild diabetics. It is possible these abnormalities occur primarily in obese subjects who are also carbohydrate intolerant. Relationships between obesity and diabetes mellitus are discussed in Sec. 16.6.

6. Increased insulin response to a glucose load (Kalkhoff et al.).
7. Decreased level of plasma growth hormone in response to falling blood glucose levels (Kalkhoff et al.).
8. Hypertriglyceridemia (Björntorp, 1974).

Are the metabolic abnormalities observed in the obese a causal factor in the development and maintenance of obesity, or are they simply a result of the obesity itself? Kalkhoff et al. evaluated six obese patients both before and after weight loss for various plasma substrate levels and responses. Before weight reduction, fasting plasma glucose, FFA, and insulin exceeded normal levels. Insulin response to oral glucose and intravenous tolbutamide was above control responses and plasma growth hormone response to intravenous insulin was subnormal. After substantial weight reduction, however, only minor differences in mean values existed between obese and control groups. Hewing et al. (1973) reinvestigated 24 patients 4 years after controlled clinical treatment with a 1000-kcal diet to determine to what extent the metabolic improvement had continued beyond the time of dietary treatment. Twelve of the patients had maintained their weight or reduced further and showed slightly improved glucose tolerance with a more normal insulin release than had been documented at the end of the previous study period. The other 12 patients, however, had returned almost to their initial weights and showed a decreased glucose tolerance compared with their previous examination. Their plasma insulin levels were still slightly elevated, with a typically delayed secretion. These findings suggest that at least some metabolic effects of obesity are reversible with weight loss and are long term. Ball et al. (1972) found that some reduced patients regained a normal growth hormone response to falling blood sugar shortly after losing weight whereas others continued to have a blunted response for up to 6 months following a return to normal body composition. Jourdan et al. (1974) reported that both weight loss and diet composition (increased carbohydrate and decreased protein) contributed independently to improved carbohydrate tolerance of obese subjects.

Adipocyte Development and Metabolism.   Excessive amounts of fat accumulating in adipose tissue depots apparently affect both the morphology and the metabolic character of this tissue. The cellular morphology and metabolic changes appear to be related and may affect other metabolic abnormalities noted in obese individuals.

Adipose tissue, as other tissues in the body, may increase in size as a result of cell replication and/or enlargement. Growth by cell replication, or increase in cell number, is called *hyperplasia,* whereas an increase in cell size is referred to as *hypertrophy.* Adipose tissue cell number and size have been measured in the obese as compared to lean controls. One useful technique for these measurements was developed by Hirsch and Gallian (1968). Fragments of human adipose tissue are obtained from subcutaneous sites by needle aspiration. The tissue is washed, weighed, and fixed in 2 percent osmium tetroxide, which combines with lipid and hardens the adipocytes. The cells then fall away from the tissue matrix, can be separated into various sizes, and counted in an electronic counter. In a duplicate adipose tissue sample, the percent lipid is determined, and the cell size can then be estimated in terms of average amount of lipid per cell (Stern and Greenwood, 1974).

In rats adipose cell numbers are essentially complete before weaning, and growth of adipose tissue after this time comes primarily from hypertrophy. The normal development of adipose tissue in the rat can be modified by overfeeding before weaning, resulting in hyperplasia. There would thus appear to be "critical periods" when nutritional influences can produce permanent changes in adipose cellularity in experimental animals (Hirsch, 1972).

From various reports of humans of various ages, it appears that fat cell number and size increase rapidly in children during the first years of life, with the cell number increasing particularly from the thirtieth week of gestation through the first year (Björntorp, 1974). The fetus accumulates a great deal of fat in the last trimester of pregnancy. Apparently after the first year or two of life, there is little increase in cell number until the preadolescent growth spurt occurs. It has been speculated that critical periods for adipocyte development in the human, at which time nutrition may have an influence on cell number, may thus be the last months of gestation, the first year of life, and during the preadolescent and adolescent growth period (Hirsch, 1972).

In general, individuals whose obesity began in childhood tend to have the most marked increase in cell number, whereas those who became obese after puberty show a greater tendency toward increase in cell size with normal cell number. Weight reduction in both cases, however, decreases adipose cell size without having any appreciable effect on cell number. Hypercellularity seems to be permanent once it occurs (Knittle, 1975; Björntorp et al., 1975; Knittle and Ginsberg-Fellner, 1972; Bray, 1970). All fat depots do not have the same mean cell size, and this must be considered in setting up a study and in comparing research reports (Duckerts and Bonnet, 1973).

The success rate for reduction of hyperplastic obesity by ordinary diet and exercise regimens would appear to be very low. *Prevention* of hypercellularity, and consequent obesity, in childhood would appear to offer a much better solution than conventional treatment of the already established obese state (Knittle, 1975; Björntorp, 1974).

Regulation of Food Intake

The desire to eat is a primitive instinct that exists in all members of the animal kingdom, although regulation of food intake is more complicated in higher than lower forms of animal life. Humans differ from other animals in that they may eat without hunger. There are many influences in addition to physiology that affect their eating habits.

The maintenance of a fairly constant body weight in a normal person without conscious effort over a lifetime suggests that some type of regulatory system is operating to control energy balance. Several hypotheses to explain this have been suggested. Feeding behavior has been variously attributed to oral and gastrointestinal sensations, body-temperature regulation (thermostatic control), utilization of glucose by cells in the hypothalamus (glucostatic theory), size of adipose tissue depots (lipostatic theory), levels of circulating amino acids (aminostatic theory), and other influences (Hamilton, 1973). The explanations involve both neurological and humoral mechanisms. Studies in the 1940s showed that when lesions were made in the *ventromedial* area of the hypothalamus of experimental animals, hyperphagia was produced with resulting obesity. When the *lateral* hypothalamus was damaged experimentally, aphagia was produced and emaciation occurred. This research was a landmark in the study of neuronal control of feeding behavior, and these ideas have dominated thinking about the regulation of feeding since that time. More recent work suggests that there are many variables in feeding behavior, and the description of mechanisms in the hypothalamus alone will not adequately explain the neuronal regulation of energy intake (Sutin, 1975). Other brain structures probably participate in feeding behavior.

Humoral hypotheses for the control of food intake are based upon the idea that substances carried in the blood coordinate feeding behavior with cell metabolism so that body weight is regulated. The glucostatic and aminostatic theories suggest primarily humoral mechanisms for short-term control of food intake, and the lipostatic theory addresses long-term control (Smith, 1975). In any mechanism, the body must have some "set point" and be sensitive to any degree of deviation from this point. There must be a detector in the feedback system to detect the deviation and initiate activity to reduce it. The brain probably serves this purpose (Hamilton, 1973).

Oral and Gastrointestinal Sensations. Taste and smell are obviously important in eating. Appetite (desire for food) may be stimulated by palatable food, and individuals may be encouraged to eat beyond the point of satisfying hunger when the flavor of food is particularly provocative. Wooley and Wooley (1973) suggested that salivary response to food stimuli may be used as a measure of appetite in the study of food regulation in humans.

Taste, olfaction, and swallowing were found not to be essential to the development of satiety in the primate (McHugh et al., 1975). In humans, Grinker (1975) and his coworkers found no differences between obese and nonobese in ability to detect sucrose in solution or in their dislike for salt solutions. However, obese subjects showed significantly *greater aversion* to concentrated sucrose solutions than did the nonobese. Grinker suggested that since a depressed taste preference has been observed in obese individuals, taste is not likely to play a major role in the etiology of obesity. In other words, an individual is evidently not made obese because of an overresponsiveness to taste stimuli. Wagner and Hewitt (1975) found that hospitalized obese subjects consumed their meals and chewed each mouthful in significantly less time than did nonobese controls and concluded that oral satiety appeared to play a less-than-meaningful role in the attainment of postprandial satiety for them.

A relationship between hunger and gastric contractions was noted in the early 1900s. One of the oldest theories to explain regulation of food intake suggested that gastric contractions regulated hunger through messages sent by the vagus nerve. Later studies, however, have demonstrated that (1) gastric motility can be greatly altered by changing the bulk of the diet without producing any lasting change in food intake, (2) vagotomy and splanchnectomy can drastically alter gastric contractions without appreciably affecting intake, and (3) patients with stomachs removed still experience feelings of hunger and satiety (Mayer, 1966; Hamilton, 1973). There are reasons to believe that the gut and the hypothalamus are associated in some way as part of a total system of food regulation. Distention of a cat's stomach by a balloon is accompanied by increased electrical activity of the ventromedial hypothalamus. Glucagon injections in rats increase blood glucose levels and also decrease gastric motility, except when the ventromedial hypothalamus has been lesioned. Apparently, neural impulses arising from filling of the stomach with food are sent to the hypothalamus for information on the extent of fill. However, gastrointestinal sensations cannot be used as the primary explanation for regulation of food intake (Hamilton, 1973).

Jordan (1975a) and his coworkers studied oral eating behavior in human subjects with liquid diets ingested through a straw from a hidden reservoir. When the caloric density of the diet was diluted, in short-term studies, subjects slightly increased the volume consumed but failed to compensate for extreme dilution and thus lost weight. In long-term studies, better compensation was observed, although adjustment was sluggish. When subjects were fed by gastric tube as well as orally, the control of caloric intake was less precise than with oral feeding alone. Wooley (1971) also found that human subjects fed a liquid diet *ad libitum* could not adequately adjust the volume to produce a constant caloric intake and maintain body weight. Results with normal weight and obese subjects were similar in both studies. However, Campbell et al. (1971) reported that five lean adult male subjects adjusted intake of a liquid diet of varied caloric density to maintain a constant energy intake, whereas four obese adult female subjects ingested a small fraction of the calories needed to maintain weight and failed to adapt volume intake to changes in caloric concentration. These studies suggest that both obese and nonobese subjects are not very sensitive to internal cues in regulating caloric intake. What the subject believes about the caloric value of the food he ingests is more important in determining his intake and hunger patterns than is the actual caloric value of the food (Wooley and Wooley, 1975).

Thermostatic Theory.   Brobeck suggested in 1948 that animals eat to keep warm and stop eating to prevent hyperthermia. The basic observation supporting this hypothesis is that most animals studied increase food intake in the cold and reduce it in the heat. When the thermosensitive area of the brain was destroyed in the rat, not only was body temperature unregulated but feeding behavior was also affected. The animals overate in the heat and underate in the cold (Hamilton, 1973). Thermostatic influences apparently play some role in the regulation of food intake but cannot explain the total system.

Glucostatic Theory.   Mayer and his coworkers suggested the glucostatic mechanism for food regulation in the early 1950s (Mayer, 1965b). This theory proposes that the ventromedial area of the hypothalamus acts as a satiety center with special glucoreceptor cells that are sensitive to blood glucose. The rate of glucose utilization by these cells is the critical factor in controlling food intake by its effect on satiety. When the cells are not using glucose, hunger develops and eating begins. It has also been suggested that the lateral areas of the hypothalamus act as feeding centers. When the ventromedial area is utilizing glucose, messages may be sent to the lateral areas to suppress their activity. When glucose is not being utilized by cells in the ventromedial area, no impulses are sent to the lateral feeding centers and they remain active, producing hunger.

It is extremely difficult to directly measure glucose utilization in the brain. Therefore, experimental evidence to test the glucostatic theory has used primarily indirect measurements, such as the capillary-venous (or arteriovenous) differences in glucose levels (Δ glucose). In general, small Δ glucose, indicating little glucose utilization by body cells, was correlated with feelings of hunger. Additional data that lend support to this theory include the (1) observation of increased food intake by rats and monkeys given injections of a competitive antagonist of glucose (2-deoxy-D-glucose) that raises blood sugar levels but inhibits glucose utilization by the brain; (2) hyperphagia and obesity in mice after injection of gold thioglucose, which destroys glucose-utilizing cells of the ventromedial area; (3) differences in uptake of radioactive phosphorus or C^{14} glucose by satiety and feeding centers of the hypothalamus in fed and fasted rats, indicating differences in metabolic activity in these two areas; and (4) differences in electrical activity of hypothalamic areas measured by implantation of electrodes in the brains of experimental animals, showing activity in the ventromedial area when blood glucose is high and activity in the lateral area when blood glucose is low (Mayer, 1965b). The satiety center apparently uses glucose in a manner similar to other insulin-sensitive tissues of the body (Debons and Krimsky, 1972).

The glucostatic theory operates over a relatively short period of time. It may explain parts of the feeding mechanism. However, the regulation of blood glucose levels is a complex process and is influenced by many hormones, including insulin and the glucocorticoids.

Lipostatic Theory. Kennedy (1953) first suggested that the mass of adipose depot fat in relation to body weight is the controlling factor for intake of food. Some unknown systemic metabolite related to the size of the adipose tissue mass supposedly supplies a signal to the central nervous system that deviation from the "set point" for amount of adipose tissue has occurred. The central nervous system then affects mechanisms that control feeding. There is some circumstantial evidence for this hypothesis, but no hard data are available. Evidence in support of the theory includes the observation that (1) rats made obese by insulin injection or excessive tube feeding ate little or nothing when these treatments were discontinued until normal body weight had been reached, and (2) rats already made obese by insulin injection were not hyperphagic after ventromedial lesions had been made. If the ventromedial lesioned obese rats were deprived of food for a sufficient period of time so that they were no longer obese, they became hyperphagic and eventually obese when food was again made available (Smith, 1975). It has been suggested that the hypothalamic lesions merely place the "set point" at a higher than usual level. Lesioned rats overeat only until they reach some stable body weight; they do not overeat indefinitely. However, the degree of obesity in lesioned rats can be enhanced to some degree by feeding a highly palatable diet. Not all observations support the lipostatic theory for regulation of body weight although the relative constancy of weight in normal man makes it plausible (Hamilton, 1973). The factor that may signal the central nervous system has not been identified.

Aminostatic Theory. The aminostatic hypothesis was suggested by Frazier et al. in 1947 to explain the rapid decrease in food intake of rats placed on a diet lacking an essential amino acid. Rats also markedly decrease their food intake when fed diets containing either an excess of one amino acid or a very high level of protein. It has been suggested that decreased ingestion of food by animals fed an amino acid imbalanced, deficient, or devoid diet may be a protective response, since force feeding a deficient diet produces pathologic lesions in some cases. The site of initiation of the mechanisms that decrease food intake may be the brain (Leung and Rogers, 1969).

Eating Patterns in Obesity. Obese individuals may differ from nonobese in terms of an inability to achieve a feeling of satiety after food intake (Linton et al., 1972). In a questionaire study of approximately 800 people, obese subjects reported that they required more will power than nonobese subjects to stop eating at the end of a meal, even though they reported more frequent sensations of discomfort (distention and nausea). They were also often preoccupied with thoughts of food half an hour after a meal, whereas this was an exceptional occurrence in nonobese subjects (Mayer et al., 1965).

Feeding Frequency

Whether eating occurs one to three times a day in meals or small amounts of food are taken throughout the day appears to influence metabolic processes that have to do with the synthesis of body fat from dietary nutrients. More fat synthesis occurs with a few large meals than with many small meals and snacks. Other factors, however, including age, total caloric intake, diet composition, and physical activity, moderate the final effects of feeding frequency (Fábry and Tepperman, 1970). When the total caloric intake is relatively high, the diet contains a large amount of carbohydrate (particularly simple forms), and physical inactivity characterizes the usual way of life, the consumption of a small number of large meals is most likely to produce excessive amounts of body fat in comparison with the same amount of food consumed in several small meals and snacks.

The metabolic effects of feeding frequency have been extensively studied in experimental animals. The rat is normally a "nibbler," eating small quantities of food more or less continuously and reaching a maximum in the night time. If food intake for the rat is restricted to 1 to 2 hours a day, he learns to eat large amounts of food at a time and becomes a "gorger." Several effects in animals of gorging in comparison to nibbling have been reported and include (1) enlargement of the stomach and small intestine, (2) increased activity of pancreatic enzymes, (3) enhanced intestinal absorption of glucose, (4) increased serum insulin response to eating, (5) increased activity of enzymes catalyzing fat synthesis in liver and adipose tissue, (6) increase in total body fat, (7) enhanced synthesis of cholesterol in the liver, (8) enhanced synthesis of protein and nucleic acids in adipose tissue, and (9) increased sensitivity to diabetogenic agents (Fábry and Tepperman, 1970). When a great flux of energy nutrients is available to the body, adaptations in metabolic pathways for handling these nutrients occur so that they can be stored for later use during the long periods between meals. A significant amount of energy can be stored as glycogen, but the large amounts coming in all at once require a more concentrated form of storage as triglycerides. The rat diet is typically high in carbohydrate which must be rapidly changed to triglyceride. Therefore, adipose tissue becomes very important in synthesizing and storing fat (Leveille, 1970; Leveille and Romsos, 1974).

Some observations have been made on meal frequency and overweight in humans. Metzner et al. (1977) found an inverse relationship between frequency of eating and adiposity index in 1000 men and 1000 women in Tecumseh, Michigan. Hejda and Fábry (1964) reported that prevalence of overweight, hypercholesterolemia, and glucose intolerance tended to decrease in Czechoslovakian men as meal frequency increased. Young et al. (1972) found that skin-fold thicknesses, average daily nitrogen retention, and percentage of fat intake excreted were not significantly different for normal male subjects on feeding regimens of six versus one meal a day, although glucose tolerance appeared to decrease on one meal a day in comparison with three or six. Young et al. (1971b) also reported that the frequency of feeding had no significant effect on losses in fat, skin-fold thicknesses, or body circumferences in moderately obese young college men on a rigidly controlled 1800-kcal diet fed either as six, three, or one meals a day. Pringle et al. (1976) fed low-kilocalorie diets to young overweight women in either a gorging or nibbling pattern for 4 weeks each. The gorging elevated the insulin response of those subjects with normal prestudy insulin levels. Nibbling lowered the insulin response of those subjects who had shown an exaggerated, delayed prestudy insulin response. Regression equations, calculated from the data, were used to predict the influence of eating frequency on weight reduction. Increasing the frequency was predicted to have no effect on the weight losses of subjects with normal prestudy serum insulin levels but was predicted to increase weight loss of the subjects with abnormal prestudy insulin responses by 22 percent. It has not yet been established whether in humans, as has been shown for rats, decreasing the frequency of food intake decreases the average caloric expenditure of the body by decreasing voluntary physical activity (Fábry and Tepperman, 1970).

Large effects on humans are not to be expected from altering eating frequency alone. However, under conditions where the demands for energy are limited by physical inactivity, diets are high in simple carbohydrates, and caloric intake is excessive, the adaptation to increased lipogenesis by large, infrequent meals may be pathogenic (Fábry and Tepperman, 1970).

Physical Inactivity

The role of physical activity in development and maintenance of obesity has been both presented as being important and dismissed as being insignificant. Differences in physical activity between groups of obese and nonobese adolescent girls were studied by Bullen et al. (1964) using motion picture sampling while subjects were participating in summer camp sports. They found the obese girls to be far less active than the nonobese, even during supervised periods. Huenemann et al. (1967) used activity and food diaries to collect information on general patterns of activity for teenagers. Their findings of poor correlation between low level of physical activity and larger amounts of body fat were not too surprising because all the teenagers studied were fairly inactive. They also found that obese teenagers tended to consume fewer calories than did their nonobese counterparts (Hampton et al., 1967). It was suggested that the low level of physical activity observed in their total teenage population, as well as that seen in adult populations, may be a major contributing factor to the high incidence of obesity in the United States. The work of Trulson et al. (1964) suggests that a more physically active population is less inclined to be obese than a sedentary one. However, Lincoln (1972), in a questionnaire study involving 867 men, found that physical activity levels of the more obese group were not lower than those of the less obese group. The more obese group consumed no more calories than the less obese group, but this was because restraint was used in food selection. He suggested that perhaps voluntary restriction of food intake depressed activity levels. Additional research is needed to clarify the role of physical inactivity in the etiology of obesity.

Sociological and Psychological Effects
The sciences of sociology and psychology are concerned with people's environment and the rewards and punishments that determine their behavior. Use of these sciences in the study of obesity has demonstrated marked influences of environment on eating patterns (Stunkard, 1968).

Social Factors in Obesity.   Goldblatt et al. (1965) investigated relationships between social class and obesity using data collected as part of a comprehensive survey of the epidemiology of mental illness in midtown Manhattan. They found an inverse relationship between obesity in women and parental socioeconomic status and also between obesity in women and one's own socioeconomic status. Obesity was six times more common among women of low status than among those of high status. In addition, they reported that upwardly mobile women in the social structure were less obese (12 percent) than downwardly mobile women (22 percent). Generation in the United States was strongly linked to obesity. The longer a woman's family had been in this country, the less likely she was to be obese. Similar trends were found for men in the study but they were less marked than for women. It was suggested that the lesser importance of relationships between social factors and body weight among men than women may arise from a lesser importance that society attaches to the physical appearance of men and from a different definition of culturally desirable weight for them.

Several ethnic groups were included in the Manhattan study. Ethnic factors were intertwined with other social factors and with each other. The sample sizes were also small within each ethnic group. However, within the low socioeconomic status, the percent obese women differed as follows: fourth generation American, 13 percent; Puerto Rican, 15 percent; Russian, Polish, Lithuanian, 18 percent; British, 23 percent; Irish, 25 percent; Italian, 32 percent; German, Austrian, 35 percent; Czech, 41 percent; and Hungarian, 44 percent (Stunkard, 1968). Some of these differences may be related to traditional patterns of eating and social values attached to eating.

The findings of the Manhattan study are not necessarily directly applicable to other areas in the United States or to other countries of the world. In fact, studies in Germany have shown an increased incidence of obesity among upwardly mobile German men, along with a decreased incidence among upwardly mobile German women (Stunkard et al., 1972). Garn et al. (1977) found skin-fold thickness to be greater in Michigan men with more than 12 years of schooling than in those with 8 years or less. The opposite trend was observed in women. However, in a Health Maintenance Clinic population, women from 40 to 59 years of age with less than 12 years of education were more likely to be overweight than similar aged women with more education (Herman, 1973).

Apparently socioeconomic influences begin early in life. A study of Caucasian school children in three eastern cities showed that obesity was far more prevalent in lower-class than upper-class girls. Similar but less striking differences were found between boys (Stunkard et al., 1972).

Psychological Factors. The universality of psychological and emotional problems among the obese population and their role in the development of obesity are sometimes subjects for considerable discussion and disagreement among professionals (Forbes, 1967). Jordan (1975b), in an attempt to identify more precisely the relationship of psychological factors and obesity, has suggested a classification into (1) factors that have etiological significance, (2) those that result from the obesity itself, (3) those that result from losing weight or attempting not to be obese, and (4) those that occur after successful weight loss.

Bruch (1975) pointed out that obesity represents a complex condition determined by many simultaneously interacting factors and, thus, simplistic answers to either-or questions about obesity may be misleading. It is true that no one single personality variable has been isolated that characterizes obese individuals, but this does not mean that emotional factors may not be important in the development of obesity for some individuals. Certainly psychopathology is not involved in the development of all cases of obesity, but it may be a major factor in some individuals and must be treated by qualified professionals before any type of nutritional counseling will be useful to the patient. In her book *Eating Disorders,* Bruch (1973) described 35 years of experience with treating a minority of the obese population for whom obesity has been an attempt to adapt to underlying psychological problems. She observed that many, though not all, individuals with early onset obesity suffer from severe personality problems and serious handicaps.

Schachter (1968) and Nisbett (1968), among others, have suggested that eating behavior of the obese is under the primary control of external cues rather than internal physiological influences. Obese subjects ate more when they thought it was their dinner hour than when they thought it was somewhat earlier, while normal weight individuals were relatively unaffected by the manipulation of time. Obese subjects ate considerably more of good-tasting food than of bad, whereas normal weight subjects were less responsive to differences in taste. This idea of externality has been modified to postulate that eating behavior of the obese is triggered only when food cues in the environment are highly potent. The obese are thought to have a heightened sensitivty to external stimuli that extends beyond eating behavior (Rodin, 1975).

Recent reports (Levitz, 1975) now suggest that normal weight individuals also respond to external cues, eat for sociological and psychological reasons, as well as biological, and are not primarily regulated by internal physiologic signals. The type of food presented and the method of presentation influence the amount consumed by normal subjects, and they use visual cues to monitor their food intake. Further clarification is needed of possible differences between the obese and nonobese in this area. Behavioral modification techniques should logically be useful in treating obese individuals who have become dependent upon external cues to determine their eating behavior.

The psychological effects of being obese may range from mild feeling of inferiority to very serious problems that may occur when the obesity bars the individual from normal socializing. Since obesity carries a stigma, many of these effects are the result of negative social views (Hirsch, 1975). In America fat people are not only discriminated against in social situations, college entrance, and job placement, but they are made to feel that they deserve such discrimination. The condemning process itself helps to create and accentuate the handicap of overweight. To expose the stigmatization of the overweight, the National Association to Aid Fat Americans, Inc., whose membership includes both fat and thin people, has been organized (Allon, 1975).

The obese adolescent girl faces particularly difficult problems in relating to her peers, since adolescents put special emphasis on body appearance. Dwyer et al. (1969) studied adolescent attitudes toward weight and appearance. Most of the girls surveyed wanted to weigh less than they actually did while most of the boys wanted to weigh more, with the exception of the obese boys. The level of discontent with the body was high in both girls and boys. The obese girls regarded themselves as both fatter and larger than other girls in their class. Hammar et al. (1972) reported finding evidence for defective body-image development, low self-esteem, depression, and social isolation in 10 obese adolescents as they were compared with 10 nonobese control subjects. The obese adolescents were often a focus of parental conflicts and a scapegoat for their siblings in the family. Infant feeding problems, food intolerances, an earlier introduction of solid foods, and a persistent use of food as reinforcer for good behavior were often reported among the obese group.

From metabolic and behavioral studies of obese subjects during weight reduction, Grinker (1973) and his coworkers concluded that there were differences in reactions to weight reduction between those subjects with juvenile-onset obesity and those whose obesity developed in adult life. The subjects with juvenile-onset obesity experienced weight reduction as a severe starvation. They felt symptoms of anxiety, depression, concern over changing body size, preoccupation with food, and decreased vigor during weight reduction. These feelings continued after caloric intake was increased to maintain their new body weight levels. On the other hand, subjects with adult-onset obesity undergoing weight reduction did not develop depressive or anxious symptoms (Grinker et al., 1973). During weight reduction, subjects with juvenile-onset obesity significantly overestimated their body size in quantitative measurements of body size perception. In spite of marked weight losses, they saw themselves as if they had lost little or no weight. In contrast, adult-onset obese subjects tended to underestimate their body size after weight reduction (Glucksman and Hirsch, 1969).

Stunkard and Rush (1974), in summarizing their conclusions drawn from a review of the literature on psychological effects of weight reduction programs, concluded that (1) short-term fasting, with a duration of 10 to 14 days or a weight loss of 7 to 9 kg, results in fewest complications; (2) persons with juvenile-onset obesity are more likely to experience psychological and physical distress than adult-onset subjects; (3) long-term treatment, whether fasting or low-kilocalorie dieting, is consistently associated with adverse psychological and physical symptoms that are often severe; (4) low-kilocalorie diets, perhaps because they revive hunger without satisfying it, may be more stressful than total fasting; and (5) outpatient treatment is more difficult to control and evaluate than inpatient treatment, partly because of very high attrition rates.

A reduced person must become accustomed to a different body and to a different set of stimuli that will come from society at large now that he or she is in the nonobese category. Close interpersonal relationships can also change. Psychological problems may occur and this could be a fruitful area of research for the social scientist (Jordan, 1975b).

It is apparent that sociological and psychological influences are intertwined with the various facets of obesity. They must be considered in attempting to understand the causes of obesity. They must be handled in any weight reduction treatment program. They will also undoubtedly be important in any attempts to prevent the development of obesity. The extent of the sociocultural and psychological influences will vary from one obese individual to another, with psychogenic factors probably playing a greater role in obesity that begins in childhood than that occurring first in adult life.

REFERENCES

1. Alexander, J. K. 1964. Obesity and cardiac performance. *Am. J. Cardiology*, **14:** 860.

2. Alexander, J. K. and K. L. Peterson. 1972. Cardiovascular effects of weight reduction. *Circulation*, **45:** 310.

3. Allon, N. 1975. The stigma of overweight in everyday life. In *Obesity in Perspective*, Part 2, G. A. Bray (Ed.). DHEW Publication No. (NIH) 75–708.

4. Anderson, E. C. and W. H. Langham. 1961. Estimation of total body fat from potassium-40 content. *Science*, **133:** 1917.

5. Ball, M. F., A. Z. El-Khodary, and J. J. Canary. 1972. Growth hormone response in the thinned obese. *J. Clin. Endocrin. Met.*, **34:** 498.

6. Bergen, W. G., M. L. Kaplan, R. A. Merkel, and G. A. Leveille. 1975. Growth of adipose

and lean tissue mass in hindlimbs of genetically obese mice during preobese and obese phases of development. *Am. J. Clin. Nutr.,* **28:** 157.

7. Björntorp, P. 1974. Effects of age, sex, and clinical conditions on adipose tissue cellularity in man. *Metabolism,* **23:** 1091.

8. Björntorp, P., G. Carlgren, B. Isaksson, M. Krotkiewski, B. Larsson, and L. Sjöström. 1975. Effect of an energy-reduced dietary regimen in relation to adipose tissue cellularity in obese women. *Am. J. Clin. Nutr.,* **28:** 445.

9. Braunstein, J. J. 1971. Management of the obese patient. *Med. Clinics No. Am.,* **55:** 391.

10. Bray, G. A. 1970. Measurement of subcutaneous fat cells from obese patients. *Ann. Int. Med.,* **73:** 565.

11. Bray, G. A. (Ed.). 1975. *Obesity in Perspective,* Parts 1 and 2. DHEW Publication No. (NIH) 75–708.

12. Brobeck, J. R. 1948. Food intake as a mechanism of temperature regulation. *Yale J. Biol. Med.,* **20:** 545.

13. Bruch, H. 1973. *Eating Disorders.* New York: Basic Books.

14. Bruch, H. 1975. The psychological handicaps of the obese. In *Obesity in Perspective,* Part 2, G. A. Bray (Ed.). DHEW Publication No. (NIH) 75–708.

15. Bullen, B. A., R. B. Reed, and J. Mayer. 1964. Physical activity of obese and nonobese adolescent girls appraised by motion picture sampling. *Am. J. Clin. Nutr.,* **14:** 211.

16. Burwell, C. S., E. D. Robin, R. D. Whaley, and A. G. Bickelmann. 1956. Extreme obesity associated with alveolar hypoventilation—a Pickwickian syndrome. *Am. J. Med.,* **21:** 811.

17. Butterworth, C. E. and G. L. Blackburn. 1975. Hospital malnutrition. *Nutr. Today,* **10** (No. 2): 8.

18. Campbell, R. G., S. A. Hashim, and T. B. Van Itallie. 1971. Studies on food-intake regulation in man. *N. Eng. J. Med.,* **285:** 1402.

19. Chlouverakis, C. 1972. Effect of caloric restriction on body weight loss and body fat utilization in obese hyperglycemic mice (Obob). *Metabolism,* **21:** 10.

20. Davidson, M. B. 1972. Glucose metabolism in human adipose tissue of obese and normal weight subjects. *Israel J. Med. Sci.,* **8:** 826.

21. Debons, A. F. and K. Krimsky. 1972. Regulation of food intake: Role of the ventromedial hypothalamus. *Postgrad. Med.,* **51:** 74.

22. Duckerts, M. and F. Bonnet. 1973. Adipose cell size differences related to the site of adipose tissue biopsy in children. *Biomedicine,* **19:** 214.

23. Dwyer, J. T., J. J. Feldman, C. C. Seltzer, and J. Mayer. 1969. Adolescent attitudes toward weight and appearance. *J. Nutr. Educ.,* **1** (No. 2): 14.

24. Edwards, D. A. W., W. H. Hammond, M. J. R. Healy, J. M. Tanner, and R. H. Whitehouse. 1955. Design and accuracy of calipers for measuring subcutaneous tissue thickness. *Brit. J. Nutr.,* **9:** 133.

25. Fábry, P. and J. Tepperman. 1970. Meal frequency—A possible factor in human pathology. *Am. J. Clin. Nutr.,* **23:** 1059.

26. Forbes, G. B. 1967. The great denial. *Nutr. Rev.,* **25:** 353.

27. Frazier, L. E., R. W. Wissler, C. H. Stefler, F. L. Woolridge, and P. R. Cannon. 1947. Studies in amino acid utilization. I. The dietary utilization of mixtures of purified amino acids in protein-depleted adult albino rats. *J. Nutr.,* **33:** 65.

28. Garn, S. M., S. M. Bailey, P. E. Cole, and I. T. T. Higgins. 1977. Level of education, level of income, and level of fatness in adults. *Am. J. Clin. Nutr.,* **30:** 721.

29. Glucksman, M. L. and J. Hirsch. 1969. The response of obese patients to weight reduction. III. The perception of body size. *Psychosom. Med.,* **31:** 1.

30. Goldberg, M. and E. S. Gordon. 1964. Energy metabolism in human obesity. *J. Am. Med. Assoc.*, **189:** 616.

31. Goldblatt, P. B., M. E. Moore, and A. J. Stunkard. 1965. Social factors in obesity. *J. Am. Med. Assoc.*, **192:** 1039.

32. Goldman, R. F., M. F. Haisman, G. Bynum, E. S. Horton, and E. A. H. Sims. 1975. Experimental obesity in man. Metabolic rate in relation to dietary intake. In *Obesity in Perspective*, Part 2, G. A. Bray (Ed.). DHEW Publication No. (NIH) 75–708.

33. Goodhart, R. S. and M. E. Shils (Eds.). 1973. *Modern Nutrition in Health and Disease*, 5th ed. Philadelphia: Lea and Febiger.

34. Gordon, E. S. 1960. Non-esterified fatty acids in blood of obese and lean subjects. *Am. J. Clin. Nutr.*, **8:** 740.

35. Grande, F. 1975. Assessment of body fat in man. In *Obesity in Perspective*, Part 2, G. A. Bray (Ed.). DHEW Publication No. (NIH) 75–708.

36. Grinker, J. 1973. Behavioral and metabolic consequences of weight reduction. *J. Am. Dietet. Assoc.*, **62:** 30.

37. Grinker, J. A. 1975. Obesity and taste: Sensory and cognitive factors in food intake. In *Obesity in Perspective*, Part 2, G. A. Bray (ed.). DHEW Publication No. (NIH) 75–708.

38. Grinker, J., J. Hirsch, and B. Levin. 1973. The affective responses of obese patients to weight reduction: A differentiation based on age at onset of obesity. *Psychosom. Med.*, **35:** 57.

39. Hamilton, C. L. 1973. Physiologic control of food intake. *J. Am. Dietet. Assoc.*, **62:** 35.

40. Hammar, S. L., M. M. Campbell, V. A. Campbell, N. L. Moores, C. Sareen, F. J. Gareis, and B. Lucas. 1972. An interdisciplinary study of adolescent obesity. *J. Ped.*, **80:** 373.

41. Hampton, M. C., R. L. Huenemann, L. R. Shapiro, and B. W. Mitchell. 1967. Caloric and nutrient intakes of teen-agers. *J. Am. Dietet. Assoc.*, **50:** 385.

42. Heald, F. P. 1972. The natural history of obesity. *Adv. Psychosom. Med.*, **7:** 102.

43. Hejda, S. and P. Fábry. 1964. Frequency of food intake in relation to some parameters of the nutritional status. *Nutr. Dieta.*, **6:** 216.

44. Herman, M. W. 1973. Excess weight and sociocultural characteristics. *J. Am. Dietet. Assoc.*, **63:** 161.

45. Hewing, R., H. Liebermeister, H. Daweke, F. A. Gries, and D. Gruneklee. 1973. Weight regain after low calorie diet: Long term pattern of blood sugar, serum lipids, ketone bodies and serum insulin levels. *Diabetologia*, **9:** 197.

46. Hirsch, J. 1972. Can we modify the number of adipose cells? *Postgrad. Med.*, **51:** 83.

47. Hirsch, J. 1975. The psychological consequences of obesity. In *Obesity in Perspective*, Part 2, G. A. Bray (Ed.). DHEW Publication No. (NIH) 75–708.

48. Hirsch, J. and E. Gallian. 1968. Methods for the determination of adipose cell size in man and animals. *J. Lipid Res.*, **9:** 110.

49. Huenemann, R. L., L. R. Shapiro, M. C. Hampton, and B. W. Mitchell. 1967. Teen-agers' activities and attitudes toward activity. *J. Am. Dietet. Assoc.*, **51:** 433.

50. Hunt, C. E., J. R. Lindsey, and S. U. Walkley. 1976. Animal models of diabetes and obesity, including the PBB/Ld mouse. *Fed. Proc.*, **35:** 1206.

51. Jordan, H. A. 1973. In defense of body weight. *J. Am. Dietet. Assoc.*, **62:** 17.

52. Jordan, H. A. 1975a. Physiological control of food intake in man. In *Obesity in Perspective*, Part 2, G. A. Bray (Ed.). DHEW Publication No. (NIH) 75–708.

53. Jordan, H. A. 1975b. Psychological factors associated with obesity. In *Obesity in Perspective*, Part 1, G. A. Bray (Ed.). DHEW Publication No. (NIH) 75–708.

54. Jourdan, M., D. Goldbloom, S. Margen, and R. B. Bradfield. 1974. Differential effects

of diet composition and weight loss on glucose tolerance in obese women. *Am. J. Clin. Nutr.*, **27**: 1065.

55. Kalkhoff, R. K., H. J. Kim, J. Cerletty, and C. A. Ferrou. 1971. Metabolic effects of weight loss in obese subjects. *Diabetes*, **20**: 83.

56. Kannel, W. B., G. Pearson, and P. M. McNamara. 1969. Obesity as a force of morbidity and mortality in adolescence. In *Adolescent Nutrition and Growth*, F. P. Heald (Ed.). Englewood Cliffs, N.J.: Prentice-Hall.

57. Kennedy, G. C. 1953. The role of depot fat in the hypothalamic control of food intake in the rat. *Proc. Royal Soc. Lond. (Biol.)*, **140**: 578.

58. Keys, A., F. Fidanza, M. J. Karvonen, N. Kimura, and H. L. Taylor. 1972. Indices of relative weight and obesity. *J. Chron. Dis.*, **25**: 329.

59. Knittle, J. L. 1975. Early influences on development of adipose tissue. In *Obesity in Perspective*, Part 2, G. A. Bray (Ed.). DHEW Publication No. (NIH) 75–708.

60. Knittle, J. L. and F. Ginsberg-Fellner. 1972. Effect of weight reduction on in vitro adipose tissue lipolysis and cellularity in obese adolescents and adults. *Diabetes*, **21**: 754.

61. Leung, P. M. B. and Q. R. Rogers. 1969. Food intake: Regulation by plasma amino acid pattern. *Life Sciences*, **8** (Part II): 1.

62. Leveille, G. A. 1970. Adipose tissue metabolism: Influence of periodicity of eating and diet composition. *Fed. Proc.*, **29**: 1294.

63. Leveille, G. A. and D. R. Romsos. 1974. Meal eating and obesity. *Nutr. Today*, **9** (No. 6): 4.

64. Levitz, L. S. 1975. The susceptibility of human feeding behavior to external controls. In *Obesity in Perspective*, Part 2, G. A. Bray (Ed.). DHEW Publication No. (NIH) 75–708.

65. Lincoln, J. E. 1972. Calorie intake, obesity, and physical activity. *Am. J. Clin. Nutr.*, **25**: 390.

66. Linton, P. H., M. Conley, C. Kuechenmeister, and H. McClusky. 1972. Satiety and obesity. *Am. J. Clin. Nutr.*, **25**: 368.

67. Lourenco, R. V. 1969. Diaphragm activity in obesity. *J. Clin. Investig.*, **48**: 1609.

68. Mayer, J. 1965a. Genetic factors in human obesity. *Postgrad. Med.*, **37**: A-103.

69. Mayer, J. 1965b. The ventromedial glucostatic mechanism as a component of satiety. *Postgrad. Med.*, **38**: A-101.

70. Mayer, J. 1966. Why people get hungry. *Nutr. Today*, **1** (June): 2.

71. Mayer, J., L. F. Monello, and C. C. Seltzer. 1965. Hunger and satiety sensations in man. *Postgrad. Med.*, **37**: A-97.

72. Metropolitan Life Insurance Company. 1959. New weight standards for men and women. *Statistical Bull.*, **40** (Nov.-Dec.): 1.

73. Metzner, H. L., D. E. Lamphiear, N. C. Wheeler, and F. A. Larkin. 1977. The relationship between frequency of eating and adiposity in adult men and women in the Tecumseh Community Health Study. *Am. J. Clin. Nutr.*, **30**: 712.

74. Miller, D. S. 1975. Overfeeding in man. In *Obesity in Perspective*, Part 2, G. B. Bray (Ed.). DHEW Publication No. (NIH) 75–708.

75. Montoye, H. J., F. H. Epstein, and M. O. Kjelsberg. 1966. Relationship between serum cholesterol and body fatness. *Am. J. Clin. Nutr.*, **18**: 397.

76. McHugh, P. R., T. H. Moran, and G. N. Barton. 1975. Satiety: A graded behavioral phenomenon regulating caloric intake. *Science*, **190**: 167.

77. National Dairy Council. 1975. Current concepts of obesity. *Dairy Council Digest*, **46**: 19.

78. Nisbett, R. E. 1968. Determinants of food intake in obesity. *Science*, **159**: 1254.

79. Pike, R. L. and M. L. Brown. 1974. *Nutrition: An Integrated Approach.* New York: Wiley.

80. Pringle, D. J., P. S. Wadhwa, and C. E. Elson. 1976. Influence of frequency of eating low energy diets on insulin response in women during weight reduction. *Nutr. Rep. Internat.,* **13:** 339.

81. Rath, R., J. Masek, H. Bittnerova, V. Kujalova, and A. Veselkova. 1970. Metabolism of the obese. *Nutr. Rep. Internat.,* **1:** 197.

82. Rauh, J. L. and D. A. Schumsky. 1969. Relative accuracy of visual assessment of juvenile obesity. *J. Am. Dietet. Assoc.,* **55:** 459.

83. Rimm, A. A., L. H. Werner, B. Van Yserloo, and R. A. Bernstein. 1975. Relationship of obesity and disease in 73,532 weight-conscious women. *Pub. Health Rep.,* **90** (No. 1): 44.

84. Rodin, J. 1975. Responsiveness of the obese to external stimuli. In *Obesity in Perspective,* Part 2, G. A. Bray (Ed.). DHEW Publication No. (NIH) 75–708.

85. Salzano, J. V., R. V. Gunning, T. N. Mastopaulo, and W. W. Tuttle. 1958. Effect of weight loss on blood pressure. *J. Am. Dietet. Assoc.,* **34:** 1309.

86. Schachter, S. 1968. Obesity and eating. *Science,* **161:** 751.

87. Schultz, R. B. 1973. Metabolic aspects of obesity. *Metabolism,* **22:** 359.

88. Seltzer, C. C. and J. Mayer. 1964. Body build and obesity—Who are the obese? *J. Am. Med. Assoc.,* **189:** 677.

89. Seltzer, C. C. and J. Mayer. 1965. A simple criterion of obesity. *Postgrad. Med.,* **38:** A-101.

90. Seltzer, C. C. and J. Mayer. 1966. Body measurements in relation to disease, Part 2. *Postgrad. Med.,* **40:** A-145.

91. Seltzer, C. C. and J. Mayer. 1969. Body build (somatotype) distinctiveness in obese women. *J. Am. Dietet. Assoc.,* **55:** 454.

92. Sheldon, W. H., S. S. Stevens, and W. B. Tucker. 1940. *The Varieties of Human Physique.* New York: Harper & Row.

93. Shenker, I. R., V. Fisichelli, and J. Lang. 1974. Weight differences between foster infants of overweight and nonoverweight foster mothers. *J. Ped.,* **84:** 715.

94. Smith, G. P. 1975. Humoral hypotheses for the control of food intake. In *Obesity in Perspective,* Part 2, G. A. Bray (Ed.). DHEW Publication No. (NIH) 75–708.

95. Stern, J. S. and M. R. C. Greenwood. 1974. A review of development of adipose cellularity in man and animals. *Fed. Proc.,* **33:** 1952.

96. Stunkard, A. J. 1968. Environment and obesity: Recent advances in our understanding of regulation of food intake in man. *Fed. Proc.,* **27:** 1367.

97. Stunkard, A., E. d'Aquili, and R. D. L. Filion. 1972. Influence of social class on obesity and thinness in children. *J. Am. Med. Assoc.,* **221:** 579.

98. Stunkard, A. J. and J. Rush. 1974. Dieting and depression reexamined. *Ann. Int. Med.,* **81:** 526.

99. Sutin, J. 1975. Neural factors in the control of food intake. In *Obesity in Perspective,* Part 2, G. A. Bray (Ed.). DHEW Publication No. (NIH) 75–708.

100. Thomas, A. E., D. A. McKay, and M. B. Cutlip. 1976. A nomograph method for assessing body weight. *Am. J. Clin. Nutr.,* **29:** 302.

101. Trulson, M. F., R. E. Clancy, W. J. E. Jessop, R. W. Childers, and F. J. Stare. 1964. Comparisons of siblings in Boston and Ireland. Physical, biochemical, and dietary findings. *J. Am. Dietet. Assoc.,* **45:** 225.

102. U.S. Department of Health, Education and Welfare, Public Health Service. 1966. *Obesity and Health.*

103. Van Itallie, T. B. and R. G. Campbell. 1972. Multidisciplinary approach to the problem of obesity. *J. Am. Dietet. Assoc.,* **61:** 385.

104. Wagner, M. and M. I. Hewitt. 1975. Oral satiety in the obese and nonobese. *J. Am. Dietet. Assoc.,* **67:** 344.

105. Waxler, S. H. and L. S. Craig. 1964. Lipid, cholesterol and triglyceride levels in obese women. *Am. J. Clin. Nutr.,* **14:** 128.

106. Weinsier, R. L., R. J. Fuchs, T. D. Kay, J. H. Triebwasser, and M. C. Lancaster. 1976. Body fat: its relationship to coronary heart disease, blood pressure, lipids and other risk factors measured in a large male population. *Am. J. Med.,* **61:** 815.

107. Wilson, R. H. L. and N. L. Wilson. 1969. Obesity and respiratory stress. *J. Am. Dietet. Assoc.,* **55:** 465.

108. Withers, R. F. J. 1964. Problems in the genetics of human obesity. *Eugen. Rev.,* **56:** 81.

109. Wooley, O. W. 1971. Long-term food regulation in the obese and nonobese. *Psychosom. Med.,* **33:** 436.

110. Wooley, S. C. and O. W. Wooley. 1973. Salivation to the sight and thought of food: A new measure of appetite. *Psychosom. Med.,* **35:** 136.

111. Wooley, O. W. and S. C. Wooley. 1975. Short-term control of food intake. In *Obesity in Perspective,* Part 2, G. A. Bray (Ed.). DHEW Publication No. (NIH) 75–708.

112. Young, C. M., L. F. Hutter, S. S. Scanlan, C. E. Rand, L. Lutwak, and V. Simko. 1972. Metabolic effects of meal frequency on normal young men. *J. Am. Dietet. Assoc.,* **61:** 391.

113. Young, C. M., S. S. Scanlan, C. M. Topping, V. Simko, and L. Lutwak. 1971. Frequency of feeding, weight reduction, and body composition. *J. Am. Dietet. Assoc.,* **59:** 466.

STUDY GUIDE

Several procedures are available for assessing the degree of obesity or fatness in humans.

1. Describe several procedures that might be used in assessing obesity and body fatness, and discuss the strengths and weaknesses of each procedure for clinical and/or research use.

The obese state may have an effect on morbidity and mortality.

2. How would you approach patients who have come for counseling on weight reduction in regard to possible health benefits from reducing? Explain why you would use this approach.

Genetic influences on obesity are sometimes difficult to separate from those produced by the environment.

3. How would you counsel a young juvenile-onset obese mother who is concerned that her children may inherit her obesity? Explain your approach.

Several metabolic and anatomic abnormalities have been observed in obese humans but their cause is not always apparent.

4. Support with research findings the statement that metabolic abnormalities in the obese are a result of the obesity itself.

5. Describe metabolic abnormalities of plasma FFA, ketones, glucose, insulin, triglycerides, and growth hormone that have been reported for obese subjects.

6. Explain why it may be particularly unwise to allow excessive weight gain during the first few months of life and at the time of the preadolescent growth spurt.

Physiologic mechanisms probably exist for both short-term and long-term regulation of food intake in animals and humans.

7. Discuss possible roles for oral and gastrointestinal sensations in the regulation of food intake.

8. Describe the glucostatic, lipostatic, aminostatic, and thermostatic theories for regulation of food intake and discuss the merits of each theory.

9. Discuss possible roles of mechanisms for regulating food intake, both short- and long-term, in the development and maintenance of obesity in humans.

The frequency of eating or the number of meals per day influences energy metabolism and synthesis of body fat in experimental animals and possibly in humans.

10. Give a probable explanation, based on research studies with "meal-eating" and "nibbling" rats, as to why more body fat is produced by single than by multiple daily meals in groups of experimental animals receiving comparable amounts of food.

11. Give concrete suggestions to a client who is following a 1200-kcal dietary program for weight reduction concerning the most appropriate spacing of her meals. Give the rationale for your suggestions.

The documented relationships between obesity and socioeconomic status, ethnic background, and social-psychological factors suggest that obesity is under a certain degree of control by environmental influences.

12. Describe several reported relationships between incidence of obesity and socioeconomic-cultural factors. Although the mechanism of influence is not known, discuss the possible effect of *fashion* and *values* on the development of obesity.

13. Describe and discuss the types of research and observation that have been interpreted to mean that the food intake of obese individuals is controlled to a very great degree by environmental factors. Also discuss controversial views concerning this idea.

Psychogenic factors may play important roles in the development and maintenance of some cases of severe obesity, particularly in children.

14. Suggest a satisfactory approach to the treatment of obesity with a probable psychogenic origin and specify the role of the dietitian in this treatment program.

5

Treatment of Obesity

Obesity is not a single disease entity but a symptom of underlying energy imbalance with many possible contributing causes. Therefore, treatment of the obese is a complex process.

Traditional methods of treatment have assumed that the law of conservation of energy holds: Energy balance = energy input − energy output. To achieve a negative energy balance, energy input is restricted by curtailing food intake. Physical exercise increases energy output. However, traditional methods for treating obesity have not been spectacularly successful. Few long-term follow-up studies have documented more than a 10 to 25 percent rate of successful weight reduction. Review of the medical literature shows that only 25 percent of those who enter therapy lose as much as 20 lb and only 5 percent lose as much as 40 lb (Young, 1975). For those who do successfully lose weight, the recurrence rate is high. No information is available about the individuals in the general population who institute their own successful weight-reduction programs and do not appear in the medical literature. According to Young (1975), a high degree of motivation, a reasonable degree of emotional stability, obesity of short duration and moderate degree, obesity beginning in adult life, no previous history of failure at weight reduction, and good management procedures in the reduction program are positive factors that contribute to successful weight reduction.

Since treatment of obesity is difficult, a number of approaches to the problem have been reported. This chapter discusses several procedures that have been used with varying degrees of success.

5.1 Diet Composition

The optimal diet for weight reduction is not known. It should, however, be low enough in kilocalories to allow a steady weight loss yet supply adequate nitrogen, minerals, and vitamins. No undesirable side effects should occur.

Protein

Low-kilocalorie diets prescribed for weight reduction usually provide protein levels surpassing the Recommended Dietary Allowance. Obese subjects are able to keep the breakdown of body protein to a minimum while they are consuming low-kilocalorie diets. Jourdan et al. (1974) found that obese women were able to maintain nitrogen equilibrium on 75 g protein daily while consuming only 50 percent of the kilocalories required for weight maintenance. Negative nitrogen balance was not marked on 20 g protein daily and 25 percent of maintenance kilocalories. Therefore, when normal levels of protein are included in a low-kilocalorie diet for an obese individual, excessive catabolism of lean body tissue should not occur.

Carbohydrate and Fat

Low-carbohydrate reducing diets have been repeatedly recommended to the public in the popular press, and the ideal proportion of kilocalories as carbohydrate and fat has been debated. Reports on effects of low-carbohydrate diets during weight reduction have differed. Hegsted et al. (1975) reported that loss in body weight and fat was similar in several groups of obese adult rats fed equally low-kilocalorie diets varying widely in protein, fat, and carbohydrate content. The only significant dietary effect observed was a modest increase in the body protein of animals fed high-protein diets. Low-carbohydrate, high-fat, high-protein diets showed no advantage as reducing diets for these animals as compared to other diets on an equicaloric basis.

Kekwick and Pawan (1957) fed 14 obese patients 1000-kcal diets containing 90 percent of kilocalories as carbohydrate, fat, or protein, with 5 to 9 days on each diet. The rate of weight loss varied markedly with the composition of the diet, being greatest with 90 percent fat and least with 90 percent carbohydrate. The weight differences did not appear to be solely the result of fluctuations in body water, nor were they caused by defective absorption from the alimentary tract. The researchers concluded that some aspects of metabolism in the obese differ from the nonobese and that this may be affected by diet composition. However, the diets used in this study were bizarre in terms of usual diet composition and the time periods were very short.

Kasper et al. (1973) compared low-carbohydrate, high-fat formula diets with a reducing diet of conventional foods and customary carbohydrate/fat ratio for 25 obese subjects. Despite a higher total kilocalorie intake (1700 versus 1000 kcal), the low-carbohydrate, high-fat formula diets produced a mean daily weight loss of 0.30 kg as compared to 0.26 kg on the low-kilocalorie diet of usual composition.

Young et al. (1971) studied eight moderately obese college men on 1800 kcal reduction diets consumed over a 9-week period. Three subgroups, matched for maintenance caloric requirement and percent body weight as fat, consumed 105, 60, or 30 g carbohydrate daily. Weight loss, fat loss, and percent weight loss as fat appeared to be inversely related to the level of carbohydrate in the isocaloric, isoprotein diets. There were no outstanding differences in nitrogen, sodium, or potassium balances among the diet groups, and no adequate explanation could be given for the weight loss differences. Urinary ketones increased markedly with decreasing dietary carbohydrate content and were excreted continuously by subjects on the 30 g carbohydrate diet.

In contrast to the three human studies which indicate there may be greater loss of body weight and fat with low-carbohydrate diets than with those of conventional composition, Kinsell et al. (1964) reported that "calories do count" and that the rate of weight loss in five subjects on isocaloric reducing diets was essentially constant throughout the study period as the composition of the diet was changed. The fat intake varied from 12 to 83 percent, protein from 14 to 36 percent, and carbohydrate from 3 to 64 percent of total kilocalories. Hood et al. (1970) also reported no significant difference in the rate of weight loss when 1000 kcal diets of graded carbohydrate content were fed to four obese women for 8 days each.

Lewis et al. (1977) fed 10 obese men on a metabolic ward two isocaloric liquid formula reducing diets (one high-carbohydrate, low-fat and one high-fat, low-carbohydrate) for 14 days. Both diets were equally effective in producing weight loss, and both decreased serum lipids without deleterious effects on glucose tolerance. However, the low-carbohydrate diet produced greater hyperketonemia and hyperuricemia as well as a more striking change in the plasma insulin/glucagon ratio than did the high-carbohydrate diet. Worthington and Taylor (1974a), comparing a balanced low-kilocalorie diet with an equicaloric high-protein, low-carbohydrate diet for 20 obese women, found more weight loss during the first week on the low-carbohydrate regimen but similar losses during the second week of the study. The variety of foods was limited on the low-carbohydrate diet, and this regimen provided inadequate amounts of vitamin A, ascorbic acid, iron, and calcium. The frequency and amount of urinary ketones was increased on the low-carbohydrate diet (Worthington and Taylor, 1974b).

Carbohydrate deprivation is associated with loss of water, sodium, and potassium from the body. Bortz et al. (1967 and 1968) varied the proportions of carbohydrate and fat in 800-kcal reducing diets for obese humans both with and without added sodium. In the absence of added salt, weight loss appeared to be constant, regardless of the proportions of fat and carbohydrate in the diet. The weight plateau that tended to occur with carbohydrate feeding when salt was added to the diet seemed to be the result of sodium and fluid retention. North et al. (1972) studied the effect of carbohydrate in patients on reduction diets and during fasts and postulated that the inability of the kidney to modify ammonium anion excretion rates rapidly enough to keep pace with changes in ketone anion excretion, which increases during fasting or in the absence of carbohydrate, was responsible for loss of sodium during the early stages of carbohydrate deprivation or fasting and was also responsible for the avid reabsorption of sodium by the kidney during refeeding, when urinary ketone levels dramatically decrease. Fluctuations in salt and water balance with carbohydrate on a low-kilocalorie diet have been widely observed. Fluid retention with carbohydrate consumption may mask the short-term effects of a reduction diet on loss of body fat and is often discouraging to the patient trying to lose weight.

Several potential hazards of low-carbohydrate reduction diets have been suggested. Hyperlipidemia may occur on low-carbohydrate diets that are also high in animal fat and protein. Elevated serum cholesterol levels were reported for 12 moderately overweight hospital employees who followed the Stillman diet, consisting almost totally of protein and animal fat, for 3 to 17 days (Rickman et al., 1974). These findings are important to consider when working with persons who may have coronary artery disease and obesity simultaneously.

Ketosis is a constant characteristic of low-carbohydrate reducing diets. On less than 50 g carbohydrate daily ketosis may be severe. Loss of ketone bodies in large amounts and over a prolonged period has the potential danger of concomitant loss of body base (Young et al., 1971). Bone calcium and connective tissue may be mobilized as a result of the mild acidosis of ketosis, thus affecting the skeleton over a period of time (Cahill, 1975). Hyperuricemia may be exaggerated by ketosis because of competition between uric acid and ketones for renal tubular excretion (Krehl et al., 1967). Symptoms of gout may be exacerbated by a low-carbohydrate reducing regimen in a patient predisposed to this disorder. Postural hypotension and fatigue have been reported for subjects on low-carbohydrate reducing diets.

The low-carbohydrate reducing diet is not new, although it is periodically heralded as an innovative discovery. An English ear surgeon, William Harvey, used it for a very obese patient in the 1800s. When his diet was published in 1863, it became a center of controversy. Variants of the diet have been described by Pennington in 1953, as the Air Force diet in 1960, by Taller of *Calories Don't Count* fame in 1961, by Stillman in 1967, and by Atkins in 1972 (Council on Foods and Nutrition, 1973). The controversy is continuing. Yudkin (1972) has become an exponent of the moderately low-carbohydrate diet for weight reduction. Grey and Kipnis (1971) reported that the hyperinsulinemia that is characteristic of obesity decreased in three obese subjects on 1500-kcal low-carbohydrate diets, in comparison to isocaloric high-carbohydrate diets. On the other hand, the Council on Foods and Nutrition of the American Medical Association (1973) severely criticized the widespread use of "ketogenic" reducing diets. An ad hoc committee on weight reduction brought together by the National Live

Stock and Meat Board in 1966 suggested that the low-carbohydrate diet for weight reduction could be potentially hazardous to health unless competently supervised by a physician or nutritionist (Young, 1975).

Good weight loss can be achieved by using low-kilocalorie diets with usual proportions of carbohydrate. The possible hazards of extremely low-carbohydrate diets should discourage their general use for weight reduction.

Cellulose

Baked products and mashed potatoes to which microcrystalline cellulose was added as a nonnutritive bulking agent in quantities up to 30 percent have been found to be acceptable by taste panels composed of both obese and normal weight judges (Lee et al., 1969; Pratt et al., 1971; Brys and Zabik, 1976). The practical value of this in long-term weight reduction has not been investigated.

5.2   Fasting and Modified Fasting

Fasting for weight reduction has been advocated by a few professionals at periodic intervals over the past 60 years and was fairly widely used during the 1960s. The report of Drenick et al. (1964) is representative of a number of studies concerned with prolonged starvation as treatment for severe obesity. Drenick et al. fasted 11 obese ambulatory patients for periods of 12 to 117 days, giving them only water and vitamins. After the first few days, hunger was virtually absent and the procedure seemed to be well tolerated. Weight losses averaged 0.41 kg (0.91 lb) daily. Reversible complications that developed during fasting included severe orthostatic hypotension in three cases, severe normocytic normochromic anemia in one, and gouty arthritis with hyperuricemia in two. Kollar and Atkinson (1966) concluded that many extremely obese individuals can be subjected to food deprivation and major weight loss without adverse psychological reactions, providing that the environment is supportive as they cope with emerging interpersonal problems. Large weight losses increased self-esteem in some fasting obese patients (Crumpton et al., 1966).

The metabolic changes taking place during fasting include decreases in blood glucose and insulin levels and an increase in serum-free fatty acids during the first few days. These levels then remain stable, and ketosis develops. As the body adapts to starvation it uses fat-based fuel almost exclusively, with even the brain burning ketones. The need for glucose, which is supplied by gluconeogenesis using amino acids from lean body tissue as substrate, gradually decreases and loss of nitrogen diminishes. However, some protein continues to be lost, since adaptation is not complete, and may be equivalent to 1250 g (about 6 kg muscle tissue) after 3 to 4 weeks of fasting (Flatt and Blackburn, 1974).

Barnard et al. (1969) reported that half of the weight lost by seven grossly obese patients fasted from 10 to 45 weeks was lean body tissue. Bolinger et al. (1966), by calculating theoretical balances, could account for only 20 percent of the weight lost by fasting obese patients as fat, whereas 35 percent of the loss was accounted for as fat-free protoplasm. With the loss of lean body mass rather than the desired loss of fatty tissue, total fasting does not appear to be an effective and satisfactory method for weight reduction in most cases (Lindner and Blackburn, 1976). In addition, the long-term results of fasting have been disappointing. Only a small number of patients have maintained their weight losses (Drenick, 1975). Since no food is consumed during the period of fasting, it is difficult to change the original eating habits that produced excessive weight gain in the first place, and weight may be easily regained as previous living patterns are resumed.

An alternative to total fasting is a protein-sparing modified fast. This reducing regimen involves the daily ingestion of 0.6 to 1.4 g protein per kg ideal body weight to compensate for the breakdown of protein tissue that occurs in complete starvation. Supplying amino acids leads to lesser insulin secretion with less inhibition of fat mobilization and also supports protein synthesis. Nitrogen balance is close to zero with protein supplementation (Bistrian et al., 1977), and ketosis is less pronounced than in starvation. Thus, lean body mass is preserved to a large extent, and adipose tissue decreases (Flatt and Blackburn, 1974).

Lean meat, fish, or fowl in amounts to provide 1.0 to 1.4 g protein per kg ideal body weight daily have been used in some modified fasting programs. The meat is taken in small amounts throughout the day and no other food is eaten. Elemental protein or amino acid mixtures have been used by others. About 5 or 6 oz of a protein preparation, containing 15 g protein per oz, is often given daily in several portions. Patients must drink at least 4 to 6 cups of water each day and usually take prescribed vitamin and mineral supplements. Some researchers have used a mixture of protein and glucose instead of nitrogen-supplying compounds alone. Genuth et al. (1974) successfully maintained 75 obese patients on 45 g of casein calcium (Casec) and 30 g of glucose for several months. They found that the glucose limited ketosis, but there was a small continuing nitrogen deficit in their patients. Body composition was not measured. Baird et al. (1974) reported good results on five extremely obese subjects with amino acids alone (30 g per day), but they found that adding a small amount of glucose reduced ketosis to a more moderate level returned the serum uric acid to normal, and reduced the amino acid requirement by half. Positive nitrogen balance was generally maintained, but there was considerable individual variation. Lindner and Blackburn (1976) suggested that carbohydrate interferes with the effectiveness of the protein-sparing process.

Lindner and Blackburn found use of the protein-sparing modified fast without a supportive regimen unsuccessful. However, they reported successful long-term weight loss when using a program that emphasized nutrition education, behavior-modification therapy, and exercise along with a well monitored protein-sparing modified fast.

5.3 Physical Exercise

Exercise is usually not popular among the obese. The frequent rationalization is that exercise will stimulate the appetite and cause increased food intake. This is not necessarily true (Jankowski and Foss, 1972), particularly when the individual is sedentary. Mechanisms for the regulation of food intake in both animals and humans appear to be reasonably effective when light to moderately heavy work is being performed. However, if physical activity decreases below a certain threshold level, a commensurate decrease in food intake does not always occur (Mayer, 1966). Figures 5.1 and 5.2 show relationships between physical activity and food intake for experimental rats and for humans in a West Bengal study by Mayer et al. (1956).

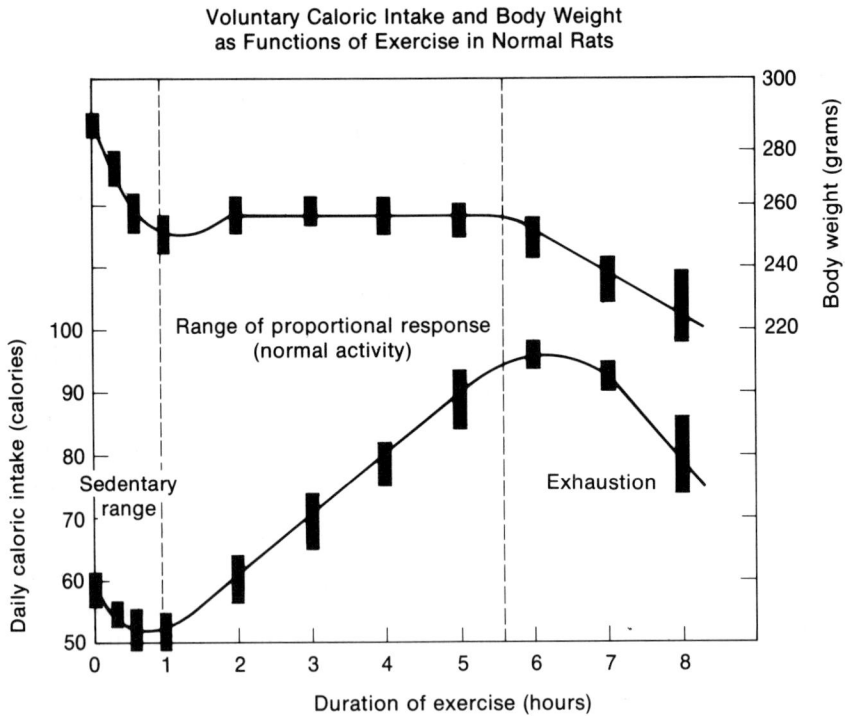

Voluntary Caloric Intake and Body Weight as Functions of Exercise in Normal Rats

Fig. 5.1 The regulation of food intake generally operates with precision only in the area of normal activity. With low levels of exercise, an increase in exercise is not accompanied by an increase in food intake. At extremely low levels of activity, voluntary food intake is greater than at moderate levels. In the range of "normal activity," the regulation of food intake is functioning: as activity increases, food intake increases correspondingly and weight is maintained. At excessively high levels of activity, both food intake and weight decrease. (Reproduced with permission of *Nutrition Today* magazine, 101 Ridgely Ave., Annapolis MD 21401 © June 1966.)

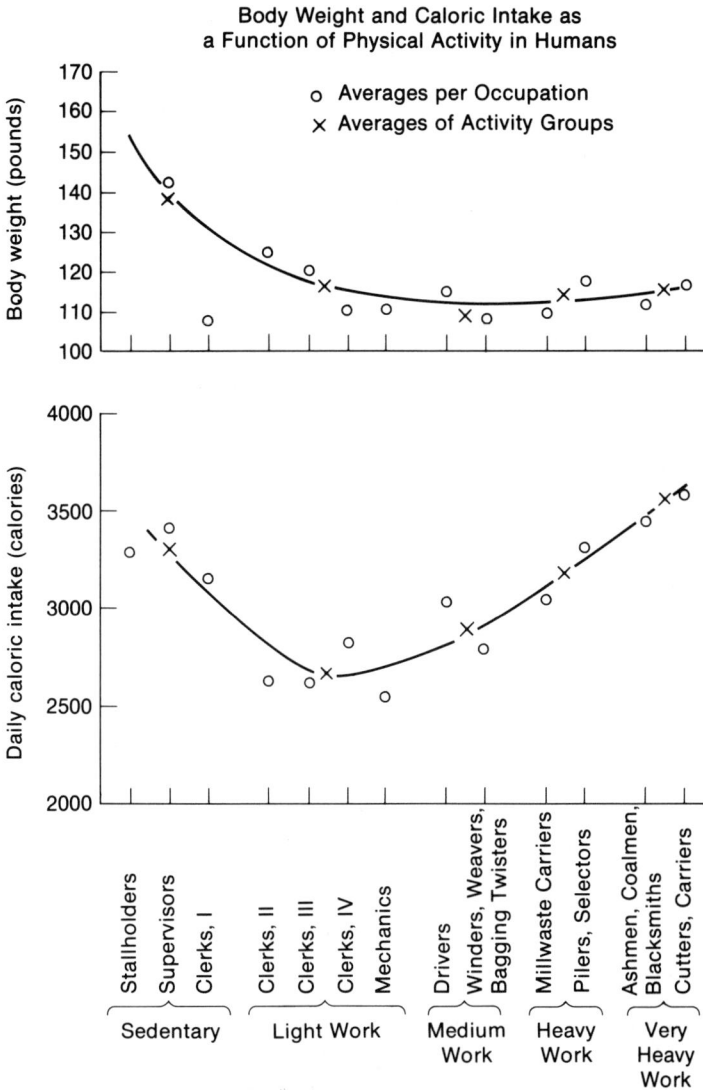

Fig. 5.2 The voluntary food intake of 300 West Bengal workers was studied by Mayer. The lowest voluntary food intake was seen in workers who engaged in light regular activity. Sedentary workers ate more and were much fatter. Workers performing heavy work ate more but their weight was still light. (Reproduced with permission of *Nutrition Today* magazine, 101 Ridgely Ave., Annapolis MD 21401 ©️ June 1966.)

It appears that moving an obese individual out of a sedentary state into at least light activity would be beneficial in terms of regulating food intake.

Benefits from exercise in treatment of obesity have been documented:

1. Obese middle-aged women on a 17-week self-determined caloric restriction and exercise program, including jogging and calis-

     thenics, had decreased body fat by 5.4 kg, which closely paralleled total body weight loss (4.2 kg). Mean heart rates and systolic blood pressures were lower after weight reduction (Lewis et al., 1976).

2. College-age women on a 1200-kcal diet plus a moderate exercise program did not lose significantly more weight than did similar subjects on diet alone, but they appeared to have a more positive attitude toward the weight reduction experience than did the nonexercising women (Dudleston and Bennion, 1970).

3. Six superobese subjects on a formal exercise protocol combined with a low-kilocalorie liquid diet showed a lower resting heart rate and a greater fat weight loss than did nonexercised controls, although motivation to exercise was a problem (Kenrick et al., 1972).

4. Lower plasma insulin values were reported in obese patients the day after exercise on a bicycle ergometer for 60 minutes (Fahlen et al., 1972). Physical training of obese subjects apparently increases insulin sensitivity of body tissues (Björntorp et al., 1970).

5. Anorexigenic substance, which is increased in plasma after exhaustive treadmill exercise in humans, may be responsible for decreased appetite and food intake following exercise (Belbeck and Critz, 1973).

6. A 14 percent increase in the basal metabolic rate of young men the morning after a doubling of physical activity was noted by Miller and Mumford (1966), demonstrating residual effects of previous exercise.

7. A program of swimming for experimental rats in very early life was effective in decreasing the number of adipose tissue cells and total body fat later in life, in comparison with sedentary control animals (Oscai et al., 1974). Apparently the exercise program must begin about the first week of life, however, to affect the adipocyte number (Booth et al., 1974).

     Exercise in a weight-reduction program, as a companion to caloric restriction, should be psychologically and physiologically beneficial to any individuals for whom activity is not contraindicated. Although its effect on increasing caloric expenditure may be small when viewed in terms of kilocalories used per day, the effect of this small increase in energy expenditure over several weeks and months may be considerable. Stuart (1975b) suggested that the exercise program should be an aerobic activity, be sufficient to produce a discernible level of fatigue, last for 15 to 45 min per session, and be executed three to five times weekly.

5.4   Behavioral Modification in Treating Obesity

Behavior therapy has been used successfully in the treatment of a variety of psychologic disorders, and some of these techniques have been applied to the problems of weight reduction and control. Both considerable weight loss and superior maintenance of weight loss after treatment with behavioral techniques have been accomplished by some researchers in comparison to weight loss reported from traditional therapy (Penick et al., 1971; Stuart, 1967). Stuart (1975a) suggested that because the behaviors of eating abnormalities and exercise insufficiencies are found in all types of obesities, regardless of their anatomic or physiologic characteristics, behavior-modification procedures have something to contribute to the clinical management of most obese individuals. In addition, the behavioral program has no known adverse side effects, so there is little to be lost and possibly much to be gained in trying it.

What is behavior therapy? Its focus is on *observable* behavior and behavior change. It is concerned with the discrete behaviors that define a problem and the specific behaviors that should be changed to solve the problem. In obesity, the behaviors that define the problem are the habits which produce excessive eating and insufficient exercising, with obesity a consequence of this behavior. Behavior therapy is characterized by measurement of the target behaviors both before and during treatment. Before therapy begins, the obese patient is asked to keep a detailed record of her activity in relation to eating and food. She records the circumstances under which she eats and how she feels at the time. From this record, specific eating problems can be identified. Behavior therapy uses a series of techniques to change undesirable behaviors. A process of *shaping* is implied throughout the therapeutic program, which provides for small, incremental changes in a behavior as the final goal is approached. A gradual weight loss for the obese subject of 1 to 2 lb/week is usually the criteria for a successful program. Since the processes of behavior monitoring and change are under the control of the client, education for self-management is important. The therapist is a teacher and also a source of social influence to the client (Levitz, 1973).

Techniques involved in behavior therapy for obesity have included (1) instructions to help the client eat more slowly, as chewing each mouthful thoroughly, putting down her eating utensil after every third bite, or planning short delays during the meal; (2) helping the client to make eating a "pure" experience so that antecedent stimuli do not control eating behavior, by eating in the same place and times each day and not doing anything else (including watching TV) while eating; (3) helping the client to program enjoyable activities other than eating in response to emotional depressions or anxieties; and (4) having the client contract for reinforcing rewards, other than food, when a desired behavior change is observed (Levitz, 1973).

In many programs, a professional therapist has been used. Jordan and Levitz (1973), however, conducted an apparently successful pilot study in which the lay leader of a self-help weight-control group was given some training in behavioral techniques to use with the group. There are books that may be used by an obese person in a self-directed program or by lay leaders (Stuart and Davis, 1972; Ferguson, 1975a,b; Ferguson, 1976).

Paulsen et al. (1976) utilized nutritionists in conducting behavior-modification programs for weight control and compared the results with a traditional approach using food exchange lists. They found that weight loss was small and similar in the two approaches when the nutritionists were not trained in behavioral techniques. In a second study, the nutritionists were trained by a behavioral psychologist before acting as therapists. The weight loss of the subjects in this case was significantly greater and longer-lasting on a 1-year follow-up than in the first study. Considerable nutrition information was systematically built into all the treatment programs so that the subjects would become knowledgeable about a variety of food and nutrition topics. Most of the subjects rated the nutrition information as relevant and helpful in an evaluation of the program.

Weisenberg and Fray (1974) found that a behavior-modification approach to weight reduction did not work well in a small clinic outpatient group with ethnically and racially mixed participants. Modifications may be necessary for particular populations. The emphasis of behavior-modification programs is on long-term change in eating habits so that excess weight may be lost and normal weight maintained. This is also the goal of the traditional approach to weight control, but success has been elusive. Behavioral techniques should be of value in any sensible approach to weight reduction, although they may not produce dramatic effects in all cases.

5.5 Drug Treatment of Obesity

Use of drugs for the primary treatment of obesity has, in general, been unsuccessful. Combinations of drugs, in the so-called diet pill program, have been criticized by the scientific and medical communities, and deaths from these pills have been documented (Jelliffe et al., 1969). The series of pills usually contains thyroid preparations, digitalis, amphetamines, and diuretics, and their use has been associated with hypokalemia and cardiac arrhythmias (Henry, 1967).

Included in the group of drugs that have been prescribed individually for weight reduction are (1) hormones, as thyroid hormones and chorionic gonadotropin; (2) anorexigenic drugs, as amphetamines and related compounds; (3) diuretics to initiate water loss; and (4) bulk fillers, as methyl cellulose.

Both thyroxine (T_4) and triiodothyronine (T_3), when administered in sufficiently high doses, will reduce body weight. However, the weight loss is transitory during treatment and consists primarily of lean body mass with relatively little body fat. There is considerable hazard associated with the use of thyroid hormones in treating obesity, including cardiovascular symptoms, palpitation, tachycardia, elevated systolic blood pressure, sweating, and increased urinary loss of calcium and nitrogen associated with bone catabolism. Thyroid hormones should be used only for obese patients in whom hypothyroidism can be clearly documented (Rivlin, 1975).

Human chorionic gonadotropin (HCG) was first used in a weight-reduction program by Simeons (1954), who gave injections of the hormone 6 days a week in combination with a 500-kcal diet for 6 weeks. Simeons claimed that HCG mobilized fat depots. A number of studies with this substance have been reported with controversial results: some claimed greater weight loss

Drug Enforcement Administration (DEA) Schedule	Chemical Structure	Generic Name	Proprietary Name(s)
	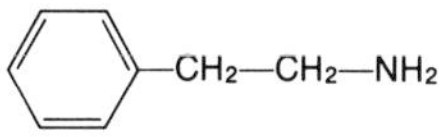	Phenylethylamine	
II	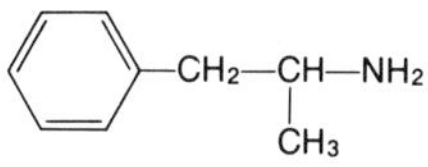	Amphetamine	Dexedrine, etc.
II	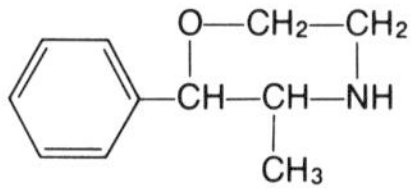	Phenmetrazine	Preludin
III	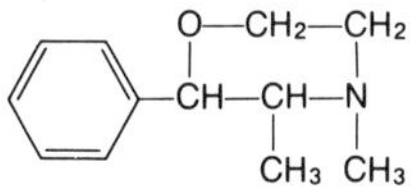	Phendimetrazine	Plegine
III	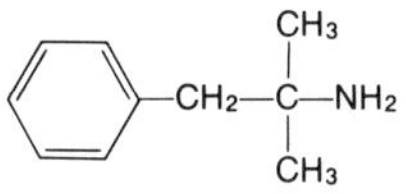	Phentermine	Ionamin, Wilpo
III	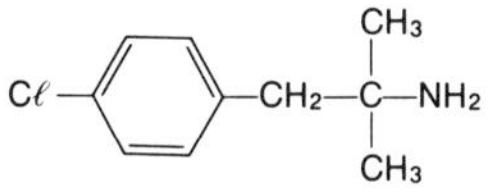	Chlorphentermine	Pre-Sate
III	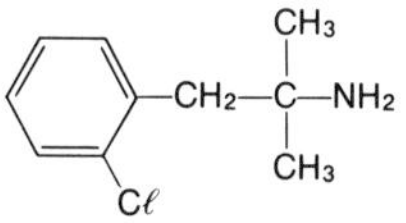	Chlortermine	Voranil
III	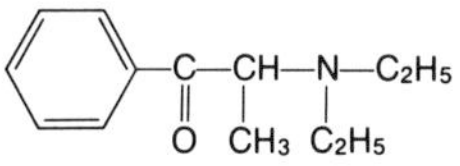	Diethylpropion	Tenuate, Tepanil
IV	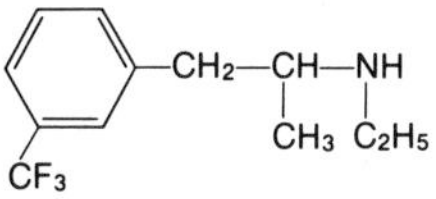	Fenfluramine	Pondimin

Fig. 5.3 Some phenylethylamine derivatives approved by the Food and Drug Administration for use as anorexigenic agents in the treatment of obesity. DEA schedules are numbered in order of decreasing potential for abuse, with II being the most dangerous. (From B. A. Scoville, "Review of Amphetamine-Like Drugs by the Food and Drug Administration: Clinical Data and Value Judgments," in *Obesity in Perspective*, G. A. Bray (ed.), DHEW Pub. No. (NIH) 75–708, Washington, D.C.: U.S. Government Printing Office, 1975.)

and decreased hunger with HCG (Asher and Harper, 1973), but others found no effect over placebo (Stein et al., 1976; Shetty and Kalkhoff, 1977).

Amphetamines and related compounds are prescribed as anorectic agents, particularly during the early stages of dietary restriction. They have been abused, and controversy has arisen as to whether or not they should be used (Fineberg, 1972). Amphetamine produces anorexia through inhibition of the activity of the lateral hypothalamus, or feeding center. However, it also has central nervous system stimulating properties (sympathomimetic) and may be addictive. There has been much research on the development of related compounds that retain anorectic activity but have less central stimulant activity than amphetamine. Several compounds that have been used as anorectic agents are shown in Fig. 5.3. Fenfluramine does not have central stimulant properties and even causes sedation. It is effective in depressing appetite when used over a period of several months (Burland, 1975).

Anorectic drugs may have a place in the treatment of obesity but should be used only as part of a total program. They may be most helpful in relieving the discomfort of hunger at the beginning of a diet program.

Methyl cellulose is a bulking agent that is said to reduce appetite by swelling in the stomach. However, it swells relatively slowly and is unlikely to reach its full bulk before leaving the stomach. Therefore, it is a better laxative than anorexiant (Samuel and Burland, 1975).

5.6 Management of the Reducing Patient

Crash diets for weight reduction include the grapefruit and egg diet, vanilla ice cream and poundcake diet, watercress and skim milk diet, grape diet, no willpower diet, Stone Age meat diet. The vast number of bizarre diets that are printed and actually followed by many people, usually for very short periods of time, emphasize the lack of nutrition knowledge among the population and the desire for a quick cure for obesity. The individual who needs and desires to lose weight requires some basic knowledge of food composition and nutrition if he or she is going to be successful on a long-term basis. Diet is an essential part of a weight-reduction program since the most likely way to achieve the necessary energy deficit required for weight loss is to decrease food intake. The limited caloric intake of the reducing patient makes it especially important that food choices are wise ones in terms of nutrient content. An important role of the nutrition counselor in working with the reducing client is that of effective teacher.

It is important to first review a client's case and determine his suitability for weight reduction. Young (1975) suggested that unless there is a reasonable possibility of success in a weight-reduction program, it may be best to help the client learn to live with his obesity rather than to develop the sense of guilt, anxiety, and frustration that goes with being unable to lose weight satisfactorily. A medical history and complete physical examination should clarify any physiological factors affecting the obesity so that they may be treated. A careful interview by the dietitian/nutritionist, in which the client is put at ease, should search into the history of his obesity, finding out when it began and under what circumstances. He should be asked about obesity among other family members, vocational and recreational interests, patterns of physical activity, and his feelings of appetite and hunger. A detailed history of his food intake is important. What are his usual eating habits; when, where, what, how much, and with whom does he usually eat? What are his food likes and dislikes? How does he feel about his weight? The interviewer should listen not only to what he says but should also get a feeling for how it is said and for what remains unsaid. What is the meaning of his life to him? How strong is his motivation to lose weight? Does he believe that he can do it, or does he have a sense of failure and hopelessness? Will he have support from others around him? With this information at the disposal of the dietitian, the instruction and counsel can be better tailored to individual needs (Young, 1975).

Sometimes several obese clients may meet together with the dietitian. Searching individual interviews are less likely to occur in a group discussion, but the interaction among group members may bring added benefits of understanding and motivation to the individual members of the group. If meetings can be scheduled at regular intervals, which is most desirable in terms of giving continuing help, support, and instruction during the weight-reduction program, the client may first be asked to keep a detailed record of his usual food intake from which his eating habits are discerned before the diet program begins.

The client needs to understand that it is loss of fatty tissue which is desired and that "scale" weight may not always be a true indication of this loss. This is particularly true in the first weeks of dieting, when water and electrolyte balance is adjusting. The rate of weight loss should be gradual. Quick weight loss in large amounts is usually caused by loss of water and lean body tissue, which is quickly replaced by normal body processes when eating is resumed. The client also needs to know basic principles of normal nutrition and be convinced that good eating habits make an important contribution to his sense of well-being.

The dietitian, as well as other therapists working with the client, should make him feel that he can talk with them without a feeling of guilt or fear of judgment. He should be given constant support, encouragement, and praise for all progress made. The client should be prepared to cope with the reactions of family and friends, which may be very helpful but also can be detrimental. However, he must realize that this is *his* problem to solve and he must do it himself. Once the desired weight is reached, he should be followed at periodic intervals until he has shown that he can maintain his new weight level (Young, 1975).

After a careful assessment of the client's situation, the dietitian may develop an individualized diet pattern. All desires cannot be satisfied, of course, since the caloric level must be restricted for weight loss to occur.

One pound of adipose tissue contains approximately 87 percent fat and is, therefore, equivalent to 3500 to 3700 kcal. Thus, decreasing the number of kilocalories required daily for weight maintenance by 500 kcal should allow a 3500-kcal deficit over a period of 1 week. A daily deficit of 1000 kcal will allow a 7000-kcal weekly deficit, which should produce a weight loss of approximately 2 lb. In most cases, a loss of 1 to 2 lb/week is desirable. This type of gradual weight loss is more likely to be largely adipose tissue and permanent than are large losses in a short period of time. Quick weight loss is usually associated with catabolism of protein tissue, in which case about 4 lb water accompanies the loss of 1 lb of body protein (Heald and Khan, 1973).

It is difficult to plan a nutritionally adequate diet and with less than 1200 kcal daily. Most women, unless they are very short and elderly or extremely inactive, should lose weight on this level. Most men will lose weight on 1500 to 1800 kcal daily. Young, active men may lose on even higher kilocalorie levels. Occasionally, in a hospitalized patient, an 800- to 1000-kcal diet may be appropriate but should not be necessary for most outpatients.

The exchange lists, discussed in Sec. 2.2, are helpful tools in instructing a client. Once a desired daily kilocalorie level has been decided upon, the total kilocalories may be divided into a suggested number of servings from each exchange list and distributed into a pattern of three or more meals and snacks. On a daily basis, the consumption of at least 1 to 2 cups of milk should be encouraged, along with adequate amounts of vegetables and fruits. The number of meat and bread exchanges may be adjusted to the preference of the client. Giving a larger number of meat exchanges will make the diet higher in protein and lower in carbohydrate than giving a minimum of meat exchanges and allowing more choices from the bread list. The daily carbohydrate level of the diet should probably not go below approximately 100 g. The minimum protein level should probably be about 70 g. Tables 5.1 and 5.2 show diet patterns and menus using the exchange lists.

Childhood obesity is more often associated with genetic, psychologic, and possibly metabolic problems, and management differs from that of adult obesity. Obese children may have developed an abnormally high number of adipose tissue cells, contributing to the resistance to weight reduction often found in this group at later stages of life. When planning diet therapy for obese children and early adolescents, it is extremely important to understand the nutritional needs for growth and to allow for them. The child should not be in negative nitrogen balance during dieting since this may limit normal growth. Negative nitrogen balance may occur with even moderate caloric restriction. Severe caloric restriction for long periods is not recommended for children or adolescents. Only a restriction of clear excesses through control of portion sizes is advisable. The obese children can eat what the rest of the family eats, but less of it, assuming that the family diet is nutritionally balanced. The most realistic goal in working with

Table 5.1 NUTRIENT COMPOSITION OF TWO ALTERNATIVE DIET PATTERNS FOR A 1200-KCAL REDUCING DIET

Exchange List	Total Daily Exchanges	Alternative A				Total Daily Exchanges	Alternative B			
		Protein	Fat	Carbo-hydrate	Kcal		Protein	Fat	Carbo-hydrate	Kcal
Milk	2	16		24	160	2	16		24	160
Vegetable	4	8		20	100	3	6		15	75
Fruit	3			30	120	3			30	120
Bread	2	4		30	140	4	8		60	280
Meat	9	63	27		495	6	42	18		330
Fat	4		20		180	5		25		225
Totals		91	47	104	1195		72	43	129	1190

Table 5.2   SUGGESTED MENUS FOR TWO ALTERNATIVE 1200-KCAL PATTERNS

Alternative A (91 g P, 47 g F, 104 g Cho)	Alternative B (72 g P, 43 g F, 129 g Cho)
Breakfast	*Breakfast*
½ cup orange juice	½ small banana on
1 poached egg on	½ cup bran flakes
1 slice whole wheat toast	1 cup skim milk
1 tsp margarine	Coffee, black
1 cup skim milk	
Coffee, black	
Lunch	*Lunch*
Fruit and vegetable plate:	Sandwich:
¾ cup low-fat cottage cheese	2 oz tuna fish
¼ small cantaloupe	2 tsp mayonnaise
1 medium peach, unsweetened	1 tsp margarine
1 medium tomato, sliced	3 slices fresh tomato
Cucumber slices	2 lettuce leaves
Celery sticks	2 slices whole wheat bread
Green pepper rings	Carrot sticks and green pepper rings
Coffee or tea, artificially sweetened	1 small fresh apple
Dinner	*Dinner*
5 oz baked fresh salmon	4 oz baked chicken breast
1 small baked potato with	1 small baked potato with
2 tbsp sour cream	4 tbsp sour cream
½ cup carrot strips, panned with	½ cup chopped broccoli
½ tsp. margarine	½ broiled grapefruit
Tossed green salad with	*Bedtime Snack*
1 tbsp French dressing	1 cup skim milk
Bedtime Snack	
1 cup skim milk	

obese children is the prevention of further gains in body fat rather than the loss of large amounts of weight. In late adolescence, especially in well-motivated girls, weight control is often successful (Heald and Khan, 1973).

The social and emotional aspects of childhood and adolescent obesity must be considered. Complete abstinence from favorite foods, such as desserts and soft drinks, produces emotional trauma and will rarely occur. Spargo et al. (1966), in working with obese adolescents, learned not to talk calories but to talk appearance; not to talk weight but to talk diversified outside interests; not to talk diets but to talk moderation at the table; not to talk special foods but to talk a sensible balance where no foods are taboo.

5.7   Surgery for Obesity

Although individuals who are 10 to 40 lb overweight will usually respond to reasonable weight-reduction programs, there is a group of massively obese patients in which failure in weight reduction is commonplace. Severe medical problems often complicate their obesity. Surgical treatment is generally aimed at this group of obese individuals, weighing 300 to 400 lb, although it has been performed on subjects who are more moderately obese.

Two types of surgery for severe obesity are the gastric bypass and the intestinal bypass. A gastric bypass is a reversible operation patterned after subtotal gastric resection and excluding about 90 percent of the stomach, as indicated in Fig. 5.4. It restricts the amount of food that can be eaten at one time; therefore less total food is consumed, leading to weight loss.

Intestinal bypass surgery removes a major portion of the small intestine and thus reduces absorbing surface by up to 90 percent. Anastomosis between the jejunum and the colon produces severe side effects, and the more moderate jejunoileostomy is usually done. End-to-side or end-to-end anastomoses are used. Some procedures are diagrammed in Fig. 5.5. The exact length of small intestine bypassed should be tailored to the individual patient. The patients apparently lose weight, in variable amounts, because of decreased intestinal absorption and loss of nutrients in the feces and decreased food intake. Most patients are unable to reach their ideal weights after surgery, however, particularly the heavier patients (Pi-Sunyer, 1976).

A number of clinical problems and complications of intestinal bypass commonly occur. Mortality rates of 2 to 10 percent have been reported. Diarrhea begins after surgery and usually continues for 3 to 6 months. Some patients have cramping abdominal pain and gastrointestinal bleeding. Electrolyte imbalance may occur, and good postoperative care is extremely important (Bleicher et al., 1974). A threefold increase in hepatic

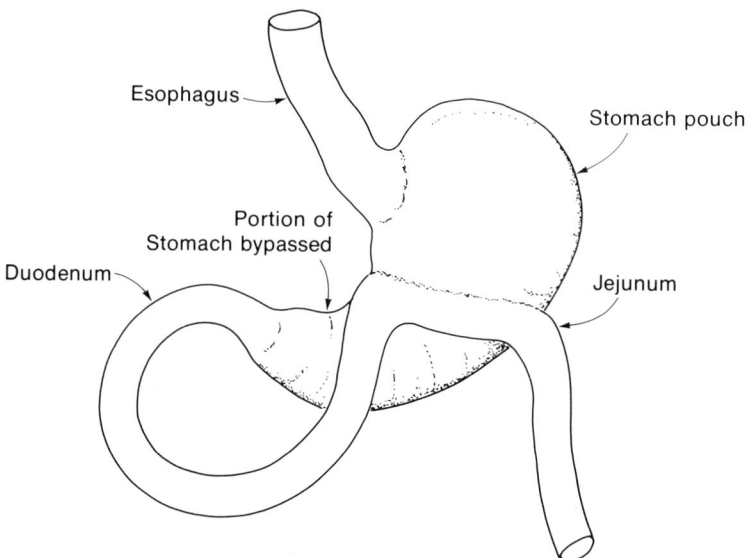

Fig. 5.4 Procedure for gastric bypass surgery in the treatment of obesity.

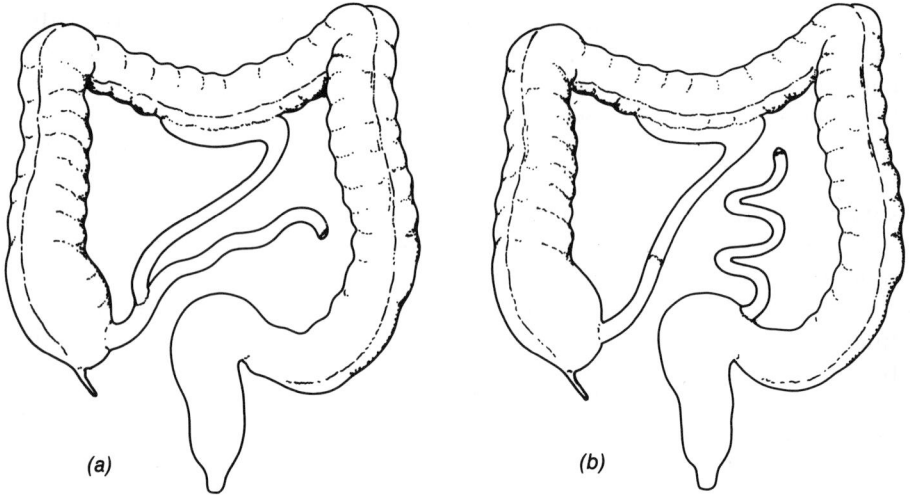

Fig. 5.5 Procedures for intestinal bypass surgery (jejunoileostomy) in the treatment of obesity. (a) End-to-side anastomosis. (b) End-to-end anastomosis; distal end of bypassed intestine anastomosed end-to-side to colon for drainage.

lipid accompanies the period of weight loss (Holzbach, 1974). Impaired liver function may occur.

Although strong opposition to surgical procedures for the treatment of obesity has been raised, jejunoileal bypass surgery is being performed frequently. It is not a benign curative surgical procedure, however. Pi-Sunyer (1976) has cautioned that (1) the procedure seems indicated only for those in whom the obesity itself is sufficiently life-threatening to justify the surgical risks; (2) life-long follow-up is essential; (3) nutritional deficiency states must be watched for and vigorously treated, and vitamin and mineral supplements are necessary; and (4) probably only larger centers with adequate supportive care facilities should perform the surgery.

5.8 Prevention of Obesity

The old adage that "an ounce of prevention is worth a pound of cure" is appropriate in a conversation about obesity. As the preceding pages emphasized, once obesity is well established the probability of treating it successfully on a long-term basis is low. The optimal time for prevention of obesity appears to be very early in life. In conducting a weight-control program for obese children in Hawaii, Matsuno et al. (1974) found that the children who failed to attain success in weight control had become obese at a younger age than had those who were successful. Research on the possible significance in the development of obesity of an increased number of adipocytes that are produced in infancy strongly suggests that programs for prevention of obesity should begin with education of the present generation for the benefit of the following generation. Young mothers need sound nutrition information both during pregnancy and as they begin to feed their new infants.

Habits are less entrenched and easier to change in childhood than in adulthood. Work with young people to develop not only sensible eating habits but patterns of living that include vigorous physical activity offer the greatest opportunity for success in the prevention of obesity. Seltzer and Mayer (1970) showed that an effective voluntary weight-control program, consisting of increased physical exercise, dietary education, and psychological support, can be introduced into a public school system. With the proper approach, motivation and support from both students and parents can be attained.

REFERENCES

1. Asher, W. L. and H. W. Harper. 1973. Effect of human chorionic gonadotropin on weight loss, hunger, and feeling of well-being. *Am. J. Clin. Nutr.*, **26:** 211.

2. Baird, I. M., R. L. Parsons, and A. N. Howard. 1974. Clinical and metabolic studies of chemically defined diets in the management of obesity. *Metabolism*, **23:** 645.

3. Barnard, D. L., J. Ford, E. S. Garnett, R. J. Mardell, and A. E. Whyman. 1969. Changes in body composition produced by prolonged total starvation and refeeding. *Metabolism*, **18:** 564.

4. Belbeck, L. W. and J. B. Critz. 1973. Effect of exercise on the plasma concentration of anorexigenic substance in man. *Proc. Soc. Exp. Biol. Med.*, **142:** 19.

5. Bistrian, B. R., J. Winterer, G. L. Blackburn, V. Young, and M. Sherman. 1977. Effect of a protein-sparing diet and brief fast on nitrogen metabolism in mildly obese subjects. *J. Lab. Clin. Med.*, **89:** 1030.

6. Björntorp, P., K. De Jounge, L. Sjöström, and L. Sullivan. 1970. The effect of physical training on insulin production in obesity. *Metabolism*, **19:** 631.

7. Bleicher, J. E., M. Cegielski, and J. A. Saporta. 1974. Intestinal bypass operation for massive obesity. *Postgrad. Med.*, **55:** 65.

8. Bolinger, R. E., B. P. Lukert, R. W. Brown, L. Guevara, and R. Steinberg. 1966. Metabolic balance of obese subjects during fasting. *Arch. Intern. Med.*, **118:** 3.

9. Booth, M. A., M. J. Booth, and A. W. Taylor. 1974. Rat fat cell size and number with exercise training, detraining and weight loss. *Fed. Proc.*, **33:** 1959.

10. Bortz, W. M., P. Howat, and W. L. Holmes. 1968. Fat, carbohydrate, salt, and weight loss. *Am. J. Clin. Nutr.*, **21:** 1291.

11. Bortz, W. M., A. Wroldson, P. Morris, and B. Issekutz, Jr. 1967. Fat, carbohydrate, salt, and weight loss. *Am. J. Clin. Nutr.*, **20:** 1104.

12. Brys, K. D. and M. E. Zabik. 1976. Microcrystalling cellulose replacement in cakes and biscuits. *J. Am. Dietet. Assoc.*, **69:** 50.

13. Burland, W. L. 1975. A review of experience with fenfluramine. In *Obesity in Perspective*, Part 2, G. A. Bray (Ed.). DHEW Publication No. (NIH) 75–708.

14. Cahill, G. F. 1975. Weight reduction diets. In *Obesity in Perspective*, Part 1, G. A. Bray (Ed.). DHEW Publication No. (NIH) 75–708.

15. Council on Foods and Nutrition. 1973. A critique of low-carbohydrate ketogenic weight reduction regimens. *J. Am. Med. Assoc.*, **224:** 1415.

16. Crumpton, E., D. B. Wine, and E. J. Drenick. 1966. Starvation: Stress or satisfaction? *J. Am. Med. Assoc.,* **196**: 394.

17. Drenick, E. J. 1975. Weight reduction by prolonged fasting. In *Obesity in Perspective,* Part 2, G. A. Bray (Ed.). DHEW Publication No. (NIH) 75–708.

18. Drenick, E. J., M. E. Swendseid, W. H. Blahd, and S. G. Tuttle. 1964. Prolonged starvation as treatment for severe obesity. *J. Am. Med. Assoc.,* **187**: 100.

19. Dudleston, A. K. and M. Bennion. 1970. Effect of diet and/or exercise on obese college women. *J. Am. Dietet. Assoc.,* **56**: 126.

20. Fahlén, M., J. Stenberg, and P. Björntorp. 1972. Insulin secretion in obesity after exercise. *Diabetologia,* **8**: 141.

21. Ferguson, J. M. 1975a. *Learning to Eat. Leader Manual.* Palo Alto, Calif.: Bull Publishing.

22. Ferguson, J. M. 1975b. *Learning to Eat. Student Manual.* Palo Alto, Calif.: Bull Publishing.

23. Ferguson, J. M. 1976. *Habits, not Diets.* Palo Alto, Calif.: Bull Publishing.

24. Fineberg, S. K. 1972. An appraisal of anorexiants in the treatment of obesity. *J. Am. Geriatrics Soc.,* **20**: 576.

25. Flatt, J. and G. L. Blackburn. 1974. The metabolic fuel regulatory system: Implications for protein-sparing therapies during caloric deprivation and disease. *Am. J. Clin. Nutr.,* **27**: 175.

26. Genuth, S. M., J. H. Castro, and V. Vertes. 1974. Weight reduction in obesity by outpatient semistarvation. *J. Am. Med. Assoc.,* **230**: 987.

27. Grey, N. and D. M. Kipnis. 1971. Effect of diet composition on the hyperinsulinemia of obesity. *N. Eng. J. Med.,* **285**:827.

28. Heald, F. P. and M. A. Khan. 1973. Teenage obesity. *Ped. Clinics No. Am.,* **20**: 807.

29. Hegsted, D. M., A. Gallagher, and H. Hanford. 1975. Reducing diets in rats. *Am. J. Clin. Nutr.,* **28**: 837.

30. Henry, R. D. 1967. Weight reduction pills. *J. Am. Med. Assoc.,* **201**: 217.

31. Holzbach, R. T., R. G. Wieland, C. S. Lieber, L. M. DeCarli, K. R. Koepke, and S. G. Green. 1974. Hepatic lipid in morbid obesity. *N. Eng. J. Med.,* **290**: 296.

32. Hood, C. E., J. M. Goodhart, R. F. Fletcher, J. Gloster, P. V. Bertrans, and A. C. Crooke. 1970. Observations on obese patients eating isocaloric reducing diets with varying proportions of carbohydrate. *Brit. J. Nutr.,* **24**: 39.

33. Janowski, L. W. and M. L. Foss. 1972. The energy intake of sedentary men after moderate exercise. *Med. and Sci. in Sports,* **4**: 11.

34. Jelliffe, R. W., D. Hill, D. Tatter, and E. Lewis, Jr. 1969. Death from weight-control pills. *J. Am. Med. Assoc.,* **208**: 1843.

35. Jordan, H. A. and L. S. Levitz. 1973. Behavior modification in a self-help group. *J. Am. Dietet. Assoc.,* **62**: 27.

36. Jourdan, M., S. Margen, and R. B. Bradfield. 1974. Protein-sparing effect in obese women fed low calorie diets. *Am. J. Clin. Nutr.,* **27**: 3.

37. Kasper, H., H. Thiel, and M. Ehl. 1973. Response of body weight to a low carbohydrate, high fat diet in normal and obese subjects. *Am. J. Clin. Nutr.,* **26**: 197.

38. Kekwick, A. and G. L. S. Pawan. 1957. Metabolic study in human obesity with isocaloric diets high in fat, protein or carbohydrate. *Metabolism,* **6**: 447.

39. Kenrick, M. M., M. F. Ball, and J. J. Canary. 1972. Exercise and weight reduction in obesity. *Arch. Phys. Med. Rehab.,* **53**: 323.

40. Kinsell, L. W., B. Gunning, G. D. Michaels, J. Richardson, S. E. Cox, and C. Lemon. 1964. Calories do count. *Metabolism,* **13**: 195.

41. Kollar, E. J. and R. M. Atkinson. 1966. Responses of extremely obese patients to starvation. *Psychosom. Med.*, **28:** 227.

42. Krehl, W. A., A. Lopez-S, E. I. Good, and R. E. Hodges. 1967. Some metabolic changes induced by low carbohydrate diets. *Am. J. Clin. Nutr.*, **20:** 139.

43. Lee, C. J., E. M. Rust, and E. F. Reber. 1969. Acceptability of foods containing a bulking agent. *J. Am. Dietet. Assoc.*, **54:** 210.

44. Levitz, L. S. 1973. Behavior therapy in treating obesity. *J. Am. Dietet. Assoc.*, **62:** 22.

45. Lewis, S., W. L. Haskell, P. D. Wood, N. Manoogian, J. E. Bailey, and M. B. Pereira. 1976. Effects of physical activity on weight reduction in obese middle-aged women. *Am. J. Clin. Nutr.*, **29:** 151.

46. Lewis, S. B., J. D. Wallin, J. P. Kane, and J. E. Gerich. 1977. Effect of diet composition on metabolic adaptations to hypocaloric nutrition: comparison of high carbohydrate and high fat isocaloric diets. *Am. J. Clin. Nutr.*, **30:** 160.

47. Lindner, P. G. and G. L. Blackburn. 1976. Multidisciplinary approach to obesity utilizing fasting modified by protein-sparing therapy. *Obes. Bar. Med.*, **5:** 198.

48. Matsuno, A. S., J. H. Hankin, and L. E. Dickinson. 1974. Four factors affect weight control for obese children. *J. Nutr. Educ.*, **6:** 104.

49. Mayer, J., P. Roy, and K. P. Mitra. 1956. Relation between caloric intake, body weight and physical work. *Am. J. Clin. Nutr.*, **4:** 169.

50. Miller, D. S. and P. Mumford. 1966. Obesity: Physical activity and nutrition. *Proc. Nutr. Soc.*, **25:** 100.

51. North, K. A. K., J. Sinn, and A. D. Woolhouse. 1972. Fluid and electrolyte changes on reduction diets. *N. Zealand Med. J.*, **76:** 413.

52. Oscai, L. B., S. P. Babirak, J. A. McGarr, and C. N. Spirakis. 1974. Effect of exercise on adipose tissue cellularity. *Fed. Proc.*, **33:** 1956.

53. Paulsen, B. K., R. N. Lutz, W. T. McReynolds, and M. B. Kohrs. 1976. Behavior therapy for weight control: Long-term results of two programs with nutritionists as therapists. *Am. J. Clin. Nutr.*, **29:** 880.

54. Penick, S. B., R. Filion, S. Fox, and A. J. Stunkard. 1971. Behavior modification in the treatment of obesity. *Psychosom. Med.*, **33:** 49.

55. Pi-Sunyer, F. X. 1976. Jejunoileal bypass surgery for obesity. *Am. J. Clin. Nutr.*, **29:** 409.

56. Pratt, D. E., E. F. Reber, and J. H. Klockow. 1971. Bulking agents in foods. *J. Am. Dietet. Assoc.*, **59:** 120.

57. Rickman, F., N. Mitchell, J. Dingman, and J. E. Dalen. 1974. Changes in serum cholesterol during the Stillman diet. *J. Am. Med. Assoc.*, **228:** 54.

58. Rivlin, R. S. 1975. Drug therapy. *N. Eng. J. Med.*, **292:** 26.

59. Samuel, P. D. and W. L. Burland. 1975. Drug treatment of obesity. In *Obesity in Perspective*, Part 2, G. A. Bray (Ed.). DHEW Publication No. (NIH) 75–708.

60. Scoville, B. A. 1975. Review of amphetamine-like drugs by the Food and Drug Administration: Clinical data and value judgments. In *Obesity in Perspective*, Part 2, G. A. Bray (Ed.). DHEW Publication No. (NIH) 75–708.

61. Seltzer, C. C. and J. Mayer. 1970. An effective weight control program in a public school system. *Am. J. Pub. Health*, **60:** 679.

62. Shetty, K. R. and R. K. Kalkhoff. 1977. Human chorionic gonadotropin (HCG) treatment of obesity. *Arch. Int. Med.*, **137:** 151.

63. Simeons, A. T. W. 1954. The action of chorionic gonadotrophin in the obese. *Lancet*, **2:** 946.

64. Spargo, J. A., F. Heald, and P. S. Peckos. 1966. Adolescent obesity. *Nutr. Today,* **1** (Dec.): 2.

65. Stein, M. R., R. E. Julis, C. C. Peck, W. Henshaw, J. E. Sawicki, and J. J. Deller, Jr. 1976. Ineffectiveness of human chorionic gonadotropin in weight reduction: a double-blind study. *Am. J. Clin. Nutr.,* **29:** 940.

66. Stuart, R. B. 1967. Behavioral control of overeating. *Behav. Res. Therapy,* **5:** 357.

67. Stuart, R. B. 1975a. Behavioral control of overeating: A status report. In *Obesity in Perspective,* Part 2, G. A. Bray (Ed.). DHEW Publication No. (NIH) 75–708.

68. Stuart, R. B. 1975b. Exercise prescription in weight management: Advantages, techniques and obstacles. *Obes. Bar. Med.,* **4:** 16.

69. Stuart, R. B. and B. Davis. 1972. *Slim Chance in a Fat World.* condensed ed. Champaign, Ill.: Research Press.

70. Weisenberg, M. and E. Fray. 1974. What's missing in the treatment of obesity by behavior modification? *J. Am. Dietet. Assoc.,* **65:** 410.

71. Worthington, B. S. and L. E. Taylor. 1974a. Balanced low-calorie vs. high-protein-low-carbohydrate reducing diets. I. Weight loss, nutrient intake, and subjective evaluation. *J. Am. Dietet. Assoc.,* **64:** 47.

72. Worthington, B. S. and L. E. Taylor. 1974b. Balanced low-calorie vs. high-protein-low-carbohydrate reducing diets. II. Biochemical changes. *J. Am. Dietet. Assoc.,* **64:** 52.

73. Young, C. M., S. S. Scanlan, H. S. Im, and L. Lutwak. 1971. Effect on body composition and other parameters in obese young men of carbohydrate level of reduction diet. *Am. J. Clin. Nutr.,* **24:** 290.

74. Young, C. M. 1975. Dietary treatment of obesity. In Obesity in Perspective, Part 2, G. A. Bray (Ed.). DHEW Publication No. (NIH) 75–708.

75. Yudkin, J. 1972. The low-carbohydrate diet in the treatment of obesity. *Postgrad. Med.,* **51:** 151.

CLIENT REFERENCES

1. Better Homes and Gardens. 1968. *Eat and Stay Slim.* New York: Better Homes and Gardens Books.

2. Black, C. 1962. *The Low-Calorie Cookbook.* New York: Collier Books.

3. Ferguson, J. M. 1976. *Habits, not Diets.* Palo Alto, Calif.: Bull Publishing.

4. Milo, M. 1972. *Diet and Exercise Guide.* New York: Family Circle.

5. Netzer, C. T. 1969. *The Brand-Name Calorie Counter.* New York: Dell.

6. Page, L. and N. Raper. 1973. *Food and Your Weight.* Home and Garden Bulletin No. 74. U.S. Department of Agriculture.

7. Stuart, R. B. and B. Davis. 1972. Slim Chance in a Fat World. condensed ed. Champaign, Ill.: Research Press.

STUDY GUIDE

Low-kilocalorie, low-carbohydrate diets have been popular for weight reduction because of quick weight loss and high satiety value.

1. Given a menu or diet pattern for a weight-reduction diet, estimate the grams of carbohydrate and the percent of total kilocalories as carbohydrate that it contains, using exchange list values. Categorize the diet as low, moderate, or high carbohydrate.

2. Explain why weight loss on a low-carbohydrate diet is often more marked on a short-term basis but probably similar on a long-term basis to any other equicaloric diet. Also explain why satiety value may be high for a low-carbohydrate diet. Discuss disadvantages and possible advantages of a low-carbohydrate diet for weight reduction.

It is important to change dietary habits and reeducate an obese individual to sound nutritional practices during the period of dieting.

3. Explain why the preceding statement about reeducation is true.

4. Given menus for a weight reduction diet and some information about an obese client's usual pattern of living and eating, decide and discuss whether or not the diet would serve well as a long-term education tool for this client.

The suggested caloric intake for weight reduction should be estimated on the basis of energy requirements and should ideally provide for a weight loss of 1½ to 2 lb/week.

5. Explain why the rate of weight loss specified is usually desirable in a long-term weight-reduction program.

6. Given the age, sex, height, present weight, and general level of physical activity, suggest an appropriate caloric level to achieve desirable weight loss.

Total and modified fasting for long periods of time have been used for weight reduction, particularly in massively obese patients.

7. Describe characteristics of an obese patient that may make him or her a likely candidate for a fasting or modified fasting program.

8. Describe and explain disadvantages or limitations to the use of fasting, both total and modified, for weight reduction in most obese clients.

9. Describe and explain the theoretical advantages of a modified fasting program over a total fasting program for severely obese subjects.

The basal metabolic rates of obese individuals do not appear to be significantly different from those of the nonobese.

10. In view of the preceding statement, discuss disadvantages and possible advantages for the use of thyroid compounds in the treatment of obesity.

Anorexigenic drugs may be successfully used or misused in treating obesity.

11. Describe the types of anorexigenic agents most commonly prescribed for obesity and the mode of their action in the body. Also discuss possible side effects and disadvantages of their use.

12. Suggest and justify guidelines for the effective use of anorexigenic drugs in weight reduction programs.

The role of physical activity in the treatment of obesity has been both presented as important and dismissed as insignificant.

13. Make and explain recommendations for type and amount of exercise in response to a question from an obese client as to whether or not exercise is worthwhile in a weight-reduction program.

Surgical procedures have been used for treatment of some patients with obesity.

14. Describe and explain gastric and intestinal bypass surgery and discuss advantages and disadvantages of these procedures for treating obesity.

15. Explain weight loss after bypass surgery for obesity and describe complications that commonly arise.

6

Malnutrition, Underweight, and Anorexia Nervosa

Protein-calorie malnutrition (PCM) has been widely documented in the developing countries of the world, particularly among young children. It may also occur in adults and appears to be one of the most common forms of hospital malnutrition (Butterworth and Blackburn, 1975; Bistrian et al., 1974). The dietitian may thus need to deal with it. This chapter discusses the characteristic features of PCM in children and adults. It also includes discussion of nutritional care for the moderately underweight individual and problems encountered in treating patients with anorexia nervosa, in which case the treatment of severe malnutrition is complicated by psychological factors.

6.1 Protein-Calorie Malnutrition (PCM)

The causes of malnutrition in a population are complex and multiple. They include (1) inadequate dietary intake as a result of poverty, agricultural problems, misinformation or lack of knowledge, and sociocultural taboos; (2) infections and chronic diseases that produce anorexia, gastrointestinal problems, and metabolic abnormalities; and (3) sociocultural factors that prescribe food preparation, consumption patterns, and child feeding practices (Jelliffe, 1969).

Mild to moderate PCM may occur in a population on a continuum of severity. In many developing countries, the majority of citizens may be at nutritional risk, although severe symptoms are observed in a smaller proportion of individuals. Two types of severe disease have been characterized: nutritional marasmus and kwashiorkor. Fig. 6.1 compares the clinical features of these forms of PCM.

Nutritional Marasmus

Nutritional marasmus is the result of a diet that is low in both protein and kilocalories; it is starvation. In developing countries this condition most often occurs when breast feeding has failed and the child is given diluted and infected breast milk substitutes. Expense of cow's milk or commercial infant formulas, unsanitary conditions for preparation and feeding of the formulas, and lack of education for mothers limits successful artificial feeding of infants. The basic marasmic condition is made worse by constant bouts with infection (Jelliffe, 1969).

Nutritional marasmus may also occur in adulthood from near starvation. Patients with chronic diseases that have interfered with adequate food intake may develop marasmus without careful nutritional care. A survey by Bistrian et al. (1976) of malnutrition among hospitalized patients on general medical wards showed the prevalence of PCM to be 44 percent or greater by use of weight/height charts, triceps skin-fold measurement, arm-muscle circumference, serum albumin, and hematocrit criteria. More marasmic malnutrition was found among medical patients and more kwashiorkor among surgical patients.

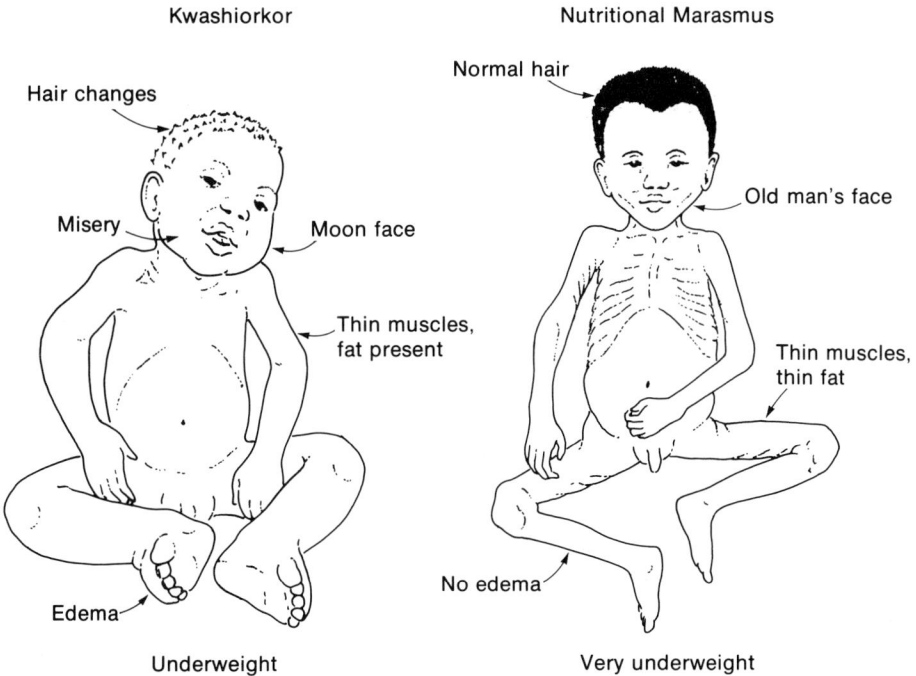

Fig. 6.1 Clinical features of kwashiorkor and nutritional marasmus. (From D. R. Jelliffe, *Child Nutrition in Developing Countries*, Washington, D.C.: U.S. Department of State, 1969.)

Clinical signs of marasmus always present include extreme growth failure in a child, with body weight only 60 percent or less of expected weight; marked wasting of muscles; and loss of subcutaneous fat. The face is thin, wizened, and has a "little old man" appearance. Signs occasionally present include associated symptoms of vitamin deficiencies, anemia, and diarrhea (Jelliffe, 1969).

Response of marasmus to treatment is often slow. In severely ill infants and children, hospitalization is desirable for control of accompanying diarrhea or infections and for biochemical tests as necessary. For young marasmic children in developing countries, Jelliffe recommended, for economy, a milk formula based upon dried skimmed milk. Alternatively, suitable formulas for treatment can be prepared from fresh cow's milk, full cream dried milk, or evaporated milk. Extra kilocalories can be added with sugar and a vegetable oil. Suggested proportions are 20 tsp dried skimmed milk powder, 4 tsp sugar, 6 tsp vegetable oil, and 20 fluid oz boiled water. The formula may at first be administered slowly through an intragastric tube. Additional foods should be added, as appropriate for the age, as soon as signs of improvement are seen. An adult patient with secondary nutritional marasmus may be maintained with total parenteral feeding, or a chemically defined diet may be given by intragastric tube. Oral food consumption should be implemented as soon as possible on an individual basis, and encouragement should be given to overcome anorexia.

Kwashiorkor

The word *kwashiorkor* was introduced into medical literature by Dr. Cicely Williams in the 1930s. It comes from the Ga language of West Africa and means "disease that occurs when displaced from the breast by another child." The disease often occurs at weaning from the breast when a source of good quality protein is no longer provided, but it may develop many months later. The cause is lack of protein, particularly good quality protein. Adequate kilocalories are present as carbohydrate or fat so that starvation does not occur. Many children in developing countries are susceptible to kwashiorkor during 1 to 3 years of age, when there are comparatively high protein requirements for growth; however, the food available for the child is largely bulky, indigestible, carbohydrate food such as starchy roots and cereal grains. Many infections are also common at this age and further deplete the body of important protein supplies (Jelliffe, 1969).

Clinical signs of kwashiorkor always present in children include edema; growth failure; psychological changes such as apathy, misery, and anorexia; and weak, wasted muscles with some overlying subcutaneous fat. Signs usually present are light, silky, sparse hair that can be easily plucked, skin changes, anemia, and loose stools. Signs occasionally present include a flaky paint rash, enlarged liver, ulcers and open sores on the skin, and associated vitamin deficiency symptoms (Jelliffe, 1969). The individual with kwashiorkor has a round "moon" face and a swollen, edematous body.

A number of cases of kwashiorkor and marasmus have been found among American Indians, and additional case reports have appeared in the medical literature of the United States. Four cases of kwashiorkor in infants under 1 year of age were reported in Arizona (John et al., 1977). The disease followed protein-deficient diets consumed for 5 weeks to 7 months. Two cases of kwashiorkor were encountered in Cleveland within a short period of time (Lozoff and Fanaroff, 1975). Both were the result of major feeding abnormalities that had been neither recognized nor corrected during contact of the patients and their parents with medical personnel. Another case of kwashiorkor was in Chicago, the result of a pure vegetarian diet (Berkelhamer et al., 1975). A balanced vegetarian diet for an infant is possible, but the parents did not receive the necessary help and encouragement from medical personnel in providing it. Adult kwashiorkor has occurred in hospitalized surgical patients who have abundant stores of adipose tissue but lack an exogenous protein source (Butterworth and Blackburn, 1975).

The treatment of kwashiorkor for children in developing countries is similar to that for nutritional marasmus. An adequate amount of good quality protein must be given. Nutrition education for parents of these children is also essential so the problem will not reoccur. A toasted full-fat soya flour formula was successfully used in the treatment of mild kwashiorkor by Rutishauser and Wharton (1968) but was less successful than a milk formula for several children with moderate and severe disease. Graham et al. (1973) reported the successful use of a lactose-free, medium-chain triglyceride-casein formula (lactose-free Portagen) and a casein hydrolysate-medium-chain triglyceride formula (Progestimil) for treatment of infants and children with PCM. MacLean and Graham (1976) found a casein-soy protein isolate blend (Isocal), which was originally designed as a complete tube feeding formula for adults, to be similar to casein in maintaining positive nitrogen balance for convalescent malnourished children after the acute treatment phase.

In an otherwise healthy person undergoing starvation, adaptation occurs. There is a gradual transition from glycogenolysis the first day to gluconeogenesis (utilizing protein tissues as substrate) the next several days to an increasingly effective protein-sparing economy where insulin output is decreased and ketones are oxidized in comparatively large quantities (see Sec. 5.2). However, some body protein continues to be lost when an exogenous source of protein is not supplied.

Previously well-nourished adults who are hospitalized for severe surgical or medical problems will break down muscle tissue when energy requirements are inadequately met during the stress of illness. If the patients have adequate supplies of adipose tissue, parenteral protein-sparing therapy may consist of giving only amino acids intravenously to decrease the catabolism of muscle tissue. Small amounts of glucose given intravenously tend to elevate blood insulin levels, are not sufficient to completely spare protein, and may inhibit the ketogenesis that is part of the body's adaptation to starvation. Thus, amino acids given parenterally do not always need to be accompanied by glucose, particularly in hospitalized patients who have adequate adipose tissue stores (Blackburn, 1973). Assessment of improvement with treatment for patients with PCM may be made by measurement of lean body mass, visceral protein, and fat stores, as discussed in Sec. 1.3.

There are major differences in the abilities of children and adults to adapt to food deprivation. The child is actively growing and thus has a greater demand for nutrients to build new tissues. He is also biochemically and immunologically immature and has had less opportunity to build resistance toward infections and to store essential nutrients. Clinical signs of deficiency will develop more quickly in children than adults with food restriction.

Plasma essential amino acids are low, whereas nonessential amino acids are variable in both children and adults with PCM (Smith et al., 1974). Diminished glucose tolerance has been reported in patients with PCM, associated with a reduced insulin secretory response and a degree of insulin resistance (Smith et al., 1975). Disturbed metabolism in the liver of patients with PCM has been reported, especially with kwashiorkor. Fatty infiltration of the liver is common and gradually disappears with treatment over several weeks (Waterlow, 1975; McLaren et al., 1968). A slower rate of metabolism of drugs in the liver has been found in children with PCM (Mehta et al., 1975). Changes in the gastrointestinal tract and effects on the body's immune system also have been studied.

Gastrointestinal Changes with PCM

The coexistence of diarrhea with severe PCM has been noted from the earliest descriptions. Postmortem studies of both children and adults with PCM show atrophy of the pancreas and the intestine. Clinical studies reveal decreased secretion of pancreatic enzymes, which return to normal with treatment. Gastric mucosal atrophy and hypochlorhydria have been described. Malabsorption frequently occurs in PCM with varying degrees of steatorrhea, although amino acids seem to be well absorbed (Viteri and Schneider, 1974). Overgrowth of bacteria in the small intestine is a common abnormality (Mata et al., 1972a).

Light microscopic studies of the small intestine in PCM show nonspecific changes that are similar to those in other enteropathies, including shortening, widening, and fusion of the villi and diminished epithelial cell height. Dense material accumulates in a subepithelial location in villi, in crypts, and around the capillaries of the lamina propria. A consistent reduction in thickness of intestinal mucosa and atrophy of the crypts appear to be specific characteristic effects of severe PCM (Duque et al., 1975a). Electron microscopy reveals nonspecific microvillar abnormalities such as shortening, diminished numbers, abnormal positioning, and branching (Duque et al., 1975b).

Lack of conjugated bile acids may affect the malnourished individual's ability to form fat micelles in the intestine. Malnourished children show an abnormally high level of secondary free bile acid, which could adversely affect intestinal cell function. Two possible explanations for bile abnormalities have been suggested: (1) the terminal ileum may function defectively in PCM, causing an increased fecal loss of bile acids and increased cycling in the free form as a consequence of increased passive absorption in the colon, or (2) bacterial overgrowth in the small intestine may cause deconjugation of bile salts, with the secondary free bile acids then being passively absorbed in the upper intestine and colon (Viteri and Schneider, 1974).

Gastrointestinal effects of PCM are widespread in some populations, particularly those in tropical countries, with a continuum in regard to severity. It is difficult to separate the effects of PCM and the environment in terms of intestinal morphology and function. Viteri and Schneider suggested that the alterations in digestive physiology with severe PCM are in many cases a synergistic combination of factors: (1) PCM itself, which reduces the production of conjugated bile acids and alters liver metabolism, pancreatic output, and intestinal cell function, and (2) a change in "intestinal ecology" precipitated by environmental contamination, which leads to bacterial overgrowth with frequent bouts of diarrhea. This reduces the disaccharidase content of the intestinal wall and is accompanied by terminal ileal dysfunction, loss of bile acids through feces, an increase in the passive diffusion of free bile acids, and an altered composition of the bile acid pool. As a consequence of synergistic action, further alteration of cell function occurs, possibly reducing normal defense mechanisms of the gut and favoring greater incidence of infections.

Immunity and Infection in PCM

A synergistic interaction between malnutrition and infection, with the two conditions producing mutual aggravation, has been described (Rosenberg et al., 1976; Scrimshaw et al., 1968; Scrimshaw, 1965). In persons whose diets are of borderline adequacy in specific nutrients, infections precipitate deficiency disease. Infectious disease also produces higher morbidity and mortality in malnourished than in well-nourished populations.

Many factors are involved in the establishment of resistance to infection, and it is difficult to separate the specific mechanisms through which nutritional factors may exert their influence (Axelrod, 1974). Studies in low-socioeconomic groups have shown that the problems of malnutrition begin very early in life. Inadequate nutrition of the mother may retard fetal growth so that some infants begin life with nutritional deficits. The high frequency of elevated values of cord blood IgM detected in a typical Guatemalan study village by Mata et al. (1972b) suggested the possibility of frequent intrauterine infection as another cause, in addition to maternal malnutrition, for poor fetal growth. Viral infections in the first 3 months of life, even with breast-fed babies, were found to be associated with a deficit in weight through the first year of life. Infectious diseases thus have negative effects on both the well- and the malnourished host, but with greater morbidity and mortality from infection in the malnourished. When the incidence of infection is high in a population, attention to nutritional measures alone is not sufficient.

Whether lower resistance to infection in malnourished individuals is caused by immunological deficiencies, decreased tissue mass, or other causes has not been clarified. The immune response of the body is an important factor in establishing resistance to infection, and extensive studies have been carried out on pathogenesis and pathophysiology of immune failure in PCM. There are many conflicting reports. In some cases, circulating antibody (humoral) responses to various antigens have been reported to be normal in individuals with PCM; in other studies, they have been found to be somewhat diminished. The same is true for measurements of serum immunoglobulin levels. Cell-mediated immunity has generally been reported to be depressed in PCM, as indicated by a failure to develop delayed cutaneous hypersensitivity to various allergens (Neumann et al., 1975). A position paper of the Food and Nutrition Board of the National Research Council (1976) stressed the importance of research on the immune response of the malnourished host to resolve conflicting data. Deficiencies of certain vitamins and minerals, particularly vitamin B_6, may also decrease immunologic competence and are being studied (Worthington, 1974).

6.2   Underweight

Body weight decreases when energy intake is not equal to energy output on a long-term basis and adaptation cannot replace food intake. A healthy nonobese adult can lose up to 25 percent of body weight without endangering life, and some persons have survived losses of 50 percent of their initial weight (Parham, 1975). An individual whose body weight is 10 percent or more below that listed in standard height/weight tables is generally classified as underweight. Persons may be slightly underweight according to these imprecise standards and still be well nourished, with satisfactory nutrient intake. They may have a genetic predisposition to leanness, participate in consistent vigorous activity, or have a natural or acquired preference for moderately low-kilocalorie foods. Other individuals who are underweight, however, may have a suboptimal or borderline nutritional status that could be improved with intake of increased amounts of energy along with optimal amounts of other essential nutrients. Underweight basically may be due to an inadequate intake or utilization of kilocalories, to excessive physical activity, or to both. Disease, both acute and chronic, may also contribute to the development of less than desirable body weight.

Nutritional Care of the Underweight Patient

Adding approximately 500 kcal/day to the maintenance energy need should result in about 1-lb gain in body weight each week since this weekly increase will be 3500 kcal, the approximate caloric value of 1 lb of adipose tissue. Greater caloric increases than this may be very difficult to achieve, especially in an anorectic patient. Individual goals for increased caloric intake and weight gain should be set, with due consideration to previous weight status, height, age, sex, activity, and sociocultural influences.

The underweight individual must be motivated to gain weight. A careful history of usual food intake, activity patterns, and general health habits is helpful in detecting patterns of living that contribute to the maintenance of a suboptimal weight level. Behavior-modification techniques may be useful in establishing improved eating and living habits. A decision for change must be made by the patient, with the support of the dietitian and other medical personnel. Economic, social, and cultural influences should be integrated into plans for change.

Extra food intake will be easier to achieve if the patient consumes at least three regular meals per day and has regular exercise, relaxation, and sleeping regimens. Between-meal snacks may be helpful if they do not depress the appetite for the next meal. Some foods with concentrated caloric value may be inconspicuously added, such as cream (on cereal), whole milk instead of low-fat milk (for drinking), salad dressings and cream sauces, margarine or butter (on breads), and properly fried foods. Hospitalized patients may be given supplementary commercial products that are high in kilocalories and protein. The type of fat and carbohydrate specified for a particular patient may regulate choices of supplemental foods; for example, the use of vegetable instead of animal fats may be mandated. The basic diet pattern should allow adequate consumption of fruits, vegetables, whole grain cereal products, good quality protein foods, and milk products to ensure optimal intake of all nutrients along with the appropriate caloric level.

6.3   Anorexia Nervosa

The independent reports of Gull in England and Laseque in France more than 100 years ago marked the beginning of anorexia nervosa as a clinical entity. Primary anorexia nervosa is a very distinctive, dramatic, and unmistakable condition, but its basic cause and effective treatment are still controversial. Bruch (1973) wrote about the history of the concept of anorexia nervosa and pointed out that even from the beginning there were differences of opinion concerning definition and etiology. Laseque in 1873 conceived the disorder as a "peripheral" disturbance, with starting symptoms being some hysterical disturbance in the digestive tract, such as vomiting, gastric pains, or hematemesis. The typical picture was seen in young girls, with onset related to an emotional upset. Gull attributed the lack of appetite in this disease to a morbid mental state with a central rather than a peripheral origin. He stressed the remarkable hyperactivity associated with this condition, commenting that "it seemed hardly possible that a body so wasted could undergo the exercise which seemed so agreeable."

Simmonds' 1914 report of pituitary lesions in an emaciated woman suggested an endocrine etiology, an idea that persisted until the 1930s, when it was again established that anorexia nervosa is a disease of psychological origin. However, it is not always recognized that the disease is a dynamic one, and patients are seen at various stages of the illness. Starvation itself is associated with marked psychological changes that are often denied by the patients. The family patterns of interaction are also dynamic and include progressively rising levels of anxiety and concern for the patient, and, at the same time, there are rising levels of annoyance and resentment. The complexity of the disease has undoubtedly contributed to the confusion on etiology and effective treatment (Bruch, 1973).

Anorexia nervosa is a relatively rare disorder, with an average annual incidence of 0.24 to 0.61 per 100,000 (Halmi, 1974). It is characteristic of young females but has also been reported in males and older women (Hasan and Tibbetts, 1977; Beumont, 1970; Bruch, 1973). It is one of the few psychiatric conditions that may lead to death, with actual causes of death sometimes unexplained (Bruch, 1971).

Characteristics of the Disease

The following criteria for diagnosis of anorexia nervosa were suggested by Feighner et al. (1972).

1. Age of onset prior to 25 years
2. Anorexia with accompanying weight loss of at least 25 percent original weight
3. A distorted, implacable attitude toward eating, food, or weight that overrides hunger, admonitions, reassurance, and threats, e.g.,
    a. Denial of illness with failure to recognize nutritional needs
    b. Apparent enjoyment in losing weight with overt manifestation that food refusal is a pleasurable indulgence
    c. A desired body image of extreme thinness with overt evidence that it is rewarding to the patient to achieve and maintain this state
    d. Unusual hoarding or handling of food
4. No known medical illness that could account for the weight loss
5. No other known psychiatric disorder
6. At least two of the following manifestations:
    a. Amenorrhea
    b. Lanugo (fine hair on body or face)
    c. Bradycardia (persistent resting pulse of 60 or less)
    d. Periods of overactivity
    e. Episodes of bulimia (insatiable hunger)
    f. Vomiting (may be self-induced)

Halmi (1974), in a review of 94 cases of anorexia nervosa, found a greater maternal and paternal age at time of the probands' birth and a greater incidence of both low and high birth weights than in the general population. Feeding histories were available for 57 of the 94 patients. Although these histories are subject to a considerable bias, a relatively high incidence of premorbid feeding problems during infancy, preadolescence, and adolescence was noted. All patients demonstrated unusual alimentative habits and attitudes. A steadfast refusal to eat was found in 90 percent of the patients, bulimia in 10 percent, regular vomiting in 33 percent, and abuse of laxatives in 11 percent. A denial of illness with failure to recognize nutritional needs was obvious in 80 percent of the patients, with hoarding of food in 31 percent.

Silverman (1974) reported his experience with 29 patients, aged 10 to 17 years, who were hospitalized for the treatment of anorexia nervosa. Each patient was previously somewhat overweight and was teased or embarrassed by family members, teachers, or peers. The patient then embarked on a routine of strict and steadfast avoidance of food that led to marked weight loss. Early weight loss was often ignored or not noted by the family. The typical patient was described as a teenage girl who was depressed, weepy, hostile, frequently agitated, and in seemingly constant motion. Usually she wore heavy sweaters and slacks, presumably not only to mask her gaunt frame but to keep her warm. She was extremely underweight, complained of severe constipation, and had small urinary output. She was an outstanding student but may have been an "overachiever" who needed to study many hours daily to maintain good grades. The skin appeared dark and dirty, despite the fact that personal cleanliness was rarely a problem. Skin texture was rough and desquamation common. Long, fine, silken hairs were found extensively over the trunk and extremities and sometimes on the face.

The state of starvation in this disorder may affect various physiologic and metabolic functions. Low levels of plasma luteinizing hormone (LH) and follicle-stimulating hormone (FSH) have been reported in anorexia nervosa, and Boyar et al. (1974) found an immature pattern of secretion that resembled that seen in prepubertal and pubertal children. Elevations of blood urea nitrogen and abnormalities of hematopoiesis have also been observed (Silverman, 1974). The rate of albumin synthesis and serum levels of valine, isoleucine, and tryptophan were found to be decreased in two adult females with anorexia nervosa (Yap et al., 1975). The reduced supply of amino acids in the blood, particularly tryptophan, was suggested as the most important factor in the decrease of albumin synthesis in these patients. Elevated serum cholesterol levels have been reported, although the range of individual values is wide. Other serum lipid levels have shown striking lability during treatment and appeared to be unrelated to variation in caloric intake or to the qualitative composition of the diet (Crisp et al., 1968). Hypercarotenemia is a common finding in anorexia nervosa. Increased intake of carotene-rich foods or an acquired defect in the utilization of vitamin A have been suggested as causal factors (Robboy et al., 1974).

Bruch (1973) emphasized that a primary form of anorexia nervosa, with relentless pursuit of thinness as the driving motivation, must be differentiated from secondary forms with unspecific atypical pictures to clarify the apparent inconsistencies in diagnosis and treatment. She pointed out that anorexia nervosa is really not a disease of anorexia since there is usually no true loss of appetite. In fact, patients often have a great desire to eat but deliberately refuse to do so. Bruch believes that in primary anorexia nervosa the lack of eating is a late manifestation secondary to disturbed underlying personality problems. The main issue is a struggle for control, for a sense of identity, competence, and effectiveness. Many patients who develop the disorder have previously struggled, sometimes for years, to make themselves over and be perfect in the eyes of others. Concern with thinness and food refusal are late steps in this maldevelopment. According to Bruch (1973) there are three areas of disordered psychological function:

1. A disturbance of delusional proportions in the body image and body concept. The often gruesome emaciation is defended as normal. The abnormality is denied and actively maintained. Without a corrective change in body concept, improvement is apt to be only temporary.
2. Disturbance in the accuracy of the perception or cognitive interpretation of stimuli arising in the body, with failure to recognize signs of nutritional needs as the most pronounced deficiency. There are many complaints about acute discomfort and fullness after the intake of even small amounts of food but also uncontrollable impulses to gorge oneself.
3. A paralyzing sense of ineffectiveness that pervades all thinking and activities. They see themselves as acting in response to demands from others. They lack awareness of their own resources and do not rely on their own feelings, thoughts, and bodily sensations.

Treatment

For effective and lasting correction of the abnormal body weight in anorexia nervosa, the nutritional program must be coordinated with psychotherapy and resolution of family conflicts. Correction of the extreme underweight condition is often a matter of great urgency since the very survival of a patient may be at stake. In cases of extreme emaciation where the patient refuses food, total intravenous feeding may be used on a temporary basis (Bruch, 1976).

The physiological principles involved in the treatment of anorexia nervosa are very simple: increase food intake and decrease physical activity. However, how to persuade, bribe, cajole, trick, or force a negativistic patient into doing this when the patient is determined not to do so has been a matter for great debate. Silverman (1974) attempted to create a protective nonpunitive environment free of stress for hospitalized patients with anorexia nervosa (27 girls and 2 boys, 10 to 17 years of age). Upon admission, each patient was supplied with hospital clothes and allowed no personal possessions nor privacy. Strict rules about fluid intake were enforced. Failure to comply resulted in at least three subsequent days of make-up intravenous fluid therapy. It was emphasized that the therapy was a hospital regulation for nondrinkers and was not to be construed as punishment. Intensive psychiatric treatment for patients was started on the day of admission, and parents were also treated by the same psychiatrist. As the patient began to make progress and to eat, she or he began to earn such privileges as possession of personal clothing. After hospitalization for about 3 months, the youngsters had corrected nearly all their metabolic abnormalities, had normal eating and drinking habits, and had made a significant start in their psychotherapy. They were followed medically and psychiatrically as outpatients.

Maxmen et al. (1974) treated hospitalized patients with anorexia nervosa under the philosophy that pragmatic, rather than etiological, considerations should determine the treatment approach, especially in the initial phase. The patient was weighed every day upon arising and after voiding. The goal was set for the patient to gain at least 113 g (0.25 lb) daily above her highest previous weight obtained within the hospital. If she gained this weight, no other procedures were instituted that day. However, if she failed to gain the 113 g, she received 236 ml of a high caloric liquid feeding every 4 hours while awake. (Any one of several commercially available liquid food supplements or a dietary department product could be used.) These feedings were dispensed by the nursing staff in a nonchalant manner, just as medications were handed out. If after 3 to 4 days the patient failed to consistently gain weight, the physician had the option of increasing the (1) expected daily weight gain from 113 to 226 g, (2) frequency of the feedings from every 4 hours to every 3 hours to every 2 hours, thereby increasing the number of feedings, or (3) caloric content of the feedings. This protocol was continued until the patient had not required supplemental feedings for at least 4 consecutive days and had gained within 10 percent of her original premorbid body weight. The medical staff was open, honest, and yet firm about implementing the treatment. Before the program began, the patient was told by the physician that anorexia nervosa is a potentially life-threatening illness and that the treatment protocol was being prescribed to prevent her "inadvertent" suicide. Patients were praised for gaining weight but not criticized for failing to do so. Psychological issues were not discussed until the patient was well on the way to gaining weight without the assistance of supplemental feedings in order to avoid excessive anxiety that might have distracted the patient from concentrating upon the primary task of gaining weight. Psychotherapy was done, as appropriate, after weight gain. These clinicians emphasized the initial stage of treatment and did not report long-term follow-up.

Hall (1975) reported the treatment of 22 patients with anorexia nervosa in three main areas: (1) hospital restoration of normal weight with bed rest, a regular diet that was gradually increased in amount, the setting of a target weight, and rewards for weight gain; (2) family intervention, with separate counseling for the parents; and (3) individual psychotherapy as the patient improved physically. Eight of the 22 patients recovered, based upon criteria of at least 1 year of maintaining normal weight, return of spontaneous menstruation, and normal eating behavior. Treatment was continued for most of the other patients.

Leitenberg et al. (1968) found verbal praise following gradual improvements in eating behavior and the granting of more tangible privileges for gradual weight gain to be effective reinforcements for two patients with anorexia nervosa. Agras et al. (1974) suggested that feedback of information to the patient as to weight gained and number of kilocalories consumed may be very important in that it sets the stage for reinforcement. Without this feedback, positive reinforcement appeared to be relatively ineffective. They suggested the following procedures to encourage weight gain in patients with anorexia nervosa:

1. The therapeutic environment should be arranged so that the patient can engage in pleasurable activities only if progress, as measured by weight gain, is being made. The reinforcements may include attention from and social interaction with staff members, other patients, and visitors; reading, writing, and using the telephone; watching television, smoking, and physical activity.

2. Measurement of weight gain should be done carefully, using metabolic scales at the same time each day under standard conditions.

3. Meals should be large and attractively served and of standard selection, the patient not being allowed to choose special items. Feedback on the success of eating should be given consistently. If immediate calculation of caloric intake is possible after each meal, this should be used. Otherwise, the patient can count the number of mouthfuls eaten for feedback information. She should be told her exact weight each day and should plot caloric intake, mouthfuls eaten, and weight each day on a graph kept on the wall of her room.

4. The entire staff must decide which problem behaviors to ignore and which adaptive behaviors to consider or treat.

Although behavior-modification techniques have been advocated with enthusiasm by a number of clinicians for the treatment of anorexia nervosa, Bruch (1976) cautioned that the long-term results are often disappointing and sometimes disastrous. Weight gain itself is not a cure for anorexia nervosa. When weight gain is achieved without satisfactory treatment of the underlying psychological problems, serious depression, psychotic disorganization, and suicidal attempts often follow. According to the experience of Bruch, behavior modification aimed primarily at increased food intake and body weight gain may undermine the last vestiges of self-esteem for the patient and destroy the crucial hope of achieving autonomy and self-determination. On the other hand, it is also dangerous not to correct the weight and to permit a patient to exist at a marginal level of physiological safety while undergoing psychotherapy. The treatment program must consider both the life-threatening aspects of starvation and the basic psychological problems. It must be comprehensive and individualized, with psychotherapy focusing on the development of autonomy for the patient.

REFERENCES

1. Agras, W. S., D. H. Barlow, H. N. Chapin, G. G. Abel, and H. Leitenberg. 1974. Behavior modification of anorexia nervosa. *Arch. Gen. Psychiatry,* **30:** 279.

2. Axelrod, A. E. 1974. Nutrition and acquired immunity. *Food and Nutr. News,* Nat. Live Stock and Meat Board, **46** (No. 1): 1.

3. Berkelhamer, J. E., F. K. Thorp, and S. Cobbs. 1975. Kwashiorkor in Chicago. *Am. J. Dis. Child.,* **129:** 1240.

4. Beumont, P. J. V. 1970. Anorexia nervosa in male subjects. *Psychother. Psychosom.,* **18:** 365.

5. Bistrian, B. R., G. L. Blackburn, E. Hallowell, and R. Heddle. 1974. Protein status of general surgical patients. *J. Am. Med. Assoc.,* **230:** 858.

6. Bistrian, B. R., G. L. Blackburn, J. Vitale, D. Cochran, and J. Naylor. 1976. Prevalence of malnutrition in general medical patients. *J. Am. Med. Assoc.,* **235:** 1567.

7. Blackburn, G. L. 1973. Adaptation to starvation. *Intake: Perspectives in Clinical Nutrition* (Eaton Laboratories), No. 5.

8. Boyar, R. M., J. Katz, J. W. Finkelstein, S. Kapen, H. Weiner, E. D. Weitzman, and L. Hellman. 1974. Anorexia nervosa. *N. Eng. J. Med.,* **291:** 861.

9. Bruch, H. 1971. Death in anorexia nervosa. *Psychosom. Med.,* **33:** 135.

10. Bruch, H. 1973. *Eating Disorders.* New York: Basic Books.

11. Bruch, H. 1976. The treatment of eating disorders. *Mayo Clin. Proc.,* **51:** 266.

12. Butterworth, C. E. and G. L. Blackburn. 1975. Hospital malnutrition. *Nutr. Today,* **10** (No. 2): 8.

13. Crisp, A. H., L. M. Blendis, and G. L. S. Pawan. 1968. Aspects of fat metabolism in anorexia nervosa. *Metabolism,* **17:** 1109.

14. Duque, E., O. Bolaños, H. Lotero, and L. G. Mayoral. 1975a. Enteropathy in adult protein malnutrition: light microscopic findings. *Am. J. Clin. Nutr.,* **28,** 901.

15. Duque, E., H. Lotero, O. Bolaños, and L. G. Mayoral. 1975b. Enteropathy in adult protein malnutrition: ultrastructural findings. *Am. J. Clin. Nutr.,* **28:** 914.

16. Feighner, J. P., E. Robins, and S. B. Guze. 1972. Diagnostic criteria for use in psychiatric research. *Arch. Gen. Psychiat.,* **26:** 57.

17. Food and Nutrition Board, National Research Council. 1976. Immune response of the malnourished child. A position paper. Washington, D.C.: National Academy of Sciences.

18. Graham, G. G., J. M. Baertl, A. Cordano, and E. Morales. 1973. Lactose-free, medium-chain triglyceride formulas in severe malnutrition. *Am. J. Dis. Child.,* **126:** 330.

19. Hall, A. 1975. Treatment of anorexia nervosa. *N. Zealand Med. J.,* **82** (No. 543): 10.

20. Halmi, K. A. 1974. Anorexia nervosa: Demographic and clinical features in 94 cases. *Psychosom. Med.,* **36:** 18.

21. Hasan, M. K. and R. W. Tibbetts. 1977. Primary anorexia nervosa (weight phobia) in males. *Postgrad. Med. J.,* **53:** 146.

22. Jelliffe, D. B. 1969. *Child Nutrition in Developing Countries.* U.S. Department of State.

23. John, T. J., J. Blazovich, E. S. Lightner, O. F. Sieber, Jr., J. J. Corrigan, and R. Hansen. 1977. Kwashiorkor not associated with poverty. *J. Ped.,* **90:** 730.

24. Leitenberg, H., W. S. Agras, and L. E. Thomson. 1968. A sequential analysis of the effect of selective positive reinforcement in modifying anorexia nervosa. *Behav. Res. Ther.,* **6:** 211.

25. Lozoff, B. and A. A. Fanaroff. 1975. Kwashiorkor in Cleveland. *Am. J. Dis. Child.,* **129:** 710.

26. MacLean, W. C., Jr. and G. G. Graham. 1976. Evaluation of an isoosmotic tube feeding formula in the diets of convalescent malnourished infants and children. *Am. J. Clin. Nutr.,* **29:** 496.

27. Mata, L. J., F. Jimenez, M. Cordón, R. Rosales, E. Prera, R. E. Schneider, and F. Viteri. 1972a. Gastrointestinal flora of children with protein-calorie malnutrition. *Am. J. Clin. Nutr.,* **25:** 1118.

28. Mata, L. J., J. J. Urrutia, C. Albertazzi, O. Pellecer, and E. Arellano. 1972b. Influence of recurrent infections on nutrition and growth of children in Guatemala. *Am. J. Clin. Nutr.,* **25:** 1267.

29. Maxmen, J.'S., P. M. Silberfarb, and R. B. Ferrell. 1974. Anorexia nervosa. *J. Am. Med. Assoc.,* **229:** 801.

30. Mehta, S., H. K. Kalsi, S. Jayaraman, and V. S. Mathur. 1975. Chloramphenicol metabolism in children with protein-calorie malnutrition. *Am. J. Clin. Nutr.,* **28:** 977.

31. McLaren, D. S., R. Faris, and B. Zekian. 1968. The liver during recovery from protein-calorie malnutrition. *J. Trop. Med. Hygiene,* **71:** 271.

32. Neumann, C. G., G. J. Lawlor, Jr., E. R. Stiehm, M. E. Swendseid, C. Newton, J. Herbert, A. J. Ammann, and M. Jacob. 1975. Immunologic responses in malnourished children. *Am. J. Clin. Nutr.,* **28:** 89.

33. Parham, E. S. 1975. Starvation. *J. Home Econ.,* **67** (Nov.): 7.

34. Robboy, M. S., A. S. Sato, and A. D. Schwabe. 1974. The hypercarotenemia in anorexia nervosa: a comparison of vitamin A and carotene levels in various forms of menstrual dysfunction and cachexia. *Am. J. Clin. Nutr.* **27:** 362.

35. Rosenberg, I. H., N. W. Solomons, and D. M. Levin. 1976. Interaction of infection and nutrition: Some practical concerns. *Ecol. Food Nutr.* **4** (No. 4): 203.

36. Rutishauser, I. H. E. and B. A. Wharton. 1968. Toasted full-fat soya flour in treatment of kwashiorkor. *Arch. Dis. Child.,* **43:** 463.

37. Scrimshaw, N. S. 1965. Malnutrition and infection. *Borden's Rev. Nutr. Res.,* **26** (No. 2): 17.

38. Scrimshaw, N. S., C. E. Taylor, and J. E. Gordon. 1968. Interactions of nutrition and infection. *World Health Org. Monograph Ser.,* No. 57.

39. Silverman, J. A. 1974. Anorexia nervosa: Clinical observations in a successful treatment plan. *J. Ped.,* **84:** 68.

40. Smith, S. R., P. J. Edgar, T. Pozefsky, M. K. Chhetri, and T. E. Prout. 1975. Insulin secretion and glucose tolerance in adults with protein-calorie malnutrition. *Metabolism,* **24:** 1073.

41. Smith, S. R., T. Pozefsky, and M. K. Chhetri. 1974. Nitrogen and amino acid metabolism in adults with protein-calorie malnutrition. *Metabolism,* **23:** 603.

42. Viteri, F. E. and R. E. Schneider. 1974. Gastrointestinal alterations in protein-calorie malnutrition. *Med. Clin. No. Am.,* **58:** 1487.

43. Waterlow, J. C. 1975. Amount and rate of disappearance of liver fat in malnourished infants in Jamaica. *Am. J. Clin. Nutr.*, **28:** 1330.

44. Worthington, B. S. 1974. Effect of nutritional status on immune phenomena. *J. Am. Dietet. Assoc.*, **65:** 123.

45. Yap, S. H., J. C. M. Hafkenscheid, and J. H. M. Van Tongeren. 1975. Important role of tryptophan on albumin synthesis in patients suffering from anorexia nervosa and hypoalbuminemia. *Am. J. Clin. Nutr.*, **28:** 1356.

STUDY GUIDE

Various factors may contribute to the development of malnutrition in populations or individuals.

1. Describe and explain several factors that may contribute to malnutrition and underweight in adults and children.

2. Explain why children develop clinical signs easily when food restriction exists for even short periods of time, whereas adults are more resistant to food deprivation.

Nutritional marasmus and kwashiorkor are types of severe PCM, each with distinguishing clinical signs and symptoms.

3. Be able to distinguish between nutritional marasmus and kwashiorkor when observing photographs of young patients with PCM. Describe characteristic clinical signs of each.

4. Describe the major causes of kwashiorkor and nutritional marasmus and give suggestions for prevention.

5. Outline a satisfactory procedure for the treatment of severe and of mild PCM in children and adults.

6. Explain a possible relationship between a decrease in the number of mothers who are breast feeding and an increase in the incidence of nutritional marasmus in developing countries.

7. Describe gastrointestinal changes that may occur in patients with PCM and discuss possible relationships between these changes and the clinical signs of the disease.

8. Discuss possible synergistic relationships between PCM and infection.

Underweight individuals may have a suboptimal nutritional status that can be improved with proper nutritional care.

9. How might the dietitian/nutritionist effectively assess the status of an underweight patient in terms of need for nutritional improvement.

10. Give suggestions that may be useful in helping an underweight patient to gain weight and improve his nutritional status.

Anorexia nervosa is a psychophysiologic disorder resulting in self-induced starvation.

11. Describe criteria that might be used in the diagnosis of anorexia nervosa.

12. Give a possible explanation for the confusion in the medical literature on etiology and effective treatment of anorexia nervosa.

13. Describe and evaluate several apparently successful approaches to treatment of anorexia nervosa that have been reported in the literature. Define a useful role of the dietitian in treatment of this disorder.

14. Suggest possible disadvantages for the use of behavior-modification techniques in the treatment of anorexia nervosa.

7

Nutritional Anemias

Anemia results from a reduction in the circulating red blood cell (RBC) mass and is usually defined in terms of a decrease in the volume of packed RBCs, hemoglobin concentration, and/or number of RBCs. Erythrocytes or RBCs are produced in the bone marrow and released to the circulation, where they survive approximately 120 days. They are then removed by the reticuloendothelial system, which breaks down the hemoglobin to bile pigments, iron, and globin. The system normally maintains a balance between RBC production and destruction so that the cell mass remains constant in size. When destruction exceed production, the cell mass decreases and anemia develops. This imbalance may result from blood loss, excessive destruction of RBCs, inadequate production of RBCs, or various combinations of these processes.

Different types of anemias have been classified in terms of the basic cause of the imbalance in RBC production and destruction. Only a few of these anemias are related to nutritional effects. Nutritional deficiencies that may result in anemia include: (1) iron, (2) vitamin B_{12} and/or folic acid, (3) protein, (4) possibly ascorbic acid, and (5) experimentally—copper, cobalt, pyridoxine, nicotinic acid, riboflavin, possibly pantothenic acid and thiamin.

The most common nutritional anemia is caused by iron deficiency, and this type of anemia is emphasized in this chapter. A macrocytic, megaloblastic anemia, which may occur with a deficiency of vitamin B_{12} or folic acid, is also discussed.

7.1 Iron-Deficiency Anemia

Assessment of Iron Nutritional Status

The quantity of iron in the body (normally about 35 to 50 mg per kg body weight in the adult) is maintained primarily by controlled absorption from the duodenum and to a lesser extent by excretion. About two-thirds of the body iron is found in hemoglobin, and most of the remainder is in storage depots. The major iron storage protein is ferritin, which occurs mainly intracellularly in the liver and reticuloendothelial system. About 1 percent of the ferritin circulates in the blood. Hemosiderin is an insoluble iron-storage protein found in bone marrow. Some iron circulates in the plasma bound to transferrin, a beta$_1$ globulin carrier protein, and a very small proportion of the total body iron is present in myoglobin and the cytochrome enzymes (Finch, 1969; Wintrobe et al., 1974, p. 1581).

The average adult diet in the United States provides about 6 mg iron/1000 kcal or 10 to 20 mg/day. However, intake is variable. Many adolescent girls and menstruating women have a borderline iron intake of 10 mg or less per day. Approximately 5 to 10 percent of iron in a mixed diet is absorbed, with up to 15 percent being absorbed in iron-deficient subjects. Adult men are generally in balance when iron loss is replaced by daily absorption of 0.5 to 1 mg. Most iron is lost from the intestinal tract by exfoliation of gastrointestinal mucosa, as blood loss, and as iron in the bile. The postmenopausal woman is probably similar to the adult man in iron balance, although she may come to menopause with deficient iron stores because of excessive menstrual losses or repeated pregnancies (Committee on Iron Deficiency, 1968).

Blood losses from menstruation are variable, having been reported to range from 0 to 540 ml with an average of 43.4 ± 2.3 ml per cycle (equivalent monthly to an iron loss of about 0.5 mg/day) (Hallberg et al., 1966). A menstruating woman must absorb about 0.7 to 2 mg iron daily to maintain iron balance. The recommended dietary allowance (RDA) of iron for a menstruating woman is 18 mg/day, whereas that for a man or postmenopausal woman is 10 mg. The pregnant woman needs additional iron, particularly during the last half of pregnancy. Iron is transferred to the growing fetus and placental structures, additional iron is needed to expand the RBC volume by about 30 percent, and iron is lost with blood at delivery. Table 7.1 summarizes iron requirements for pregnancy. An iron supplement is usually prescribed for the pregnant woman.

Because of rapid growth during infancy, iron requirements in proportion to food intake exceed those during any other period of life. The RDA of iron for infants up to 6 months of age is 10 mg/day and 15 mg for those 6 months to 1 year of age. There is variation in the amount of iron stored by the fetus, and several studies have shown no clear relationship between iron intake and hematologic findings in infants and preschoolers (National Dairy Council, 1972; Beal and Meyers, 1970). The Committee on Nutrition of the American Academy of Pediatrics (1969) emphasized the

Table 7.1 IRON REQUIREMENTS OF PREGNANCY*

	Mean (mg)	Range (mg)
Usual external iron loss	170	150–200
Expansion of RBC mass	450	200–600
Fetal iron	270	200–370
Iron in placenta and cord	90	30–170
Total requirement	980	580–1340
Additional loss from blood at delivery	150	90–310
Cost of pregnancy (not including iron for expansion of RBC mass, which returns to stores after delivery)	680	440–1050

* Adapted from Committee on Iron Deficiency, 1968.

value of iron-fortified milk formulas for the prevention of iron-deficiency anemia in infancy. Fomon (1970) recommended the use of iron-fortified foods (i.e., formula or cereal) or medicinal iron for all infants by 4 to 6 weeks of age and continued use of these products until at least 18 months of age to maintain concentrations of hemoglobin at or above 10 g/100 ml blood.

Iron depletion exists in varying degrees, from the mild depletion of iron stores to the development of severe anemia. With a continuing negative iron balance, body stores of ferritin and hemosiderin gradually decrease. Simultaneously, iron absorption is enhanced, and there may be some increase in the iron binding capacity of the plasma as the body adapts to the deficiency. During this phase, plasma iron is not appreciably altered, nor is blood hemoglobin level. When iron stores become exhausted, however, plasma iron falls and erythropoiesis is decreased (Committee on Iron Deficiency, 1968).

Certain laboratory tests are used to assess the status of iron nutrition before anemia occurs. In iron-deficient subjects, smears of aspirate from bone marrow examined under the microscope show little or no stainable iron. It has been observed that serum ferritin concentration is directly related to the level of available storage iron. The average serum ferritin values in men have been reported to be 53 to 112 ng/ml and 27 to 43 ng in women. Serum ferritin between 12 and 300 ng/ml is considered normal (Bowering et al., 1976).

The adequacy of iron supplied to the bone marrow for erythropoiesis is reflected in the level of plasma iron and in iron-binding capacity or transferrin saturation. Plasma iron values of less than 50 mcg/100 ml are usually found in iron-deficiency anemia (normal values 75 to 175). Total iron binding capacity (transferrin) may be increased in iron-deficiency anemia to greater than 400 to 450 mcg/100 ml (normal 150 to 400). Dividing plasma iron by the total iron-binding capacity gives the percent saturation of transferrin. A figure of 10 percent or less transferrin saturation indicates iron-deficiency anemia. Values between 10 and 16 percent imply an inadequate supply of iron to the marrow. These low saturation values may be produced by infection as well as by iron-deficiency anemia, however. The presence or absence of Prussian blue stained siderotic granules of iron in RBC precursors of bone marrow is another indication of iron supplies. Normally about one-third of the bone marrow normoblasts contain such granules and are called sideroblasts. With iron deficiency, these granules virtually disappear. As iron stores are depleted, the synthesis of hemoglobin is affected, and a decreased amount is found in each RBC. The volume of the RBC usually decreases, and a microcytic, hypochromic anemia results (Committee on Iron Deficiency, 1968).

Iron depletion may thus be identified in decreased or absent bone marrow hemosiderin or subnormal serum ferritin levels. Iron deficiency without anemia is characterized by absent iron stores and transferrin saturation of 15 percent or less. Iron-deficiency anemia includes, in addition, abnormally low levels of serum iron, hemoglobin, and packed RBC volume. Lower limits of normal for hemoglobin and packed RBC volume are listed in Table 7.2.

It is difficult to assess the prevalence of iron deficiency and iron-deficiency anemia. Much of the information available has come from people in the health care system rather than from representative normal populations. However, it has been suggested that certain population groups, particularly infants, young children, the elderly, menstruating women, and pregnant women, are at risk of developing anemia (WHO Scientific Group, 1968; U.S. Department of Health, Education and Welfare, 1968–1970; O'Neal et al., 1976; Paine et al., 1974).

Iron Absorption and Availability

Iron absorption is the primary physiological control point for iron balance, with the upper gastrointestinal mucosa acting as the major site. Many factors appear to participate in control of this process. Anemia itself plays a

Table 7.2 LOWER LIMITS OF NORMAL FOR HEMOGLOBIN AND PACKED RED BLOOD CELL VOLUME (AT SEA LEVEL)*

Age	Sex	Hemoglobin, g/100 ml	Packed Cell Volume %
0.6–4	Both sexes	11	33
5–9	Both sexes	11.5	34.5
10–14	Both sexes	12	36
Adults	Men	14	42
	Women	12	36
	Pregnant women	11	33

* Committee on Iron Deficiency, 1968.

role since an increased proportion of dietary iron is absorbed by anemic individuals. Absorption is also greater than normal when the body stores of iron are low yet hemoglobin concentration is normal. Changes that increase the rate of erythropoiesis, such as hemorrhage or hemolysis, tend to increase iron absorption, even if stores are adequate. Normally the mucosal cell takes up iron from the intestinal lumen, transports it across the cell, and releases it from the serosal side. Some iron may be sequestered within the cell. In iron deficiency or under conditions when absorption is increased, the amount of iron taken up by the mucosal cell is increased, very little iron is sequestered in the cell, and transport to the plasma is rapid. In addition, little endogenous iron is secreted back into the mucosal cell. In cases of iron overload, the reverse is true. Uptake by the mucosal cell may be depressed, very little is transported to the plasma, and much of the iron is apparently sequestered by the mucosal cell, to be returned to the lumen of the intestine when the cell is sloughed off (Van Campen, 1974). Much speculation has occurred as to possible feedback mechanisms involved in intestinal mucosal cell response to the body's need for iron, but further clarification is needed (Crosby, 1969).

Generally, as the level of iron in the diet is increased, the proportion absorbed is decreased, although the absolute amount increases. Absorption of iron is sensitive to changes in the intestinal milieu. It has been theorized that some substances improve absorption because of their ability to maintain iron in a soluble state, either by forming a complex with it or reducing it from ferric to ferrous form. Ascorbic acid has been shown to increase iron absorption under a variety of conditions (Grebe et al., 1975; Sayers et al., 1974; Van Campen, 1972). Cook and Monsen (1977) found that when given with a semisynthetic meal, increase in iron absorption was directly proportional to amount of ascorbic acid up to doses of 1000 mg. The relative contributions of the ascorbic acid as a reducing agent or as a chelating agent in affecting iron absorption have not been resolved. A number of other organic acids as well as amino acids also increase iron absorption. They may act as chelating agents in increasing iron solubility (Van Campen, 1973). Some researchers have reported that complexes of ferric iron with fructose are more efficiently absorbed than is ferrous sulfate, which is a usual standard for comparison (Bates et al., 1972). However, this effect of fructose could not be demonstrated by Heinrich et al. (1974). Phytates, when added to the diet as soluble salts, have been shown to depress iron absorption. However, the effect of endogenous phytate in foods such as wheat is less clear. Morris and Ellis (1976) isolated a soluble and stable monoferric phytate from wheat bran and found its biological availability in rats similar to that of ferrous ammonium sulfate. Monoferric phytate accounted for about one-half the iron in whole wheat.

The absorption of iron from foods has been reported to vary widely as different methods have been used to measure availability. Bing (1972) suggested that the availability of iron in any food is not an inherent property that is characteristic of that food but an experimentally determined value that shows the absorption and utilization of the iron under conditions of the test only. When different workers report different ratings for the availability of iron in the same food substance, it is likely that the conditions of the testing varied.

Bowering et al. (1976) reviewed information on iron availability. *In vitro* tests have included the chemical determination of ionizable iron in foods and quantitation of the iron liberated by *in vitro* digestion with pepsin and hydrochloric acid. A bioassay of iron availability involves a hemoglobin repletion procedure in which experimental animals are made anemic and the response of hemoglobin levels to test doses of food or iron compounds measured in the depleted animals, using ferrous sulfate or ferric chloride as a standard for comparison. An absolute method of bioassay has also been used with analysis for iron of the entire body of the experimental animal (Bing, 1972). Iron availability in humans has been studied with the use of radioactive tracers and balance studies. Radioisotopes of iron, ^{55}Fe or ^{59}Fe, either have been introduced biologically into food so that they are incorporated into tissues by the plant or animal (intrinsic label) or mixed with food before ingestion (extrinsic label). Both RBC and whole body counting procedures have been used to follow the radioactive labels. Most human studies have used fasting subjects who were given either a dose of the single iron compound and/or food being tested or a well-defined test meal (Bowering et al., 1976).

It has been postulated that there are common pools of either heme iron or nonheme iron in the intestinal lumen to which all food sources and iron salts consumed in a meal contribute. Iron from hemoglobin is more available to human subjects than is nonheme iron from food sources (Bowering et al., 1976).

Animal sources of iron (with the exception of egg) appear to be better absorbed than plant sources. Although egg yolk was thought to be a well-utilized source of iron on the basis of early bioassay studies with experimental animals (Bing, 1972), more recent reports using radioisotopes with human subjects indicate that eggs are a relatively poor dietary source. Absorption of iron from biologically labeled eggs has been reported to be about 3 percent in most cases, although 20 percent absorption was found in some iron-deficient subjects. It has been suggested that the iron in egg yolk is tightly bound to the phosphoprotein, phosvitin, and is thus unavailable for absorption. The iron in meat has been shown in some studies to be equally as available as standard ferrous salts (Bowering et al., 1976). Layrisse (1975) reported that mean iron absorption from animal foods ranges from 6 percent in purified ferritin to 22 percent in veal muscle and liver, with intermediate values of 11 percent in fish and 12 percent in purified hemoglobin. The work of Cook et al. (1972) and Layrisse and Martinez-Torres (1972) found that the mean iron absorption in seven vegetable foods ranged from 1 percent in rice and spinach to 7 percent in soybean, with intermediate values of 3 percent in maize and black beans and 4 to 5 percent in lettuce and wheat.

Iron absorption from veal muscle was not reduced when the veal was administered with a vegetable, and absorption from vegetable foods was enhanced approximately twofold when these foods were combined with veal or fish. However, iron absorption from liver was reduced when it was given with vegetables, even though the liver increased absorption of iron from the vegetables (Layrisse, 1975).

Most bread and cereal enrichment in the United States is accomplished with four iron sources: ferrous sulfate, reduced iron, ferric orthophosphate, and sodium iron pyrophosphate (Fritz et al., 1975). Great differences in the bioavailability of these compounds have been documented, with ferric orthophosphate and sodium iron pyrophosphate appearing to be of little value to the consumer. The largest single iron source used in enrichment of foods is reduced iron. The availability of this compound appears to be very dependent upon the method of manufacture and the physical characteristics, particularly the size of the particles. Use by the food industry of water soluble iron salts or reduced iron with most of the material in particles of 10 μm or less has been suggested to improve the availability of iron in enriched products (Waddell, 1974; Fritz et al., 1975).

Diagnosis and Clinical Features of Anemia

Iron-deficiency anemia may result from a decreased intake or utilization of dietary iron or from chronic blood loss. Kasper et al. (1965) reported that chronic, occult bleeding from the gastrointestinal tract was the usual cause of iron loss in 100 hospitalized older patients with iron-deficiency anemia. Women with heavy menstrual flow may find it difficult to consistently consume a diet that is high enough in utilizable iron to maintain iron balance. In the infant whose blood volume is expanding rapidly, an iron-deficient milk diet is a common cause of anemia.

Certain erythrocyte indices are useful in defining anemia and determining its characteristics. They are calculated from the three measures—number of RBCs, volume of packed red cells (VPRD) or hematocrit (Hct), and hemoglobin (Hb). The indices, with normal values, are:

Normal Values

Mean corpuscular volume (MCV) $= \dfrac{\text{Hct}}{\text{RBC (millions)}} \times 10 \ \mu^3$ $80-94 \ \mu^3$

Mean corpuscular hemoglobin concentration (MCHC) $= \dfrac{\text{Hb}}{\text{Hct}} \times 100$ $33-38\%$

Mean corpuscular hemoglobin (MCH) $= \dfrac{\text{Hb}}{\text{RBC}}$ $27-32$ pg

In iron-deficiency anemia, which is a hypochromic and usually a microcytic type, MCH and either MCV or MCHC, or both, are reduced (Wintrobe et al., 1974, p. 296). Hemoglobin will always be decreased below normal concentrations. However, iron-deficiency anemia may sometimes be present in adults when RBCs are of normal size (Kasper et al., 1965).

Iron-deficiency anemia develops insidiously, and clinical symptoms are not usually present with mild to moderate forms of the disease. With more severe iron-deficiency anemia the clinical manifestations are those common to all chronic anemias and include fatigability, headache, anorexia or capricious appetite, heartburn, palpitation, dyspnea, ankle edema, vasomotor disturbances, and numbness or tingling. Abnormalities in epithelial tissues, including sore tongue, sore mouth, angular stomatitis, thinning or spooning of the nails (koilonychia), may occur in an occasional patient with iron-deficient anemia. Menstrual disturbances are also common (Wintrobe et al., 1974, pp. 1582–1583). Gardner et al. (1977) showed that physical work capacity during treadmill testing was significantly decreased by iron-deficiency anemia.

Werkman et al. (1964) observed feeding practices, mother-child interactions, socioeconomic constellations, and behavioral sequelae in 28 children with iron-deficiency anemia who had been hospitalized. In comparison to a control group who did not have anemia but were either in- or out-patients at the hospital, the anemic children had more illnesses, more feeding difficulties, and more behavioral problems. They were less often breastfed, remained on the bottle a relatively long time, drank excessive amounts of milk, and were more difficult to wean. The central core of the syndrome seen in the anemic children seemed to be a lack of psychological availability of the mother to the child and substitution of the milk bottle for gratification. The syndrome was associated with lower socioeconomic groups and related to depression and apathy in the mothers. A screening by Karp et al. (1974) of inner-city school children 5 to 8 years of age revealed an incidence of 5.5 percent iron-deficiency anemia, based on a MCV less than 77 μ^3. Families of these children were also evaluated, with the indication that when a school-age child of inner-city families was iron deficient, the mother and siblings were also likely to be deficient.

Treatment

Although it is commonly believed that anemia causes symptoms, there is little valid evidence that many of the symptoms are closely related to changing levels of circulating hemoglobin or that iron therapy has a beneficial effect on the feeling of well-being. Berry and Nash (1954) found no significant differences in mean hemoglobin levels of housewives who complained of symptoms and those who did not. Several other studies also failed to show an association between circulating hemoglobin level and the severity of symptoms, although there was some indication that symptoms occur when hemoglobin levels are approximately 7 or 8 g/100 ml. Elwood (1973) summarized a number of published studies concerning morbidity, mortality, and impairment of working capacity with anemia and found little evidence for harmful effects of low hemoglobin levels. It has been sug-

Table 7.3 FOOD SOURCES OF IRON*

Food	Weight (g)	Measure	Kilocalories	Iron (mg)
Apricots, dried, sulfured	35	10 medium halves	91	1.9
Beans, kidney, dried, cooked	93	½ cup	109	2.2
Beef, chuck, lean, cooked	86	3 oz	182	3.3
Beet greens, cooked	73	½ cup	13	1.4
Bread, enriched, white	28	1 slice	76	0.7
Bread, whole wheat	28	1 slice	67	0.8
Cereals, dry, prepared, enriched	28	⅓ to 1 cup	80–90	4.5
Chard, cooked, leaves and stalks	50	½ cup	13	1.3
Chicken, cooked, boneless, dark meat	70	2½ oz	120	1.3
Dandelion greens, cooked	53	½ cup	18	1.0
Egg, whole, cooked	57	1 large	82	1.2
Halibut, broiled	84	3 oz	144	0.6
Heart, beef, cooked	56	2 oz	106	3.4
Lamb, leg, lean, cooked	85	3 oz	158	1.4
Liver, beef, fried	85	3 oz	195	7.5
Liver sausage	28	1 oz	87	1.5
Maple syrup	60	3 tbs	150	0.6
Molasses, medium extraction	20	1 tbs	46	1.2
Oatmeal, cooked	120	½ cup	66	0.7
Oysters, fried	28	1 oz	68	2.3
Peaches, canned, sliced, in heavy syrup	128	½ cup	100	0.4
Peaches, dried, sulfered	65	5 medium halves	170	3.6
Peas, dried, cooked	100	½ cup	115	1.7
Pork, fresh ham, lean, cooked	70	2½ oz	155	2.7
Peanuts, roasted, salted	38	¼ cup	210	0.8
Prunes, dried, softened, with pits	38	5 medium	82	1.3
Prune juice	128	½ cup	99	5.3
Raisins, dried	41	¼ cup, packed	119	1.5
Sardines, drained solids	56	2 oz	116	1.6
Shrimp, cooked	56	2 oz	128	1.2
Spinach, frozen, cooked	103	½ cup	23	2.2
Strawberries, raw	149	1 cup	55	1.5
Tomato juice, canned	122	½ cup	23	1.1
Tuna, canned, drained	80	½ cup	158	1.5
Turkey, cooked, light meat	70	2½ oz	123	0.9
Veal, chuck, boneless, cooked	70	2½ oz	168	2.5
Watermelon, diced	160	1 cup	42	0.8
Wheat germ	12	2 tbs	46	1.0

* C. F. Adams, 1975.

gested that when anemia develops slowly, physiologic adjustment may be so effective that few clinical symptoms develop. On the other hand, Gardner et al. (1975 and 1977) found that physical performance requiring high oxygen delivery was significantly affected by hemoglobin levels. They divided 29 adult iron-deficient subjects into an iron treatment and a placebo group. Hemoglobin levels improved in the treatment group, whereas the placebo group showed no change over an 80-day period. Peak exercise heart rates were also significantly reduced in the treatment group, whereas the placebo group remained unchanged. A measurement by Andersen and Staven (1972) of respiratory gases during exercise in two anemic subjects showed more marked acid-base variations before than after iron therapy.

Iron-deficiency anemia is treated by the administration of iron. However, the basic cause of the anemia must be determined and provision made for treating the cause if long-range results are to remain positive. Oral iron therapy is usually sufficient, unless the iron is poorly absorbed, in which case it may be given parenterally. Several oral iron preparations are available, but none seems to be better than ferrous sulfate. Gastrointestinal side effects may sometimes occur with iron therapy. Mitchell (1974) compared the acceptability of equivalent doses of elemental iron as ferrous sulfate tablets, given before or after meals, sustained release preparations of this compound, ferrous fumarate, ferrous succinate, ferrous gluconate, ferrous calcium citrate, or a placebo. A liquid mixture of ferrous gluconate was also given. The palatability of ferrous sulfate given before meals was not improved by administration after meals, by sustained release formulation, or by substituting other ferrous salts. The liquid preparation was the least acceptable of the substances tested. Ferrous sulfate tablets were the least expensive preparation used.

The individual with iron-deficiency anemia or low iron stores should be counseled concerning food sources of iron. Although a concentrated iron compound is necessary to treat frank anemia, intake of an adequate amount of dietary iron over a period of time should be helpful in maintaining a normal hemoglobin level once it is achieved and in building an adequate supply of storage iron. Takkunen and Seppänen (1975) reported that the mean intake of meat products was lower in anemic women with hemoglobin levels less than 12.0 g/100 ml or hematocrits less than 36 percent than it was in other subjects surveyed. The intake of liquid milk products was also higher in the anemic women. The meat product intake was lower in iron-deficient men and women (serum iron level < 50 mcg/100 ml or total iron-binding capacity ≥ 400 mcg/100 ml) than in men and women who were not iron deficient. This supports the suggestion that dietary habits are a significant factor in the etiology of iron-deficiency anemia. Table 7.3 lists foods that are reasonably good sources of dietary iron.

7.2 Megaloblastic Anemias

Megaloblastic anemia occurs when erythrocyte maturation does not proceed normally. The erythroblastic cells of the bone marrow, which are the precursors of mature erythrocytes, not only fail to proliferate rapidly but become larger than usual since hemoglobin synthesis continues at a normal rate. These abnormally large erythrocyte precursors are called *megaloblasts* and develop into abnormally large adult erythrocytes called *macrocytes*. The macrocytes may enter the circulating blood and are capable of carrying oxygen. However, they have flimsy membranes, are often irregular and oval in shape, and are fragile. Their life is shortened in relation to that of normal cells. The production of mature effective erythrocytes is not adequate for the needs of the body and anemia is the result (Guyton, 1971, pp. 99–102).

Disordered synthesis of deoxyribonucleic acid (DNA) is the basic metabolic defect that produces megaloblasts. When DNA synthesis is impaired, the cells cannot divide normally and maturation is affected. Both vitamin B_{12} and folacin are essential to DNA synthesis. Thus a deficiency of one or both vitamins is the underlying abnormality in most patients with megaloblastic anemia.

The exact role of vitamin B_{12} in DNA synthesis has not been clarified but it is probably related to certain functions of folacin. Figure 7.1 depicts some possible relationships between vitamin B_{12} and folacin in the synthesis of DNA thymine. The diagram indicates that 5,10-methylenetetrahydrofolic acid (5,10-MeTHFA), one of the active coenzymes of folic acid, is necessary for methylation of deoxyuridylate (dUMP) to form deoxythymidylate (dTMP) for incorporation into DNA. Therefore, a deficiency of folate will directly affect DNA synthesis. It is probable that in subjects who are deficient in vitamin B_{12}, synthesis of methionine is blocked. As a result, folate tends to accumulate in the form of 5-methyltetrahydrofolate (5-MeTHFA) since this compound is normally converted to tetrahydrofolate (THFA) during methionine synthesis. Because of this accumulation,

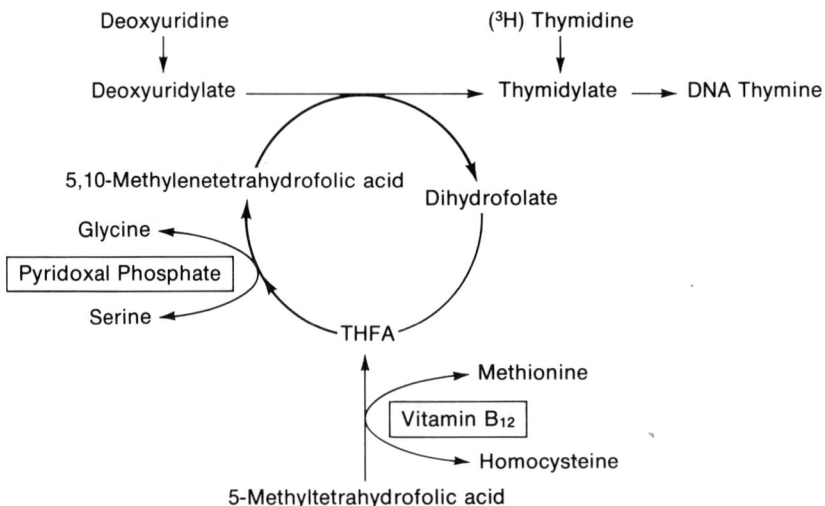

Fig. 7.1   Relationships between folic acid and vitamin B_{12} coenzymes in DNA synthesis. (From S. Waxman, J. Corcino, and V. Herbert, "Aggravation or Initiation of Megaloblastosis by Amino Acids in the Diet," *Journal American Medical Association*, **214:** 40, 1970. Copyright 1970, American Medical Association.)

Table 7.4 CLASSIFICATION OF MEGALOBLASTIC MACROCYTIC ANEMIAS*

	Main Abnormality	Probable Pathogenesis
Pernicious anemia	Deficiency of vitamin B_{12}	Lack of intrinsic factor
Total gastrectomy	Deficiency of vitamin B_{12}	Lack of intrinsic factor
Fish tapeworm infestation	Deficiency of vitamin B_{12}	Competition for vitamin
Blind loops; strictures; diverticuli	Deficiency of vitamin B_{12} and sometimes folate	Small intestine bacterial overgrowth; competition for vitamin
Nutritional macrocytic anemia	Deficiency of folate and sometimes vitamin B_{12}	Inadequate diet
Sprue and other malabsorption syndromes	Deficiency of folate and sometimes vitamin B_{12}	Defective intestinal absorption
Pregnancy; infancy	Deficiency of folate	Increased need; inadequate diet
Chemotherapeutic agents	Inhibition of folate metabolism	Administration of methotrexate
	Inhibition of purine metabolism	Administration of 6-mercaptopurine
	Inhibition of pyrimidine metabolism	Administration of cytosine arabinoside
Anticonvulsant therapy	Folate deficiency	Inhibition of intestinal conjugase
Contraceptives	Folate deficiency	Impairment of folate absorption

* Adapted from Wintrobe et al., 1974, p. 1586.

a relative deficiency of other folate coenzymes develops, including THFA and 5,10-MeTHFA, the cofactor essential for the synthesis of the DNA precursor, dTMP. Thus either vitamin B_{12} or folate deficiency may affect the maturation of erythrocytes (Wintrobe et al., 1974, pp. 1588–1589; Waxman et al., 1970).

Pernicious anemia is the most common megaloblastic anemia in North America and Europe, although it is uncommon in developing and tropical countries where other types predominate. Many of the clinical features of pernicious anemia are also those of other megaloblastic anemias. A classification of megaloblastic macrocytic anemias is in Table 7.4.

Pernicious Anemia

History. Pernicious anemia is characterized by megaloblastic anemia, achylia gastrica (absence of HCl and enzymes in gastric secretions), and neurologic damage. It was described as early as 1823 and was an ultimately fatal condition for many years. In 1926, stimulated by the early investigations of Whipple and his associates concerning the effects of various foods on experimental anemia in animals, Minot and Murphy showed that large amounts ($\frac{1}{2}$ lb/day) of fresh liver consistently produced remission of the symptoms of pernicious anemia (Wintrobe et al., 1974, p. 1587). In an early issue of the *Journal of the American Dietetic Association,* Tubbs and Bellinger (1926), hospital dietitians in Boston, presented recipes for liver that could be used by pernicious anemia patients at home (Table 7.5).

Table 7.5   EARLY RECIPES FOR LIVER IN THE TREATMENT OF
PERNICIOUS ANEMIA*

Liver Juice

Score the raw liver and sear slightly in a pan, for less than 1 min. Place the seared liver in a square made of gauze (several folds) and squeeze out the juice. About 150 ml of juice from 2 lb of liver. Serve cold. Orange juice may be taken after it.

Scraped or Sieved Liver

Dash liver in hot water and remove the skin. Broil the liver 5 to 10 min (until cooked through) and scrape through sieve, or press through potato ricer.

Liver Soup

Add 90 g of scraped or sieved liver to 200 ml of clear tomato or chicken broth with fat removed. Season with onion if desired.

Liver Soup (Creamed)

120 g chopped liver, 220 ml milk, 4 tsp flour, 10 g butter. Make white sauce and add liver.

* Tubbs and Bellinger, 1926.

In 1929 Castle demonstrated the lack of a substance that he called an "intrinsic factor" in the stomach which normally acts with an "extrinsic factor" present in beef muscle and other foods. The two factors were thought to combine to form an "anti-pernicious anemia principle" that was stored in the liver. The intrinsic factor has since been identified as a thermolabile glycoprotein, secreted by gastric mucosa, which forms a complex with vitamin B_{12}, attaches to specific receptors in the wall of the distal ileum, and facilitates absorption of the vitamin. The extrinsic factor of Castle was apparently vitamin B_{12} itself, which was present in large amounts in liver. Enough vitamin was absorbed from $\frac{1}{2}$ lb of liver daily to ameliorate the symptoms of the disease. The anti-pernicious anemia principle stored in the liver was really vitamin B_{12} but could not be absorbed without intrinsic factor. Pernicious anemia was treated with liver extract before vitamin B_{12} was isolated in the 1940s. The prognosis of pernicious anemia has changed dramatically from fatal to very favorable with vitamin B_{12} treatment (Wintrobe et al., 1974, p. 1587).

Pathogenesis and Clinical Features.   The average age for onset of pernicious anemia is 60 years, and it is rarely found in patients under the age of 30. There is an exception, however, in congenital pernicious anemia, a very rare form observed in children, which differs from that seen in adults because it does not show gastric atrophy and achylia gastrica (Lampkin and Schubert, 1968). The relatively high familial incidence of pernicious anemia suggests that the defect in secretion of intrinsic factor may be genetically determined, particularly in congenital disease. It has been suggested that pernicious anemia is produced by autoantibodies directed against the gastric mucosa so that intrinsic factor is not effectively produced and that the tendency to form such antibodies may be genetically determined (Goldberg and Bluestone, 1970).

The onset of pernicious anemia is insidious. Nonspecific symptoms include anorexia, weight loss, weakness, palpitations, lightheadedness, syncope, and headache. Elderly patients may have angina pectoris and mild ankle edema from fluid retention. More specific symptoms include sore tongue, paresthesias in extremities, disturbances of gait, disorders of bowel or urinary bladder function, and disturbances of memory or affect (forgetfulness, irritability, paranoia, hallucinations). Unfortunately, these symptoms in an older person may be attributed to aging and may lead to hospitalization in a mental or custodial institution without recognition of the underlying anemia (Sullivan, 1970). Upon examination the patient usually will be found to be pale, with a flabby rather than wasted appearance, to have a slight or pronounced yellowish color of the skin, a tongue that is often glazed and sometimes red and sore, and a rapid pulse with slight cardiac enlargement. In the nervous system, loss of vibratory sense and incoordination in lower extremities, loss of finer coordination of fingers, and evidence of peripheral nerve degeneration are common findings. The biochemical basis for the neurologic changes is not known (Wintrobe et al., 1974, p. 1587).

Anemia of a moderate to severe degree is almost always present. Since large RBCs predominate, the mean corpuscular volume (MCV) is greater than normal (usually $>100\mu^3$). There is a corresponding increase in the hemoglobin content of the RBCs so that the concentration of hemoglobin in the corpuscles (MCHC) is normal. The RBCs in pernicious anemia and other macrocytic anemias are not "hyperchromic" (Wintrobe et al., 1974, p. 1587).

Diagnosis.   When the physician begins with the knowledge that the patient is anemic, it is a simple matter to diagnose pernicious anemia. The problem is one of separating it from other megaloblastic anemias. The cause is often suggested by the situation, as in pregnancy, malnutrition, malabsorption, or after total gastrectomy. Serum vitamin B_{12} may serve as a screening test (Hall, 1967), normally being 200 to 900 pcg/ml, most of which is bound to the specific protein carrier, transcobalamin. Tests of radiovitamin B_{12} absorptive capacity are used in the differential diagnosis of megaloblastic anemias. These include measurement of the amount of radiovitamin B_{12} excreted in the feces after an oral dose or the uptake of the radioisotope by the plasma, liver, or whole body. The most widely used absorption test is the urinary excretion test devised by Schilling (Sullivan, 1970).

In the standard Schilling procedure, an oral dose of vitamin B_{12} (cyanocobalamin) tagged with a radioactive isotope of cobalt is given, followed $\frac{1}{2}$ hour later by a parenteral injection of 1000 mcg of nonradioactive vitamin B_{12} to "flush" absorbed radioactive vitamin into the urine. A 24-hour urine sample is collected and counted for radioactive vitamin. If vitamin B_{12} absorption is normal, the radioactive compound will be found in the urine. When vitamin B_{12} absorption is poor, the test must be repeated with intrinsic factor being given orally along with the radioactive vitamin. If the malabsorption of vitamin B_{12} is corrected by giving intrinsic factor, the diagnosis of pernicious anemia can be made (McCurdy, 1966). Differentiation from bacterial overgrowth causing the anemia can be made by repeating the test after a course of antibiotics.

Treatment.   With appropriate treatment, it is possible to restore the blood to normal and to promote a return to optimal nutritional status. Changes in the nervous system can be halted and, in some cases, are reversible. Adequate amounts of vitamin B_{12} are administered parenterally, usually intramuscularly. A positive response to treatment will usually occur within 48 hours, although neural symptoms do not change as quickly as does the blood picture. Therapeutic doses of vitamin B_{12} initially range from 30 to 1000 mcg daily for 7 to 14 days to replenish body stores. With doses larger than 50 mcg daily, a large percentage of the vitamin given is excreted in the urine. After initial replacement therapy, monthly injections of 50 to 1000 mcg vitamin B_{12} must be given for life to maintain normal hematocrit and neurologic functions. Additional supportive treatment may include adequate hydration, eradication of infection, and physiotherapy for patients with significant neurologic dysfunction (Sullivan, 1970). As appetite returns to normal, the patient should be counseled on an individual basis, after appropriate assessment of usual eating habits, to ensure adequate dietary intake and maintenance of an optimal nutritional state.

The total body vitamin B_{12} content in the normal adult is approximately 5000 mcg (range 2000 to 10000 mcg), of which about 1700 mcg are stored in the liver. Stores are usually adequate for 3 to 4 years. Biochemical evidence of deficiency is not seen until the total body content drops to less than 500 mcg. The RDA of vitamin B_{12} for an adult is 3 mcg, but the requirement is increased during periods of rapid growth and in pregnancy. Vitamin B_{12} is synthesized by some microorganisms and is available to humans principally in products from animals, such as meat and milk, where the animals have had access to the products of bacterial action. It is not present in higher plants.

Other Megaloblastic Anemias

Megaloblastic anemia may result from a dietary deficiency of folate or vitamin B_{12}, from increased requirements for these vitamins, or from faulty absorption and metabolism. Since vitamin B_{12} is stored in the body, a pure dietary deficiency is rare. Some cases of deficiency and consequent megaloblastic anemia have been reported in strict vegetarians (vegans), but even here it is not common. A possible explanation for this is their increased folate intake. As body stores of vitamin B_{12} are decreased, daily loss from the body becomes less and the amount of vitamin B_{12} needed daily may be smaller. Another possibility is the absorption from the colon or last part of the small intestine of vitamin B_{12} synthesized by bacteria. However, many vegans now take supplements of vitamin B_{12} to guard against the development of a deficiency. Treatment for megaloblastic anemia caused by a dietary deficiency of vitamin B_{12} involves giving vitamin B_{12} supplements or making sure that animal products are included in the diet as a source of the vitamin (Ellis, 1974). Vitamin B_{12} content of selected foods is listed in Table 7.6.

A dietary deficiency of folate producing nutritional macrocytic anemia is most common in pregnant women, infants, and the aged. Complaints include weakness, shortness of breath, sore mouth and tongue, diarrhea, and edema. Achlorhydria is usually not present, and degenerative changes in the nervous system are seldom found. Nutritional macrocytic anemia has been detected in as many as 40 percent of alcoholics who become ill enough to be hospitalized. In addition to dietary deficiency, effects of alcohol on folate absorption and hepatic metabolism may contribute to the development of the anemia (Wintrobe et al., 1974, pp. 1590–1591).

The term *folic acid* is often used to refer only to the single chemical substance, pteroylglutamic acid (PGA), and *folate* or *folacin* is used to designate a group of conjugated as well as unconjugated compounds with vitamin activity. About 90 percent of natural folic acid is conjugated with two to seven glutamate residues. These must be converted to the monoglutamate by intestinal conjugases for absorption to occur. Folates are synthesized by higher plants as well as by microorganisms and are found in many vegetables, particularly green leafy plants, and in liver. Folate content of selected foods is listed in Table 7.6. This vitamin in natural foods is heat labile, and from 50 to 95 percent may be destroyed by cooking (Wintrobe et al., 1974, p. 1589; Ellis, 1974).

Inadequate absorption of folate and/or vitamin B_{12} is the usual cause of megaloblastic anemia in malabsorption syndrome. Patients with tropical sprue have a megaloblastic anemia that usually responds to folic acid and/or vitamin B_{12} supplementation. Megaloblastic anemia following total gastrectomy may develop because of lack of the intrinsic factor essential for vitamin B_{12} absorption. It may also follow partial gastrectomy, but the incidence is much lower in this case. The macrocytic anemia seen in association with intestinal strictures, diverticula, and blind loops may be due to colonization of the small intestine by large masses of bacteria that divert vitamin B_{12} from the host (Wintrobe et al., 1974, pp. 1590–1591).

Patients with megaloblastic anemia caused by folate deficiency respond rapidly to oral folic acid therapy, even in the presence of disease of the small intestine. Although the absorption of food folates (primarily polyglutamic forms) may be suppressed by diseases causing steatorrhea, the absorption of PGA may be only slightly affected, if at all. Responses to oral doses of 50 to 100 mcg folic acid daily are often satisfactory. Daily doses of 300 mcg or more may be needed in pregnant patients because of an increased requirement. However, folate-deficient patients are commonly given larger dosages in treatment. The RDA of folacin for adults is 400 mcg

Table 7.6 FOLACIN AND VITAMIN B_{12} CONTENT OF SELECTED FOODS IN 100-G EDIBLE PORTIONS

Food	Total Folacin* in 100-g edible portion (mcg)	Vitamin B_{12}† in 100-g edible portion (mcg)
Meat, Poultry, and Fish		
Beef, without bone, lean		
Raw	7	1.80
Cooked	4	
Liver, beef		
Raw	219	80.00
Cooked	145	
Pork, without bone, lean		
Raw	8	0.60
Cooked	5	
Liverwurst	30	13.90
Chicken, without skin		
Dark meat		
Raw	11	0.40
Cooked	7	
Light meat		
Raw	6	0.45
Cooked	4	
Halibut, frozen	12	1.00
Tuna, canned	15	2.20
Dairy Products and Eggs		
Milk, cow, fluid		
Whole, pasteurized	5	0.40
Yogurt	11	0.11
Cheese		
Cheddar	18	1.00
Cottage	12	1.00
Ice cream, vanilla	2	
Eggs, whole		
Raw	65	2.00
Hardboiled	49	
Cereals and Legumes		
Rice, uncooked		
Brown	16	
White	10	
Wheat, whole grain	52	
Oatmeal, uncooked	52	
Bread		
White	39	
Whole wheat	58	
Beans, red		
Raw, dry	133	
Cooked	37	
Peanuts, roasted	106	
Peanut butter	79	
Soybeans, mature, dry	171	

Table 7.6 FOLACIN AND VITAMIN B$_{12}$ CONTENT OF SELECTED FOODS IN 100-G EDIBLE PORTIONS (*cont'd.*)

Food	Total Folacin* in 100-g edible portion (mcg)	Vitamin B$_{12}$† in 100-g edible portion (mcg)
Vegetables		
Beans, snap		
Cooked, drained	40	
Beets, cooked	78	
Broccoli, spears, cooked	56	
Cabbage		
Raw	66	
Cooked	18	
Carrots		
Raw	32	
Cooked	24	
Cauliflower		
Raw	55	
Cooked	34	
Endive, raw	49	
Lettuce		
Leaf or head	37	
Romaine	179	
Potatoes		
French fried	22	
Mashed	10	
Spinach		
Raw	193	
Cooked	91	
Tomatoes, raw	39	
Fruits		
Apples	8	
Apricots, dried	14	
Avocados, raw	51	
Bananas, raw	28	
Grapefruit juice	21	
Muskmelon or cantaloupe	30	
Oranges, raw	46	
Orange juice	55	
Peaches, raw	8	
Prunes, dried, softened, raw	4	
Raisins	4	
Strawberries, raw	16	
Watermelon, raw	8	

* Perloff and Butrum, 1977.
† Orr, 1969.

from a mixed diet. Folate in foods may be less available for absorption than a supplement of PGA. Therapy should be continued for 7 to 14 days to replenish stores. Equally important to the folate supplement is effective nutrition instruction for the patient, particularly in nutritional macrocytic anemia caused by inadequate dietary intake. The patient should be taught basic nutrition principles and how to choose an adequate diet and be given specific instruction concerning food sources of folate. Attention to social and psychological problems is also helpful in alcoholic patients and those with food fetishes. Long-term therapy with folic acid is not necessary if the underlying problem that led to the development of folate deficiency can be corrected and an adequate nutritional status maintained on a normal diet (Sullivan, 1970).

REFERENCES

1. Adams, C. F. 1975. *Nutritive Value of American Foods.* U.S. Department of Agriculture.

2. Anderson, H. T. and P. Stavem. 1972. Iron deficiency anaemia and the acid-base variations of exercise. *Nutr. Metabol.*, **14:** 129.

3. Bates, G. W., J. Boyer, J. C. Hegenauer, and P. Saltman. 1972. Facilitation of iron absorption by ferric fructose. *Am. J. Clin. Nutr.*, **25:** 983.

4. Beal, V. A. and A. J. Meyers. 1970. Iron nutriture from infancy to adolescence. *Am. J. Pub. Health*, **60:** 666.

5. Berry, W. T. C. and F. A. Nash. 1954. Symptoms as guide to anaemia. *Brit. Med. J.*, **1:** 918.

6. Bing, F. C. 1972. Assaying the availability of iron. *J. Am. Dietet. Assoc.*, **60:** 114.

7. Bowering, J., A. M. Sanchez, and M. I. Irwin. 1976. A conspectus of research on iron requirements of man. *J. Nutr.*, **106:** 985.

8. Committee on Iron Deficiency. 1968. Iron deficiency in the United States. *J. Am. Med. Assoc.*, **203:** 119.

9. Committee on Nutrition. 1969. Iron balance and requirements in infancy. *Pediatrics*, **43:** 134.

10. Cook, J., M. Layrisse, C. Martinez-Torres, R. Walker, E. Monsen, and C. A. Finch. 1972. Food iron absorption measured by an extrinsic tag. *J. Clin. Invest.*, **51:** 805.

11. Cook, J. D. and E. R. Monsen. 1977. Vitamin C, the common cold, and iron absorption. *Am. J. Clin. Nutr.*, **30:** 235.

12. Crosby, W. H. 1969. Intestinal response to the body's requirement for iron. *J. Am. Med. Assoc.*, **208:** 347.

13. Department of Health, Education and Welfare. 1968–1970. Ten-state nutrition survey. DHEW Publication No. (HSM) 72–8134.

14. Ellis, F. R. 1974. Nutritional megaloblastic anaemia. *Practioner*, **212:** 503.

15. Elwood, P. C. 1973. Evaluation of the clinical importance of anemia. *Am. J. Clin. Nutr.*, **26:** 958.

16. Finch, C. A. 1969. Iron-deficiency anemia. *Am. J. Clin. Nutr.*, **22:** 512.

17. Fomon, S. J. 1970. Prevention of iron-deficiency anemia in infants and children of preschool age. DHEW Publication No. (PHS) 2085.

18. Fritz, J. C., G. W. Pla, and C. L. Rollinson. 1975. Iron for enrichment. *Bakers Dig.*, **49** (Apr.): 46.

19. Gardner, G. W., V. R. Edgerton, R. J. Barnard, and E. M. Bernauer. 1975. Cardiorespiratory, hematological and physical performance responses of anemic subjects to iron treatment. *Am. J. Clin. Nutr.,* **28:** 982.

20. Gardner, G. W., V. R. Edgerton, B. Senewiratne, R. J. Barnard, and Y. Ohira. 1977. Physical work capacity and metabolic stress in subjects with iron deficiency anemia. *Am. J. Clin. Nutr.,* **30:** 910.

21. Goldberg, L. S. and R. Bluestone. 1970. Hidden gastric autoantibodies to intrinsic factor in pernicious anemia. *J. Lab. Clin. Med.,* **75:** 449.

22. Grebe, G., C. Martinez-Torres, and M. Layrisse. 1975. Effect of meals and ascorbic acid on the absorption of a therapeutic dose of iron as ferrous and ferric salts. *Current Therapeu. Res.,* **17:** 382.

23. Guyton, A. C. 1971. *Textbook of Medical Physiology,* 4th ed. Philadelphia: Saunders.

24. Hall, C. A. 1967. Pernicious anemia. *Geriatrics,* **22** (Oct.): 109.

25. Hallberg, L., et al. 1966. Menstrual blood loss, a population study: Variation at different ages and attempts to define normality. *Acta Obstet. Gynec. Scand.,* **45:** 320.

26. Heinrich, H. C., E. E. Gabbe, J. Brüggemann, and K. H. Oppitz. 1974. Effects of fructose on ferric and ferrous iron absorption in man. *Nutr. Metab.,* **17:** 236.

27. Karp, R. J., W. S. Haaz, K. Starko, and J. M. Gorman. 1974. Iron deficiency in families of iron-deficient inner-city school children. *Am. J. Dis. Child.,* **128:** 18.

28. Kasper, C. K., D. Y. E. Whissell, and R. O. Wallerstein. 1965. Clinical aspects of iron deficiency. *J. Am. Med. Assoc.,* **191:** 359.

29. Lampkin, B. C. and W. K. Schubert. 1968. Pernicious anemia in the second decade of life. *J. Ped.,* **72:** 387.

30. Layrisse, M. 1975. Dietary iron absorption. *Proc. 9th Int. Congr. Nutr., Mexico 1972,* **1:** 141.

31. Layrisse, M. and C. Martinez-Torres. 1972. Model for measuring the dietary absorption from heme iron. Test with a complete meal. *Am. J. Clin. Nutr.,* **25:** 401.

32. McCurdy, P. R. 1966. Megaloblastic anemia. *GP,* **34** (No. 4): 89.

33. Mitchell, A. B. S. 1974. Oral iron tolerance. *Postgrad. Med. J.* **50:** 702.

34. Morris, E. R. and R. Ellis. 1976. Phytate as a carrier for iron. *Bakers Dig.,* **50** (June): 28.

35. National Dairy Council. 1972. Iron-deficiency anemia in infants and preschool children. *Dairy Council Dig.,* **43** (No. 1): 1.

36. O'Neal, R. M., O. G. Abrahams, M. B. Kohrs, and D. L. Eklund. 1976. The incidence of anemia in residents of Missouri. *Am. J. Clin. Nutr.,* **29:** 1158.

37. Orr, M. L. 1969. Pantothenic acid, vitamin B_6, and vitamin B_{12} in foods. Home Economics Research Report No. 36, Agric. Res. Ser., U.S. Department of Agriculture.

38. Paine, C. J., A. Polk, and E. R. Eichner. 1974. Analysis of anemia in medical inpatients. *Am. J. Med. Sci.,* **268:** 37.

39. Perloff, B. P. and R. R. Butrum. 1977. Folacin in selected foods. *J. Am. Dietet. Assoc.,* **70:** 161.

40. Sayers, M. H., S. R. Lynch, R. W. Charlton, T. H. Bothwell, R. B. Walker, and F. Mayet. 1974. Iron absorption from rice meals cooked with fortified salt containing ferrous sulfate and ascorbic acid. *Brit. J. Nutr.,* **31:** 367.

41. Sullivan, L. W. 1970. Differential diagnosis and management of the patient with megaloblastic anemia. *Am. J. Med.,* **48:** 609.

42. Takkunen, H. and R. Seppänen. 1975. Iron deficiency and dietary factors in Finland. *Am. J. Clin. Nutr.,* **28:** 1141.

43. Tubbs, T. and E. Bellinger. 1926. Preparation of calves' liver for pernicious anemia diets. *J. Am. Dietet. Assoc.,* **2:** 165.

44. Van Campen, D. 1974. Regulation of iron absorption. *Fed. Proc.*, **33**: 100.

45. Van Campen, D. 1973. Enhancement of iron absorption from ligated segments of rat intestine by histidine, cysteine, and lysine: Effects of removing ionizing groups and of stereoisomerism. *J. Nutr.*, **103**: 139.

46. Van Campen, D. 1972. Effect of histidine and ascorbic acid on the absorption and retention of ^{59}Fe by iron-depleted rats. *J. Nutr.*, **102**: 165.

47. Waddell, J. 1974. The bioavailability of iron sources and their utilization in food enrichment. *Fed. Proc.*, **33**: 1779.

48. Waxman, S., J. Corcino, and V. Herbert. 1970. Aggravation or initiation of megaloblastosis by amino acids in the diet. *J. Am. Med. Assoc.*, **214**: 39.

49. Werkman, S. L., L. Shifman, and T. Skelly. 1964. Psychosocial correlates of iron deficiency anemia in early childhood. *Psychosom. Med.*, **26**: 125.

50. WHO Scientific Group. 1968. Nutritional anaemias. World Health Organization Technical Report Series No. 405. Geneva, Switzerland.

51. Wintrobe, M. M., G. W. Thorn, R. D. Adams, E. Braunwald, K. J. Isselbacher, and R. G. Petersdorf (Eds.). 1974. Harrison's Principles of Internal Medicine, 7th ed. New York: McGraw-Hill.

STUDY GUIDE

Anemia may result from various causes, some of which are nutritional in nature.

1. List several nutritional deficiencies that may produce anemia.

2. Describe and explain differences in the characteristics of RBCs found in iron-deficiency anemia, pernicious anemia, and other megaloblastic anemias.

Iron depletion exists in varying degrees, from mild decreases in iron stores to severe anemia.

3. Describe, explain, and evaluate the usefulness of several methods for evaluating the iron nutritional status of an individual.

4. Explain why it is often difficult to maintain iron balance in a menstruating woman, and give suggestions that might help the problem.

5. Explain why the presence or absence of iron stores may be of particular importance during pregnancy.

6. Compare the usual dietary intake of iron among various groups in the United States with the RDAs of iron for these groups and discuss possible consequences of the findings.

Intestinal absorption of iron is influenced by several factors.

7. Give the proportion of dietary iron that is usually absorbed in normal adults and discuss possible effects of each of the following on that absorption: decrease in iron stores or development of iron-deficiency anemia, blood loss, increased dietary iron, ascorbic acid, amino acids, phytates.

8. Describe several methods for measuring iron absorption, and discuss problems involved in these types of measurements.

9. Compare the apparent availability of iron from animal and vegetable foods and from usual iron-enrichment compounds.

Iron-deficiency anemia may not always be easy to define or diagnose.

10. Suggest criteria for defining or diagnosing iron-deficiency anemia, and explain why these criteria are often arbitrary.

11. Describe clinical symptoms that may accompany iron-deficiency anemia, and discuss research that has attempted to correlate symptoms and severity of anemia as determined by blood measurements.

Iron-deficiency anemia is generally treated by iron administration and a nutritionally balanced diet.

12. Compare, in terms of acceptability and effectiveness, various iron compounds that are available for the treatment of iron-deficiency anemia.

13. List several foods that are generally considered good sources of dietary iron, and explain how this information might be used in nutritional counseling.

14. Recommend and justify general procedures for the prevention of iron-deficiency anemia in infants and young children.

A deficiency of vitamin B_{12} or folate produces megaloblastic anemia.

15. Describe metabolic relationships between vitamin B_{12} and folic acid that may affect erythrocyte maturation in deficiencies of either vitamin.

16. List several conditions that include megaloblastic anemia as one clinical sign, and describe the probable pathogenesis in each.

17. Give and justify dietary suggestions to a patient with nutritional megaloblastic anemia caused by dietary folate deficiency.

18. Explain why vegans may sometimes develop megaloblastic anemia, and suggest possible reasons why many of them do not.

Pernicious anemia is characterized by megaloblastic anemia, achylia gastrica, and neurologic damage.

19. Explain why large quantities of liver were used with some success in the early days of treating patients with pernicious anemia.

20. Describe and explain the use of the Schilling test in the diagnosis of pernicious anemia.

21. Outline an effective treatment for pernicious anemia, and explain why the treatment is effective.

Nutrition in Times of Stress

Nutritional Implications of Trauma and Surgery

Patients hospitalized for surgery or treatment of severe injury are subjected to (1) varying degrees of stress, (2) bed rest, and (3) starvation or semistarvation. Stress may include psychological adjustments to the hospital environment, illness, or loss of function, as well as the physiological effects of anesthesia, incisions for surgery or the repair of injury, and the injury itself. An understanding of the metabolic effects produced by stress, bed rest, and starvation is important in planning nutritional support for hospitalized patients. This chapter discusses the nutritional implications of stress and metabolic responses to trauma. Appropriate nutritional care for patients undergoing surgery is also discussed in general terms. Special nutritional problems that may occur with gastrointestinal surgery are discussed in Secs. 12.5 and 13.5.

8.1 Stress, Illness, and Nutrition

"Stress" is a common word, with different meanings for various ind - viduals. Selye (1973) has said that "everybody knows what stress is and nobody knows what it is." It is part of the daily vocabulary for most of the population, but only a few specialists have really tried to define it. According to Selye (1973 and 1970), stress is the nonspecific response of the body to any demand made upon it. Many different stimuli— heat, cold, physical trauma, drugs, athletic competition, psychological shock—may produce unique specific effects on the body. However, in addition to their specific effects, the stimuli have in common a nonspecific demand for the body to adapt and maintain homeostasis.

Kinney defined stress (Nelson et al., 1976) as any stimulus or condition that threatens the body homeostasis. In the hospitalized patient, this threat may range from mild to severe. The uncomplicated, elective postoperative patient might represent a relatively mild level of stress. Body adaptive changes are self-limited and not severe enough to threaten convalescence. A more serious stress would result from multiple injuries, such as those of an automobile accident victim. A severe infection, such as generalized peritonitis, represents a third level of stress because of the considerable destruction of tissue and duration of illness. An example of an extreme level of stress is the major third-degree burn, with severe and prolonged tissue loss.

Selye (1973 and 1970) suggested the *General Adaptation Syndrome* (G.A.S.) as an all-comprising term that includes three stages of general response to stressor agents. The initial stage is called an *alarm reaction* and includes, in stressed experimental animals, (1) an enlargement of the adrenal cortex; (2) a shrinking of the thymus, spleen, lymph nodes, and all other lymphatic structures; and (3) the development of deep, bleeding ulcers in the stomach and upper gut. There is discharge of adrenal cortex secretions into the blood, stimulated by increased levels of ACTH, along with hemoconcentration, hypochloremia, and general tissue catabolism. If the alarm reaction is extremely severe and prolonged, death may occur at this stage since no organism can be maintained continuously in a state of alarm. In most cases, however, the alarm reaction is followed by the second stage of resistance, which is an adaptive phase. The adrenal cortex becomes particularly rich in secretory granules, there is hemodilution, hyperchloremia, and anabolism, with a return toward normal body weight. After still more exposure to the stressor, the acquired adaptation is lost and the third stage of exhaustion develops.

Life-events research has demonstrated some associations between the onset of illness and a recent increase in the number and intensity of stressful events that require socially adaptive responses. The impact of these events, which may include such things as death of spouse, marriage, vacation, change in job, and change in recreation, is presumed to be additive. This type of research is complex, however, since illness onset is undoubtedly the outcome of multiple characteristics of the individual interacting with a number of interdependent factors in the social environment and a disease agent. In a review of published research in this area, Rabkin and Struening (1976) emphasized the importance of considering this complexity in designing additional research studies.

Mutter and Schleifer (1966) reported that the families of 42 ill children were more disorganized and exposed their children to a greater number of psychological and social changes than did families of 45 well children. These researchers suggested a multifactorial concept of disease, implicating psychological, social, and biological factors. Roghmann and Haggerty (1973) reported more illness than would ordinarily be expected in mothers of young children on the first day of a stress episode, as documented by daily diaries.

The stress of illness itself has been studied from a psychosocial standpoint. Psychological responses to physical illness include coping, use of defense mechanisms, and emotional reactions subjectively experienced as "feelings." The type and intensity of these reactions depend upon the interaction of many factors, including stresses pertinent to the physical illness per se, certain characteristics of the ill person, and various situational factors (Verwoerdt, 1972; Kiely, 1972).

According to Selye (1970), dietary factors, such as fat, cholesterol, and vitamin overdosage, can act as stressors that are capable of producing the typical manifestations of the G.A.S. In experimental animals that have been specially conditioned by giving corticoid hormones and sodium salts to induce the cardiotoxic effects of stress, the addition of large amounts of dietary fat or cholesterol can produce fatal myocardial necroses. These findings suggest that in preexisting conditions of stress, faulty diet can be the final disease-precipitating factor.

Various stresses may interact differently with nutritional factors. The stress of starvation or semistarvation, for example, does not predispose an individual to cardiac damage. It may, in fact, have a beneficial effect on an overburdened heart. Starvation produces other manifestations of disease, including changes in the gastrointestinal mucosa and the development of ulcers. Environmental stress may influence the utilization of nutrients in the body. Baltimore children living in stressful environments showed more signs of nutritional deficiency than did other children under less stressful conditions, even though the apparent nutrient intake was similar in both groups. In each case the diet was borderline in terms of nutritional adequacy. Interactions between the stress of infection and malnutrition were discussed in Sec. 6.1. In a prisoner who volunteered for a study of experimental scurvy, Hodges (1970) reported that emotional stress produced a markedly increased rate of utilization of ascorbic acid in the body. Many other nutritional factors may be involved in the body's reaction to stress.

Prolonged bed rest, which occurs in many hospitalized patients, has metabolic or physiologic effects (Chobanian et al., 1974; Heath et al., 1972), including:

1. Exaggerated responses of heart rate and cardiac output
2. Negative sodium balance and reduction in plasma volume
3. Decrease in muscle mass with loss of nitrogen, sulfur, and potassium
4. Loss of calcium and phosphorus in the urine from decrease in bone substance, with dangers of renal calculi and osteoporosis

5. Ulcers from pressure (bed sores)
6. Various gastrointestinal complaints such as heartburn, constipation, and anorexia
7. Venous stasis leading to thrombosis and potentially fatal embolism

These changes cannot be corrected by increased consumption of nutrients above normal, although their severity may be increased by a nutritconally inadequate diet.

Metabolic effects of starvation or semistarvation, discussed in Secs. 5.2 and 6.1, include:

1. Negative nitrogen balance with loss of lean body mass
2. Decreased basal metabolism
3. Changes in the gastrointestinal mucosa
4. Immune deficiencies
5. Eventual development of several nutrient deficiency signs

Cells of the gastrointestinal epithelium are particularly sensitive to starvation and severe malnutrition since this is a rapidly proliferating tissue. In humans the colon is the primary site of starvation-induced ulceration, with lesions appearing in the ileum in severe cases (Pfeiffer, 1970).

8.2   Metabolic Response to Trauma

Trauma produces significant alterations in body metabolism, as indicated in the discussion of G.A.S. A knowledge of these changes is important when developing a rationale for nutritional therapy following injury. Many of the changes are mediated by hormone secretions triggered by the body's response to trauma. Loss of blood volume activates the renin-angiotensin mechanism, which effects the release of aldosterone and thus increases sodium retention and potassium excretion. Increased secretion of antidiuretic hormone causes retention of body water. A group of catabolic hormones, including epinephrine, norepinephrine, glucocorticoids, and growth hormone, are secreted in larger than normal amounts and exert profound effects on many metabolic processes (Trunkey et al., 1973; Nelson et al., 1976).

The initial metabolic changes reflect the nature of the injury. In very severe injuries, such as massive crushes and extensive burns, there is a rapid loss of fluid and electrolytes from the body, creating a number of metabolic imbalances. Hemorrhage results in hypovolemia. Shock causes decreased perfusion of organs and cells with resultant organ failure, acidosis, and the release of toxic substances from damaged cells. Inflammation and abscess formation can later affect body function. The psychic stress of physical trauma can further increase hormonal release (Trunkey et al., 1973).

Major injury or trauma places a great stress on endogenous energy sources. Energy requirements following injury have been estimated to increase by 10 to 20 percent in skeletal injuries, 15 to 50 percent in infections, and 40 to 100 percent after burns (Trunkey et al., 1973).

A catabolic phase is common to all types of trauma with mobilization of metabolic reserves. Glycogen stores are rapidly depleted. Triglycerides are mobilized from adipose tissue. Hyperglycemia and diabeticlike glucose tolerance tests have been commonly observed in immediate posttrauma patients despite normal or increased insulin secretion. Injected insulin does not produce the expected decline in blood glucose after severe trauma. Glucose does not have its usual protein-sparing action (Ryan, 1976). The glucocorticoids released in the early response to trauma reduce the sensitivity of peripheral tissues to insulin and the catecholamines inhibit its release. Thus preservation of body cell mass by action of the anabolic insulin appears to be sacrificed in favor of supplying an abundance of circulating substances that will meet the energy and synthetic needs of body cells (Blackburn and Bistrian, 1976).

A characteristic metabolic effect of serious injury and infection is negative nitrogen balance. Body protein components are rapidly hydrolyzed, and nitrogen is excreted in the urine primarily as urea. The magnitude of the response depends to a large extent upon body stores of labile protein, with protein-depleted patients losing less total nitrogen (Cuthbertson and Tilstone, 1968). Urinary nitrogen loss may be large, attaining levels as high as 25 g/day. The deaminated amino acids can be used for energy, either directly or after conversion to glucose through gluconeogenesis. The energy available from the amount of utilized amino acids, indicated by the degree of negative nitrogen balance, roughly corresponds to the heat produced as a result of the increased metabolic rate after trauma. It has been suggested that the rapid mobilization of body protein may be necessitated, at least in part, by increased energy demands during the hypermetabolic period of the response to major injury (National Dairy Council, 1969). It may also provide amino acids for the synthesis of needed blood proteins, structural proteins, and enzymes (Blackburn and Bistrian, 1976). The source of most of the mobilized body protein is muscle. Creatinuria and urinary loss of sulfur, phosphorus, and potassium also occur. Visceral protein is spared to a great degree. In fact, protein synthesis in the liver of surgically treated dogs has been reported in the early postoperative period even while muscle protein was being broken down (National Dairy Council, 1969).

The catabolic protein response to trauma has been deplored classically. However, it has been realized recently that it provides for synthesis of needed body proteins as well as supplying energy demands (Blackburn and Bistrian, 1976).

The catabolic phase following minor injury or uncomplicated surgery is usually brief, lasting only a few days, and no serious consequences result for the normal, well-nourished patient. However, if this catabolic state occurs in individuals who are already malnourished or weakened by age and disease and if the catabolic period is prolonged by a complicated injury or infection, then the large loss of body protein may become a threat to the individual's survival. Prolonged protein catabolism results in muscle weakness, reduced immune system potency, and eventually leads to problems with wound healing (Ryan, 1976).

An adaptive phase follows the acute catabolic phase with decreased blood glucose levels, normal blood urea nitrogen, decreased urinary urea nitrogen, ketosis, and ketonuria. A fall in blood glucose helps to identify the transition from acute to adaptive phase. Effective nutritional support can occur at this phase, whereas during the acute catabolic phase unnecessary intake of protein and calories contributes to hypermetabolism and can be considered detrimental. When the hormonal environment is favorable, administered protein can be retained, as long as an adequate caloric supply is also available (Blackburn and Bistrian, 1976).

Changes in gastrointestinal function result from severe injury and infection. Adynamic ileus is common. Some parts of the gastrointestinal tract may return to normal motility more slowly than others. Delayed emptying of the stomach and the colon appear to be limiting factors in the ability of the gastrointestinal tract to normally propel secretions or ingested materials after severe trauma. Normal gastric and colonic function sometimes does not return for as long as 5 to 6 days, although some orally ingested food can often be handled. Mild jaundice with elevated serum bilirubin levels is also common after severe trauma or infection (Silen and Skillman, 1976).

8.3   Nutritional Care in Surgery and Trauma

The patient's nutritional state will affect her metabolic response to surgery or injury, influence her ability to survive the stress without significant morbidity, and determine the urgency of early postoperative nourishment. In elective surgery every reasonable effort should be made to correct preoperative nutritional deficits. Chronic malnutrition is commonly present in a patient with prolonged illness who has been unable or unwilling to eat an adequate diet. If a patient is malnourished because of a disease condition that may be corrected only by surgery, such as ulcerative colitis and gastrointestinal cancer, little will be gained by postponing surgery while attempting to improve nutritional status. However, it is important before surgery to bring about the greatest improvement possible in hydration, restoration of blood volume, and correction of protein, caloric, vitamin, and mineral deficits (Bacharach and Richardson, 1965). Preoperative weight reduction of an obese patient is desirable since obesity increases the usual stress on the cardiovascular system during surgery and contributes to a prolonged recovery period. A large amount of abdominal adipose tissue may also cause difficulties in suturing and wound healing.

The well-nourished patient who is subjected to an uncomplicated surgical procedure or moderately severe trauma usually does well postoperatively without complex nutritional intervention. Malt (1971) recommended that after an operation the major nutritional objective should be to get the patient to eat a full diet as soon as possible and made a plea for using logical procedures that are relatively simple in giving appropriate nutritional care. For the well-nourished patient, the surgeon may use a relatively simple program of parenteral infusion that is designed to maintain circulatory volume and to provide water, salt, and potassium to prevent dehydration or electrolyte imbalance in the immediate postoperative period (Goodhart and Shils, 1973, p. 950).

According to Malt (1971), the usual patient with cholecystectomy or major surgery of a similar type should be permitted 30 ml of clear liquids hourly by the morning after surgery. The same amount, or 60 ml, is allowed the next day. Sometime between the second and fifth days, Malt recommended that soft-cooked eggs, cereal gruels, and toast be added. The diet is progressed rapidly from this point, regulated by appetite. Clear fluids commonly used for hospitalized surgical patients include tea, coffee, clear broth, clear fruit juices, liquid gelatin mixtures, fruit-flavored drinks, and water. Carbonated beverages are allowed in some cases, depending upon the philosophy of the medical and dietetic staff.

The presence of audible bowel sounds and the absence of gastrointestinal symptoms after the stress of surgery are helpful criteria in determining the speed with which the diet may be advanced. According to Hayes (1959), there is no rational basis for providing patients with only nutritionally inadequate liquids for several days postoperatively. Although there is inhibition of upper gastrointestinal secretions in the first 24 to 48 hours after surgery, these secretions soon return to normal composition and volume, along with the return of peristaltic activity. The secretions of the stomach, duodenum, pancreas, and biliary system total many liters in a day, and the reabsorption of these materials actually imposes a greater physiologic burden on a gastrointestinal tract than does the usual oral intake given in the immediate postoperative period. Hayes recommended the provision to the patient of an attractively served, well-balanced, nutritionally sound general diet as soon as gastrointestinal activity approached normal.

Postinjury nutrition is important in compensating for the body's catabolic response and replacing lost tissue. Blackburn and Bistrian (1976) recommended the optimal protein intake for the injured patient as 16 percent of calculated caloric needs. The remaining kilocalories from non-protein sources should ideally yield a nitrogen-to-calorie ratio of 1 : 150 for anabolism in stressed patients.

Experimental animals fed low-protein diets have been reported to suffer from retarded healing of abdominal wounds when compared with animals fed an adequate level of protein (National Dairy Council, 1969). A relationship between wound healing and ascorbic acid nutrition has been established, probably because of this vitamin's role in collagen formation (Schwartz, 1970). Zinc is also involved in the processes of wound healing. A general impairment of protein synthesis with a secondary defect in the biosynthesis of collagen has been observed in zinc-deficient rats (Fernandez-Madrid et al., 1973). Pories et al. (1967) reported that oral zinc supplementation for young men significantly increased the rate of wound healing as compared to no supplementation. Hallböök and Lanner (1972) found that venous leg ulcers in patients with an initial serum zinc level higher than 110 mcg/100 ml, or after giving 200 mg of oral zinc sulfate three times a day, healed significantly faster than did those in patients with a low serum zinc level. However, several studies with rats and guinea pigs showed no differences in rate of healing for excised granulating wounds or development of tensile strength in incised wounds when supplementary zinc salts were added to a normal adequate diet with unsupplemented wounded animals being used as controls (Norman et al., 1975a,b; Quarantillo, 1971).

Postoperative convalescence is delayed and mortality rates are higher in malnourished than in well-nourished surgical patients. Patients in a poor nutritional state are more inclined to develop decubitus ulcers with prolonged bed rest. These sores may develop even within a short period of time if proper nursing care is not instituted along with improvement of nutritional state. Hypoproteinemia may be associated with increased susceptibility to hemorrhagic shock and decreased production of antibodies with changes in resistance to infection (Webb, 1964). Anemia may limit the supply of oxygen to tissues. In the patient who was severely malnourished preoperatively, vigorous measures need to be taken immediately following surgery to improve nutritional status. In any case, constant evaluation of nutritional status should be made on an individual basis so that not only is deterioration during hospitalization prevented but optimal nutritional support is provided. When a physician anticipates that a period of stress will last more than a few days, he or she should plan early for adequate nutritional care (Nelson et al., 1976).

The optimal procedure for providing nourishment is to use the gastrointestinal tract. If food cannot be taken orally, tube feeding may be instituted. A small feeding tube may be introduced into the stomach or duodenum by way of the nasopharynx and a nutrient fluid delivered by gravity drainage or by pump. A jejunostomy or gastrostomy is sometimes made at the time of surgery in a patient who, for special reasons such as esophageal damage, will be unable to eat normally for a long period of time. A gastrostomy will also avoid the nasal and esophageal erosions and gastroesophageal reflux that sometimes accompany prolonged use of nasogastric tubes. Various mixtures for tube feeding are discussed in Sec. 10.3. Whatever feeding formula is used, it should be relatively dilute at first, delivering about 0.75 kcal/ml. If diarrhea or other signs of intolerance appear, the formula should be diluted further. The feeding should be started slowly and the rate adjusted to the individual (Trunkey et al., 1973; Malt, 1971). Elemental diets may be well absorbed in the upper gastrointestinal tract even in immediate postoperative periods (Nelson et al., 1976).

When oral or tube feeding is inadequate, parenteral nutrition is necessary. The intravenous route is commonly used by way of a peripheral vein. This can be helpful as an adjunct to oral or tube feeding but is limited in terms of total kilocalories. Concentrated solutions cannot be given in peripheral veins since they cause severe phlebitis and thrombosis (Webb, 1964). One liter of a 5 percent glucose solution contains only 200 kcal. Nelson et al. (1976) suggested that there is little advantage to giving crystalline amino acids for the first few days after surgery. After that, the provision of amino acids plus glucose by peripheral vein has some advantages over isotonic glucose infusion since it lessens the degree of negative nitrogen balance. Flatt and Blackburn (1974) found that intravenous administration of amino acid mixtures without glucose is more effective in replenishing body pools of amino acids for protein synthesis. The amino acid infusion does not elicit an insulin response and thus does not discourage mobilization of triglycerides from adipose tissue as an energy source. The protein-sparing concept is discussed in Secs. 5.2 and 6.1.

Total parenteral feeding may be accomplished in severely malnourished patients for whom other forms of nourishment are not possible. Hyperosmolar nutrient solutions are administered by a catheter usually placed in the subclavian vein. The concentrated solution is tolerated in the large central vein because dilution is rapid and hyperosmolarity is decreased. The process of total parenteral feeding is more complex than that of any other method of nourishing the patient and should, therefore, be used only when other methods are not feasible. Amino acids, sugars, a fat emulsion, vitamins, and electrolytes may be given in total parenteral feeding to adequately nourish the patient (Trunkey et al., 1973).

The surgical patient should be evaluated at least daily in terms of nutritional needs. When changes are being made from parenteral to tube or oral feedings, there should be an overlapping of feeding routes, perhaps for several days, to allow adaptation and avoid periods of inadequate nutrient intake. When a patient begins to eat from a tray, it should not be assumed without checking that he will eat everything that he is served. Actual dietary intake should be assessed regularly (Nelson et al., 1976). At discharge from the hospital, the patient should be instructed concerning the importance of adequate nutrition during his convalescent period and afterward.

REFERENCES

1. Bacharach, B. and F. M. Richardson. 1965. Preoperative nutrition. *Med. Sci.,* July, 54.

2. Blackburn, G. L. and B. R. Bistrian. 1976. Nutritional care of the injured and/or septic patient. *Surg. Clin. No. Am.,* **56:** 1195.

3. Chobanian, A. V., R. D. Lille, A. Tercyak, and P. Blevins. 1974. The metabolic and hemodynamic effects of prolonged bed rest in normal subjects. *Circulation,* **49:** 551.

4. Cuthbertson, D. P. and W. J. Tilstone. 1968. Nutrition of the injured. *Am. J. Clin. Nutr.,* **21:** 911.

5. Fernandez-Madrid, F., A. S. Prasad, and D. Oberleas. 1973. Effect of zinc deficiency on nucleic acids, collagen, and noncollagenous protein of the connective tissue. *J. Lab. Clin. Med.,* **82:** 951.

6. Flatt, J. and G. L. Blackburn. 1974. The metabolic fuel regulatory system: implications for protein-sparing therapies during caloric deprivation and disease. *Am. J. Clin. Nutr.,* **27:** 175.

7. Goodhart, R. S. and M. E. Shils (Eds.). 1973. *Modern Nutrition in Health and Disease,* 5th ed. Philadelphia: Lea and Febiger.

8. Hallböök, T. and E. Lanner. 1972. Serum-zinc and healing of venous leg ulcers. *Lancet* **2:** 780.

9. Hayes, M. A. 1959. Postoperative diet therapy. *J. Am. Dietet. Assoc.,* **35:** 17.

10. Heath, H., III, J. M. Earli, M. Schaaf, J. T. Piechocki, and T. Li. 1972. Serum ionized calcium during bed rest in fracture patients and normal men. *Metabolism,* **21:** 633.

11. Hodges, R. E. 1970. The effect of stress on ascorbic acid metabolism in man. *Nutr. Today,* **5** (No. 1): 11.

12. Kiely, W. F. 1972. Coping with severe illness. *Adv. Psychosom. Med.,* **8:** 105.

13. Malt, R. A. 1971. Keep it simple. *Nutr. Today,* **6** (No. 3): 30.

14. Mutter, A. Z. and M. J. Schleifer. 1966. The role of psychological and social factors in the onset of somatic illness in children. *Psychosom. Med.,* **28:** 333.

15. National Dairy Council. 1969. Nutrition in illness. *Dairy Council Dig.,* **40** (No. 5): 25.

16. Nelson, R. A., C. F. Gastineau, J. M. Kinney, and J. Metcoff. 1976. Nutrition in stress and starvation. *Dialogues in Nutrition, Mayo Clinic,* **1** (No. 3): 1.

17. Norman, J. N., A. Rahmat, and G. Smith. 1975a. Effect of supplements of zinc salts on the healing of granulating wounds in the rat and guinea pig. *J. Nutr.,* **105:** 815.

18. Norman, J. N., A. Rahmat, and G. Smith. 1975b. Effect of supplements of zinc salts on the healing of incised wounds in the rat and guinea pig. *J. Nutr.,* **105:** 822.

19. Pfeiffer, C. J. 1970. Gastrointestinal response to malnutrition and starvation. *Postgrad. Med.,* **47** (No. 4): 110.

20. Pories, W. J., J. H. Henzel, C. G. Rob, and W. H. Strain. 1967. Acceleration of wound healing in man with zinc sulphate given by mouth. *Lancet,* **1:** 121.

21. Quarantillo, E. P., Jr. 1971. Effect of supplemental zinc on wound healing in rats. *Am. J. Surg.,* **121:** 661.

22. Rabkin, J. G. and E. L. Struening. 1976. Life events, stress, and illness. *Science,* **194:** 1013.

23. Roghmann, K. J. and R. J. Haggerty. 1973. Daily stress, illness, and use of health services in young families. *Ped. Res.,* **7:** 520.

24. Ryan, N. T. 1976. Metabolic adaptations for energy production during trauma and sepsis. *Surg. Clin. No. Am.,* **56:** 1073.

25. Schwartz, P. L. 1970. Ascorbic acid in wound healing—a review. *J. Am. Dietet. Assoc.,* **56:** 597.

26. Selye, H. 1973. The evolution of the stress concept. *Am. Scientist,* **61:** 692.

27. Selye, H. 1970. On just being sick. *Nutr. Today,* **5** (No. 1): 2.

28. Silen, W. and J. J. Skillman. 1976. Gastrointestinal responses to injury and infection. *Surg. Clin. No. Am.,* **56:** 945.

29. Trunkey, D., S. Grzyb, and G. F. Sheldon. 1973. Nutrition and trauma. *Intake: Perspectives in Clinical Nutrition (Eaton Laboratories),* No. 6.

30. Verwoerdt, A. 1972. Psychopathological responses to the stress of physical illness. *Adv. Psychosom. Med.,* **8:** 119.

31. Webb, R. S., Jr. 1964. Correction of malnutrition in surgical patients. *Surg. Clin. No. Am.,* **44:** 141.

STUDY GUIDE

Patients hospitalized for surgery or injury are usually subjected to (1) stress, (2) bed rest, and (3) starvation.

1. Define stress and describe common stressor agents for hospitalized patients.

2. Outline the General Adaptation Syndrome (G.A.S.) postulated by Selye.

3. Describe and explain the usual metabolic response of the body to severe stress, and discuss its implications for nutritional care of surgical or injured patients.

4. Describe undesirable physiological effects of prolonged bed rest and starvation, and explain the effect of dietary intake on these changes.

Stress may take many different forms, with interactions between stress and nutritional factors compounding the effects of stress.

5. Cite several examples of interactions between stress and nutritional factors in humans or experimental animals.

6. Discuss possible effects of social factors and life events on the onset of illness in humans.

Preoperative nutritional inadequacies and/or postoperative nutritional deterioration enhance the usual physiological problems for a surgical patient.

7. Describe and explain several clinical problems that may be associated with malnutrition in a surgical patient.

8. Describe and explain the possible effect of each of the following on morbidity and mortality of surgical patients:
   (a) Obesity
   (b) Protein deficiency and hypoproteinemia
   (c) Anemia
   (d) Subclinical ascorbic acid deficiency
   (e) Zinc deficiency

Since adequate nutrition is important for the surgical patient in avoiding complications and encouraging rapid recovery, it should be supplied soon after surgery.

9. Recommend an appropriate general procedure for giving nutritional care to surgical patients, giving rationale for the recommendations.

10. Explain why oral food intake is contraindicated immediately following major surgery, and describe physiological criteria that indicate when food may be given.

11. Describe and explain a usual sequence of nourishment procedures for a well-nourished patient after surgery, and explain why it is important for the patient to progress to a full diet as soon as possible.

12. Discuss and explain the role of tube and parenteral feeding, both peripheral and total, in the surgical patient.

Nutrition and Fevers; Burns

Fevers—particularly those resulting from infection—and severe burns on a sizeable portion of the body both represent stresses on the metabolic systems. They each elicit the general responses to stress and trauma discussed in Chap. 8. This chapter discusses nutritional implications of fevers and burns.

9.1 Fevers

Body temperature is normally maintained within a narrow range despite wide variations in environmental conditions and physical activity. The control of body temperature integrates various physical and chemical processes for heat production or loss and is a function of cerebral centers located in the hypothalamus. A disturbance in temperature regulation, usually an increase in body temperature, is a sensitive and reliable indicator of the presence of disease. In fever, the body's temperature-regulating mechanism still functions and retains its sensitivity but is "set" at a higher level (Wintrobe et al., 1974, pp. 48–49).

Fever accelerates all metabolic processes and contributes to the wasting of body nitrogen and energy. Weight loss usually occurs. Increased synthesis of special body proteins, such as antibodies, may utilize amino acids in greater than normal quantities (Goodhart and Shils, 1973, p. 609). Basal energy metabolism is increased by about 13 percent for each degree Celsius rise in temperature above normal (7 percent for each °F). Fever affects basal water requirements of the body largely through hyperventilation and increased evaporation (Goodhart and Shils, 1973, p. 955).

Most fevers are remittant, showing diurnal characteristics, with the body temperature rising and falling each day but not returning to normal. Some fevers, however, may be "sustained," continuing over relatively long periods of time without diurnal variation. Typhoid fever may show this characteristic. Malaria is an example of a relapsing fever that is distinguished by short febrile periods between one or several days of normal temperature.

Acute febrile illnesses of short duration (less than 10 days) are common and include influenza, pneumonia, tonsillitis, measles, and other bacterial or viral infections. In most instances the fever is of infectious origin, with characteristic symptoms including (1) high fever (30 to 41°C or 102 to 105°F) of abrupt onset, with or without chills; (2) respiratory symptoms; (3) severe malaise with muscle or joint pain, photophobia, headache; (4) nausea, vomiting, or diarrhea; (5) acute enlargement of lymph nodes or spleen; and (6) leukocyte count above 12,000 or below 5000 per mm^3 (Wintrobe et al., 1974, p. 57). Synergistic interaction between infection and malnutrition, increasing the severity of the stress, is discussed in Sec. 6.1. In a previously well-nourished patient an acute fever of short duration will usually create few nutritional problems, even though intake of kilocalories and protein may be inadequate to balance body losses during the acute stage.

Prolonged fever illness requires careful attention to nutritional needs, particularly when the metabolic rate is markedly increased by high temperatures. Examples of this type of illness include tuberculosis, upper abdominal infections, renal infections, bacterial endocarditis, neoplasms, and rheumatic fever (Wintrobe et al., 1974, p. 58).

Nutrition and Fevers of Short Duration

Both elevated basal energy requirements and the restlessness that often accompanies acute febrile disease contribute to increased energy needs. An acutely ill patient is usually anorectic and is not likely to voluntarily consume more than 600 to 1200 kcal daily, often primarily in the form of liquid foods. Increased water intake is extremely important to prevent dehydration.

An experimentally induced mild acute viral illness in 10 normal men was reported by Rayfield et al. (1973) to significantly alter carbohydrate metabolism with elevated fasting serum glucose levels, diminished glucose tolerance, and mild hyperinsulinemia. These alterations were associated with increases of serum glucagon, glucocorticoids, growth hormone, and free fatty acids. The deterioration in carbohydrate metabolism apparently resulted from interrelated factors.

Protein catabolism is increased during acute fever disease, and changes occur in amino acid metabolism. Wannemacher et al. (1972 and 1975) reported that fasting plasma concentrations of most individual free amino acids were depressed in volunteers experimentally infected with sandfly fever virus in comparison to baseline values obtained prior to infection. Plasma concentrations of phenylalanine were increased. Despite the decline of most plasma amino acid levels during the illness, only the urinary excretion of phenylalanine and 3-methylhistidine were significantly increased. These results supported the concept that unusually large quantities of most plasma amino acids are taken up by hepatic cells during acute fever disease. The skeletal muscle appeared to be the major source of amino acids shunted to the liver. An additional study with rats (Wannemacher et al., 1976) suggested that larger amounts of phenylalanine than tyrosine were released from skeletal muscle of infected animals as compared with control animals, and that the serum phenylalanine to tyrosine ratio may have potential value for estimating the presence of an inflammatory disease and a catabolic state. Wannemacher et al. (1975) also found a depression in serum zinc levels and a significant hypozincuria during febrile illness in humans. Pekarek and Beisel (1974) suggested a redistribution and sequestering of various essential trace elements in the body during acute infection.

The nutritional needs of the usual patient with fever of short duration thus include increased kilocalories, protein, water, and possibly vitamins and minerals. Balanced proportions of protein, carbohydrate, and fat in the diet are desirable. Soft, bland, easily digested foods usually will be most acceptable to the ill patient during the acute stage and may be offered at 2- to 3-hour intervals. Although it is not likely that total caloric needs will be met during the first few days, increased food intake should be encouraged as soon as possible to avoid excessive depletion of body nutrients.

Nutrition and Typhoid Fever

Typhoid fever is an acute systemic disease resulting from infection with *Salmonella typhi* and is unique to human beings. Since this organism is usually ingested with contaminated food, water, or milk, the disease has steadily decreased in the United States with improvement in socioeconomic conditions, pure water supplies, effective sewage disposal, and widespread pasteurization of milk. Typhoid fever still occurs on a large scale in countries where sanitation is suboptimal.

If typhoid fever is not treated with antibiotics, the illness lasts about 4 weeks. The body temperature gradually increases for 5 to 7 days and then plateaus as a sustained or mildly remittent fever at 39 to 40°C (102 to 104°F) for 2 to 3 weeks. Along with anorexia and weakness, the elevated temperature often leads to general debility. During the fourth week the fever gradually decreases. A characteristic feature of the disease is the enlargement of lymphoid tissues in the intestines, particularly Peyer's patches of the terminal ileum. Necrosis in hyperplastic Peyer's patches may be associated with erosion of blood vessels and hemorrhage. Lesions may extend deep into the intestinal wall and cause perforation of the bowel (Wintrobe et al., 1974, p. 805).

Nutritional and nursing care were extremely important for the typhoid patient before the use of antimicrobial agents in treatment. High-calorie (3000 to 5000 kcal daily) and high-protein (up to 1½ g/kg) diets were found to bring benefits in lower mortality, shorter convalescence, and fewer complications. The foods were generally low in residue, including cooked refined cereals, toast, puddings, strained fruits and vegetables, and 1 to 2 quarts of milk and two to six eggs daily. Meat was avoided in the early stages of the illness.

With appropriate antibiotic treatment, the usual course of typhoid fever has been greatly shortened; improvement begins within 48 hours. The temperature often returns to normal in 2 to 5 days after beginning treatment (Wintrobe et al., 1974, p. 807). The nutritional care of the typhoid patient treated with antibiotics, therefore, is similar to that of patients with other acute fever diseases of relatively short duration, with the additional precaution of low-residue foods because of inflammation in the intestinal tract. Dietary protein and kilocalorie levels should be relatively high, estimated on an individual basis, to prevent excessive wasting of body tissues.

Nutritional Needs in Tuberculosis

Tuberculosis is a necrotizing infection of the bacillus *Mycobacterium tuberculosis*. The lungs are most often affected, but lesions may occur in the kidneys, bones, and lymph nodes or be disseminated throughout the body. In 1971 there were about 34,000 new cases of clinical tuberculosis in the United States, an incidence of 17 per 100,000. Primary tuberculosis results when the tubercle bacilli invade the host that has no specific immunity. At this stage the disease usually heals spontaneously. Postprimary tuberculosis is the result of progression of infection, usually years later, in spite of specific immunity and after a latent or dormant stage (Wintrobe et al., 1974, pp. 858–860).

Chronic pulmonary tuberculosis has an insidious onset as symptoms develop gradually. Fever is often low grade and present only in the late afternoon or evening. Body weight may be well maintained until late in the course of the illness. When abdominal symptoms predominate, loss of weight may be rapid. Malaise, exhaustion, and cough are often present. Treatment with isoniazid (isonicotinic acid hydrazide) inhibits DNA synthesis and intermediary metabolism of the tuberculin bacillus (Wintrobe et al., 1974, p. 861). This drug causes increased urinary excretion of pyridoxine (vitamin B_6), and clinical evidence of pyridoxine deficiency, including peripheral neuritis, has been reported in patients undergoing treatment for tuberculosis (Roe, 1976). A daily supplement of 50 mg vitamin B_6 is recommended for these patients. Although pellagra from niacin deficiency is a rare complication of isoniazid therapy among well-nourished patients, poorly nourished ones receiving the drug may develop this deficiency disease.

The nutritional care of a patient with chronic pulmonary tuberculosis includes supplying calories to achieve and maintain normal body weight. Dietary protein should be provided in only slightly higher amounts than those recommended for the healthy individual, to ensure adequate amounts for healing and maintenance of normal serum proteins. Serum levels of vitamin A and ascorbic acid are often low in patients with chronic tuberculosis, so liberal amounts of these vitamins should be included in the diet. Calcium is apparently involved in the healing of lesions and should be emphasized (Brewer et al., 1954), along with an adequate amount of vitamin D to aid in its absorption. Iron should be supplied in sufficient amounts to prevent anemia and build iron stores in the body. This is particularly important if hemorrhage occurs. Brewer et al. (1954) found that the metabolism of women with active tuberculosis with respect to phosphorus, riboflavin, and thiamin was similar to that of women free from the disease.

Foods to supply the essential nutrients should be easily digested, attractive, and appropriate for the preferences of the individual patient. Regularity of meals is important in maintaining a constant food intake.

9.2 Burns

The severity of body burns varies from minor injuries to severe trauma requiring long periods of hospitalization. The extent of the burn is expressed as percent total body surface involved. This is important information in evaluating the severity of the injury and anticipated fluid requirements. As a rough estimate of burned area, the head and neck and each arm may be considered 9 percent body surface area; the anterior trunk, posterior trunk, and each lower extremity may be twice 9 percent, or 18 percent body surface area; and the perineum 1 percent, making a total of 100 percent. Various charts may also be used in estimating percent burn.

First-degree burns are superficial injuries involving only the epidermis. Complete healing usually occurs in 5 to 10 days. Second-degree burns extend through the epidermis into the underlying corium. They have intact dermal appendages (sweat glands, hair follicles) that can regenerate the epidermis in time but may need grafting to prevent extensive fluid loss and sepsis. Third-degree burns extend through and destroy all dermal elements. Coagulation necrosis of the skin then produces a dry, leathery, inelastic coagulum called an *eschar* on the surface of the burn (Artz and Gibson, 1976). These burns cannot regenerate skin and must granulate in from borders of the wound or be grafted.

Physiologic Effects of Severe Burns

Burn shock describes the profound changes in dynamics of the body's circulation during the immediate postburn period. A marked, transient reduction in cardiac output is the first effect, compounded by a decrease in plasma volume with characteristic hemoconcentration. This is caused by an increased vascular permeability, particularly in the immediate area of the burn, which allows large quantities of interstitial fluid to accumulate in this area. Protein and sodium escape from the capillaries and become sequestered in the extracellular space. The decrease in blood volume is roughly proportional to the extent and depth of burn. Thermally damaged collagen-producing cells avidly take up salt and water, creating a characteristic burn edema. Water loss from the burned surface by evaporation may be more than 10 times the normal rate and requires a large expenditure of body heat (0.58 kcal/ml). A sharp increase in basal metabolic rate (BMR) helps to meet this increased energy need. Red blood cell hemolysis does not usually exceed 10 percent (Artz and Gibson, 1976; Crenshaw, 1973; Moncrief, 1973).

The increase in BMR in response to trauma of extensive second- and third-degree burns is marked, and nitrogen losses are also far in excess of those resulting from other types of injury. Weight loss is characteristic of the early posttrauma period. A comparison of the starving burn patient and a starving normal person may emphasize the hypermetabolism and nitrogen wastage. With resting starvation, the normal individual could survive approximately 2 months without food intake. However, in the patient with third-degree burns who is losing 30 g nitrogen and up to 1 kg in body mass per day, fatal starvation may occur in 3 to 4 weeks (Wilmore, 1974). The increased BMR peaks between the sixth and tenth postburn days, but returns to normal only as the burn completely closes (Artz and Gibson, 1976).

Hyperglycemia frequently occurs in burn patients during the early stages. Glucose tolerance tests are abnormal and serum insulin levels depressed while serum glucagon is elevated. These hormonal changes contribute to the catabolic state (Artz and Gibson, 1976).

Gastrointestinal complications following thermal injury include adyamic ileus and Curling's ulcer, life-threatening gastrointestinal ulceration occurring in about 11 percent of hospitalized burn patients. Czaja et al. (1976) measured total titratable acidity of fasting gastric secretion in 34 hemodynamically stable patients within 5 days after receiving third-degree burns. Acid output was not predictive of gastroduodenal disease. However, acute duodenal ulcers were not found in patients with acid secretion less than 3.11 meq/hour. Clinically significant gastrointestinal complications developed in 9 of the 34 patients. However, 31 patients showed acute gastroduodenal disease of some degree. Artz and Gibson (1976) suggested that the primary consideration in the treatment of Curling's ulcer is prevention and that all patients with more than 30 percent of the body surface burned may appropriately be given a liquid antacid preparation to maintain gastric contents at a pH of 7 or above. Lack of peristalsis, as well as other effects of posttrauma shock, limit oral feeding in the early postburn stage, although attempts should be made to initiate this as rapidly as possible to meet nutrient needs.

Management of the Burn Patient

Fluid and electrolyte balance takes first priority in the initial treatment of burn patients unless there are pulmonary problems associated with burns of the face and inhalation injury, which must be handled immediately. Fluid is given intravenously until the patient is able to take adequate amounts by mouth. Optimum therapy probably includes rapid fluid resuscitation with only isotonic salt or buffered electrolyte solutions in the first 8 to 24 hours after a burn to increase plasma volume and encourage the return of normal cardiac output. In the second 24-hour period, when capillary permeability improves, intravenous administration of a colloid solution such as plasma or albumin is more effective than electrolyte solutions in maintaining plasma volume, with salt solutions merely aggravating the edema at this time. An estimate of the usual need for sodium ion during the first 24-hour period after the burn is 0.5 to 0.7 meq per kg body weight for each 1 percent of body surface burned. Large volumes of fluid are required to carry this quantity of sodium in isotonic solution and are sufficient to meet water needs. Hypernatremia occurs if water needs are not met. Potassium supplements should be given as indicated by serum potassium determinations (Artz and Gibson, 1976; Crenshaw, 1973; Moncrief, 1973).

Artz and Gibson (1976) suggested that after the burn patient has been stabilized, the general objectives of management are (1) preservation of dermal elements spared by the original injury, (2) provision of an optimal environment for epithelial regeneration, (3) safe and rapid removal of devitalized tissue, (4) rapid skin graft closure of full thickness defects, and (5) accomplishment of these objectives without overcoming already depressed body reserves.

Infection is an ever-present threat to the burn patient. The vascular supply to a full thickness burn is completely occluded, and no appreciable circulation is reestablished to this area until approximately 3 weeks after the injury. In a partial thickness burn, circulation to the burn area is restored within 24 to 48 hours. The presence of large amounts of nonviable tissue in the burn wound provides an excellent medium for bacterial growth. Topical application of antibacterial substances has significantly reduced the fatal outcome due to burn wound sepsis (Moncrief, 1973).

Therapy will vary, depending upon depth and extent of injury. It may involve excision of devitalized skin and subcutaneous tissue and early grafting. Skin obtained from cadaver donors may be used as a biologic dressing to protect the wound until the host skin is available. This procedure diminishes evaporative water loss, and the homograft skin may be frequently changed to avoid a period of rejection by the host. Heterograft skin obtained from other species (usually pigs) is replacing the use of cadaver skin (Artz and Gibson, 1976; Moncrief, 1973).

Nutritional Care of Burn Patients

The increase in BMR appears to be directly proportional to the magnitude of burn injury up to 60 percent total body surface burn (Curreri et al., 1974). Adequate provision of nutrients and energy is essential to effective wound healing and successful skin grafting. Normal eating is not possible during the first few days postburn because of the gastrointestinal changes that include nausea, adynamic ileus, and distention. Within 7 to 10 days, however, adequate oral intake should be attained.

Estimates of energy and protein needs for burned adult patients have included 50 to 70 kcal with 2 to 3 g protein per kg body weight by Artz and Gibson (1976) and 40 to 60 kcal per kg by Curreri et al. (1974). Crenshaw (1973) suggested that a minimum of 2800 kcal daily is required to spare protein for restorative processes. Curreri et al. used a formula for estimating the individual energy requirements of an adult burn patient based upon both body size and magnitude of injury as:

Ideal caloric intake = 25 × weight (kg) + 40 × % total body surface burn

From regression analysis of data on nutrient intake and weight changes in nine adult patients with total body surface burns between 40 and 73 percent, over a period of 20 days, they produced a regression line that fit this empirical formula. In this study, a high-protein, high-caloric selective house diet was served. Average daily caloric content of the food offered was 5000 kcal, but actual mean consumption varied from 296 to 2279 kcal. In addition, the intake of high caloric oral supplements was encouraged at frequent intervals, and liquid high-protein, high-caloric solutions were given via an indwelling nasogastric feeding tube. Dextrose, with or without protein hydrolysate, was administered parenterally at varying levels. Combined mean daily intake by all nutritional pathways was 2513 kcal (range 1230 to 3206). Voluntary enteral intake of food was relatively poor in this group in spite of their understanding of increased nutritional requirements.

Since balancing the caloric equation by increasing food intake is sometimes difficult to accomplish, efforts to reduce caloric expenditure have been made and are usually directed toward reducing evaporative water loss from the burned area. However, burn hypermetabolism is evidently the result of multiple mechanisms and will probably require more than reduction of evaporative water loss for successful control (Gump and Kinney, 1971).

Patients with extensive second- and third-degree burns require increased amounts of essential nutrients in addition to protein and kilocalories. Crenshaw (1973) suggested for adults that the basic daily regimen of peroral vitamin therapy should include at least 2 g ascorbic acid, 50 mg thiamin, 50 mg riboflavin, and 500 mg nicotinamide. Children should receive about one-third of these amounts. In addition, vitamins A and D are essential for children and probably important for optimum healing in adult patients. Folic acid, vitamin B_{12}, vitamin K, pyridoxine, pantothenic acid, and vitamin E also require special consideration in burn patients.

Nutritional support of burned patients begins with fluid resuscitation, given intravenously. Hypertonic solutions by a central vein including glucose and amino acids may then be given in early treatment to overcome the deficiency of kilocalories inherent in peripheral intravenous feeding and the inability of the patient to take food orally. With total parenteral feeding, patients may begin to gain weight after about 1 week, and nitrogen balance becomes positive. However, complications such as hyperosmolarity coma, sepsis, vena cava thrombosis, and pneumothorax may develop unless great care is used in the preparation and administration of the feeding solutions. The greatest danger to the burn patient is catheter-related sepsis (Crenshaw, 1973).

If a patient cannot ingest enough food orally to prevent a substantial amount of body weight loss within a reasonable period of time, tube feeding through a small polyethylene tube may be given, continuously or intermittently. From a study with burned rats, Langlois et al. (1972) concluded that feeding an elemental diet prior to and immediately after burning significantly reduced the mortality rate and the incidence of gastrointestinal lesions in the experimental animals. Great care must be exercised, however, in feeding burned children and seriously ill adults by tube to avoid aspiration, respiratory infection, and gastric dilation (Crenshaw, 1973).

The most desirable feeding route is oral, even though it is difficult for patients with major burns to consume the needed 5000 to 6000 kcal daily. Most patients require constant encouragement and psychological support. Pennisi (1976) reported on the use of a Nutritional Management Record Sheet in a team approach to diet therapy for burn patients. This provides a systematic approach to patient care. The first section of the sheet identifies the patient, the percent total body surface burned, initial weight, and calculated weight loss limit (10 percent). Another section contains energy and protein requirements calculated according to the following formulas:

Energy requirement = 20 kcal × kg body weight + 70 kcal × % burn   adults
                 = 60 kcal × kg body weight + 35 kcal × % burn   children

Protein requirement = 1 g × kg body weight + 3 g × % burn   adults
                 = 3 g × kg body weight + 1 g × % burn   children

Body weight is recorded by the nurses at least twice a week. If the weight limit is approached or reached, the physician, nurse, and dietitian must respond with appropriate changes in the delivery of nutritional therapy. On the sheet, the dietitian describes the methods of feeding being used, keeps the nutritional record updated, and is available to help the physician make changes where desirable.

Holli and Oakes (1975) described a procedure for individualized nutritional care of hospitalized burned children; it involves a selective menu and concerted efforts of the care team to encourage food intake. Multidisciplinary patient care conferences are held twice a week to discuss all aspects of care. Caloric intakes and weight records are noted and changes in nutritional care plans discussed. Tube feeding, intravenous feeding, oral intake, or a combination of approaches may be emphasized, and the burned child's mother is frequently involved in nutritional counseling.

Nutritional support is thus an extremely important part of the treatment of burn patients, although it is one of the most difficult aspects of care. Nutritional requirements are increased beyond those in other kinds of trauma, and a combination of intravenous therapy, tube feeding, and oral feeding at frequent intervals must usually be employed to meet these needs.

REFERENCES

1. Artz, C. P. and T. Gibson. 1976. Management of burns. *Military Med.,* **141:** 673.

2. Brewer, W. D., D. C. Cedarquist, B. Cole, H. Tobey, M. A. Ohlson, and C. J. Stringer. 1954. Calcium and phosphorus metabolism of women with active tuberculosis. *J. Am. Dietet. Assoc.,* **30:** 21.

3. Crenshaw, C. 1973. Nutritional support for burn patients. *Intake: Perspectives in Clinical Nutrition* (Eaton Laboratories), No. 2.

4. Curreri, P. W., D. Richmond, J. Marvin, and C. R. Baxter. 1974. Dietary requirements of patients with major burns. *J. Am. Dietet. Assoc.,* **65:** 415.

5. Czaja, A. J., J. C. McAlhany, and B. A. Pruitt, Jr. 1976. Gastric acid secretion and acute gastroduodenal disease after burns. *Arch. Surg.,* **111:** 243.

6. Goodhart, R. S. and M. E. Shils (Eds.). 1973. *Modern Nutrition in Health and Disease,* 5th ed. Philadelphia: Lea and Febiger.

7. Gump, F. E. and J. M. Kinney. 1971. Energy balance and weight loss in burned patients. *Arch. Surg.,* **103:** 442.

8. Holli, B. B. and J. B. Oakes. 1975. Feeding the burned child. *J. Am. Dietet. Assoc.,* **67:** 240.

9. Langlois, P., H. B. Williams, and F. N. Gurd. 1972. Effect of an elemental diet on mortality rates and gastrointestinal lesions in experimental burns. *J. Trauma,* **12:** 771.

10. Moncrief, J. A. 1973. Burns. *N. Eng. J. Med.,* **288:** 444.

11. Pekarek, R. S. and W. R. Beisel. 1974. Redistribution and sequestering of essential trace elements during acute infection. *Proc. IX Nutrition Congress,* **II:** 183.

12. Pennisi, V. M. 1976. Monitoring the nutritional care of burned patients. *J. Am. Dietet. Assoc.,* **69:** 531.

13. Rayfield, E. J., R. T. Curnow, D. T. George, and W. R. Beisel. 1973. Impaired carbohydrate metabolism during a mild viral illness. *N. Eng. J. Med.,* **289:** 618.

14. Roe, D. A. 1976. *Drug-Induced Nutritional Deficiencies.* Westport, Conn.: Avi Publishing.

15. Wannemacher, R. W., Jr., R. E. Dinterman, R. S. Pekarek, P. J. Bartelloni, and W. R. Beisel. 1975. Urinary amino acid excretion during experimentally induced sandfly fever in man. *Am. J. Clin. Nutr.,* **28:** 110.

16. Wannemacher, R. W., Jr., A. S. Klainer, R. E. Dinterman, and W. R. Beisel. 1976. The significance and mechanism of an increased serum phenylalanine-tyrosine ratio during infection. *Am. J. Clin. Nutr.,* **29:** 997.

17. Wannemacher, R. W., Jr., R. S. Pekarek, P. J. Bartelloni, R. T. Vollmer, and W. R. Beisel. 1972. Changes in individual plasma amino acids following experimentally induced sand-fly fever virus infections. *Metabolism,* **21:** 67.

18. Wilmore, D. W. 1974. Nutrition and metabolism following thermal injury. *Clin. Plast. Surg.,* **1:** 603.

19. Wintrobe, M. M., G. W. Thorn, R. D. Adams, E. Braunwald, K. J. Isselbacher, and R. G. Petersdorf (Eds.). 1974. *Harrison's Principles of Internal Medicine,* 7th ed. New York: McGraw-Hill.

STUDY GUIDE

Basal energy metabolism is increased, with concomitant alterations in carbohydrate and protein metabolism, during febrile illness.

1. Estimate the approximate caloric requirement above normal basal needs for an individual patient with a specified temperature elevation.

2. Describe effects of fever disease on carbohydrate and amino acid metabolism, and discuss nutritional implications of these effects.

In acute fever diseases, the body temperature may be very high, resulting in a greatly increased energy need, but the fever is usually of relatively short duration.

3. Suggest appropriate diet prescriptions and menus for the acute stage and for the convalescent period of fever diseases with short duration, and justify your suggestions.

The diet for a patient with typhoid fever should usually be high in kilocalories and protein but low in residue or fiber.

4. Explain why the diet described above is recommended for patients with typhoid fever, and suggest appropriate foods that may be used.

5. Name the organism causing typhoid fever, and explain why patients with this disease usually will be isolated in hospital procedure.

In the nutritional care of patients with tuberculosis the intake of several nutrients should be carefully monitored.

6. Explain why each of the following nutrients is particularly important in the treatment of patients with tuberculosis: calcium, iron, vitamin D, ascorbic acid, and vitamin A.

7. Suggest appropriate menus to meet the nutrient needs for a patient with tuberculosis.

8. Explain why pyridoxine supplementation should accompany the antibiotic isoniazid.

Dramatic physiological changes occur in an extensively burned patient and require intensive therapy.

9. Describe the major physiological changes occurring during the initial phase of thermal injury and the usual immediate treatment.

The form of therapy for major burns is individualized and based upon the depth and extent of injury.

10. Outline general objectives for management of the burned patient.

11. Explain why sepsis is a common problem in a burn patient, and describe precautions that may be taken to avoid this problem.

Nutrition is a critical problem for severely burned patients because of the high demands for kilocalories and essential nutrients.

12. Compare the relative water-vapor transmitting properties of normal and burned skin, and discuss possible relationships between this property and the large caloric requirements after burns.

13. Suggest and discuss some appropriate ways of estimating the energy and protein needs of extensively burned patients.

14. Explain advantages of maintaining adequate caloric and essential nutrient intake in burned patients, and suggest possible ways in which satisfactory alimentation may be accomplished.

10

Parenteral and Tube Feeding

The most appropriate route of supply for energy and essential nutrients is the gastrointestinal tract and, whenever possible, food should be given orally. When this is not feasible, yet the gastrointestinal tract can effectively handle food, tube feedings may be appropriately employed, i.e., nasogastric tube, esophagostomy, gastrostomy, and jejunostomy.

Parenteral feeding is an acceptable method of providing nutrients when there are abnormalities of the gastrointestinal tract that do not allow feeding by this route, and during other periods, such as after surgery or trauma, when the alimentary canal is not functioning effectively. In a strict definition, parenteral feeding includes any route other than the gastrointestinal tract. Subcutaneous or intramuscular injections have been used for electrolytes, vitamins, or iron. The intraperitoneal route has been used in special cases. However, intravenous feeding is the most satisfactory method and is essentially synonymous with parenteral feeding. Although it is not possible to supply all nutritional needs by feeding through peripheral veins, total parenteral feeding through a central vein may provide complete nourishment for an individual.

This chapter reviews briefly some elements of fluid, electrolyte, and acid-base balance in the body in preparation for the study of parenteral and tube feeding. The uses of tube and parental feeding are then discussed. The nutritional care of the patient who is no longer able to take food by mouth is often managed entirely by the physician. However, the dietitian should be able to effectively contribute to the management of intravenous nutrient regimes (Allen and Lee, 1969).

10.1 Body Fluid and Electrolytes

Water accounts for 45 to 75 percent of total body weight, the percentage varying with the body-fat content. Since fatty tissue contains little water, the fatter the individual the smaller the proportion of water to total weight. Water balance is usually maintained in the body, with intake equaling output, except for periods of growth and recovery from illness where water is retained to build tissues. Body water is replenished by ingestion, either alone or as part of foods that may contain 10 to 98 percent water, and also by water released in the body from oxidation of energy nutrients. One gram protein, carbohydrate, or fat gives 0.41, 0.60, or 1.07 ml water, respectively (Consolazio et al., 1963). Water leaves the body through the kidneys, lungs, skin, and gastrointestinal tract. The kidneys are the principal ultimate regulators of internal environment, regulating loss of not only water (approximately 1500 ml/day) but also electrolytes and hydrogen ion (H^+). Average daily water loss through the skin and lungs is about 1000 ml. Loss of water is influenced by respiratory rate, fever, environmental temperature and humidity, and injury to the skin, e.g., large evaporative losses in severe burns. Thirst is important in the regulation of water balance.

Water moves freely from one body compartment to another, sometimes by simple diffusion. Two major compartments are described as (1) intracellular and (2) extracellular. The extracellular compartment may be further divided into intravascular (plasma within the blood vessels) and interstitial (fluid within spaces between cells). Osmotic pressure is produced by the activity of solute particles (ions or small nonionized molecules) in water solution. The most important force pulling water between intra- and extracellular compartments is osmotic pressure of electrolyte solutions.

The concentration of electrolytes in body fluids is often expressed as milliequivalents per liter (meq/l). This may be calculated from milligrams per liter as follows:

$$meq/l = \frac{mg/l \times valence}{atomic\ weight}$$

The milliequivalents per liter of plasma electrolytes varies within a relatively narrow range for healthy individuals. This range for sodium is 136 to 145 meq/l, and for potassium it is 3.5 to 5.0 meq/l.

The osmotic activity of a solution is measured in osmols or milliosmols (mOsm). Osmotic pressure is an indication of the work done in drawing fluid through a semipermeable membrane from an area of low concentration to an area of high concentration. Osmotic activity depends upon the number of particles present in solution without regard to the amount of charge they carry. The osmolarity of a solution may be estimated by determining the concentration, in millimoles per liter, of each different type of particle in the solution and adding these together for the total concentration, expressed as milliosmols. Osmotic activity may sometimes be expressed as osmolality, rather than osmolarity, then being mOsm per 1000 g solvent instead of mOsm per liter of solution. Normal human blood serum has an osmolarity of 285 to 295 mOsm/l.

Some electrolytes are found predominantly in intracellular fluid while others are in extracellular fluid. Table 10.1 gives an approximate indication of the electrolyte content of body fluid compartments. Active transport of solute across cell membranes is an important activity in body tissues. Sodium, the chief cation of extracellular fluid, is probably kept out of cells by means of an energy-requiring sodium pump. Potassium is the dominant intracellular cation.

Sodium ion is a key factor in maintaining osmotic equilibrium between intra- and extracellular fluids and thus affects distribution of body water. An increase in serum sodium concentration stimulates the release of antidiuretic hormone (ADH) with subsequent retention of water. ADH secretion is inhibited when serum sodium concentration is decreased below normal levels and diuresis results. A decrease in blood volume, intracellular water volume, or total body water leads to increased sodium reabsorption in the kidney tubules, under the influence of the renin-aldosterone system. When sodium is lost or retained by the body, it is accompanied by water. Sodium ion also functions as a buffer base in conjunction with bicarbonate and phosphate, and also aids in conduction of nerve impulses and muscle contractility.

Potassium is the most abundant electrolyte in the body and the chief regulator of intracellular osmolarity and electroneutrality. It supplies cations for organic anions of cell protoplasm. The small proportion of total body potassium (approximately 1.5 percent) in the extracellular compartment is extremely important for the function of cells, particularly neural

Table 10.1 ELECTROLYTE DISTRIBUTION IN BODY FLUID COMPARTMENTS*

		Extracellular (Approximate meq/l)		
Intracellular (Approximate meq/l)		Plasma	Interstitial Fluid	
Cations (205 meq)		Cations (154 meq)		Cations (154 meq)	
Na^+	10	Na^+	142	Na^+	145
K^+	160	K^+	4	K^+	4
Mg^{++}	35	Mg^{++}	3	Mg^{++}	2
		Ca^{++}	5	Ca^{++}	3
Anions (205 meq)		Anions (154 meq)		Anions (154 meq)	
Cl^-	2	Cl^-	103	Cl^-	115
HCO_3^-	8	HCO_3^-	27	HCO_3^-	30
HPO_4^{--}	140	HPO_4^{--}	2	HPO_4^{--}	2
$Protein^-$	55	SO_4^{--}	1	SO_4^{--}	1
		Organic acids⁻	5	Organic acids⁻	5
		$Protein^-$	16	$Protein^-$	1

* Adapted from Abbott Laboratories, 1973.

and muscle cells, since it is the ratio of the concentration of potassium in cells to that in the extracellular fluid that is the major determinant of the transmembrane potential (Suki, 1976). Either elevated or depressed levels of potassium in extracellular fluids block nerve impulses and interfere with muscle cell contraction, particularly heart muscle. Potassium levels are maintained within a relatively narrow range by renal mechanisms that include passive reabsorption of most of the filtered K^+ in the proximal tubule and secretion of K^+ in the distal tubule. An extrarenal mechanism involving aldosterone aids in adapting to chronic potassium loading with rapid uptake of K^+ by muscle (Suki, 1976). Aldosterone also influences potassium excretion by the colon.

Maintaining or establishing adequate composition of fluid and electrolytes in patients who suffer from a variety of diseases has become one of the most important functions of modern hospitals (Bruck, 1972). For effective management of fluid and electrolyte (osmolar) disturbances, an etiological diagnosis needs first to be established. According to Eklund et al. (1972) the general guiding principles for treatment include (1) providing an adequate supply of water and osmols, giving consideration to the mode of administration, the osmolarity of the solution given, and the time interval; (2) normalizing metabolism with a proper balance between anabolism and catabolism; (3) reducing or adequately replacing pathological extrarenal losses; and (4) constantly checking renal osmoregulation and the influence of treatment, if any, on it.

A fluid and electrolyte disturbance is affected by treatment the patient receives. In fact, treatment can fully determine the type of disturbance. For example, hypoosmolarity will develop in a burned patient treated mainly with electrolyte-free solutions, whereas he may become hyperosmolar if he is given hyperosmolar solutions in excess. Parenterally administered fluids must always contain some osmols to avoid hemolysis of blood cells. The water in these solutions does not become available to the body as free water until the osmolar substances in the solutions are removed. Giving isotonic glucose solutions will provide free water to the body after the glucose has been taken up and metabolized by body cells (Eklund et al., 1972).

10.2 Acid-Base Balance

Acid-base balance should be evaluated in conjunction with electrolyte status. A number of commonly measured physiological parameters, for example, P_{CO_2} (partial pressure of carbon dioxide), pH, and HCO_3^- (bicarbonate) concentration, give an indication of the acid-base status of the body when properly interpreted. The normal acid-base regulating mechanisms usually maintain the pH of blood within a precise range (7.35 to 7.45). However, a number of disease states can markedly affect these mechanisms and produce imbalance. These include (1) congestive heart failure with hypoxemia, sodium and water retention, and complications of potassium loss from use of certain diuretics; (2) cor pulmonale with hypoxemia and respiratory acidosis or alkalosis; (3) myocardial infarction with hypoxemia that is variably associated with metabolic acidosis; (4) strokes causing dehydration and hyperventilation; (5) peptic ulcer with severe vomiting, resulting in hypochloremic alkalosis and dehydration, and electrolyte depletion; (7) lactic acidosis resulting from impaired glucose oxidation, hypoxia, and circulatory insufficiency; and (8) kidney infection with impaired renal function resulting in acidosis, dehydration, and azotemia (Fleischer, 1974).

The principal acid-base regulating mechanisms of the body are (1) buffer systems; (2) respiratory regulation of oxygen-carbon dioxide exchange between cells, lungs, and external environment; and (3) selective elimination of ions by the kidneys. The body's first line of defense in adjusting an acid-base imbalance is buffering and dilution. Respiratory compensation might be called the second line of defense, with renal compensation following and acting on a long-term basis.

In the Bronsted-Lowry classification, any substance that can function as a proton donor is considered an acid and those substances that act as proton acceptors are considered bases. Buffers are substances that, in solution, can resist change in H^+ concentration by combining with certain amounts of either added acid or alkali. The buffer systems of the body can be divided into two groups: (1) the bicarbonate system which involves H_2CO_3 (carbonic acid) and HCO_3^- as its buffer pair; and (2) the nonbicarbonate system which consists mainly of hemoglobin, plasma proteins, and organic and inorganic phosphates. The bicarbonate system differs from the others since its acid member, H_2CO_3, is in equilibrium with a volatile gas, CO_2. In addition, CO_2 differs from the other fixed or nonvolatile acids in several respects. It readily permeates cell membranes and thus influences intracellular H^+ concentration; large amounts of CO_2 are being produced continuously by metabolic processes; and CO_2 is rapidly and continuously excreted by the lungs (Siegel, 1973).

Carbon dioxide is transported in the body chiefly as bicarbonate. It diffuses from the tissue cells to the interstitial fluid and then to the plasma. In the plasma, a small amount of CO_2 slowly forms H_2CO_3 which ionizes to produce H^+ and HCO_3^-, and the H^+ is then buffered by systems in the blood. Most of the CO_2, however, diffuses into the red blood cells where H_2CO_3 is rapidly formed by the action of carbonic anhydrase. The H_2CO_3 dissociates and the H^+ is taken up by hemoglobin as oxygen is released from this molecule to the tissues. While H^+ is being held by the hemoglobin molecule, much of the HCO_3^- moves out of the red blood cell to the plasma and Cl^- moves in. In the lungs, H^+ is released from hemoglobin, as the heme is oxygenated, and combines with HCO_3^- again to form H_2CO_3. The H_2CO_3 is rapidly broken down by carbonic anhydrase and the resulting CO_2 excreted through the lungs.

The kidneys aid in maintaining acid-base balance through the processes of HCO_3^- reabsorption, generation of H^+, and production of ammonia (NH_3). In the renal tubule cell, H_2CO_3 is formed and the H^+ dissociated from it may be exchanged for Na^+ coming in from the lumen of the tubule. The Na^+ is returned, along with HCO_3^-, to the plasma. Excreted H^+ acidifies buffer salts, particularly phosphates, in the urine. The tubule cell also forms ammonia, from deamination of certain amino acids, which diffuses into the tubular urine and reacts with H^+ to form NH_4^+ which is excreted.

Acid-base imbalances result from physiologic or metabolic derangements and are not simple biochemical abnormalities of the blood. Acidosis and alkalosis may refer to conditions where the total buffer base is decreased or increased, respectively. They become clinically detectable when one or more of the body's compensatory mechanisms are no longer able to resist a change in pH. Four basic forms of acid-base imbalance have been described on a clinical basis. Metabolic acidosis or alkalosis result from metabolic problems, whereas respiratory acidosis or alkalosis are of pulmonary origin (Fleischer, 1974; Siegel, 1973), as follows:

1.   Respiratory acidosis is caused primarily by the inability of alveolar ventilation to excrete CO_2 as rapidly as is required. The direction of change in plasma parameters is given in Table 10.2. The most common causes of respiratory acidosis are chronic obstructive pulmonary diseases and overuse of respiratory depressant drugs. A renal mechanism, taking days to develop fully, responds to respiratory acidosis with an increased reabsorption of Na^+ and HCO_3^- and an increased secretion of Cl^- and H^+.

2.   Metabolic acidosis may be caused by increased production, ingestion, or infusion of noncarbonic acid; decreased renal excretion of H^+; loss of HCO_3^- or other conjugate base from extracellular fluid; or an ingress of H^+ from the intracellular to the extracellular fluid. Diabetic acidosis is a cause of increased production of organic acids. Excess production of lactic acid occurs in severe hypoxemia. Severe diarrheas and fistulas causing loss of bowel content result in loss of HCO_3^- and other conjugate bases. Acidosis results from uremia because renal H^+ excretion is deficient. Ingestion of NH_4Cl may cause acidosis because it is metabolized to urea by the liver with a net yield of one mole of H^+ per mole of metabolized NH_4^+.

Table 10.2   PLASMA PARAMETERS INDICATING ACID-BASE IMBALANCE*

	P_{CO_2} (arterial)	$[H^+]$	pH	HCO_3^-	Total CO_2 Content
Normal range	38–42 mm Hg	38–42 nmoles/l	7.37–7.42	23–25 meq/l	26–28 meq/l
Respiratory acidosis	↑	↑	↓	(↑)†	↑
Respiratory alkalosis	↓	↓	↑	(↓)	↓
Metabolic acidosis	(↓)	↑	↓	↓	↓
Metabolic alkalosis	(↑)	↓	↑	↑	↑

* Adapted from Fleischer, 1974; Siegel, 1973.
† Compensatory changes are in parentheses.

Hydrogen ion concentration increases in metabolic acidosis and pH decreases. The buffer systems of the blood act immediately to reduce the acid load and there is a decrease in HCO_3^-. Compensatory hyperventilation lowers the P_{CO_2}. The kidney compensates by increased excretion of H^+.

3. Respiratory alkalosis may result from alveolar ventilation in excess of the existing need of the body for CO_2 elimination. Alveolar hyperventilation may be produced by certain drugs and may occur in anxious or tense patients for no apparent reason. Fever and shock may also cause hyperventilation. The direction of change in plasma parameters is shown in Table 10.2. Renal compensatory mechanisms operate if respiratory alkalosis persists for several days.

4. Metabolic alkalosis may be caused by excessive loss of noncarbonic acid from the body, such as loss of acid gastric juice in severe or prolonged vomiting. This may also occur with certain types of external fistulas and in patients receiving gastric suction. When too much Na^+ and HCO_3^- are retained by the kidney, as during excessive use of mineralocorticoid hormones or in diseases where these hormones are produced in excess, metabolic alkalosis may result, as also with excessive intake of conjugate bases such as $NaHCO_3$ or $CaCO_3$.

Any excess of conjugate base added to the extracellular fluid will rapidly lead to a relatively large increase in HCO_3^- concentration and a decrease in H^+ concentration. The pH increases as buffering mechanisms become inadequate. Compensatory retention of CO_2 through respiratory response is variable. In uncomplicated acute metabolic alkalosis the kidney rapidly excretes excess HCO_3^-. The renal response is subject to many other influences in chronic metabolic alkalosis that complicate its compensatory response.

10.3   Tube Feeding

When efforts to ensure an adequate oral intake have been unsuccessful and the patient's gastrointestinal tract is still functioning normally, a tube feeding may be appropriately initiated. Reasons why patients may be unable to consume food orally include problems in swallowing due to facial injuries, fractures of the jaw, stricture of the esophagus, weakness of the muscles of mastication from various neurological disorders, or the presence of a tracheostomy (Peaston, 1967). Radical surgery of the upper alimentary tract, neck, upper respiratory system, and oral pharynx may limit oral food intake, as do paralysis, unconsciousness, and mental disturbances. Some patients, for various reasons, may simply refuse to eat. A survey of 121 patients in Hawaii, California, and Washington who had received nasogastric tube feedings for at least four days each, with a total of 1730 days of tube feeding, revealed the most common diagnoses to be head and neck carcinoma (40 percent) and disorders of the central nervous system (32 percent). Nearly half of all study subjects were confused, semiconscious, or comatose (Walike, 1975).

Tube feeding is most commonly administered via a pliable, nonirritating nasogastric tube of the smallest gauge that will allow the feeding to flow freely. The tube may be inserted through the mouth when there is a nasal injury or a grossly deviated nasal septum (Kaminski, 1973). In special cases where tube feeding will be long term or when the esophagus is severely damaged, gastrostomy feedings may be employed. Jejunostomy feedings may also be used.

Types of Tube Feedings

As early as 1598, indication was recorded for the use of nasogastric tube feeding as an alternative to oral alimentation. Milk, broth, and wine were the first substances given (Walike, 1975). In the 1950s Barron reported on the use of blenderized natural whole foods, including a mixture of meat, vegetables, fruits, complex carbohydrates, eggs, fats, and oils prepared in the hospital dietary department. Since these mixtures were too viscous to flow through tubes by gravity force, use of the Barron food pump was introduced (Schuman, 1972). The food industry has since developed nutritionally balanced blenderized formulas for use in tube feeding. Table 10.3 lists several commercial products that are suitable for tube and sometimes oral feeding. In addition to blenderized formulas, they include milk-based formulas, lactose-free formulas, protein hydrolysates or amino acid mixtures, formulas containing medium-chain triglycerides, and chemically defined formulas.

Nutritionally complete liquid diets made with nutrients in purified form are available commercially. They have commonly been called "chemically defined" or "elemental" diets. Since they are not elemental in a strict sense and vary widely in composition, the alternative designation of "defined-formula" diets has been suggested (Chernoff and Bloch, 1977). The osmolarity of many of these products is high because of the small molecules in true solution. The use of complex oligosaccharide decreases the tendency of the high simple sugar mixtures to cause diarrhea or the dumping syndrome. Symptoms of dumping syndrome include weakness, palpitation, and pallor and occur when a hyperosmolar mixture rapidly pours into the small intestine. The nutrients provided in defined-formula diet mixtures require little or no digestion, are readily absorbed by a relatively small portion of the gut, and have a low residue for excretion (Kark, 1974). Defined-formula diet mixtures with high-nitrogen content are also available.

Miller and Taboada (1975) tested the use of an "elemental" diet of defined composition and simple chemical form on a variety of surgical patients. The complete absorption in the upper gastrointestinal tract and minimal fecal residue were especially advantageous for patients undergoing abdominal surgery. Haddad et al. (1974) reported on a patient who had recurrent subacute intestinal obstruction, weight loss, and malnutrition following intensive radiation therapy for peritoneal carcinomatosis. Her symptoms resolved and her nutritional status improved while she was maintained for more than 8 months on a defined-formula diet exclusively. Successful use of a defined formula diet has been reported in the nutritional management of fistulas of the alimentary tract (Bury et al., 1971).

Problems and Complications of Tube Feeding

Gastrointestinal problems associated with tube feeding may range from mild distress to incapacitating diarrhea. Diarrhea may be caused by bacterial contamination, a formula high in osmolarity, excessive lactose in the formula, too rapid introduction of the feeding, improper insertion of the feeding tube, and administration of cold feedings. A formula with high osmolarity is rapidly diluted to a more isotonic solution in the gastrointestinal tract by fluid shifting from the blood to the intestine. Excessive fluid movement can stimulate peristalsis and diarrhea if the patient has not been gradually introduced to a relatively concentrated formula (Gormican and Liddy, 1973).

In a double-blind experiment, Walike and Walike (1973) administered by nasogastric tube two diets, differing only in the presence or absence of 7 percent lactose, to 11 patients. Each diet was given to each patient for approximately 10 consecutive days. Increased frequency of stools and more liquid stools were noted in nine patients while on the lactose-containing diet. Only two of these patients showed classical lactose intolerance. The others had a relative lactose intolerance that was clinically apparent only when they ingested a large quantity of lactose in the milk-based tube feeding.

Goldenberg and Saperstein (1976) used a presterilized milk-based formula with relatively low osmolarity (400 mOsmol per liter) as a tube feeding for 21 postoperative or post-trauma patients over a period of 2 to 3 weeks. Good tolerance to this formula was noted in all patients. Only one subject displayed a loose stool. There were no indications of dumping syndrome or regurgitation. Measurement of stool pH, with either neutral or slightly alkaline reactions, indicated that lactose was not being fermented in the intestinal tract. The low osmolarity and freedom from bacterial contamination were probably important factors in the successful use of this milk-based formula.

Hypernatremia, hyperchloremia, azotemia, and dehydration have been described as complications of nasogastric tube feeding, and this combination of clinical findings has sometimes been called the *tube-feeding syndrome* (Walike, 1969). Symptoms may be minimal. Thirst is often masked because of the body's adaptation to the hypertonicity. Weight loss, increased hematocrit, and increased serum osmolarity may be noted. Progression of this syndrome will lead to mental deterioration, fever, and tachycardia. Walike (1969) described a case of the syndrome in a 70-year-old man who underwent surgery for carcinoma of the larynx and was started on a nasogastric tube feeding the third postoperative day. By the

Table 10.3 SELECTED TUBE AND ORAL LIQUID DIET PREPARATIONS*

Product	Kcal/ml	mOsm/kg	Protein Sources	g Protein per 1000 kcal	Carbohydrate Sources	g Carbohydrate per 1000 kcal	Fat Sources	g Fat per 1000 kcal
Meat-containing Formulas								
Compleat B† (Doyle)	1.00	490	Beef Nonfat milk	40.0	Sucrose Maltodextrin Vegetables Fruits Orange juice	120.0	Corn oil	40.0
Formula 2† (Cutter)	1.00	435–510	Nonfat milk Beef	37.5	Sucrose Vegetables Orange juice Farina Dextrose	122.5	Corn oil Egg yolk	40.0
Milk-base Formulas								
Meritene (liquid) (Doyle)	1.00	700–750	Concentrated skim milk Casein	60.0	Corn syrup solids Sucrose	115.0	Vegetable oil	33.3
Sustacal (liquid) (Mead Johnson)	1.00	625	Concentrated skim milk Casein Soy protein	60.3	Sucrose Corn syrup solids	137.8	Soy oil	23.0
Nutri-1000 (Syntex)	1.06	500	Skim milk	38.0	Sucrose Corn syrup solids	95.6	Corn oil	52.0

Table 10.3 SELECTED TUBE AND ORAL LIQUID DIET PREPARATIONS* (cont'd.)

Product	Kcal/ml	mOsm/kg	Protein Sources	g Protein per 1000 kcal	Carbohydrate Sources	g Carbohydrate per 1000 kcal	Fat Sources	g Fat per 1000 kcal
Low Lactose Formulas								
Ensure (Ross)	1.06	450	Casein Soy protein	35.0	Corn syrup solids Sucrose	136.7	Corn oil	35.0
Mull-soy (Syntex)	0.66	252	Soy flour	48.0	Sucrose Invert sugar	79.5	Soy oil	55.5
Hydrolyzed Protein or Amino Acid Formulas								
Nutramigen (Mead Johnson)	0.66	443	Hydrolyzed casein	32.5	Sucrose Tapioca starch	130.0	Corn oil	39.0
Vivonex (Eaton)	1.00	500	Crystalline amino acids	20.4	Glucose oligo-saccharides	226.3	Safflower oil	1.4
Flexical (Mead Johnson)	1.00	723	Hydrolyzed casein Amino acids	22.4	Sugar Dextrin Citrate	154.0	Soy oil (27.4) MCT (6.6)	34.0
Medium-chain Triglyceride (MCT) Formulas								
Portagen (Mead Johnson)	1.00	357	Casein	35.0	Malto-dextrin Sucrose	115.0	MCT (41.0) Corn oil (5.5) Lecithin (1.3)	47.8
Progestimil (Mead Johnson)	0.66	590	Hydrolyzed casein	32.5	Glucose Tapioca starch	130.0	MCT (36.6) Corn oil (5.2)	41.8

* Adapted from Shils et al. (1976).
† Moderate residue; all other formulas listed are low residue.

sixth day he was somnolent and was in a confused state by the seventh day. Treatment consisted of withdrawal or reduction of the tube feeding with its high content of protein and the administration of adequate water to remove the solute load. Gault et al. (1973) also reported on three cases of hypernatremia, azotemia, and severe dehydration in elderly men resulting from the use of a high-protein tube feeding. The hypernatremia in these cases was due predominantly to dehydration and not to excess salt intake.

The important constituent of tube feedings that is implicated in development of the tube-feeding syndrome is protein. Diets containing more than 70 g per liter of protein should be given with care. Fat cannot be incorporated during the processing of a dehydrated mixture because of problems with rancidity and, therefore, protein and carbohydrate content tends to be high in these products. Tube-fed patients must be given enough fluid so that acceptable urinary output is maintained and dietary waste products from protein metabolism can be excreted (Gormican and Liddy, 1973). Particularly in tube-fed patients who are unconscious or who, for other reasons, cannot experience thirst, monitoring would ideally include serial determinations of the level of blood urea nitrogen, creatinine, electrolytes, hematocrit, urine specific gravity, and body weight (Gault et al., 1973).

Special attention should be given to providing all essential nutrients in tube feedings. Gormican et al. (1973) reported on successful use of a nutritionally balanced, fortified, milk-based tube feeding for three persons over a period of 2 years or longer. A clinical study of eight immobilized patients tube-fed the same type of preparation showed positive nitrogen balances in all subjects and excellent absorption of seven essential inorganic elements (Gormican and Catli, 1972). The caloric content of a tube feeding should be adjusted to meet the needs of the individual patient, and immobilized patients may require lower caloric levels than active ones. As calories are reduced, however, care must be taken to maintain adequate levels of essential nutrients.

The placement of the feeding tube and the rate of flow through the tube are factors that may cause problems for the patient. Markings placed on the tubes by the manufacturers are helpful in determining proper placement. A rapid delivery rate may produce distention, nausea, cramps, and diarrhea (Gormican and Liddy, 1973).

Selection of Tube-Feeding Formulas

Gormican (1975) suggested that commercial products may be advantageously used over hospital-prepared products because (1) commercial processing reduces the probability of gross bacterial contamination at the time of feeding; (2) hospital food service labor costs are reduced; (3) commercially available tube feedings provide some certainty about diet standardization and known nutrient composition, and they contain essential nutrients in which institutionally prepared diets may be lacking; (4) osmolarity of the mixture can be controlled more effectively; and (5) individualized concentrations can be furnished for the patient who has digestive and absorptive insufficiency. However, commercial products may still be inappropriately chosen and used under unsanitary conditions or in inadequate amounts. Chernoff and Block (1977), on the other hand, pointed out that "fixed" commercial formulas are limited in adaptability to individual needs, and, in some cases, dietitians may need to cooperate with physicians in designing special feeding formulas.

Decisions as to what commercial products will be used in a hospital should be made after careful review of available products and input from all involved members of the health care team. Cost, packaging, shelf life, nutrient composition, nutritional precautions required with use, nutrient omissions, and osmolarity should all be evaluated. Palatability may be important if some tube feedings are used as oral supplements. The unpleasant aftertaste that occurs from some tube feedings should also be considered in the selection process (Gormican, 1975).

Several factors should be considered when deciding upon the individual prescription for a tube feeding, including (1) the digestive and absorptive capacity of the patient's alimentary tract; (2) the adequacy of renal function; (3) the effect of various forms of therapy, past or present, on tolerance and utilization of the formula; (4) medications; (5) present nutritional status; (6) present or anticipated problems with electrolyte balance; (7) underlying disorders such as atherosclerosis and coronary heart disease that might influence composition of the feeding; and (8) how the prescription may be translated into a well-tolerated, nutritionally adequate diet that may be administered through a small tube (Gormican and Liddy, 1973).

Gormican and Liddy (1973) have suggested characteristics of an ideal tube feeding as:

Low cost

Bacteriologic safety

Relatively low osmolarity

Caloric density equivalent to 1 kcal/ml

Suitable protein-calorie ratio

Adequate but not excessive nutrient intake with nutrients present in nontoxic ratios and amounts

Balanced nutrient composition, including electrolyte content, proper balance of amino acids, and well-utilized supplementary sources of nutrients

Nutritional adequacy for short-term use and, when indicated, for long-term feeding

Convenience and ease of administration

Suitable viscosity and homogenization

[handwritten notes in top margin: 1-2 read; 2-4 notes Com Bal; 4-6 old notes; 6-8 sleep; 8-10 review]

10.4   Parenteral Nutrition

The primary purpose of parenteral feeding is to maintain an adequate nutritional state in patients who cannot utilize food through the alimentary tract. Meng (1975) suggested the following indications for parenteral nutrition:

1. Abnormality of gastrointestinal tract
    (*a*) Ingestion of food impossible or unwise, e.g., obstruction, peritonitis
    (*b*) Inability to retain ingested food, e.g., vomiting, diarrhea, fistula
    (*c*) Impaired digestion and absorption, e.g., malabsorption syndromes
    (*d*) Trauma or elective surgery
    (*e*) Edema due to severe malnutrition

2. Preparation for surgery in nutritionally depleted and emaciated patients

3. After surgery or trauma, especially burns and multiple fractures

4. Congenital anomalies in the neonate before and after surgery

5. Coma, anorexia nervosa, or refusal to eat

6. Supplementation of inadequate oral feeding in patients with cancer, especially those receiving chemotherapy or radiation therapy and those with renal or hepatic failure

History

During the 1800s some injections into the blood stream of certain salts were reported and, in 1873, three cholera patients were treated by giving milk intravenously (Allen and Lee, 1969). The concepts of sterility and asepsis had to be accepted, however, before the circulatory system could become a feasible route for nutrient administration. Physiological principles regulating water and electrolyte overload, hemolysis, and immune response were also limiting factors to the practical use of intravenous feeding. Dextrose and water solutions have been given intravenously throughout much of the twentieth century and they are the basis of most parenteral infusion programs. The preparation of nontoxic protein hydrolysates as nitrogen sources became available in the 1930s and pure amino acid preparations were subsequently developed. Fat emulsions have more recently been used (Michener and Law, 1970).

Parenteral nutrition entered a new era in the late 1960s when infusions of hyperosmolar solutions containing glucose, amino acids, vitamins, and electrolytes were given via an indwelling catheter in a central vein. Although side effects of lipid infusions limited their use in the United States for several years, a lipid emulsion for intravenous use is now available and can contribute to the complete nutritional maintenance of a patient (Meng, 1975).

Nutrients for Intravenous Feeding

The body can tolerate a loss of fluid for only a short period of time before symptoms of dehydration appear, and intravenous infusions are commonly used to maintain a proper state of hydration. Many factors influence the loss of fluid from the body and make it difficult to estimate the minimum need for water. In the absence of fever and abnormal losses, total daily water intake should be 1.5 to 2.0 liters for adults and 0.5–2.0 liters for infants and children. In calculating fluid balance, consideration must be given to the water produced by metabolism in body cells (Wretlind, 1972).

Several sources of nitrogen have been used in intravenous feeding. From a nutritional standpoint, whole blood is not the most effective source of nutrients and should be reserved for correction of blood loss. Plasma is also a source of protein (about 60 g per liter) but it is not as efficiently converted to other forms of tissue protein as are amino acid preparations (Allen and Lee, 1969). Protein hydrolysates of casein and blood fibrin are available commercially for intravenous feeding. The loss via urine of amino acids and low molecular weight peptides from casein hydrolysate is about 10 percent (Wretlind, 1972). Ghadimi et al. (1971) have shown that the intravenous administration of protein hydrolysates produces a distorted plasma amino acid pattern. This has also been shown to be true for an amino acid preparation (Ghadimi, 1973). The significance of these findings has not been clarified.

Crystalline amino acid mixtures are widely used in parenteral feeding and appear to be reasonably well utilized for the synthesis of body protein when the requirement of essential amino acids is met. Amino acid requirements for parenteral therapy are not well defined, however. It appears, because of the role of the liver in selective catabolism of some amino acids given orally, that the optimal amino acid pattern for intravenous feedings may differ from that for oral consumption. For example, parenteral mixtures should possibly have higher levels of the branched-chain amino acids (isoleucine, leucine, and valine) relative to the other essential amino acids because the amino acid spectrum emerging from the liver into the general circulation for an individual on oral feedings tends to be richer in these amino acids (Munro, 1972). According to Wretlind (1972), some of the most satisfactory results in humans have been obtained when the parenteral amino acid mixture contains all of the essential and 10 to 12 of the nonessential amino acids. He has further suggested that an optimal amino acid preparation for intravenous feeding should contain the essential as well as the nonessential amino acids in the L form and in the same proportions as found in the aminogram of body proteins or other proteins with high biological value, with the essential amino acids making up about 45 to 50 percent of the total amino acids. More research is needed to provide authoratative answers to many questions concerning optimal parenteral amino acid nutrition.

The total kilocalories infused depend upon individual needs. They must cover the requirements of basal metabolism plus physical activity, with allowance for growth in infants and children. When the feeding solution contains more than 20 to 25 percent glucose or is infused at too rapid a rate, there is some loss of calories in the urine due to osmotic diuresis. Carbohydrate and fat are the important sources of energy. The extent to which parenterally administered amino acids are utilized is directly proportional to the caloric supply. Chen et al. (1974) reported that the required caloric intake for complete utilization of 1 g nitrogen is approximately 450 total kcal or 425 nonprotein kcal.

Glucose is often used in intravenous infusions. Fructose may also be used, although rapid infusion of this sugar has been reported to produce lactic acidemia. The sugar alcohols, sorbitol and xylitol, have been used instead of the sugars in intravenous feeding. There seems to be no advantage to their use from a nutritional standpoint (Wretlind, 1972).

Fat is the most concentrated source of kilocalories and greatly increases the ease with which adequate kilocalories can be supplied intravenously, allowing a large amount of energy in a small volume of isotonic fluid. These infusions do not cause diuresis with nutrient losses in urine and thrombophlebitis occurs very infrequently. Fat is a source of essential fatty acids, without which deficiency symptoms may develop.

A fat emulsion for intravenous nutrition contains a vegetable oil in water and emulsifiers to stabilize the emulsion. Several products containing either cottonseed oil or soybean oil are available internationally. However, only one product, Intralipid, is available in the United States. It contains soybean oil with egg yolk phospholipids as emulsifiers and glycerol to obtain isotonicity. The fat emulsions appear to be utilized in much the same way as fat from food taken orally (Wretlind, 1972).

Sufficient controlled clinical studies on the safety and efficacy of 10 percent Intralipid have been completed to allow its approval by the U.S. Food and Drug Administration. Minor side effects that have been reported in adults include sleepiness, nausea, and elevated serum enzyme levels. Side effects observed among pediatric patients were somewhat more numerous and severe, occurring in 12 out of 177 children, and included hepatosplenomegaly, hyperlipidemia, and thrombocytopenia (Hidalgo, 1976). Studies on normal subjects infused with 10 percent Intralipid indicated that serum triglyceride concentration increased to maximal levels of 339 ± 102 mg/100 ml at the completion of the infusion and returned to basal levels in most subjects within 4 hours (Greene et al., 1976). Freund et al. (1975) cautioned against the administration of Intralipid in daily doses exceeding 2 g of fat per kg body weight, particularly to patients with impaired liver function. They reported the presence at autopsy of free fat droplets and extreme foamy swelling of the cytoplasm of the reticuloendothelial cells in all examined organs for a 44-year-old severely mal-nourished male who had been infused with Intralipid as the main source of kilocalories in long-term therapy. Careful monitoring of patients on Intralipid by liver function tests and serum lipid levels was recommended.

Sodium is of special importance in maintaining appropriate electrolyte concentrations of extracellular fluid for patients receiving intravenous solutions. Body losses of sodium will vary considerably and need should be met on an individual basis. Wretlind (1972) recommended for complete intravenous nutrition in adults a basal daily sodium supply of between 1 and 1.4 $m$mol per kg body weight. Potassium must also be supplied on a daily basis for patients receiving total parenteral nutrition (TPN). Hypophosphatemia may occur with TPN and phosphate must be included. Requirements for minerals, including trace minerals, in ill patients receiving parenteral feedings have not been extensively studied. However, all essential minerals must be provided when parenteral feeding is long term. Jeejeebhoy et al. (1977) reported a chromium deficiency, corrected by supplementation, in a patient on TPN for more than 5 years.

All essential vitamins must be provided in TPN. Arbitrary amounts of vitamins generally have been used in clinical practice and are available in water-soluble dispersions. The water soluble ones, particularly, should be given to any patient if his or her nutrition is dependent solely on clear liquids or parenteral fluids for more than a few days. Thiamin hydrochloride is often administered prophylactically to alcoholic patients but may be omitted for poorly nourished hospitalized nonalcoholic patients. Nadel and Burger (1976) reported two cases of Wernicke encephalopathy, a disorder of thiamin deficiency manifested by confusion, ataxia, ophthalmoplegia, coma, and death, in nonalcoholic female patients who were maintained for several weeks on 5 percent dextrose and 0.45 percent saline solutions intravenously and only clear liquids by mouth. No vitamins were given, although requirements for thiamin increase in proportion to the carbohydrate content of the diet (Shils, 1964).

Limitations of Conventional Intravenous Feeding

It is important not to substantially change the osmotic pressure of the blood when intravenous infusions are given. Therefore, solutions given in peripheral veins should be isotonic. This limits infusions to 5 percent or 10 percent glucose and electrolyte solutions. Higher concentrations may lead to inflammation and occlusion of the veins as well as blood clotting. Some amino acids can be given. However, it is impossible with these limitations on glucose concentration to provide sufficient kilocalories to permit effective utilization of the administered amino acids for protein synthesis unless very large volumes of water are infused. The body cannot usually handle more than approximately 3 liters of water daily. Giving 3 liters of a 5 percent glucose solution provides only 600 kcal and a similar amount of 10 percent solution yields 1200 kcal. Therefore, conventional intravenous feeding, as usually given, cannot maintain a patient in an optimal nutritional state. Conventional parenteral feeding is incapable of improving the condition of the already malnourished patient for similar reasons (Shils, 1972).

With the availability of fat emulsions for intravenous feeding, it may be possible to give, by peripheral vein, sufficient kilocalories in isotonic form to spare protein and achieve adequate nourishment. Coran (1972) described successful treatment of infants using a crystalline amino acid solution as the nitrogen source and a soybean oil emulsion as the major source of kilocalories with the mixture being given in a peripheral vein.

Total Parenteral Nutrition (TPN)

Although the term *hyperalimentation* appeared in the early literature concerned with the process of providing a patient total nutrition by an intravenous route, the preferred terms are *total parenteral nutrition* or *total parenteral alimentation*. Hyperalimentation may give the impression that kilocalories and essential nutrients should be provided in larger amounts than those indicated for maintenance of normal body weight and nutrition (Shils, 1972).

The use of TPN is indicated only when oral or tube feeding is contraindicated or is inadequate and when conventional parenteral support is not sufficient for the needs of the patient. Under these circumstances, this form of nutrition may be lifesaving for a variety of clinical situations, including obstructive lesions of the gastrointestinal tract where surgical intervention must be delayed; massive bowel resections prior to use of tube or oral feeding; gastrointestinal fistulas; hypermetabolic states associated with extensive burns, major trauma, and severe infections; acute stages of inflammatory bowel disease; severe uncontrolled malabsorptive states with undernutrition; congenital anomalies in the neonate prior to surgery; and prolonged coma where hope for recovery is entertained and the danger of aspiration negates tube feeding (Shils, 1972).

In the 1960s a group of researchers at the University of Pennsylvania (Wilmore and Dudrick, 1968; Dudrick et al., 1968) demonstrated, on both humans and experimental animals, that adequate nutrition and normal growth could be maintained by exclusive use of the intravenous route. This is achieved by use of an indwelling central venous catheter for the infusion of hypertonic solutions of glucose and amino acids. The catheter is inserted into the right subclavian vein and pushed along until the tip of the catheter is in the superior vena cava, as shown in Fig. 10.1. The catheter can also be inserted through the left subclavian vein or one of the jugular veins (Dudrick and Rhoads, 1972). Sterile concentrated hyperosmolar solutions of glucose and amino acids may be administered via a central vein because the large blood flow in this area allows rapid dilution.

The greatest hazard associated with indwelling catheters is infection, the incidence of infection being correlated with the length of time the catheter is in place. Aseptic techniques and proper maintenance will minimize the danger of infection (Shils, 1972). Other complications of cen-

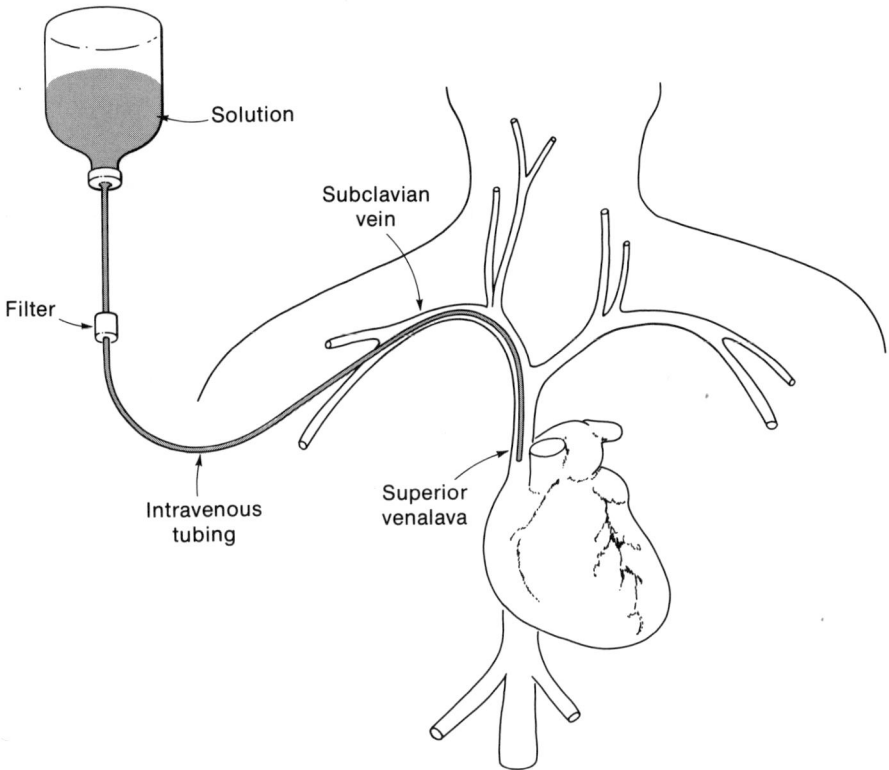

Fig. 10.1 A catheter is inserted into the right subclavian vein with the tip pushed to the superior vena cava. The high volume of blood flowing in this vein rapidly dilutes a concentrated solution given intravenously.

tral venous catheters include perforation of the heart and major vessels, with extravasation of blood or solutions; obstruction of the major vessels; pneumothorax; and air embolism. Thrombophlebitis may also develop around the catheter (Meng, 1975).

Hyperglycemia may be a problem when concentrated glucose solutions are given, particularly in patients with some degree of glucose intolerance. Hyperglycemia may lead to osmotic diuresis, dehydration, and nonketotic hyperosmolar syndrome progressing to coma. Insulin may be given, although hypoglycemia has been observed with excessive insulin administration when technical failure of the infusion system occurs. Elevation of blood urea nitrogen may result from excessive administration of nitrogen or from dehydration. Hyperammonemia may also occur as a result of free ammonia in protein hydrolysates or an inadequate amount of arginine in amino acid solutions. Too much glycine in amino acid mixtures may also cause hyperammonemia (Meng, 1975). Essential fatty acid deficiencies in both adults and children on TPN for 6 to 23 weeks have been reported (Caldwell et al., 1972; Richardson and Sgoutas, 1975; Fleming et al., 1976). Zinc deficiency was observed by Arakawa et al. (1976) in two infants receiving TPN for chronic diarrhea. Treatment with zinc resulted in a rapid decrease in deficiency signs.

To achieve optimal results with TPN, all essential nutrients must be supplied in amounts needed by the individual patient. Electrolyte imbalance may result from administration of a standard solution without consideration of individual needs (Meng, 1975). Kilocalories should be adequate to maintain ideal weight (adults normally about 30 kcal per kg) or increased to achieve weight gain where desirable. Shils (1972) recommended that prior to beginning TPN, the patient's nutritional requirements should be evaluated and her tolerance for fluid, nitrogen, glucose, and minerals (especially sodium and potassium) be reviewed in light of cardiovascular, renal, gastrointestinal, and endocrine status. Reevaluation should be made daily during treatment. He has used a daily basic formula with casein hydrolysate that contains 2150 kcal, 134 meq sodium, 100 meq potassium, 160 meq chloride, 295 mg calcium, 20 meq magnesium, and 350 mg phosphorus. A trace element solution includes 0.62 g zinc chloride, 0.60 g cupric sulfate $\cdot$ $5H_2O$, 0.20 g manganous sulfate $\cdot$ H_2O, and 0.01 g sodium iodide. Daily average vitamin intake for adults with the basic formula includes:

Thiamin, mg	18.6	Biotin, μg	57.0
Riboflavin, mg	7.1	Ascorbic acid, mg	215.0
Niacin, mg	33.6	Vitamin A, IU	2,860.0
Pyridoxine, mg	10.7	Vitamin D, IU	286.0
Pantothenate, mg	14.3	Vitamin E, IU	1.4
Folic acid, mg	0.4	Vitamin K, mg	0.7
Vitamin B_{12}, μg	2.1		

Adjustments to the basic formula may be made on an individual basis. Commercially available materials can be used in a sterile closed system to prepare individual formulas (Shils, 1972). As more information becomes available concerning the specific nutrient requirements for intravenous feeding, formulation of TPN solutions may be made on a more rational basis. In the meantime, TPN has proven to be of undisputed value in improving and maintaining the nutritional status of patients who cannot ingest food orally or by tube. Safe application of TPN for patients living at home has been described by Shils (1975).

REFERENCES

1. Abbott Laboratories. 1973. Fluid and electrolytes.

2. Allen, P. C. and H. A. Lee. 1969. *A Clinical Guide to Intravenous Nutrition.* Oxford, Eng.: Blackwell Scientific Publications.

3. Arakawa, T., T. Tamura, Y. Igarashi, H. Suzuki, and H. H. Sandstead. 1976. Zinc deficiency in two infants during total parenteral alimentation for diarrhea. *Am. J. Clin. Nutr.,* **29:** 197.

4. Barron, J. 1956. Preparation of natural foods for tube feeding. *Henry Ford Hosp. Med. Bull.,* **4:** 18.

5. Barron, J. 1953. Tube feedings with liquified natural foods. *Henry Ford Hosp. Med. Bull.,* **1:** 21.

6. Bruck, E. 1972. Fluid and electrolyte therapy. *Ped. Clin. No. Am.,* **19:** 193.

7. Bury, K. D., R. V. Stephens, and H. T. Randall. 1971. Use of a chemically defined, liquid, elemental diet for nutritional management of fistulas of the alimentary tract. *Am. J. Surg.,* **121:** 174.

8. Caldwell, M. D., H. T. Jonsson, and H. B. Othersen, Jr. 1972. Essential fatty acid deficiency in an infant receiving prolonged parenteral alimentation. *J. Ped.,* **81:** 894.

9. Chen, W., E. Ohashi, and M. Kasai. 1974. Amino acid metabolism in parenteral nutrition: With special reference to the calorie : nitrogen ratio and the blood urea nitrogen level. *Metabolism,* **23:** 1117.

10. Chernoff, R. and A. S. Bloch. 1977. Liquid feedings: Considerations and alternatives. *J. Am. Dietet. Assoc.,* **70:** 389.

11. Consolazio, C. F., R. E. Johnson, and L. J. Pecora. 1963. *Physiological Measurements of Metabolic Functions in Man.* New York: McGraw-Hill.

12. Coran, A. G. 1972. The intravenous use of fat for the total parenteral nutrition of the infant. *Lipids,* **7:** 455.

13. Dudrick, S. J. and J. E. Rhoads. 1972. Total intravenous feeding. *Sci. Am.,* **226** (May): 73.

14. Dudrick, S. J., D. W. Wilmore, H. M. Vars, and J. E. Rhoads. 1968. Long-term total parenteral nutrition with growth, development, and positive nitrogen balance. *Surgery,* **64:** 134.

15. Eklund, J., P. O. Granberg, and D. Hallberg. 1972. Clinical aspects of body fluid osmolality. *Nutr. Metabol.,* **14** (Supplement): 74.

16. Fleischer, W. R. 1974. Laboratory assessment of acid-base imbalance. *Geriatrics,* **29** (Jan.): 96.

17. Fleming, C. R., L. M. Smith, and R. E. Hodges. 1976. Essential fatty acid deficiency in adults receiving total parenteral nutrition. *Am. J. Clin. Nutr.,* **29:** 976.

18. Freund, U., Y. Krausz, I. S. Levij, and M. Eliakim. 1975. Iatrogenic lipidosis following prolonged intravenous hyperalimentation. *Am. J. Clin. Nutr.,* **28:** 1156.

19. Gault, M. H., M. E. Dixon, M. Doyle, and W. M. Cohen. 1973. Hypernatremia, azotemia, and dehydration due to high-protein tube feeding. *Ann. Int. Med.,* **68:** 778.

20. Ghadimi, H. 1973. A review: Current status of parenteral amino acid therapy. *Ped. Res.,* **7:** 169.

21. Ghadimi, H., F. Abaci, S. Kumar, and M. Rathi. 1971. Biochemical aspects of intravenous alimentation. *Pediatrics,* **48:** 955.

22. Goldenberg, I. S. and S. Saperstein. 1976. Nutritional management of hospitalized patients: An evaluation of a nutritionally complete milk-base tube feeding. *Nutr. Rep. Internat.,* **13:** 149.

23. Gormican, A. 1975. Tube feeding overview. *Dietet. Currents* (Ross Laboratories), **2** (No. 2): 1.

24. Gormican, A. and E. Catli. 1972. Nutritional and clinical responses of immobilized patients to a sterile milk-base feeding. *J. Chron. Dis.,* **25:** 291.

25. Gormican, A. and E. Liddy. 1973. Nasogastric tube feedings. *Postgrad. Med.,* **53** (No. 7): 71.

26. Gormican, A., E. Liddy, and L. B. Thrush, Jr. 1973. Nutritional status of patients after extended tube feeding. *J. Am. Dietet. Assoc.,* **63:** 247.

27. Greene, H. L., D. Hazlett, and R. Demaree. 1976. Relationship between Intralipid-induced hyperlipemia and pulmonary function. *Am. J. Clin. Nutr.,* **29:** 127.

28. Haddad, H., G. Bounous, W. T. Tahan, G. Devroede, R. Beaudry, and R. Lafond. 1974.

Long-term nutrition with an elemental diet following intensive abdominal irradiation: Report of a case. *Dis. Colon Rect.*, **17:** 373.

29. Hidalgo, J. 1976. Current status of the fat emulsions in the United States. In *Fat Emulsions in Parenteral Nutrition.* Meng, H. C. and D. W. Wilmore (Eds.). Chicago: American Medical Association. p. 122.

30. Jeejeebhoy, K. N., R. C. Chu, E. B. Marliss, G. R. Greenberg, and A. Bruce-Robertson. 1977. Chromium deficiency, glucose intolerance, and neuropathy reversed by chromium supplementation, in a patient receiving long-term total parenteral nutrition. *Am. J. Clin. Nutr.*, **30:** 531.

31. Kaminski, M. V., Jr. November 1973. Tube feeding tips and techniques. Eaton Laboratories.

32. Kark, R. M. 1974. Liquid formula and chemically defined diets. *J. Am. Dietet. Assoc.*, **64:** 476.

33. Meng, H. C. 1975. Parenteral nutrition: Principles, nutrient requirements, and techniques. *Geriatrics*, **30** (Sept.): 97.

34. Michener, W. M. and D. Law. 1970. Parenteral nutrition: The age of the catheter. *Ped. Clin. No. Am.*, **17:** 373.

35. Miller, J. M. and J. C. Taboada. 1975. Clinical experience with an elemental diet. *Am. J. Clin. Nutr.*, **28:** 46.

36. Munro, H. N. 1972. Basic concepts in the use of amino acids and protein hydrolysates for parenteral nutrition. In *Symposium on Total Parenteral Nutrition.* Chicago: American Medical Association. p. 7.

37. Nadel, A. M. and P. C. Burger. 1976. Wernicke encephalopathy following prolonged intravenous therapy. *J. Am. Med. Assoc.*, **235:** 2403.

38. Peaston, M. J. T. 1967. Nasogastric feeding and metabolic balance. *Nursing Times,* Mar. 24, p. 372.

39. Richardson, T. J. and D. Sgoutas. 1975. Essential fatty acid deficiency in four adult patients during total parenteral nutrition. *Am. J. Clin. Nutr.*, **28:** 258.

40. Schuman, B. M. 1972. Tube feeding using a food pump. *Am. Fam. Physician,* **5** (Mar.): 85.

41. Shils, M. E. 1975. A program for total parenteral nutrition at home. *Am. J. Clin. Nutr.*, **28:** 1429.

42. Shils, M. E. 1972. Guidelines for total parenteral nutrition. *J. Am. Med. Assoc.*, **220:** 1721.

43. Shils, M. E. 1964. Intravenous feeding—nutritional aspects. *Postgrad. Med.*, **36** (No. 4): A-99.

44. Shils, M. E., A. S. Bloch, and R. Chernoff. 1976. Liquid formulas for oral and tube feeding. *Clin. Bull. Memorial Sloan-Kettering Cancer Center,* **6** (No. 4): 151.

45. Siegel, P. D. 1973. The physiologic approach to acid-base balance. *Med. Clin. No. Am.*, **57:** 863.

46. Suki, W. N. 1976. Disposition and regulation of body potassium: an overview. *Am. J. Med. Sci.*, **272:** 31.

47. Walike, B. C. 1975. Nasogastric tube feeding: The nursing perspective *Dietet. Currents* (Ross Laboratories), **2** (No. 5): 1.

48. Walike, B. and J. W. Walike. 1973. Lactose content of tube feeding diets as a cause of diarrhea. *The Laryngoscope,* **83:** 7.

49. Walike, J. W. 1969. Tube feeding syndrome in head and neck surgery. *Arch. Otolaryng.*, **89:** 117.

50. Wilmore, D. W. and S. J. Dudrick. 1968. Growth and development of an infant receiving all nutrients exclusively by vein. *J. Am. Med. Assoc.*, **203:** 860.

51. Wretlind, A. 1972. Complete intravenous nutrition. *Nutr. Met.*, **14** (Supplement): 1.

STUDY GUIDE

Fluid and electrolyte balance is maintained in the body by complex mechanisms.

1. Describe the overall distribution of electrolytes in body fluid compartments and their role in maintaining normal osmotic pressures.

2. Discuss major factors operating in the control of water and electrolyte balance in the body.

Normal acid-base regulating mechanisms usually maintain the pH of body fluids within a precise range.

3. Describe relationships among the three major acid-base regulating mechanisms of the body—buffer systems, respiratory regulation, and renal regulation.

4. Indicate several disease states that commonly are associated with acid-base imbalances.

5. Differentiate between respiratory and metabolic acidosis; between respiratory and metabolic alkalosis.

When it is not possible for a patient to take food by mouth, yet gastrointestinal function is normal, tube feeding may appropriately be initiated.

6. List conditions where tube feeding might effectively be used.

7. Discuss possible considerations for the use of nasogastric tubes, gastrostomy, or jejunostomy when tube feeding is to be initiated.

8. Describe and explain several factors that should be considered when deciding upon an individual prescription for a nasogastric tube feeding.

9. List several characteristics of an ideal tube feeding.

10. Discuss probable advantages and/or disadvantages for the use as tube feedings of blenderized natural foods, milk-based formulas, defined formula diets, and formulas containing medium-chain triglycerides.

11. Give possible explanations for the development of diarrhea, dehydration, hypernatremia, azotemia, and malnutrition in patients receiving tube feedings over a period of time. Be able to calculate the approximate osmolarity of a given tube feeding mixture.

12. Outline a procedure that might appropriately be followed in deciding what commercial tube feeding products should be purchased by a hospital dietary department.

The primary purpose of parenteral feeding is to maintain an adequate nutritional state in patients who cannot utilize food through usual gastrointestinal mechanisms.

13. List conditions for which parenteral feeding is appropriate.

14. Describe substances that might satisfactorily be given intravenously and discuss limitations of use for each.

15. Explain the nutritional limitations of conventional intravenous feeding, particularly for previously malnourished patients and those who must depend on parenteral feeding for relatively long periods of time.

An effective technique developed in recent years for feeding a patient exclusively by vein is called total parenteral nutrition (TPN).

16. List conditions for which TPN is appropriate.

17. Outline a satisfactory method for initiating TPN and describe nutrient substances that may be used. Also, explain how this procedure overcomes the limitations of conventional intravenous feeding.

18. Describe and explain several problems or complications that may be associated with TPN.

11

Cancer and Nutrition

Malignant tumors or neoplasms are collectively known as cancer and interact with nutrition in several ways. Diet is one environmental factor that has been implicated in the causation of 50 to 90 percent of all human cancers. Other factors include excessive use of tobacco, occupational hazards, and radiation. Food contaminants, such as mycotoxins and nitrosamines, have been suggested as potential carcinogens. In animal studies, dietary variations have caused marked differences in the incidence and type of tumors that develop spontaneously. Epidemiological studies in human populations have shown a varying incidence of certain malignancies in different geographical areas. Associations between dietary protein, fat, sugar, fiber, or beef and colon cancer have been suggested and are discussed in Sec. 13.8. However, evidence for specific roles of diet in cancer development is still fragmentary (Shils, 1976; Wynder, 1976; Alcantara and Speckmann, 1976).

In addition to possible causative effects of diet, malignant disease influences the nutritional status of the host, particularly through the development of anorexia and dysgeusia (impaired sense of taste) with consequent weight loss and cachexia. The cancer itself and the complications of its development may cause marked derangements in body metabolism leading to catabolism and increased energy expenditure (Theologides, 1977a). The treatment of cancer by radiation, chemotherapy, and surgery may create nutritional problems. These interrelationships, as they influence the nutritional care of cancer patients, are discussed in this chapter.

11.1 Effects of Cancer on Nutritional Status

In a significant number of patients, malignant processes have a systemic influence that is associated with anorexia, hypermetabolism, and progressive wasting of tissues. Although these effects are most apparent in patients with advanced and disseminated cancer, profound anorexia may occur while the tumors are relatively small. Unexplained anorexia and weight loss in an apparently healthy patient is a signal to the physician to search for a hidden neoplasm. Such complaints should also alert the dietitian, to whom an individual with such symptoms comes for nutritional counseling, that caution should be exercised and the patient referred for further medical workup (Shils, 1976). About 15 percent of patients have significant anorexia at the time of recurrence or spread of their cancer. Another 25 percent complain of easy filling, or early satiety, despite a feeling of hunger at the beginning of a meal. The incidence and degree of anorexia and early satiety increase with progression of cancer (Theologides, 1977a).

It has been proposed that the systemic effect of cancer on anorexia is a result of peptides, oligonucleotides, and other small metabolites produced by the cancer and the host. These substances may exert a direct effect on the hypothalamic and other central nervous system sensor and responder cells and also a peripheral effect on neuroendocrine cells and neuroreceptors (Theologides, 1976).

Secondary complications of weight loss and malnutrition in cancer patients may include weakness, often necessitating prolonged bed rest; breakdown of skin with decubitus ulcers; fluid and electrolyte abnormalities that may mask true wasting of tissues by fluid retention; decreased resistance to infections; impaired absorption from the intestine; apathy; and a vicious cycle of further disinterest in foods with attendant continued weight loss. As in other conditions, prevention of malnutrition is a much more effective approach than rehabilitation of an already malnourished cancer patient (Shils, 1976). A conditioned aversion to eating may develop in patients who experience nausea and discomfort during or after eating. This conditioned aversion may be mistaken for anorexia because it can persist even after the causative factor has been removed or alleviated. It may require behavior modification therapy (Theologides, 1977b).

11.2 Nutritional Effects of Cancer Treatment

Specific treatment for cancer may produce nutritional problems for the patient. Surgery is the most frequently used treatment currently available. The 5-year survival period has been increased by this procedure in at least 85 percent of patients with skin cancer, in about 60 percent of women with breast cancer and 70 percent with uterine cancer, and in about 40 percent of cases of colon cancer. Radiotherapy has also been widely used with considerable success. Neither surgery nor radiotherapy can cure a patient unless the tumor is locally or regionally confined. However, they can decrease the tumor burden so that the systemic forms of treatment, chemotherapy and immunotherapy, may be more effective (Carter, 1976).

A variety of drugs is now available for use in chemotherapy and a significant number of patients have been cured by this type of treatment. Immunotherapy is the newest form of cancer treatment. This therapy assumes that there are characteristic antigens in or on tumor cells that distinguish them from normal host cells. The antigens are capable of eliciting humoral and cell-mediated immune responses and therapy is aimed at manipulating these responses to reject tumors. Immunotherapy has great potential for treating cancer patients but is presently primarily a clinical art (Carter, 1976).

Surgery

Radical surgery of the head and neck area frequently produces swallowing defects that may range from mild impairment to total disability. Usually the removal of up to 50 percent of the functioning tongue can be done without creating significant disability. Total laryngectomy generally does not produce swallowing problems unless the patient has also had extensive preoperative irradiation. A puréed or liquid diet may be required if there has been extensive resection of the pharynx, as well as the larynx, or if reconstruction flaps have been used (Fleming et al., 1977). Dysphagia usually occurs when a supraglottic laryngectomy is done. For these patients, liquids are often the most difficult to swallow without aspiration. Fleming et al. (1977) have suggested beginning with nonsticky custard, puréed fruits, or vegetables. To retrain the swallowing mechanism, the patient should be encouraged to inhale, swallow, and then exhale. This is a normal sequence of events and should be reinforced as it serves to clear food from the laryngeal aditus following deglutition. Most patients will swallow better from a semireclining position with the head and back on the same plane, maximizing the effects of gravity without increasing aspiration. Deglutition therapists are used in some institutions and work closely with the dietitian to provide the frequent diet modifications required during therapy (Fleming et al., 1977). Nutritional problems associated with resection of the stomach and small intestine are discussed in Secs. 12.5 and 13.5, respectively.

Radiation

Radiotherapy to the head and neck area may produce severe inflammation with ulceration and edema of the oral and pharyngeal mucosa. This may be so severe as to prevent the use of oral feedings for a period during which tube feedings can be used. Radiation usually permanently disables salivary glands with resulting xerostomia (dryness of the mouth), which contributes to difficulties in mastication and the development of dental caries. Intake of sucrose should be decreased. Some synthetic salivas may be of benefit in lubricating the mouth before eating. Providing adequate quantities of liquid foods and food lubricants, such as gravy, butter, and sauces, is helpful.

Table 11.1 SELECTED DRUGS USED IN CHEMOTHERAPY FOR CANCER*

Drug	Classification	Stomatitis	Anorexia	Toxicity vomiting	Nausea	Diarrhea	Other
Actinomycin D (Cosmegen[R])	Antibiotic	x	x	x	x	x	Oral ulceration
Bleomycin (Blenoxane[R])	Antibiotic	x	x	x	x		Fever, pulmonary toxicity
Cyclophosphamide (Cytoxan)	Alkylating agent		x	x	x		Hemorrhagic cystitis
Melphalan (Alkeran)	Alkylating agent			x	x		
Nitrogen mustard	Alkylating agent		x	x	x	x	Metallic taste, headache, fever
Cytarabine (Cytosar)	Antimetabolite		x	x	x	x	Oral inflammation and/or ulcerations, abdominal pain
5-fluorouracil	Antimetabolite	x	x	x	x	x	Oral ulcerations
Hydroxyurea	Antimetabolite	x	x	x	x	x	Constipation, ulceration of buccal mucosa, renal dysfunction
6-mercaptopurine (Purinethol)	Antimetabolite	x	x	x	x		Fever, liver dysfunction
Methotrexate	Antimetabolite	x	x	x	x	x	Hepatic toxicity, oral ulcerations, gingivitis
Vinblastine (Velban)	Vinca alkaloid	x	x	x	x	x	Constipation, abdominal pain, glossitis, numbness in extremities

The "Toxicity Affecting Nutrition" heading spans the Stomatitis, Anorexia, vomiting, Nausea, and Diarrhea columns.

* Adapted from Hegedus and Pelham, 1975.

Anorexia may also develop during radiation treatment and the senses of taste and smell may be inhibited (Fleming et al., 1977).

Altered intestinal function often occurs during radiation therapy to the abdominal area. The epithelium of the small intestine is second only to bone marrow in its sensitivity to radiation. Changes may include flattening and ulceration of the mucosa, fibrosis, endarteritis of small vessels, and stenosis of the bowel. Obstruction may require bowel resection which complicates preexisting diarrhea and malabsorption (Shils, 1972).

Hegedus and Pelham (1975) suggested that the dietitian should start contact with the patient when radiation therapy begins, even though he may not have eating problems at that time. This early contact will help the dietitian develop the needed rapport and confidence for giving assistance as problems develop. A program of between-meal supplemental feedings should be started at this time, in order to develop a nutritional "cushion" and as training for problems encountered later during therapy. Eating a good breakfast before treatment is also important.

Chemotherapy

Drugs used in therapy for cancer may influence the patient's ability to eat. A combination of drugs is often used, each with different side effects. Antineoplastic agents are thought to produce their effects by varying degrees of preferential destruction or inhibition of neoplastic tissue. They have been classified broadly as alkylating, antimetabolite, antibiotic, and miscellaneous. Some of those that are of concern in nutritional care because their side effects influence eating are listed in Table 11.1 (Hegedus and Pelham, 1975). Alkylating agents interfere with cell growth by binding to important sites, such as DNA strands, in the cell. The antimetabolites interfere with the biosynthesis of purine or pyrimidine bases by inhibiting the production of normal precursors. Since the epithelial cells of the small intestine have a relatively rapid turnover rate, it is to be expected that they will be adversely affected by many of the drugs used. The mechanism of action of antitumor antibiotics is not well understood.

Based on experience in a cancer hospital, Hegedus and Pelham suggested that soft, mechanically soft, or elemental diets may be used for patients undergoing chemotherapy, depending on individual need. Acid foods are extremely irritating to the mouth and should be avoided. The odors of hot foods sometimes aggravate nausea. Cold meat plates, fruit plates, sandwiches, and cottage cheese are better accepted. Popsicles have been accepted when a patient cannot tolerate food and vomiting occurs. The coldness tends to numb the pain from mouth ulcerations, the taste is pleasing, and they help to increase fluid intake.

11.3   Taste Abnormalities with Cancer

Cancer itself apparently induces changes in taste, as do some treatment procedures. DeWys and Walters (1975) and DeWys (1974), studying abnormalities of taste in cancer patients, found the sweet-taste threshold elevated, but the sour taste normal. Both abnormally high and low bitter-taste thresholds were found among the subjects tested, who had a variety of types of malignancy. Significant abnormalities in salt threshold were not present. It was suggested that the low bitter-taste threshold might be responsible for a dislike of meat.

Carson and Gormican (1977) measured the taste acuity of selected patients with either breast or colon cancer both before and after treatment with 5-fluorouracil. The taste abnormalities observed before treatment involved decreased salt and sweet sensitivity, with some differences in degree noted between men and women and between patients with colon or breast cancer. Slight increases in thresholds for sour detection and bitter recognition were observed after 2 weeks of treatment. Changes in taste could not be correlated with changes in food preferences as determined by a questionnaire.

Based on observation of taste abnormalities in cancer patients, Carson and Gormican recommended:

1. Differences in responses of patients with cancer to food must be recognized and each patient viewed individually.
2. Cold protein items, such as cheese, luncheon meats, deviled eggs, meat salads, and sandwiches with large portions of meat may be served with cold fruit or raw vegetables.
3. The use of cold snacks high in protein may also be beneficial, such as celery stuffed with cheese, ice cream, gelatin salad with cottage cheese, and salted nuts.
4. The use of fresh fruits may increase the appeal of such protein-containing desserts as ice cream, milkshakes, puddings, and custards.
5. The smaller meat portions in casseroles and the decreased desirability of casseroles imply that use of other meat sources is wise.
6. If coffee or other beverages become unenjoyable, substitutions with nutritious beverages, such as hot chocolate or fruit juices, can be suggested.
7. Patients should be encouraged to experiment with seasonings to improve flavors. Some may appreciate the use of additional salt or sugar. Lemon juice and a variety of spices may improve flavor for patients who report food to be tasteless.

11.4 Nutritional Management of Cancer Patients

The tendency, particularly as cancer progresses, is for the failure of food intake to meet the demands of the body. Anorexia contributes toward a decreased intake, and some increase in body metabolism increases the energy deficit. The major problem in maintaining an adequate nutritional status is getting the patient to eat while surgery, chemotherapy, and radiotherapy cure the cancer.

A complete nutritional history should be obtained early in the management period as a basis for assessing changes in food consumption and giving counsel. Patients with anorexia and early satiety should be told that they will not be able to enjoy large meals and that they should take small, rather frequent highly nutritious feedings. Maintenance of a relatively good nutritional state may be presented as a challenge, requesting the patient's cooperation. Nevertheless, the patient should be prepared psychologically for the likelihood of weight loss (Theologides, 1977a).

If oral intake is not adequate to sustain normal nutrition, tube feeding should be initiated early so that significant malnutrition will not occur; defined-formula diets may be useful in some cases. If feeding by tube is not possible, total parenteral nutrition offers an alternative feeding route. Aggressive nutritional support should be given. It will support the various therapies being used. Even if it does not contribute to longer survival, it may at least improve the quality of life (Theologides, 1977a).

REFERENCES

1. Alcantara, E. N. and E. W. Speckmann. 1976. Diet, nutrition, and cancer. *Am. J. Clin. Nutr.*, **29:** 1035.

2. Carson, J. A. S. and A. Gormican. 1977. Taste acuity and food attitudes of selected patients with cancer. *J. Am. Dietet. Assoc.*, **70:** 361.

3. Carter, S. K. 1976. Immunotherapy of cancer in man. *Am. Sci.*, **64:** 418.

4. DeWys, W. D. 1974. Abnormalities of taste as a remote effect of a neoplasm. *Ann. N.Y. Acad. Sci.*, **230:** 427.

5. DeWys, W. D. and K. Walters. 1975. Abnormalities of taste sensation in cancer patients. *Cancer*, **36:** 1888.

6. Fleming, S. M., A. W. Weaver, and J. M. Brown. 1977. The patient with cancer affecting the head and neck: Problems in nutrition. *J. Am. Dietet. Assoc.*, **70:** 391.

7. Hegedus, S. and M. Pelham. 1975. Dietetics in a cancer hospital. *J. Am. Dietet. Assoc.*, **67:** 235.

8. Shils, M. E. 1976. Nutritional problems in cancer patients. *Nutrition in Disease* (Ross Laboratories).

9. Shils, M. E. 1972. Nutritional problems arising from the treatment of cancer. *Nutrition and Cancer*, American Cancer Society, p. 10.

10. Theologides, A. 1977a. Nutritional management of the patient with advanced cancer. *Postgrad. Med.*, **61** (No. 2): 97.

11. Theologides, A. 1977b. Cancer and anorexia. *Contemporary Nutrition* (General Mills, Inc.), **2** (No. 4).

12. Theologides, A. 1976. Anorexia-producing intermediary metabolites. *Am. J. Clin. Nutr.*, **29:** 552.

13. Wynder, E. L. 1976. Nutrition and cancer. *Fed. Proc.*, **35:** 1309.

STUDY GUIDE

Cancer itself, as well as treatment modalities, may affect a patient's nutritional status.

1. Describe and explain probable effects of cancer on nutritional status.

2. Discuss eating problems that may result from surgery and from radiation for treatment of cancer, particularly when these treatment procedures involve the head and neck area.

3. Suggest possible measures that may help to alleviate the eating problems discussed in (2) and thus avoid the development of severe malnutrition.

4. Describe and explain side effects of several drugs used in the treatment of cancer as they affect food intake of the patient receiving them and offer suggestions for minimizing the detrimental nutritional effects of this form of treatment.

5. Describe possible effects of cancer and its various treatments on taste and discuss implications of these abnormalities in the nutritional care of cancer patients.

It is preferable to prevent than to cure malnutrition in a cancer patient.

6. Discuss the problems involved in nutritional rehabilitation of a cancer patient, the advantages of maintaining the patient in a satisfactory state of nourishment, and give general suggestions for nutritional care throughout the course of the illness.

UNIT 4

Gastrointestinal Disorders

12

Oral Cavity and Gastric Disorders

When a study committee of the American Medical Association's Council on Foods and Nutrition reported in 1961 on diet as related to gastrointestinal function, they concluded that relatively few of the common dietary recommendations for gastrointestinal disorders could qualify as "rational" on the basis of criteria stated as reasonably well-accepted knowledge of (1) how a dietary regimen changes gastrointestinal contents and function, and (2) how such changes, in turn, affect the mechanisms underlying the disorder (Weinstein et al., 1961). Since 1961 additional research has been reported and some traditional dietary practices changed in the treatment of gastrointestinal disease. The present status of knowledge in diet and gastric disorders, as well as some nutritional implications for problems in the oral cavity and esophagus, are discussed in this chapter. A review of normal physiology and diagnostic procedures is given first. Intestinal disorders are discussed in the following chapter.

12.1 Digestive-Absorptive Process

The ease and efficiency of chewing influences food intake. Chewing is of particular importance in the digestion of foods such as fruits and vegetables because the grinding force of chewing helps to disrupt indigestible cell walls and release nutrients. However, it is beneficial to the digestion of all solid food because it increases the surface area on which digestive enzymes may act and subdivides the mass into finer particles that will move through the digestive tract.

The teeth are normally well designed for effective chewing, providing both cutting and grinding actions. Muscles of the jaw are capable of closing the teeth with a force as great as 55 pounds on the incisors and 200 pounds on the molars (Guyton, 1971, p. 742).

The major parts of the digestive system are shown in Fig. 12.1. Food moves from the mouth to the stomach through the esophagus. Fig. 12.2 is a diagram of the swallowing process called *deglutition*. Food that is ready for swallowing is voluntarily squeezed posteriorly by pressure of the tongue upward and backward against the palate. The tongue forces the bolus of

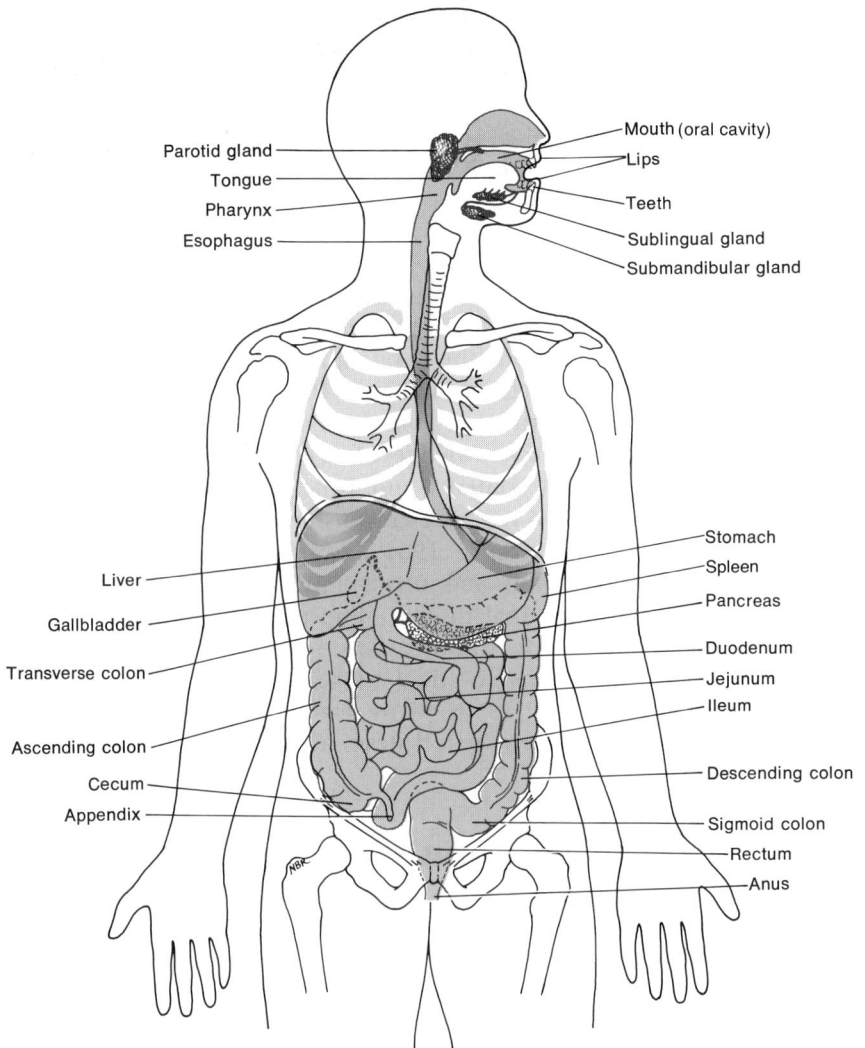

Fig. 12.1 The organs of the digestive system and related structures. (From Gerard J. Tortora and Nicholas P. Anagnostakos, *Principles of Anatomy and Physiology,* 2d ed., New York: Harper & Row, 1978: by permission of the publisher.)

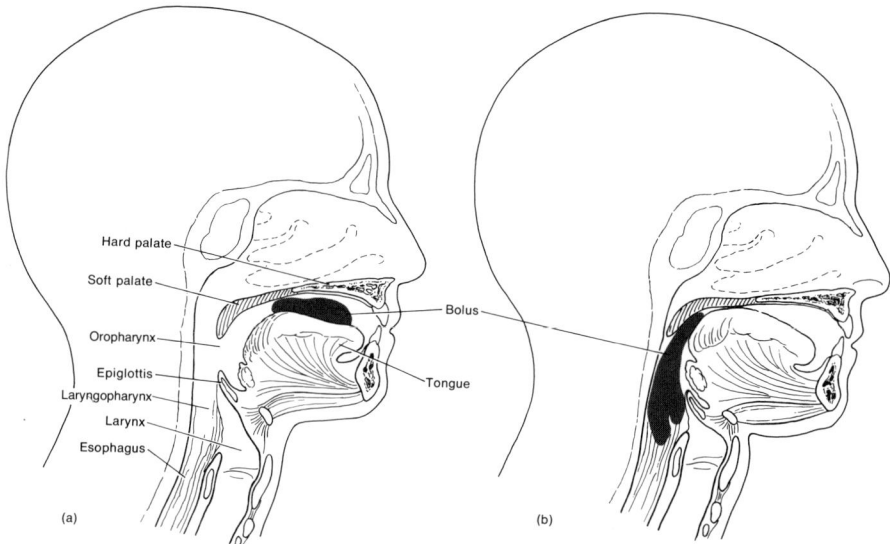

Fig. 12.2 Deglutition. (*a*) Position of structures prior to swallowing. (*b*) During swallowing, the tongue rises against the palate, the nose is closed off, the larynx rises, the epiglottis seals off the larynx, and the bolus is passed into the esophagus. (From Gerard J. Tortora and Nicholas P. Anagnostakos, *Principles of Anatomy and Psysiology*, 2d ed., New York: Harper & Row, 1978; by permission of the publisher.)

food into the pharynx, a funnel-shaped tube. From this point, swallowing enters the pharyngeal stage and becomes involuntary. When the food is pushed backward in the mouth, it stimulates swallowing receptor areas around the opening of the pharynx and impulses are sent to the brain stem to initiate a series of automatic pharyngeal muscular contractions. The soft palate is pulled tightly up against the hard wall at the rear of the throat and seals off the passage between the throat and the nose so that food does not go into the nasal cavity. The size of the particles of food to be swallowed is controlled by a brief stage in the swallowing process in which the palatopharyngeal folds on either side of the pharynx are pulled toward each other and form a slit of limited size leading into the posterior pharynx. A switching mechanism then operates whereby muscular contractions in the neck quickly move the laryngeal-pharyngeal assembly upward to close the opening of the larynx and prevent entry of food to the larynx and trachea. The pharynx is a common passageway both for food and for air passing through the larynx and trachea. During these first and second stages of swallowing, all inspiration and expiration movements are inhibited. At the same time that the larynx is being pulled upward and forward, the hypopharyngeal sphincter around the esophageal entrance, which normally prevents air from going into the esophagus during respiration, relaxes, thus allowing food to move from the posterior pharynx into the upper esophagus. The superior constrictor muscle of the pharynx contracts and gives rise to a rapid primary peristaltic wave passing downward over the pharyngeal muscles and into the esophagus. The pharyngeal stage of swallowing is a reflex action (Guyton, 1971, p. 743).

The third stage of swallowing involves the passage of food through the esophagus and into the stomach. Liquids are squirted to the lowest part without any further muscular action by the esophagus. Solid and semisolid food, however, is pushed downward by the secondary peristaltic contraction of the circular muscles in the walls of the esophagus. The musculature of the pharynx and the upper third of the esophagus is skeletal muscle, the lower third is smooth muscle, and the middle third is a mixture of the two types.

At the lower end of the esophagus is a slightly hypertrophied circular muscle, called the lower esophageal sphincter (LES) which prevents reflux of stomach contents into the upper esophagus, since the esophageal mucosa is generally not capable of resisting the digestive action of gastric secretions. When the peristaltic wave reaches the cardia, where the esophagus and stomach join, the LES relaxes and food enters the stomach (Guyton, 1971, pp. 742–744; Inglefinger, 1973).

The gastrointestinal (GI) tract is well supplied with nerve receptors, with main stimulation through the parasympathetic system. Sacral outflow from this system empties the bladder and bowel. Cranial outflow, including a number of branches of the vagus nerve, regulates gastric and intestinal secretions and salivation. Stimulation of the sympathetic nervous system inhibits motor activity of the GI tract, in general, while the parasympathetic system increases activity. In addition, the GI tract has its own primitive system of innervation controlling tone and motility.

Epithelial cells lining the GI tract are very active metabolically and are rapidly replaced, with an average half-life for gastric cells of 3 to 4 days. The half-life of small intestinal mucosal cells is about 1½ days.

Gastrointestinal Secretions
The flow of GI secretions may be stimulated or inhibited by the action of several hormones produced by cells in the stomach and small intestine, as well as by psychogenic stimuli and the presence of food in the digestive tract. Major components of various GI secretions, including the major digestive enzymes, are listed in Table 12.1.

Saliva flow is stimulated by the sight, smell, or thought of food, as well as by the presence of food in the mouth. The sight, smell, or taste of food is also important in the cephalic or neurogenic phase of gastric secretion. Vagal stimulation to the stomach during this phase is responsible for one-tenth to one-fifth of the gastric secretion normally associated with a meal and causes greater secretion of pepsin than acid.

The gastric phase of gastric secretion is initiated when food enters the stomach as distention stimulates a vagovagal reflex going to the brain stem and back to both the parietal cells that secrete acid and cells in the pyloric glands that secrete the hormone, gastrin. Gastrin is then carried by the blood to the parietal cells where it stimulates additional acid output. There

Table 12.1 MAJOR COMPONENTS OF VARIOUS GASTROINTESTINAL
SECRETIONS

Secretion	Major Digestive Enzymes (secreted as zymogens)	Other Substances
Saliva	Amylase (ptyalin)	Electrolytes; mucoproteins; blood-group substances; antibodies
Gastric juice	Pepsins; other proteolytic enzymes; lipase (tributyrase)	HCl; electrolytes; mucoproteins; gastrin; intrinsic factor; blood-group substances; serum proteins; miscellaneous enzymes
Pancreatic juice	Trypsin; chymotrypsin; carboxypeptidase A and B; aminopeptidase; lipase; amylase; ribonuclease; deoxyribo-nuclease; phospholipase; cholesterol esterase; collagenase; elastase	Bicarbonate and other electrolytes
Intestinal juice	Alpha amylase; brush border enzymes—aminopeptidase; dipeptidase; tripep-tidase; lipase; lactase; sucrase; maltase; isomaltase	Electrolytes; mucoproteins; secretin, cholecystokinin; serotonin; histamine; enterokinase
Bile		Bile salts and acids, conjugated and unconjugated; bilirubin; mucopro-teins; serum proteins; cholesterol; phospholipids; triglycerides; fatty acids

are also short intramural reflexes, completed within the wall of the stomach and initiated by distention or by chemical stimulants such as ethanol and peptides, which cause acid secretion. Ethanol and peptides, in addition, cause secretion of gastrin directly. Thus, both nervous and hormonal mechanisms act to stimulate secretion of acid gastric juice, the gastric phase accounting for two-thirds of the total gastric juice secreted during a meal. A pH below 2 in the gastric antrum exerts a negative feedback influence on the secretion of gastrin. The total daily volume of gastric juice is approximately 2000 ml (Guyton, 1971, pp. 758–759). A diagram of a typical gastric gland with secreting cells is shown in Fig. 12.3.

Saint-Hilaire et al. (1960) and Kotrba and Code (1969), in investigating the gastric acid secretory effects of some common foods in dogs, found that equicaloric meals of sucrose, methylcellulose (inert control), olive oil, and egg albumin produced 25, 31, 40, and 42 percent, respectively, of the acid produced by lean meat. The isolated proteins, lactalbumin, gluten, and casein, stimulated acid production 60 to 92 percent of that produced by lean meat. Except for egg albumin, the buffering capacity of the test meal was significantly and positively correlated with the total output of gastric acid. In other words, the greater the buffering power, the more acid secreted. This may reflect the lack of negative feedback because the pH remains above 2 when effectively buffered.

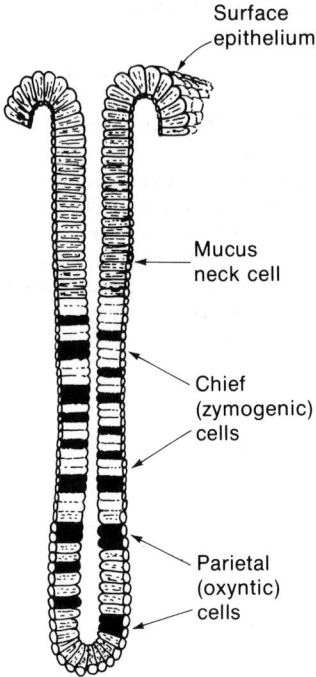

Fig. 12.3 A gastric gland.

Ippoliti et al. (1976) studied the effect on gastric acid secretion of various forms of milk in comparison to 0.15 M NaCl as a control solution. They found a significant increase in acid secretion, in both normal subjects and patients with duodenal ulcer in remission, by ingestion of 240 ml whole, low-fat, and nonfat milk. The acid secretory responses to milk were equivalent to those produced by a 300 ml 10 percent peptone meal and were approximately 20 to 35 percent of maximal pentagastrin-stimulated acid output. This effect of milk has been attributed in part to its content of readily absorbable calcium. Elevated serum calcium apparently directly stimulates the parietal cells to secrete acid.

The GI hormone, gastrin, is a peptide containing 17 amino acids, with hormone activity concentrated in the terminal four. Different molecular weight forms have also been identified. A synthetic compound with gastrin activity, containing 5 amino acids and called pentagastrin, is now used to replace histamine compounds in tests for gastric acid secretion since it is a more potent stimulator of acid and its side effects are minimal (Hiatt and Wells, 1974; Cleator et al., 1972). The major physiological effect of gastrin is the stimulation of gastric acid secretion. In fact, it is the most potent acid stimulant known. It also stimulates the growth of gastric mucosa, increases gastric motility, weakly stimulates water and bicarbonate secretion by the pancreas, strongly stimulates pancreatic enzyme production, increases bile flow, causes contraction of the LES, and probably enhances relaxation of the ileocecal valve. Approximately 10 percent of the cells found in the antral area of the stomach secrete gastrin (Hiatt and Wells, 1974). Gastrin secretion is inhibited by high acidity (low pH) in the antrum.

Probably the most important function of the stomach in the digestive-absorptive process is to act as a reservoir for retaining food until the mixture in the stomach is nearly isotonic with the rest of the tissues. A balance is created between the inpouring of fluid secretions and the absorption of water from the stomach in order to produce isotonicity. The food mixture is then, over a period of time, released to the small intestine.

As chyme enters the duodenum from the stomach, the acid stimulates secretion of the GI hormone, secretin, by cells in the intestinal mucosa. Secretin is carried to the pancreatic cells by the blood and causes them to secrete large quantities of fluid containing a high concentration of bicarbonate (HCO_3^-) but a low concentration of chloride (Cl^-). This is an important mechanism in neutralizing the acid contents coming from the stomach. The pH of this pancreatic fluid averages 8. Secretin is a strongly basic polypeptide containing 27 amino acids. The release of secretin into the blood also inhibits gastrin production (Katz, 1973).

The presence of food in the upper small intestine, particularly emulsified fats and peptides or amino acids, stimulates the release of another hormone from the mucosa, cholecystokinin-pancreozymin (CCK). This hormone was previously thought to be two different hormones, cholecystokinin stimulating gallbladder contraction and pancreozymin causing enzyme release from the pancreas. It now appears that there is only one hormone substance and that the gallbladder and pancreatic effects represent different biologic actions of the same chemical compound. CCK is a polypeptide containing 33 amino acids. It acts on the pancreas primarily to increase enzyme output. Gastrin, as previously noted, also increases the pancreatic enzyme production. CCK causes contraction of the gallbladder so that bile is released into the duodenum and may, in addition, stimulate bile flow and relax the sphincter of Oddi. As does secretin, CCK inhibits gastrin secretion in the stomach. Other GI hormones have been identified. Several of them are capable of stimulating insulin secretion. A substance called enteroglucagon, found in the GI tract, has hyperglycemic properties and glucagon-like immunoreactivity (Katz, 1973). Interrelationships among GI hormones are apparent.

Large quantities of mucus are secreted by Brunner's glands, located in the first few centimeters of the duodenum, in response to both direct tactile effects and vagal stimulation. Some intestinal hormones probably also stimulate this secretion. The mucus secreted by these glands helps to protect the duodenal wall from digestion by the gastric juice. Secretion by Brunner's glands is strongly inhibited by sympathetic stimulation, leaving the duodenal bulb unprotected. Mucus is also secreted in large amounts by goblet cells located extensively over the surface of the intestinal mucosa.

Small crypts, called crypts of Lieberkuhn, are located over most of the surface of the small intestine at the base of the villi and secrete intestinal juices at the rate of about 3000 ml per day. The secretions are almost pure extracellular fluid, with a pH of 6.5 to 7.5, and are rapidly reabsorbed by the intestinal villi thus supplying a source of water for nutrient absorption. The only enzymes that have been found in cell-free secretions of the small intestine are enterokinase, which activates trypsinogen, and a small amount of amylase. The epithelial cells of the mucosa, however, contain large quantities of digestive enzymes and presumably digest food substances as they are being absorbed through the brush border of the villi. The most important means of regulating small intestinal secretion is various local intramural nervous reflexes or direct stimuli, such as distention of the small intestine by food materials (Guyton, 1971, pp. 762–763).

The Gastric Mucosal Barrier

The gastric mucosa has a remarkable ability to resist damage from strong acid, proteolytic secretions. Although the reasons why the stomach does not usually digest itself are not completely understood, several factors contribute to the maintenance of gastric mucosal integrity. Mucus production by cells distributed throughout the mucosa plays some part in the resistance to injury. An adequate blood supply to the cells also helps keep the tissue intact. The epithelium is rapidly replaced and gastrin has a trophic or growth effect on the mucosa. There may also be some unidentified protective factors.

The normal mucosa presents a complex physical-chemical barrier to the diffusion of acid in the lumen of the stomach back into the mucosal cells. The membranes of epithelial cells lining the stomach are apparently similar to those of other cells in the body in construction and properties, including an ordered array of lipids and proteins. However, under some circumstances, detergent-like substances can break the mucosal barrier and allow greater than usual back-diffusion of acid into the cells with a simultaneous reverse movement of Na^+ into the lumen of the stomach. Ivey et al. (1970) showed that bile salts in the stomachs of human volunteers increased the back-diffusion of H^+ and Cl^- out of the lumen while Na^+ and K^+ concentrations increased in the stomach contents. Davenport (1972 and 1975) reported that salicylic acid or acetylsalicylic acid (aspirin) can break the mucosal barrier with resulting damage to the tissue. Ethanol can readily get through the mucosa and may have a damaging effect. Steroids in large doses may predispose to injury by causing secretion of abnormally thin mucus. With mild injury, the mucosa appears to rapidly and effectively repair itself. However, repair does not always occur and ulceration and/or bleeding may result. Knowledge of the physical and chemical mechanisms by which the stomach avoids digesting itself should be helpful in preventing breakdown of the mucosal barrier and in treating individuals where mucosal repair has not occurred (Davenport, 1972).

Absorption

Crane (1969) suggested that digestion and absorption have a close functional relationship, based upon integration at every level, and it is appropriate to think of digestion and absorption as two aspects of a single, overall process that might be called digestive-absorptive function. The individual events in the process, from gross to fine levels, are so arranged and integrated that each step benefits from the preceding step. For example, a "pumping" action of the individual villi that create the tremendous absorptive surface of the small intestine (Fig. 12.4) improves mixing at the surface of the mucosal epithelial cell and may also improve blood flow. This movement is sympathetically innervated, in contrast to other intestinal

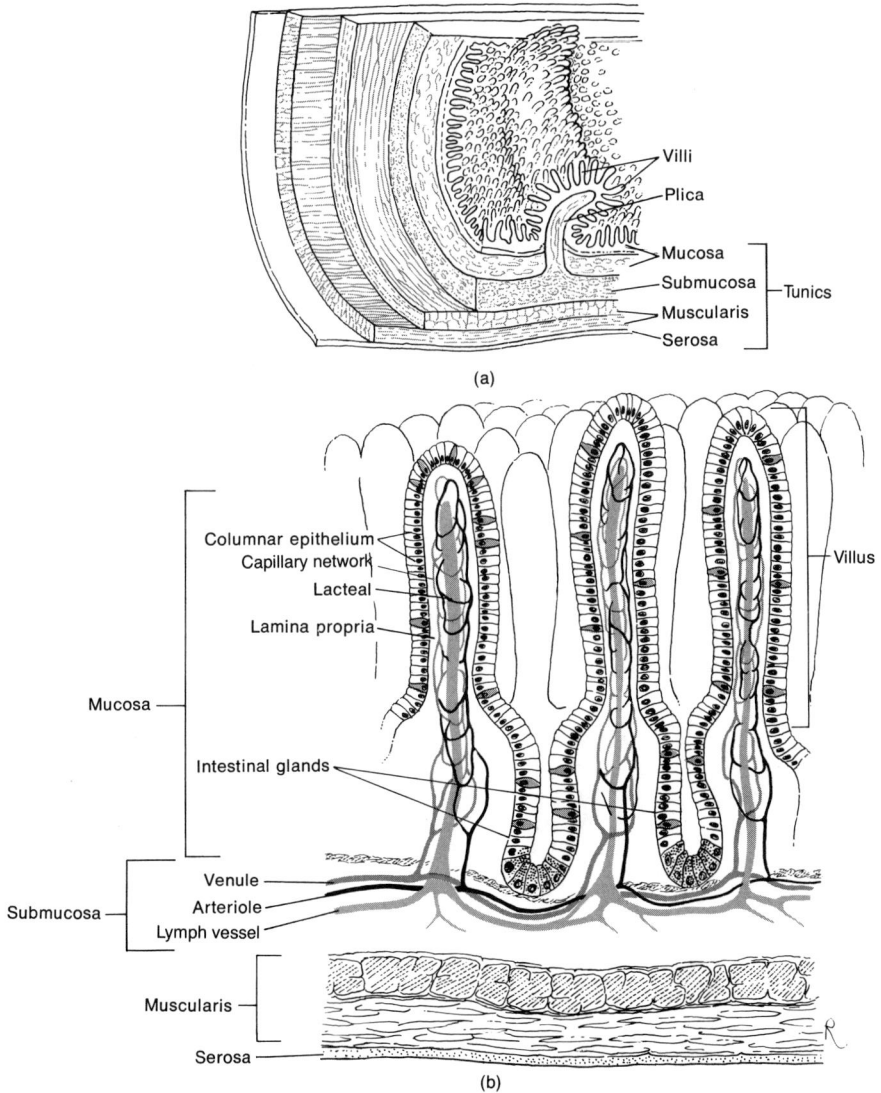

(a)

(b)

Fig. 12.4 The small intestine. (a) Villi in relation to the coats of the small intestine. (b) Enlarged aspect of several villi. (From Gerard J. Tortora and Nicholas P. Anagnostakos, *Principles of Anatomy and Psysiology*, 2d ed., New York: Harper & Row, 1978; by permission of the publisher.)

movements that are parasympathetically innervated. At the level of the cell (Fig. 12.5), the structurally elaborate brush border, the organized components of the cell, and the basal or lateral membrane of the cell all appear to be functionally polar. Diffusion back into the intestinal lumen is prevented by cellular organization to handle the molecules being absorbed and move them through the cell into the blood or lymph stem.

Some substances are actively transported, with energy involved in moving them against an electrochemical potential. Passive transport is by diffusion which is a result of molecular movement with, rather than against, an electrochemical gradient. The essentially one-way movement of materials from the small intestine to the blood is apparently facilitated by sharing processes that utilize energy. For example, Na^+ is actively transported out of the mucosal cell into the subepithelial spaces, and glucose transport into the cell is coupled with this reaction. The concepts of pores in the epithelial membrane, through which water and other small molecules may passively travel, and carrier molecules, that help to shuttle substances across the cell membrane, have been suggested (Ingelfinger, 1967). A discussion of pancreatic enzymes that play important roles in digestion-absorption is found in Sec. 14.1.

Carbohydrate. Essentially all dietary carbohydrates are absorbed as monosaccharides, only a fraction of a percent being absorbed as disac-

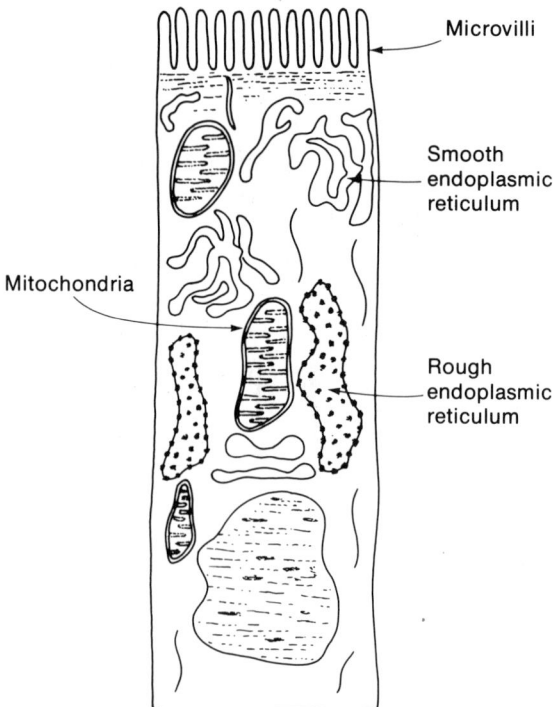

Fig. 12.5   An intestinal epithelial cell.

charides, and almost none as larger compounds. The polysaccharides, starch and glycogen, are incompletely hydrolyzed by pancreatic amylase within the lumen of the upper small intestine. The remainder of digestion, which eventually yields glucose, occurs at the surface membrane of mucosal cells where membrane-bound disaccharidases hydrolyze both the products of starch digestion and dietary disaccharides such as sucrose and lactose. The monosaccharide products are thus in an ideal position for transport into mucosal cells, from which they diffuse into capillaries and are carried in the portal blood system to the liver. It is thought that the monosaccharides move across the cell membrane by combination with carrier molecules, although specific carriers have not been identified. Both glucose and galactose are preferentially and actively absorbed in an energy-requiring process that is coupled to the sodium pump. There is little reason to believe that glucose phosphorylation is part of the glucose transport mechanism in the small intestine. Although fructose is not actively transported, its absorption is rapid and carriers probably exist for its transport. Within the mucosal cell, some fructose is converted to glucose and galactose, but in humans most appears in the portal blood as fructose (Olsen, 1974).

Protein. Proteins are split into large polypeptides and some amino acids by pepsin in the stomach. The pancreatic proteolytic enzymes attack these partially hydrolyzed products in the upper small intestine, yielding mostly dipeptides and amino acids. Amino acids are mainly absorbed in the duodenum and jejunum, but some absorption occurs in the ileum. Peptidases are present in the brush border of the mucosal cell and hydrolyze oligopeptides. Peptide hydrolases in the cytoplasm of the mucosal cell apparently hydrolyze only di- and tripeptides. Free amino acids, dipeptides, and some tripeptides are taken up by mucosal cells. Absorption of free amino acids is a highly selective process with the rate of absorption varying for different amino acids (Adibi, 1976). At least two distinct carrier systems have been demonstrated in human intestinal cells, one for basic and one for neutral free amino acids. A carrier for acidic and one for imino acids and glycine have also been suggested (Newcomer, 1973).

Absorbed amino acids diffuse into the portal blood and are taken to the liver. Small amounts of peptides and even a few intact dietary proteins may pass through the mucosal cell unhydrolyzed and appear in the portal blood. In infants, whole proteins (Colostrum antibodies) are absorbed intact during the first 36 hours after birth. Absorption of whole protein molecules or large peptides has been implicated in the development of food allergies (Newcomer, 1973).

Lipids. Fat in the duodenum retards gastric emptying and thus reduces the rate at which fat is presented to the intestine (Holt, 1972). Dietary fat is about 90 percent triglyceride which, after emulsification, is hydrolyzed in the upper small intestine by the action of pancreatic lipase to

2-monoglycerides, fatty acids, and glycerol. These more hydrophilic substances, at the moderate pH of 4.5 to 6.8, interact with bile acids and water to form micelles which are soluble in the aqueous phase of the intestinal juice. It is generally believed that much of the dietary lipid in normal humans is absorbed in the first 100 cm of the small intestine. The process of fat absorption is usually efficient and minimal amounts of dietary lipid remain for absorption by the distal intestine (Mansbach, 1976). However, Wollaeger (1973) concluded that the ileum plays an important role in fat absorption since this portion of the intestine is capable of absorbing fat and is regularly exposed to ingested fat in healthy humans eating mixed diets. It is not surprising, therefore, that even short resections of the terminal ileum may produce mild degrees of steatorrhea despite apparent maintenance of a normal enterohepatic circulation of bile acids. Cholesterol absorption probably occurs throughout the small intestine. Bile acids are reabsorbed in the ileum.

Micelles apparently release single lipid molecules at the brush border, primarily at the villous tips, for movement through the cell membrane. Bile salts enhance mucosal absorption of long-chain fatty acids, which make up more than 90 percent of the fatty acid of food fat in the United States, and also fat soluble vitamins (Holt, 1972).

Within the smooth endoplasmic reticulum of the mucosal cell the hydrolyzed products of triglycerides (long-chain fatty acids and 2-monoglycerides) are resynthesized in several enzymatic steps to triglycerides. Phospholipids are also resynthesized and cholesterol reesterified. The following steps are involved in triglyceride resynthesis (Isselbacher, 1966).

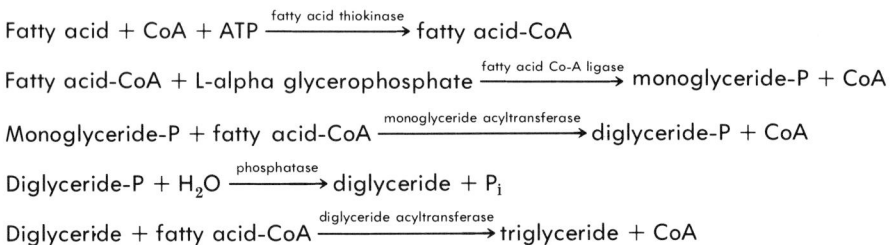

$$\text{Fatty acid} + \text{CoA} + \text{ATP} \xrightarrow{\text{fatty acid thiokinase}} \text{fatty acid-CoA}$$

$$\text{Fatty acid-CoA} + \text{L-alpha glycerophosphate} \xrightarrow{\text{fatty acid Co-A ligase}} \text{monoglyceride-P} + \text{CoA}$$

$$\text{Monoglyceride-P} + \text{fatty acid-CoA} \xrightarrow{\text{monoglyceride acyltransferase}} \text{diglyceride-P} + \text{CoA}$$

$$\text{Diglyceride-P} + \text{H}_2\text{O} \xrightarrow{\text{phosphatase}} \text{diglyceride} + \text{P}_i$$

$$\text{Diglyceride} + \text{fatty acid-CoA} \xrightarrow{\text{diglyceride acyltransferase}} \text{triglyceride} + \text{CoA}$$

Monoglycerides may also be acylated directly without being hydrolyzed to fatty acid and glycerol.

Triglycerides containing long-chain fatty acids are incorporated into chylomicrons in the rough endoplasmic reticulum of the mucosal cell before being released into the lacteals which are part of the lymph system. The chylomicron consists of an outer coating of protein, cholesterol, and phospholipid. The central core is primarily triglyceride (Isselbacher, 1967).

The digestion and absorption of medium-chain triglycerides (MCT), containing primarily fatty acids with 8 to 10 carbon atoms, differs from that of long-chain triglycerides (LCT). MCT are hydrolyzed by pancreatic lipase several times more rapidly than are LCT (Desnuelle and Lavary, 1963).

Bile salts have little influence on the hydrolysis of MCT. The rate of absorption of trioctanoin has been demonstrated in *in vivo* loops of intestine to be about twice as great as that of tripalmitin (Isselbacher, 1967). When the products of hydrolysis of MCT enter the mucosal cell, there is little reesterification to triglyceride. It has also been shown that MCT are able to enter the mucosal cells without prior hydrolysis and can be hydrolyzed by a lipase within the cell (Isselbacher, 1965). Medium-chain fatty acids are carried from the intestines as free fatty acids in the portal vein and do not participate in chylomicron formation. Because of these differences in digestion and absorption, MCT may be of clinical value under conditions where the handling of LCT is impaired, such as deficiency of pancreatic lipase or bile salts, defect in chylomicron formation, and problems with the lymphatic system. MCT, supplying about 38 percent of the kilocalories, are available in powdered formula products and also as MCT oil for use in food preparation (Harkins and Sarett, 1968).

12.2   Diagnosis of Gastrointestinal Disease

Procedures that are valuable in diagnosing disorders of the GI tract include radiography or roentgenography, endoscopy, secretory studies, absorptive studies, and peroral biopsy.

Radiography

The entire outline of the GI tract may be visualized by using X-ray and barium sulfate suspension as a radiopaque contrast material. Direct examination with use of a fluoroscope may also be used. A barium swallow may visualize the esophagus, and a barium "meal" may be followed through the stomach and upper intestine. Motility, gastric emptying, general muscle tone, and outlines of niches and craters can be seen.

For diagnosis of peptic ulcer disease, a barium meal is usually given in the morning, at least 12 hours after eating or drinking. Approximately 85 percent of gastric ulcers occur in pyloric gland mucosa and on the lesser curvature of the stomach. Gastric ulcers may not be seen if (1) they are shallow and barium does not collect within them; (2) there is mucus or blood within the ulcer; (3) there is edema in the margins around the ulcer that occludes the mouth of the ulcer; or (4) the positions of the body during the X-ray procedure do not allow its profile to be shown. Differences in appearance by radiography are often noted between benign and malignant gastric ulcers. Most duodenal ulcers are located within the duodenal bulb, although they may sometimes be found beyond this point in the more distal duodenum and proximal jejunum (Beeson and McDermott, 1975, pp. 1203–1204).

Radiographic studies may show changes in the small intestine such as strictures, fistulas, blind loops, dilatation, or marked stasis. Some of these changes may be indications of bacterial overgrowth. Differential diagnosis for various intestinal malabsorption states by roentgenographic examination alone is usually difficult.

A barium enema is used to visualize the colon. The patient is prepared for this procedure by enemas or by a clear fluid diet for 48 to 72 hours plus enemas so that the bowel is free of fecal material. Strictures, diverticuli, polyps, and cancerous growths may be observed with radiography.

Endoscopy

An endoscope is a flexible tube with a light and mirror apparatus that can be inserted through the mouth and esophagus into the stomach, allowing visualization of most ulcers in the esophagus and stomach and about 85 percent of radiographically demonstrated duodenal ulcers. Also, some duodenal ulcers not seen by radiography may be seen by endoscopy. This procedure is valuable in diagnosing esophagitis, gastritis, and duodenitis and also in differentiating benign from malignant gastric ulcers (Beeson and McDermott, 1975, p. 1204).

Secretory Studies

The secretion of acid in the stomach, both basal and stimulated by pentagastrin, histamine, or betazole injection, may be measured by passing a tube from the mouth to the stomach and withdrawing gastric contents. This procedure is usually done in the morning before food has been consumed. Average normal basal gastric acid secretion is approximately 2.5 and 1.3 meq per hour for males and females, respectively, but may range from 0 to 6 meq per hour. Average basal secretion in patients with gastric ulcer apparently is similar to normal, but for males and females with duodenal ulcer it is approximately 5 and 3 meq per hour, respectively. The wide overlapping range of basal secretion limits its value in diagnosing peptic ulcer (Beeson and McDermott, 1975, p. 1205).

Stimulated hypersecretion of gastric acid is uncharacteristic of gastric ulcer disease. Patients with duodenal ulcer tend to secrete more acid than control subjects in response to any stimulus. The upper limit of normal gastric acid response to maximal stimulation is 42 meq per hour. In about one-third of male duodenal ulcer patients, maximal acid output is greater than this. If no acid is secreted (achlorhydria), an ulcer shown with radiographic means is undoubtedly cancerous since ulcer disease does not occur in the absence of gastric acid. However, achlorhydria is not always present with gastric cancer (Beeson and McDermott, 1975, p. 1205).

The acid secreted by parietal cells of the stomach is present in gastric juice in both dissociated (H^+) and undissociated (buffered) forms. Both may be measured by use of the pH meter and titration (Makhlouf et al., 1970). Measurement of gastric secretion in response to test meals, such as a 10 percent peptone meal, may give additional information on gastric function. Gastric acid outputs are decreased after vagotomy (cutting fibers of the vagus nerve). Greenall et al. (1975) reported a permanent reduction of about 80 percent in basal acid output and 50 percent in maximal acid output for 21 patients who had had selective vagotomy 5 years previously.

Absorptive Studies

A fat balance study may be done when steatorrhea is suspected. The patient ingests a known amount of fat (usually 80 to 100 g per day) and stools are collected for a 72-hour period. Normal excretion of fat is 7 percent or less of intake. Shafer and Onstad (1975) eliminated many of the practical problems inherent in the total collection of feces and the chemical determination of fecal fat in humans by use of a radioactive marker (Ba^{131}) combined with a labeled fat (I^{131}—triolein) and calculating the ratio of these two substances in a stool sample.

The absorption of D-xylose, a pentose, is measured as an indication of malabsorption. Xylose (25 g) is given orally. Normally, about 50 percent of the oral dose is absorbed and 4.5 g or more will be excreted in a 5-hour collection of urine. Xylose is absorbed actively but its metabolism is not as rapid as that of glucose and its renal excretion does not depend upon a threshold. With some intestinal diseases, xylose excretion over a 5-hour period is significantly decreased (less than 3 g) (Beeson and McDermott, 1975, p. 1224).

Tests for vitamin B_{12} absorption are discussed in Sec. 7.2. Abnormal absorption may occur after resection or severe disease of the terminal ileum where this vitamin is usually absorbed.

A lactose tolerance test consists of administering an oral dose of lactose (usually 0.75 to 1.5 g per kg body weight) and obtaining blood samples for the measurement of glucose at periods of time after ingestion. In a positive test, the blood glucose increases less than 25 mg/100 ml above the fasting level since much of the lactose will not have been digested and absorbed. In addition, intestinal symptoms, such as cramping and bloating, usually occur. False positive tests occur in about 20 percent of normal subjects and the test may thus require confirmation by direct measurement of lactase in the intestinal mucosa (Wintrobe et al., 1974, p. 1471).

Peroral Biopsy

This procedure is used to obtain GI samples of tissue for analysis of enzyme activity or histological observation. A tube system with suction may be inserted, through the mouth, esophagus, and stomach, to the duodenum, jejunum, and ileum.

12.3 The Oral Cavity

The functions of chewing and swallowing and the condition of the mouth affect food consumption. When an individual loses teeth without satisfactory replacement, his or her food intake is often nutritionally inadequate.

In a clinical study of 160 edentulous patients, incidence of malnutrition was found to be high among those having only one or no dentures. Those wearing dentures who had a decreased vertical dimension to the face, indicating poorly fitting dentures, had greater evidence of malnutrition and complained more of GI symptoms than did patients with a normal vertical dimension. With poorly fitting dentures the consumption of adequate amounts of a variety of foods was either difficult or impossible (Goodhart and Shils, 1973, pp. 764–765). Until adequately fitting dentures can be obtained, a variety of soft, pureed, and liquid foods should be provided for edentulous patients. A nutritionally adequate diet, except for lack of fiber, may be supplied in liquid form in cases where jaws are wired shut in order to facilitate healing of broken bones.

Oral Lesions from Nutritional Deficiencies

Lesions and inflammation of the tongue, palate, and buccal membranes make eating difficult. Lack of food containing essential nutrients may itself produce lesions of the lips and mouth, thus creating a vicious circle. The tongue is particularly sensitive to nutritional disease. Riboflavin deficiency may cause the tongue to turn a magenta color. Atrophy of filliform papillae, hypertrophy of fungiform papillae, erythema, pain, loss of taste, and fissure formation on the tongue may result from a deficiency of iron, zinc, folacin, vitamin B_{12}, pyridoxine, niacin, or riboflavin (Goodhart and Shils, 1973, p. 583). Filiform papillae are small and white, do not contain taste buds, and cover the entire surface of the tongue. The somewhat larger fungiform papillae have one to eight taste buds along their edges. They are often raised, sometimes red in color, and are located on the anterior two-thirds of the tongue. A few large circumvallate papillae, containing larger numbers of taste buds, are found in a wide V formation on the posterior one-third of the tongue (Henkin, 1967).

Nonnutritional abnormalities, including a condition called geographic atrophy of the tongue papillae, may also affect the surface of the tongue. It is, therefore, important to look at dietary intake, as well as clinical signs, before making a final judgment on nutritional effects. If it is reasonably clear that lesions are caused by nutrient deficiencies, appropriate dietary supplements should be given.

Riboflavin deficiency produces edema accompanied by flaking, crusting, and cracking of the epithelium of the lips (cheilosis) in humans. This lesion has also been observed in patients who lack niacin or iron and may be a nonnutritional consequence of exposure to the elements or constant breathing through the mouth. Angular stomatitis (inflammation and fissuring at the angles of the mouth) may occur when there is a deficiency of riboflavin, pyridoxine, or iron. Other causes of this lesion include herpes stomatitis and poorly fitting dentures. When caused by nutrient deficiency, the lesions are usually bilateral (Goodhart and Shils, 1973, pp. 582–583).

Scurvy, from lack of ascorbic acid, produces marginal bleeding of the gums and hemorrhagic interdental papillae. Putrefaction of the gum, with destruction of bone and loss of teeth, occasionally occurs in scurvy. Similar loss of teeth may occur in individuals with periodontal disease due to poor hygiene (Goodhart and Shils, p. 583).

Taste and Disease

There is a growing interest in taste and smell abnormalities and their relationship to various disease states. The body of research on this topic points to the need to consider taste and smell abnormalities when giving nutritional care.

Taste and smell abnormalities have been demonstrated in a variety of disorders. Sometimes there is a loss of taste (hypogeusia) and sometimes a heightened taste acuity (hypergeusia), as shown by decreased taste

Table 12.2 FACTORS INFLUENCING TASTE SENSITIVITY

Factor	Effect
Dentures covering palate	Decreased sensitivity for sour and bitter
Surgical removal of palate with prosthesis	Decreased taste sensitivity
Turner's syndrome (gonadal dysgenesis; high arched palate)	Decreased sensitivity for sour and bitter
Adrenal cortical insufficiency	Increased sensitivity for salt, sweet, sour, and bitter
Panhypopituitarism	Increased taste sensitivity
Hypothyroidism	Decreased taste sensitivity
Cancer	Decreased sensitivity for sweet and salt; altered bitter sensitivity
Familial dysautonomia	Decreased taste sensitivity (lack taste buds)
Renal failure	Decreased sensitivity for sweet, salt, and sour
Cystic fibrosis	Possibly an increased taste sensitivity
Hepatitis	Altered taste sensitivity
Direct nerve damage	
Tongue lesions	Decreased detection levels for salt and sweet
Facial paralysis	Decreased taste sensitivity
Trauma—gunshot wounds, head injuries, burns	Decreased taste sensitivity
Zinc deficiency	Decreased taste sensitivity; pica (eating metal)
Idiopathic hypogeusia (after acute respiratory illness)	Decreased taste sensitivity
Drugs—cocaine, lignocaine, clofibrate, dinitrophenol, d-penicillamine, griseofulvin, phenindione, phenytoin, methylthiouracil	Decreased taste sensitivity
Drugs—benzocaine	Increased sensitivity to sour
Drugs—amphetamines	Increased sensitivity to bitter
Drugs—fluorouracil	Increased sensitivity to sweet; some alterations in bitter and sour
Radiotherapy to head and neck area	Decreased taste sensitivity

thresholds. The term *dysgeusia* describes an altered taste acuity. *Hyposmia* means loss of smell acuity, whereas *dysosmia* refers to an altered smell acuity. Table 12.2 lists several factors that have been reported to influence taste (Carson and Gormican, 1976; Desor and Maller, 1975; Hambidge and Silverman, 1973; Hambidge et al., 1972; Henkin et al., 1971; Henkin, 1967; Hussey, 1974; McConnel et al., 1975).

The loss of taste and smell often produces behavioral change in an individual. A first reaction of dismay is followed by food foraging and self-imposed dietary limitations. Altered social activities and depression may occur when dysgeusia continues over a long period of time. An understanding of possible reasons for observed anorexia can aid those who work with patients having this problem. More highly flavored foods may be helpful in increasing food intake. Additional salt or sugar may be suggested on an individual basis. In order to avoid nutrient deficiencies that, in the case of zinc, copper, niacin, vitamin A, and possibly other substances, may themselves cause decreased taste acuity, it is important to do all that is possible to increase food intake in patients with dysgeusia (Carson and Gormican, 1976).

The mechanism for loss of taste in zinc deficiency has been suggested by Henkin to involve a zinc-containing protein actively secreted in saliva that appears to be responsible for growth and differentiation of taste buds. This protein is decreased or absent in zinc-deficient individuals (Anonymous, 1976).

12.4 Esophageal Problems

Dysphagia

Disorders that include traumatic, nervous, or vascular lesions may be accompanied by some degree of dysphagia (difficulty in swallowing). In partially paralyzed patients, assistance may need to be given in swallowing. Experimentation may be done to determine the food texture, consistency, and temperature that best stimulate the salivary glands and swallowing reflex.

Dysphagia may result when the lumen of the esophagus is narrowed by a tumor or development of scar tissue. Inelasticity from repeated episodes of mucosal inflammation may also make swallowing difficult. The patient with these problems may not be able to swallow solid foods and eventually the swallowing of liquids is difficult. Surgical treatment is possible in some cases.

Achalasia refers to a condition where the LES maintains too high a resting tone and either does not relax or relaxes only partially upon swallowing. In most cases of achalasia the failure of relaxation in the LES is accompanied by a deficiency in the normal peristaltic movement of the esophagus so that a dilated, baggy esophagus tapers down at its lower end to a narrow channel connecting the esophagus to the stomach. It is difficult to swallow either solids or liquids. Treatment is aimed at stretching or cutting the muscle in the area of the LES. Normal peristalsis is not restored by this procedure, but the patient is nevertheless symptomatically improved. The damage to the LES must be carefully controlled so that too much reflux from the stomach back into the esophagus will not occur (Inglefinger, 1973).

Gastroesophageal Reflux

The LES normally maintains a pressure zone that is higher than the pressure within the stomach, thus preventing regurgitation of the acid gastric contents into the esophagus. If the pressure is lowered, a reflux of gastric contents into the lower esophagus may produce a burning sensation behind the sternum, commonly called heartburn. Control of LES pressure is maintained by a complex interplay of neural, hormonal, and mechanical factors. It has been observed that injection of the hormone, gastrin, causes a dramatic increase in lower esophageal pressure while other GI hormones, secretin and CCK, decrease pressure.

The effect of consumption of various foods on LES pressure has been studied. High-protein meals increased the pressure, possibly because protein stimulates gastrin release in the stomach. Fatty meals caused dramatic decreases in pressure and tended to produce gastric acid reflux. Part of the mechanism for this effect may be that fat stimulates the release of CCK from the small intestinal mucosa (Castell, 1975). Orange juice and a mixture of tomato paste and water caused only transient lessening of pressure with a gradual return to baseline, and there were considerable pressure variations during the testing. However, because of its mild acidity, orange juice may have a direct irritating effect on the lower esophagus, especially when the mucosa is inflamed. Slight, but significant, decreases in LES pressure occurred after the ingestion of 240 ml whole milk but nonfat milk produced significant increases in pressure (Babka and Castell, 1973).

Wright and Castell (1975) reported that ingestion of 120 ml chocolate syrup, diluted 1 : 1 with distilled water to a volume of 240 ml, caused the mean basal LES pressure of 14.6 ± 1.1 mmHg to decrease significantly to 7.9 ± 1.3 mmHg. Dennish and Castell (1972) found that coffee produced a slight decrease in pressure although it did not have the marked effect of chocolate. On the other hand, Cohen and Booth (1975) found sphincter pressure to be increased by both regular and decaffeinated coffee. Minimal changes in pressure were recorded in response to caffeine. Coffee, both regular and decaffeinated, stimulated gastric acid secretion, whereas the effect of caffeine, on a cup-equivalent basis, was much less. If coffee has even a slight effect on lowering sphincter pressure, this effect may be enhanced by the simultaneous increase in acid secretion. Alcohol may also reduce esophageal pressure and contribute to the likelihood of acid reflux (Hogan et al., 1972). Certain volatile oils, including peppermint and spearmint, apparently decrease LES pressure (Castell, 1975). Vagotomy, anticholinergic drugs, cigarette smoking, estrogen, and progesterone have all been shown to lower LES pressure, with implications for oral contraceptive users and pregnant women.

This line of research is clarifying some of the generally recognized relationships between eating and heartburn. Not all foods have been systematically studied, but an individual who is susceptible to gastroesophageal reflux with resulting heartburn would be well advised to avoid large amounts of fatty food, chocolate, or alcohol (Castell, 1975). Medical treatment for reflux usually concentrates on relieving patient symptoms. Small meals are recommended to reduce the volume of gastric contents. Eating during the 2 to 3 hours before bedtime is to be avoided as well as smoking or reclining immediately after a meal. Sleeping with the head of the bed elevated may decrease the tendency for reflux to occur. Antacid preparations may be taken to decrease stomach acidity and encourage the secretion of gastrin. Weight loss in obese patients is beneficial. Continued reflux over a period of time can lead to changes in the esophageal mucosa and chronic esophagitis may develop. In this case, slightly acid foods, as well as hot or cold foods, may be painful to swallow (Wintrobe et al., 1974, p. 1426).

Hiatal Hernia

A *hiatal hernia* is defined as herniation of a portion of the stomach into the chest through the esophageal hiatus of the diaphragm. The most common type of hiatal hernia is a sliding one in which the gastroesophageal junction and a portion of the stomach adjacent to it both slip up into the chest (Wintrobe et al., 1974, p. 1427). This process is illustrated in Fig. 12.6. The incidence of sliding hiatal hernia increases linearly with age. It may be

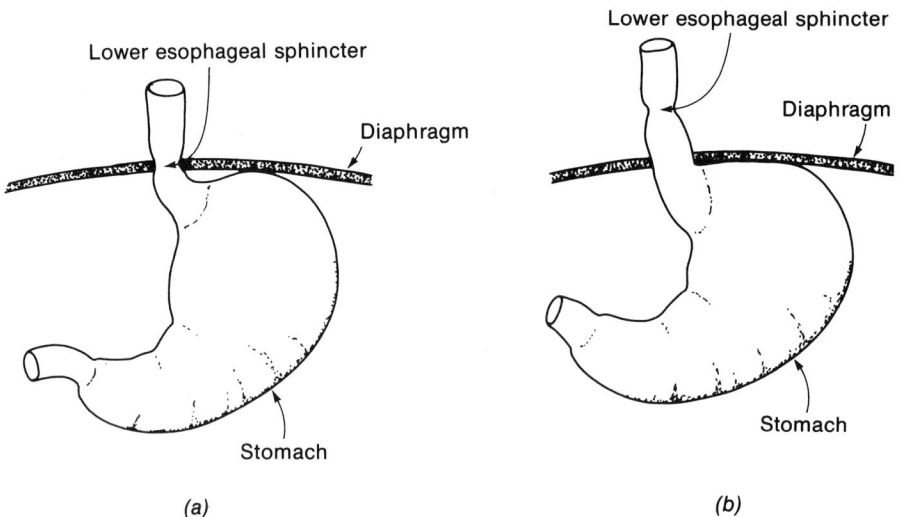

Fig. 12.6 (a) Diagram of normal structural relationships in the lower esophagus. (b) A sliding hiatal hernia.

found in more than half of the population of the United States over age 50. However, symptoms are not always present when hernias have been demonstrated radiographically, and apparently the LES is still competent in these cases.

The major symptoms attributed to a sliding hiatal hernia are the same as those associated with gastroesophageal reflux, with heartburn being the most specific, clear-cut indication. The LES apparently does not function properly, and gastric acid juice refluxes into the esophagus when symptoms are present with hiatal hernia. Many patients with reflux esophagitis have sliding hiatal hernia. However, others may have gastroesophageal reflux and esophagitis without having hiatal hernia. The relationship between hernia and sphincter incompetence is not clear.

Medical treatment of the symptoms of uncomplicated hiatal hernia is aimed at reducing reflux and neutralizing acid in the stomach. Dietary recommendations, as with gastroesophageal reflux without hernia, include frequent small feedings; avoidance of fatty foods that stimulate the production of CCK and secretin, reducing LES pressure; avoidance of chocolate, alcohol, and other foods that may aggravate the symptoms; and weight loss in the obese patient. The wearing of tight garments, such as girdles, should be avoided because of increased abdominal pressure that limits sphincter competence. The neutralization of gastric acid with antacids should encourage gastrin secretion and, thereby, increase sphincter pressure, as well as decrease the acidity of the material that may reflux into the esophagus (Katz and Pitchumoni, 1973). When medical treatment fails, surgical intervention to repair the hernia may be successful (Woodward, 1975).

12.5 Peptic Ulcer Disease

Peptic ulcer is a sharply circumscribed loss of the tissue lining those parts of the digestive tract that are exposed to pepsin-containing acid gastric juice. This includes the lower esophagus, the stomach, the first part of the duodenum, and the small intestine next to a surgically produced connection with the stomach (Beeson and McDermott, 1975, p. 1198). An ulcer is called a gastric ulcer if it is located in the wall of the stomach or a duodenal ulcer if found in the duodenum, but both are peptic ulcers. They are similar pathologically although there are differences between them.

Dietary habits have long been implicated in both the etiology and treatment of peptic ulcer. However, many of the traditional ideas concerning diet have not been founded on scientific data. They are gradually being evaluated in light of newer research findings.

Pathogenesis
The etiology of peptic ulcer is unknown. However, both acid and pepsin are required for ulcer formation. Ulcers seem to occur when there is an

imbalance between the acid-pepsin production and mucosal resistance with increased acid-pepsin secretion, decreased mucosal resistance, or both (Beeson and McDermott, 1975, p. 1198).

Gastric ulcers are less common in the United States than are duodenal ulcers by a ratio of about 1 to 4. Peptic ulcer occurs more frequently in United States males than females, with the sex difference being somewhat more pronounced in duodenal than gastric ulcer incidence. Although gastric ulcers may appear at any age, they tend to occur between 45 and 55 years, whereas the maximal incidence for duodenal ulcer is about 10 years earlier. Theories to explain the development of gastric ulcer have included the suggestions that (1) prolonged or excessive secretion of gastric juice or gastric stasis produces gastric ulceration (Dragstedt, 1963), and (2) injury of the mucosal epithelium, by regurgitation of bile acids into the stomach or by the action of certain drugs, allows back diffusion of H^+ eventually causing destruction of blood vessels and ulceration (Davenport, 1972). Few data show that gastric hypomotility or stasis is more prevalent in patients with gastric ulcer than in the normal population. George (1968) reported that the mean gastric emptying time after a test meal was longer in gastric ulcer patients than in either normal controls or patients with duodenal ulceration, but the wide range indicated that stasis was not a factor in all cases of gastric ulcer.

Acid secretion in gastric ulcer patients is usually within the normal range as commonly determined, although loss of acid by back-diffusion is not taken into account in these measurements. Excessive gastric acid secretion is found in 25 to 50 percent of duodenal ulcer cases. However, Fiddian-Green et al. (1976b) reported that only in ulcer patients who had had symptoms for more than 3 years was maximal acid output abnormally increased. Duodenal ulcer is extremely frequent in the Zollinger-Ellison syndrome, in which there is a high rate of gastric secretion. Other arguments supporting a relationship between acid-peptic juice and duodenal ulcer are: (1) duodenal ulcers are produced in dogs by introducing exogenous hydrochloric acid (HCl) into the duodenum in concentration equal to, or greater than, that secreted by the stomach at maximal secretory rates; (2) duodenal ulcers are produced in experimental animals by the administration of histamine in beeswax, which acts as a continuous and powerful stimulus to gastric acid secretion, and these ulcers can be prevented by removal of the acid-secreting mucosa; (3) duodenal ulcers often heal when gastric secretory capacity is reduced by medical or surgical means; (4) diversion of acid gastric juice into the jejunum by a gastroenterostomy frequently causes an ulcer in the jejunum; and (5) the risk in healthy humans of developing ulcer was found to increase as maximum acid output increased. In spite of these arguments, the fact that many duodenal ulcer patients have normal gastric secretory rates strongly suggests that some factor other than the ulcerogenic action of acid-peptic secretion is responsible for duodenal ulceration (Menguy, 1964; Fiddian-Green et al., 1976a and b).

Cooke (1976) examined epidemiological evidence associated with gastric damage by drugs. From this review, he concluded that caffeine and alcohol do not cause peptic ulcer. Phenylbutazone probably does not cause peptic ulcer, but there is not enough evidence to judge whether indomethacin is ulcerogenic or not. These drugs, along with adrenal corticosteroids, have been used in the treatment of rheumatoid arthritis. In a retrospective study without controls, Sun et al. (1974) found a high prevalence of peptic ulcer among patients with rheumatoid arthritis receiving indomethacin or phenylbutazone together with adrenal corticosteroids. The available evidence does not allow the conclusion that adrenal corticosteroids are ulcerogenic, but most data suggest that they are not. All these drugs, except caffeine, have little effect on gastric acid secretion, although steroids affect mucus secretion. Cooke further concluded that smoking is undoubtedly associated with peptic ulcer. Smokers have more ulcers and higher death rates from ulcers than do nonsmokers. However, none of the studies indicates whether or not smoking is a cause of peptic ulcer. Aspirin appears to be a cause of gastric ulcer, possibly by altering the permeability of epithelial cells and breaking the gastric mucosal barrier. Jacobs and Pringot (1973) reported that three patients with no history of GI disease developed acute gastric ulcers of the antral region apparently as a result of taking potassium chloride in enteric-coated tablets.

There is evidence for increased familial incidence of peptic ulcer, although a familial tendency is often absent on an individual basis. Persons with blood group O are 1.4 times as liable to have duodenal or prepyloric ulcers as are those with groups A, B, or AB, and persons who are nonsecretors into the intestinal tract of blood group substances (mucopolysaccharides with antigenic properties, present in the red blood cell) are 1.5 times as liable to these ulcers as are secretors. It has been postulated that the blood group substances may give some type of protection against ulceration. Group O nonsecretors are 2.5 times more liable to ulcer development than secretors of groups A, B, and AB. However, the inheritance of acid-peptic glandular mass and its capacity to secrete may be the most important genetic factor in ulcer development (Beeson and McDermott, 1975, p. 1199).

The frequency of occurrence of peptic ulcer varies throughout the world. Although duodenal ulcer is reported to be more common than gastric ulcer in most countries, including the United States, gastric ulcer is more common in a few populations. Duodenal ulcer was a rare disease before 1900. By 1914 it had become common in Europe and North America and gastric ulcer incidence had also increased moderately. From 1914 to 1955 these disorders remained at a relatively constant level and then began to decrease (Beeson and McDermott, 1975, p. 1199). A survey in black populations of Africa by Tovey and Tunstall (1975) revealed that the incidence of ulcer is low in areas with low rainfall where the diet is either unrefined white grain, millet, or maize. High incidence occurs where the staple diet is either refined or starchy and where there is good rainfall.

No etiologic effect was found for alcohol, caffeine, smoking, refined carbohydrate intake, spices, hookworm, infrequent meals, malnutrition, vitamin deficiencies, and stress. Yodfat (1972), from a survey of 4552 adults living in Israel and being treated at a medical center, reported that the highest risk group for duodenal ulcers was composed of males between the ages of 50 and 59 years in the high-income and educational level.

Psychological Factors. Conventional wisdom has described the typical ulcer patient as a hard-driving, ambitious executive under psychic tension or stress. Relationships between emotional or psychological factors and ulcer development require further testing, however. In 1958 the term *executive monkey* was coined by Brady and Porter at the Walter Reed Research Institute as they trained rhesus monkeys, using a red light stimulus, to avoid receiving an uncomfortable series of body shocks by pulling a lever above a certain speed. The monkeys were paired, one having no control and the other full control to prevent, by use of his lever, the shocks to himself and his partner. The executive monkey, with the real responsibility, soon showed evidence of agitation and personality change and either died in a few weeks from peptic ulcer perforation or, after being sacrificed, was found to have ulcers. The second monkey, who could supposedly not influence his own environment, did not develop ulcers. Other researchers have not been able to achieve the same results as did Porter and Brady, although some studies have suggested similarly that producing ulcers by response of an animal to a stressful environment may involve physiological pathways that activate cerebral systems (Foltz, 1964).

Weiss (1972), in reporting on ulcer development in rats placed under stress, suggested that if an animal can effectively cope with a stressful situation and receives relevant feedback that tells him he is coping successfully, he does not develop ulcers. Thus, ulcer development may be the result of lack of coping or adapting behavior rather than stress produced by responsibility. Weiss further suggested that the responding rate required for the executive monkey was extremely high (every 20 seconds) and that feedback for avoiding body shocks was low. Therefore, the animal could not cope effectively with his stressful situation and developed ulcers. Something like "emotional conflict" or inability to adapt may be involved in the development and maintenance of ulcers in humans. An ulcer patient usually responds very well to hospitalization regardless of the medical treatment used—whether rigid and controlled or very flexible. Possibly the attention and security that the patient receives in the hospital and removal from his or her stressful environment are responsible for much of this improvement.

Symptoms and Diagnosis

Peptic ulcer is a chronic disease characterized by remissions and exacerbations. Symptoms may last for a few days, weeks, or months and disappear for variable amounts of time. Ulcers, particularly gastric, may occur without symptoms in some cases. The symptoms of duodenal ulcer have a

uniform pattern. A localized, steady, gnawing, burning pain in the epigas-
trium is relieved after the ingestion of food or alkali. The pain usually
begins 2 to 2½ hours after a meal and may awaken a patient between midnight and 3:00 A.M. but, for unknown reasons, is almost never present upon
awakening before breakfast. It is thought that the gastric acid bathing the
ulcer causes discomfort and pain. This pattern of pain-food-relief is more
variable with gastric ulcers. Nausea, anorexia, and vomiting are not infrequent symptoms in gastric ulcer and may occur in the absence of
obstruction. Weight loss is frequent. In duodenal ulcer, a variety of other
GI symptoms may occur, including heartburn, regurgitation, and constipation or diarrhea. The appetite of duodenal ulcer patients is usually good
and weight gain common because of the frequent eating to avoid discomfort (Wintrobe et al., 1974, pp. 1435 and 1439).

Acute lesions of the stomach and duodenum are often multiple and
superficial erosions. They rarely extend through the muscularis mucosa.
The term ulcer is applied to a chronic ulcer. The average diameter is 5 to 25
mm, although the range in size is wide. Chronic ulcers destroy the mucosa,
muscularis mucosa, a variable amount of submucosa, and even some of the
muscular coat (Fig. 12.7). The majority of gastric ulcers occur in the pyloric
antrum of the stomach on the lesser curvature. Since the antral mucosa
occupies a variable percentage of total gastric mucosal surface, gastric ul-

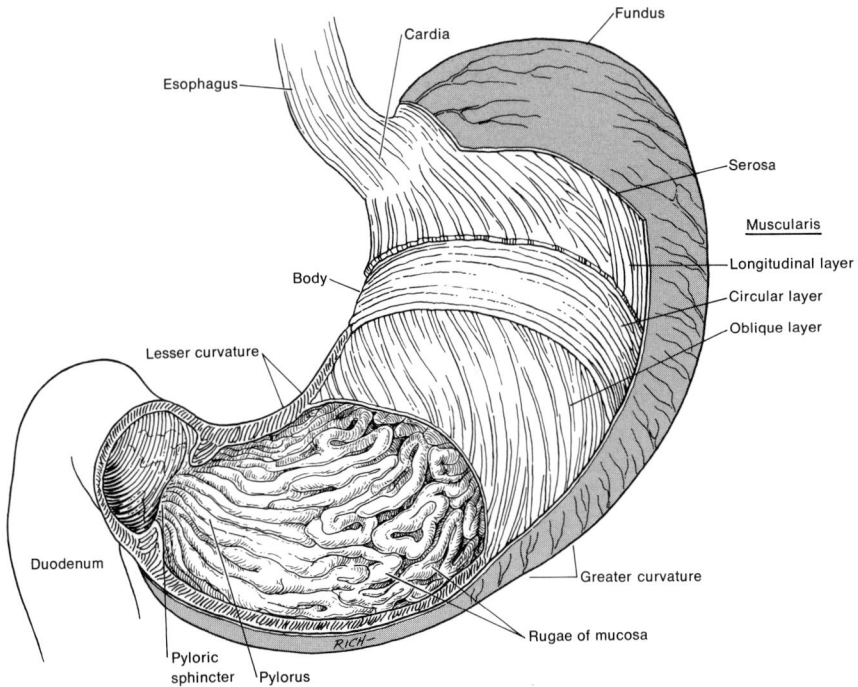

Fig. 12.7 The stomach, external and internal anatomy. (From Gerard J. Tortora, *Principles of Anatomy and Psyiology*, 2d ed., New York: Harper & Row, 1978; by permission of the publisher.)

cers can appear at widely differing distances from the pylorus in specific patients and still be in the antral region. Gastric ulcers are commonly associated with gastritis. It is not certain if the gastritis precedes or follows development of the ulcer, but it may persist after the ulcer has healed (Trier, 1976).

The diagnosis of duodenal ulcer considers the typical periodic sequence of pain-food-relief. X-ray examination with barium demonstrates the crater and gastric analysis is usually not necessary. The history is less diagnostic in gastric ulcer since symptoms are frequently vague, the diagnosis here depending more on gastroscopic examination and radiography. It is imperative that differentiation be made between benign and malignant gastric ulcer.

Complications of benign peptic ulcer include perforation, obstruction, and hemorrhage. Hemorrhage affects about 15 to 20 percent of ulcer patients. Almost all patients with hemorrhage show melena and many experience hematemesis. Gastric outlet obstruction is seen in 5 to 10 percent of ulcer patients and is usually a complication of long-standing duodenal ulcer disease. Perforation occurs when the ulcer erodes through the muscular and serosal walls and allows spillage of luminal contents into the surrounding body cavity.

Medical Management

The rate of healing of peptic ulcers seems to be little affected by the usual medical treatment. There is a tendency for ulcers to heal regardless of the therapy and even if no therapy is used (Bevan, 1975). However, medical therapy does relieve symptoms in most cases and this is one of the important goals of treatment. Antacids and anticholinergic drugs are the primary therapeutic agents used in duodenal ulcer management. Medical treatment of gastric ulcer is similar to that of duodenal ulcer; however, anticholinergic drugs are usually not used since they prolong gastric emptying (Wintrobe et al., 1974, p. 1041). Bland diets have been used traditionally in treatment, but there is no evidence that a bland diet is more effective than a regular diet in ulcer healing, prevention of complications, or recurrence. The prognosis for a patient with peptic ulcer is usually good for the immediate attack but less favorable for the long range since ulcers tend to reoccur after healing.

Antacids. The rationale for treatment with antacids to neutralize gastric contents to at least pH 5 is that (1) ulcers do not occur in the absence of acid and pepsin; (2) peptic activity decreases markedly at a pH greater than 3.5; (3) the incidence of experimental ulcers in animals is decreased by antacids; and (4) ulcer disease usually resolves with surgical therapy which decreases acid and pepsin secretion. However, there are few data indicating that use of antacids improves healing, decreases recurrences, or decreases complications in humans (Beeson and McDermott, 1975, p. 1206).

Most available antacids are mixtures of magnesium, aluminum, or calcium salts. The ideal antacid preparation does not exist. Sodium bicarbonate is potent and rapid acting, but it leaves the stomach quickly, is completely absorbed, and may present too great an alkaline load to the body. Calcium carbonate is a potent, rapidly acting antacid and less than 10 percent of the calcium is absorbed. However, repeated doses in some cases may cause elevated serum calcium levels which produce increased gastric acid stimulation, probably mediated in part by increased serum gastrin. Use of calcium carbonate may cause constipation. Magnesium hydroxide is more potent than magnesium trisilicate or magnesium carbonate and approximately 5 to 10 percent of the magnesium is absorbed. Magnesium salts act as cathartics and can seldom be used as the sole antacid. The neutralizing capacity of aluminum hydroxide preparations varies widely and some are ineffective. Prolonged use of aluminum hydroxide can decrease serum and total body phosphate since it produces nonabsorbable aluminum phosphate in the gut. It may also produce severe constipation, especially in the aged. The high sodium content of many alumina preparations may be a problem for individuals requiring a low-sodium intake. In the acutely ill patient, antacids are usually given at hourly intervals during the day and evening. When symptoms decrease, they are often given 1 and 3 hours after each meal and at bedtime (Beeson and McDermott, 1975, pp. 1206–1207; Wintrobe et al., 1974, pp. 1436–1437).

Diet. Dietary measures have been used empirically in the treatment of peptic ulcer for centuries. An hourly milk-cream feeding schedule, alternating with antacids, was first introduced into the United States by Sippy in 1915 and was widely used thereafter. In 1961 a committee composed of members from the American Dietetic Association and the American Medical Association reported on a review of published research and practice in diet therapy for GI disorders (Weinstein et al., 1961). Among other things, they pointed out that the effect of foods on the stomach must be evaluated on the basis of both their immediate direct and their delayed indirect effects on gastric contents. For example, the pH of foods ranges from about 2 (lime juice) to 8 (egg whites and graham crackers), but most foods have a pH between 5 and 7. The pH of orange or grapefruit juice is about 3.2 to 3.6, considerably less acid than normal gastric juice (pH 1.5 to 2.0). Diluting fruit juices with water affects pH negligibly. On the basis of the direct effect of their acidity, acid fruit juices should theoretically be harmful only to oral, esophageal, and perhaps gastric lesions, especially if achlorhydria is present. Otherwise the pH of a food before ingestion has little significance in diet therapy.

Weinstein et al. (1961) further stated that the immediate direct effect of food proteins is to buffer gastric acidity. Milk may very briefly elevate the pH of the stomach contents, but does not achieve a level of 3.5, which is usually defined as the minimum level desirable for healing. Proteins, especially fish and meat, are among the most potent dietary stimulants of gastric secretion, with carbohydrates and fats having a lesser effect. This delayed stimulating effect on gastric acid secretion by food proteins, therefore, may counterbalance their direct buffering effects. Rebound hyperacidity may also occur with milk ingestion because of its calcium content. Fats depress gastric motility and delay emptying, and a case may be made for moderate amounts of dietary fat to lessen the secretory and motor response to meals. However, frequency and regularity of food intake are probably more important than the type of food ingested. Controlled studies in people have shown that the so-called blandness of the diet does not affect the rate of duodenal ulcer healing (Doll et al., 1956).

Schneider et al. (1956) administered various spices along with food to 50 patients with active ulcers and observed the rate of healing, clinical symptomatology, gastroscopic appearance of the stomach before and after ingestion, and the effect on pepsin secretion for periods up to 180 days. Black pepper produced the greatest irritating effect. Chili pepper, cloves, mustard seed, and possibly nutmeg were lesser irritants. Cinnamon, allspice, mace, thyme, sage, paprika, and caraway seed exerted no harmful influence. Black pepper is usually specifically excluded from the diet for patients with peptic ulcer. Caffeine is a moderately strong stimulant of acid secretion, but there are apparently additional substances in coffee, both regular and decaffeinated, that may stimulate acid secretion to an even greater extent than does caffeine. Thus, coffee may be limited for a patient with peptic ulcer. Because of the possible effect of alcohol on the gastric mucosal barrier, it may be limited.

Because of the lack of research evidence that a bland diet (traditionally defined as one that is chemically and mechanically nonirritating to the GI tract) is effective in the treatment of peptic ulcer disease, a liberal diet is now generally advocated. The American Dietetic Association, in a position paper on Bland Diet in the Treatment of Chronic Duodenal Ulcer Disease (1971), recognized that the traditional rationale for a bland diet is not sufficiently supported by scientific evidence, and cited the following:

1. Spices, condiments, and highly seasoned foods are usually omitted on the basis that they irritate the gastric mucosa. This does not generally appear to be true, although exceptions are black pepper, chili powder, caffeine, coffee, tea, cocoa, alcohol, and drugs.
2. Milk has been used to reduce secretions and neutralize acid. While milk does relieve duodenal ulcer pain, the acid neutralizing effect is slight and its buffering effect could be outweighed by its ability to stimulate acid production. Extensive use of milk may have side effects and allergic reactions. Strict insistence on its use during remission is unwarranted.
3. Roughage, or coarse food, has been excluded from the diet on the basis that it aggravates the inflamed mucosa. There is no evidence

that such foods as fruit skins, lettuce, nuts, and celery, when they are well masticated and mixed with saliva, will scrape or irritate the ulcer. Grinding or puréeing of foods is necessary only when the teeth are in poor condition or missing.

4. Results of studies on the effect of a bland diet on the healing of duodenal ulcer indicate that it makes no difference when compared to regular or free-choice diets.

The position paper further states the belief that (1) scientific investigation supports the validity of frequent, small feedings for duodenal ulcer patients because they offer the most comfort to the patient and keep the gastric acidity relatively low, and (2) individualization should be paramount in developing a dietary plan for ulcer patients.

That certain beliefs about the diet for ulcer are traditional and widely held throughout the community was demonstrated by Caron and Roth (1972) in a survey that requested subjects to designate foods on a list as "good" or "bad" for an ulcer diet. Ulcer patients' beliefs were strikingly similar to those of a small sample of physicians and dietitians interviewed in 1958. The patients showed marked agreement on most foods and their selections did not change during a 7-year period. The food restrictions they described were excessive and could interfere with the learning of a more liberal therapeutic diet by obscuring the real nutritional requirements with many inappropriate rules. A survey by Welsh (1977) of hospital dietitians throughout the United States revealed that a bland diet was used for peptic ulcer disease in 77 percent of the hospitals. On discharge, dietitians in one-half of the hospitals instructed patients on a bland diet.

Caron and Roth (1971) found that when hospitalized patients were observed under conditions that permitted them to choose a more lenient diet by using an unauthorized diet card in a cafeteria, the median patient with peptic ulcer took his prescribed diet on only 76 percent of all observed days. One fourth of the patients cooperated on less than 60 percent of all days. Thus, many individuals with ulcers may believe that the diet should be restricted to bland foods but choose not to practice their beliefs consistently.

Although milk has traditionally been referred to as an ideal agent for neutralizing gastric acid, Ippoliti et al. (1976) reported that gastric acid secretion was significantly increased by ingestion of whole, low-fat, and nonfat milk. The stimulatory effect of milk persisted for at least 3 hours after ingestion. Doll et al. (1956) found that alkaline milk drip did not affect the healing rate of gastric ulcer.

For several reasons, excessive use of milk in ulcer therapy may be detrimental. The milk-alkali syndrome results from excess ingestion of calcium along with absorbable alkali. The combination of sodium bicarbonate and/or calcium carbonate as antacid preparations and consumption of large quantities of milk can produce hypercalcemia, alkalosis, azotemia, and hyperphosphatemia, which may lead to the development of renal calculi and permanent renal damage. Symptoms of the milk-alkali syndrome include anorexia, malaise, nausea, vomiting, weakness, muscle pain, polydipsia, and polyuria and are similar to those of hypercalcemia from other causes (Beeson and McDermott, 1975, p. 1206). At least in the early stages of this syndrome, abnormalities will disappear with discontinuance of the high calcium intake.

Clinical and autopsy records for 1940 to 1959 were examined by Hartroft (1964) in order to collect information on possible relationships between coronary heart disease and peptic ulcer. A clear association between a high incidence of myocardial infarction and the consumption of a Sippy-type (high milk) diet was found in both the United States and Great Britain. In the United States, the incidence of myocardial infarction was 15 percent in ulcer patients not treated with Sippy diets and in nonulcer controls, whereas it was 36 percent in the ulcer group treated with a Sippy diet. This incidence increased to 42 percent if the patients who had been on a Sippy diet for 1 year or less were eliminated from the study. No cause and effect could be shown from this study, but data pointed out a possible relationship between milk consumption and coronary heart disease.

Serum cholesterol levels of peptic ulcer patients may be decreased with the feeding of polyunsaturated fatty acid milk preparations as substitutes for whole milk or milk-cream mixtures (Kaplan et al., 1965; Berkowitz, 1964; Cayer and Ruffin, 1964; McHardy et al., 1964). Laureta et al. (1964) reported that a preparation of skim milk to which soy oil, vitamins, and minerals were added was slightly more effective in buffering gastric acidity than was the use of a milk and cream mixture.

In summary, research data do not support severe dietary restriction for peptic ulcer patients. Coffee, caffeine, alcohol, black pepper, and chili powder are contraindicated. Small, frequent meals that are nutritionally well balanced should be provided. Individualization of the nutritional care is important and foods that are not tolerated by an individual may be eliminated for her comfort. Moderate amounts of protein for some immediate buffering effect and moderate amounts of fat to control gastric motility may be helpful. However, antacids are usually relied on for buffering during acute stages of the disease. In initial stages, frequent, small feedings of milk (which may be skim or low-fat) or soft bland foods, such as cream soups, cooked, refined cereals, soft-cooked eggs, cottage cheese, white potato, and custards, may be useful.

In general, food should be consumed slowly and in a pleasant, congenial atmosphere. Educational materials to aid the patient in understanding and achieving appropriate nutritional objectives should be provided on an individual basis.

Drugs. Anticholinergic drugs block the action of acetylcholine on postganglionic nerve sites and are used to decrease acid and pepsin secretion in peptic ulcer patients. Although they have additional side effects, they are useful in many cases.

Carbenoxolone sodium, an extract of licorice that increases the production and viscosity of gastric mucus and decreases mucosal cell turnover, has been reported to be of value in the healing of gastric ulcers among outpatients. This compound is similar in structure to the hormone, aldosterone, and produces salt and water retention (Beeson and McDermott, 1975, p. 1207). A potential agent for treatment of peptic ulcer is prostaglandin E_2 since it is a potent inhibitor of acid secretion (Isenberg, 1975). H_2-histamine-receptor antagonists (cimetidine) may have value in ulcer treatment since the final common local chemostimulator of the acid-secreting cell may be histamine (Debas, 1977).

Hemorrhaging Peptic Ulcers. It is generally believed that feeding should be commenced as soon as nausea and hematemesis have stopped in the case of hemorrhaging from the upper GI tract. Lenhartz, in 1904, was one of the first to recommend early feeding when he suggested the use of small feedings hourly during the first day after hemorrhaging. Meulengracht reinforced this regimen in 1934 when he recommended the use of somewhat larger meals composed of soft or puréed foods with between-meal feedings of milk. With a relatively liberal diet, a good nutritional state could be maintained. The mortality rate is lower with feeding than under the previously used starvation method (Goodhart and Shils, 1973, p. 778). A soft or regular diet with frequent, small feedings should be appropriate for most patients being treated for bleeding peptic ulcers.

Surgical Management

Few patients are considered for surgical treatment until the physician is satisfied that medical treatment has been conscientiously applied and that, in spite of these measures, relapses of typical ulcer symptoms are becoming more frequent, severe, and prolonged. The majority of duodenal ulcer patients approaching surgery have had symptoms for between 5 and 10 years and sometimes longer (Gillespie, 1968). The complications of intractable bleeding, obstruction, and perforation usually necessitate surgery.

Surgical Procedures. A major goal for surgery in the treatment of peptic ulcer is to produce a large and lasting decrease in the secretion of HCl and pepsin. The type of surgery to be performed in accomplishing this and other goals will depend upon many factors. The approach will be individualized with consideration of the patient's peculiar preoperative problems, the physiological basis for each operative procedure, and the expected postoperative physiological effects. Preoperative tests, including secretory tests and measurement of serum gastrin levels, may aid the physician in planning for surgery. Three types of surgical procedures are most frequently used in treatment of peptic ulcer disease. The dietitian needs to be aware of the procedure performed on an individual patient in order to give effective nutritional care postoperatively (Behm et al., 1974), as follows:

1. Subtotal gastrectomy. A high gastric resection of the distal 75 to 80 percent of the stomach removes both the antrum where gastrin is secreted and much of the parietal cell mass. A Billroth II procedure is usually used to join the proximal jejunum to the remnant of the stomach (Fig. 12.8). This procedure may be used for patients with distal gastric carcinoma, proximal gastric ulcers, or duodenal ulcers. Since there is a major loss of gastric reservoir, individuals who are preoperatively underweight may have difficulty in maintaining normal weight postoperatively.

2. Antrectomy. The distal 40 to 50 percent of the stomach is removed and anastomosis made to the intestine either by a Billroth I procedure, which joins the remnant of the stomach to the duodenum (Fig. 12.9), or by a Billroth II procedure involving a gastrojejunostomy. Antrectomy may be used for treatment of distal gastric ulcer. It is usually combined with vagotomy in the treatment of duodenal ulcer.

3. Vagotomy and drainage procedure. The vagus nerves are cut in order to reduce gastric acid production and drainage is provided, by either pyloroplasty or gastrojejunostomy (Fig. 12.10), to avoid retention secondary to the decreased gastric motility. The vagotomy may be a truncal vagotomy, with cutting of the two main trunks and any subsidiary fibers of the vagus nerve at the level of the esophageal hiatus so that the whole gut as far as the transverse colon, the biliary system, and the pancreas are completely deprived of parasympathetic innervation. A selective vagotomy divides all vagal fibers running to the stomach but the hepatic and celiac branches are spared, preserving vagal innervation of all other abdominal organs. A highly selective vagotomy affecting only part of the stomach has also been used in recent years (Kennedy, 1974). Pyloroplasty involves plastic surgery of the pylorus to allow easier movement of food from the stomach. Vagotomy with drainage procedure is frequently used for the control of duodenal ulcer disease.

Zollinger-Ellison Syndrome. A syndrome was originally described by Zollinger and Ellison in 1955 that consisted of a triad: (1) fulminant recurrent

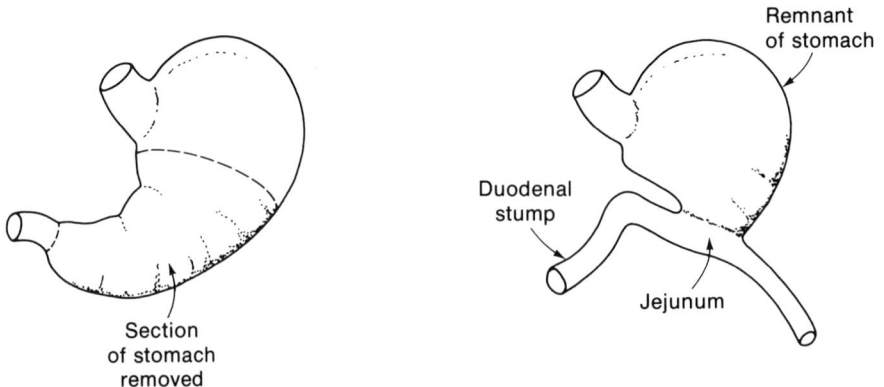

Fig. 12.8 A subtotal gastrectomy with a Billroth II procedure.

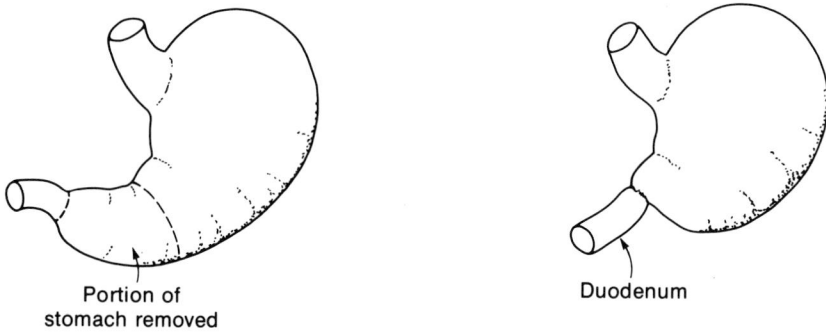

Portion of
stomach removed

Duodenum

Fig. 12.9 An antrectomy with a Billroth I procedure.

peptic ulcer disease despite "adequate" surgery, (2) gastric hypersecretion, and (3) nonbeta cell islet tumors of the pancreas. The term *gastrinoma* has also been applied to this syndrome since there is an excessive release of gastrin from the tumor. All features of the triad need not be present and diagnosis is often difficult (Dodsworth and Fischer, 1974).

Symptoms of the Zollinger-Ellison syndrome are often similar to those of the usual duodenal ulcer, but the tendency toward fulminant ulceration with severe complications is great. Ulceration rapidly recurrs after surgery that would be adequate for most peptic ulcers. Diarrhea and malabsorption are additional clinical features of this syndrome. The best treatment is total gastrectomy. The mortality rate in cases without total gastrectomy is as high as 90 percent, whereas when this surgical procedure is performed, the mortality is 10 to 15 percent (Wintrobe et al., 1974, p. 1442).

Nutritional Problems after Gastric Resection. Since nutrition-related problems such as weight loss, anemia, hypoproteinemia, and fluid and

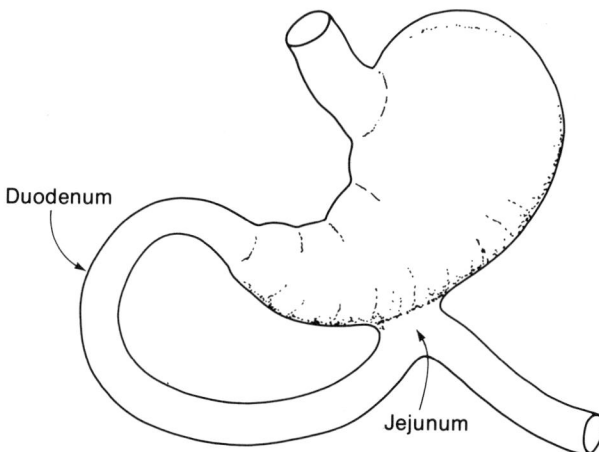

Duodenum

Jejunum

Fig. 12.10 A gastrojejunostomy is one type of drainage procedure that may be used with vagotomy in the treatment of duodenal ulcer.

electrolyte imbalance, are common among candidates for peptic ulcer surgery, provision of optimal nutritional care during the postoperative period is extremely important for maximal benefit to the patient. Immediately following gastric surgery, the patient is given nothing by mouth (NPO). The length of time an individual remains NPO and on nasogastric suction is variable, some being able to take food or liquid orally within hours after surgery while others may require nasogastric suction for a week or more. In general, surgeons order the first postoperative feeding when bowel sounds are detectable or flatus is passed (Behm et al., 1974).

The feeding procedure immediately following gastric surgery may vary from one institution to another. Clear liquids in small portions are sometimes used as the first regimen, gradually augmented with full liquids. In other cases, the feeding of choice is small amounts of dry, low fiber foods, with the rationale that liquids may cause distention and dumping. Behm et al. (1974) reported that the initial postoperative diet served at Ohio State University Hospital consists of 120 ml of broth or bouillon and dry toast or crackers at each meal. This diet is low in fluid volume, contains no concentrated carbohydrate, and provides stimulants to increase GI function. It is offered for one or two meals or until the diet can be progressed to an individualized postgastrectomy regimen.

The major goal of nutritional care for the patient following gastric surgery is to avoid symptoms of postgastrectomy syndrome while supplying optimum nutrition in a form that can be tolerated. Postgastrectomy syndrome includes dumping syndrome, reactive hypoglycemia, and diarrhea. Nutritional problems that may develop at a later time include anemia and bone disease.

Dumping syndrome, sometimes referred to as the early syndrome, is characterized by the development of weakness, nausea, a feeling of warmth, palpitation, pallor, perspiration, apprehension, diarrhea, and abdominal distention 10 to 30 minutes after a meal. The patient usually has an urgent desire to lie down and this may produce significant relief. The symptoms disappear after 30 to 60 minutes. The dumping syndrome apparently results from loss of the reservoir function of the stomach. Hyperosmolar chyme from the stomach is "dumped" rapidly into the small intestine, which causes an outpouring of fluid from the plasma to produce an isoosmotic intestinal content. The upper small intestine is distended by the large amount of material suddenly placed in it and by the fluid entering from the plasma to equalize the osmotic pressures.

It was previously thought that a sudden decrease in blood volume produced by this sequence was responsible for the clinical symptoms. However, the lack of correlation between decreases in plasma volume and the severity of the symptoms has led to a search for other causes of the early postprandial dumping syndrome. The release of serotonin or other vasoactive amines from the small intestine has been implicated in the development of the vasomotor symptoms. The diarrhea may be caused by the effect on peristalsis of the large amount of fluid in the small intestine and also by the release of enteric glucagon in response to glucose in the gut, since glucagon inhibits sodium absorption by the small intestine (Behm et al., 1974; Wintrobe et al., 1974, p. 1446).

There are large individual differences in ability to adapt to changes produced by gastric surgery, the majority of patients having minimal symptoms and only 5 to 10 percent having significant problems. However, careful medical and nutritional management immediately after surgery have a great influence on whether or not symptoms will develop. Careful and slow introduction of oral nutrition should occur on an individual basis. Ross (1971), who reported an incidence of dumping syndrome of less than 2 percent of the patients operated on by surgeons in his institution, has suggested that the patient should be gradually introduced to extremely small quantities of noncaloric liquids and then be given soft solids, restricting liquids to 15 to 30 minutes after frequent small meals, to allow the jejunum to adjust. His experience has been that by approximately the eighth to tenth postoperative day, small meals of solid foods can be assimilated without incident.

The early postgastrectomy dietary regimen should avoid sugar and concentrated sweets (puddings, ice cream, milkshakes, etc.). Dietetic canned fruits and juices may be given. Fluids, if served with meals, should be restricted, with a maximum of 120 ml being taken at the end of each meal. If this amount of fluid taken with meals causes GI symptoms, the meals may need to consist completely of nonliquid foods. Table 12.3 gives suggested menus for the early stages of the regimen. The dietitian should visit the hospitalized patient regularly to assess progress in tolerating the types of foods, portion sizes, and total volume of food offered, and the diet progressed according to the individual's needs. Portion sizes and variety of foods are increased once the patient is free of symptoms or the feeling of fullness. Moderate amounts of sugar in regular canned fruits and juices and simple desserts may be added to the diet as tolerated. Raw fruits and vegetables may not be included for the first few weeks postoperatively until the healing process is more complete (Behm et al., 1974). Five or six small feedings daily and avoidance of high fluid intake with meals should be continued after discharge from the hospital.

Biggar et al. (1960) evaluated the nutritional status of 100 postgastrectomy patients at least 1 year after surgery and found that 67 percent were at or above their desirable weight level while 33 percent were below. Five of the underweight patients had never reached their desirable weight at any time preoperatively, however, and would not be likely to do so after a gastrectomy. Seventy-four percent of the individuals reported that they were able to eat anything they desired or had only a few aversions. Willis and Postlewait (1962) interviewed 51 patients with gastric resection 2 to 7 years previously. Caloric intakes ranged from 1200 to 4000 kcal daily, with a mean of 2600. One-third of the patients were within 10 lb of ideal weight, 18 percent were overweight, and 49 percent were 10 lb or more underweight. Eight of the underweight patients had consistently high daily caloric

Table 12.3 SUGGESTED MENUS FOR EARLY PHASE POSTGASTRECTOMY DIET

	Day 1 or 2		Day 3 or 4
Breakfast	Scrambled egg, 1 Buttered toast, 1 slice	Breakfast	Soft cooked egg, 1 Crisp bacon, 2 strips Buttered toast, 1 slice Unsweetened orange juice, ½ cup
Mid-morning	Cornflakes, ¾ cup Milk, ⅓ cup	Mid-morning	Flaked wheat cereal, ¾ cup Milk, ½ cup
Lunch	Macaroni and cheese, ½ cup Soda crackers, 2 Unsweetened applesauce, ½ cup Milk, ½ cup	Lunch	Baked halibut, 2 oz Buttered rice, ½ cup Buttered peas, ½ cup Soft roll with butter or margarine, 1 Milk, ½ cup
Mid-after- noon	Cottage cheese, ¼ cup Ritz crackers, 2	Mid-after- noon	Dietetic baked custard, ½ cup Ritz crackers, 4
Dinner	Roast chicken, 2 oz Buttered noodles, ½ cup Unsweetened orange juice, ½ cup	Dinner	Roast beef, 2 oz Creamed potatoes, ½ cup Baked squash, ½ cup Ripe banana, ½ Milk, ½ cup

Evening	Cheese sandwich, ½
	Unsweetened canned pears,
	  ½ cup
		Evening	Turkey sandwich, ½
			Unsweetened canned cherries,
			  ½ cup

intakes, but often had a high fluid intake as well, particularly with meals. Weight gain occurred in some of these patients when liquid was eliminated from meals. Pittman and Robinson (1962) reported that 30 outpatients following a diet consisting of frequent small "dry" feedings low in carbohydrate, high in protein, and high in fat had no marked nutritional deficiencies or other complications. Their diets included a caloric ratio of 1.0 carbohydrate, 1.5 protein, and 5.0 fat. In spite of the high fat intake, 95 percent of the patients remained within normal prescribed limits for serum cholesterol and 50 percent had values below initial findings. It would thus appear that the majority of postgastrectomy patients are able to maintain at least normal weight over a long period of time but that underweight is a problem with some. Follow-up nutritional counseling is of particular importance where there are weight problems. Steatorrhea was reported in 14 of 15 patients undergoing fat-balance studies immediately following subtotal gastrectomy (Lewis et al., 1958). This may be a factor contributing to the inability to maintain normal weight in some patients.

Postprandial postgastrectomy hypoglycemia (alimentary or reactive) may develop as a late syndrome 2 to 3 hours after a meal. Symptoms include weakness, sweating, nervousness, tachycardia, and hunger. Etiological mechanisms have been suggested as (1) an excessive insulin output in response to an initial hyperglycemia which results from the rapid absorption of simple sugars, and (2) an increased responsiveness to normal levels of circulating insulin. Shultz et al. (1971) studied nine patients with documented postprandial hypoglycemia following subtotal gastrectomy. They reported that the patients showed early hyperglycemia and late hypoglycemia following oral administration of glucose. Insulin secretion was exaggerated. Plasma insulin and glucose responses to intravenously administered glucose were either low or normal as compared to control subjects. Two patients restricted dietary carbohydrate to 50 g daily for several months. On this regimen they gained weight and had a striking amelioration of their hypoglycemic symptoms. Oral glucose tolerance tests after the diet showed no late hypoglycemia and decreased insulin secretion, although the early plasma glucose curve was unchanged from that before the diet began. One patient voluntarily resumed a high-carbohydrate diet and her hypoglycemic symptoms returned after several months on this program. The data suggested that postgastrectomy hypoglycemia is inducible by a high-carbohydrate diet and may be caused by a GI factor that potentiates glucose-mediated insulin release.

A hypochromic microcytic anemia frequently follows gastric surgery in 4 to 8 years, particularly if the operative procedure employed resulted in bypassing the duodenum (gastrojejunostomy) where much of the iron absorption occurs. Gastrointestinal bleeding may contribute to the development of anemia. Macrocytic anemias have also been observed in postgastrectomy patients.

Hines et al. (1967) found anemia in 153 (53 percent) of 292 patients who had undergone partial gastrectomy 1 to 20 years previously. In 100 of the patients, treatment with orally or parenterally administered iron resulted in restoration of normal hemoglobin concentrations, whereas in 35 the anemia responded partially to treatment with iron but either vitamin B_{12} or folic acid was required to achieve a normal hemoglobin value. Twelve patients had vitamin B_{12} deficiency and six patients folate deficiency. Anemia was documented by Shafer et al. (1973) in 69 of 142 (48 percent) male patients. In 16 the anemia appeared to be solely the result of iron deficiency, in 14 it was due to vitamin B_{12} deficiency, to folic acid deficiency in six, and to a mixed deficiency of vitamin B_{12}, iron, or folic acid in 33 patients. It is, therefore, important that postgastrectomy patients be followed over long periods of time in order to detect and treat anemias.

Diarrhea may be a problem in some patients after gastric resection with production of a gastrojejunostomy. Several mechanisms could be involved. (1) There may be inadequate stimuli to the secretion of bile and pancreatic juice by gastric chyme since the stomach contents go directly into the jejunum, affecting emulsification and hydrolysis of fats. MCT may be substituted for LCT in the diet. (2) There may be proliferation of intestinal bacteria in the duodenum with deconjugation of bile salts which exerts an inhibitory effect on the action of pancreatic and intestinal enzyme systems.

Treatment with antibiotics should be helpful. (3) An augmented gastroenterocolic reflex mechanism may develop that results in faster intestinal transit. Treatment with antispasmodics should be effective (Ross, 1971).

Eddy (1971) reported that 30 percent of 342 postgastrectomy patients exhibited metabolic bone disease, particularly osteomalacia, as compared with only 5 percent of peptic ulcer patients of similar age and sex who had not undergone surgery. Statistical correlation between amount of fecal fat and calcium abnormalities suggested that malabsorption of fat with accompanying loss of calcium may be a causative mechanism in the development of bone disease. Faulty absorption of vitamin D may also contribute to bone problems after gastrectomy.

Nutritional Effects of Vagotomy and Drainage Procedures. When vagotomy is performed without a drainage procedure, subsequent gastric stasis leads to ulceration in some patients. Therefore, drainage procedures are usually used with vagotomy to promote gastric emptying. Cobb et al. (1971) found a very rapid initial liquid emptying phase in 19 patients who had had a vagotomy and pyloroplasty, followed by emptying at a rate somewhat faster than that of either 12 patients with duodenal ulcers or nine patients with normal upper GI tracts. Patients with vagotomy and pyloroplasty who complained of postprandial fullness and dumping had extremely rapid initial gastric emptying of liquids. The handling of liquid and semisolid food is apparently different, however, since Buckler (1967), using potato mash and enteric-coated barium granules, found gastric emptying to be considerably delayed after vagotomy and pyloroplasty, more so than after any other gastric operation. Symptoms of dumping syndrome may occur in some patients with vagotomy and drainage procedure when large amounts of fluid are taken with meals. It is possible that the consistency of a meal has a marked effect on gastric emptying rate in these patients.

Cox et al. (1964) performed laboratory tests and interviews on 120 consecutive patients with duodenal ulcer 4 years after vagotomy and jejunostomy. The majority of patients reported a gain in weight between the time of surgery and follow-up, although the weight of the majority of patients 4 years after surgery remained below their estimated best weight before the operation. The number of patients seriously below their ideal weights was much smaller than before. The incidence of anemia was low. Serum vitamin B_{12} levels were almost all within the normal range but a small though statistically significant reduced mean level of vitamin B_{12} absorption was found in these patients. Some impairment of fat absorption was also found but the small associated caloric loss would be unlikely to have a recognizable effect on nutrition. The incidence of troublesome diarrhea in patients with vagotomy and gastrojejunostomy is probably about 5 percent, and the mechanism of its development has not been adequately explained. The postoperative nutritional effects of vagotomy with drainage procedure are generally not large and patients manage reasonably well.

12.6 Gastritis

Gastritis, involving inflammation of the mucosal lining of the stomach, is common, the reported incidence of the chronic variety starting at 28 percent in childhood and rising to 96 percent of the population past age 60 (Wintrobe et al., 1974, p. 1452). Gastric mucosa is exposed continuously to a wide variety of stimuli that are conducive to irritation or injury, including ingestion of drugs, condiments such as black pepper, and extremes of pH and temperature. The diagnosis of "gastritis" has been popular as a plausible and convenient label for diverse GI symptoms. For a period of time, overdiagnosis led to disrepute of gastritis as a clinical entity. However, much progress has recently been made in characterizing gastritis from histological and secretory measurements and in defining its relationships with gastric ulcer and cancer (Phillips, 1972; Ivey, 1973). Gastritis is usually present with gastric ulcer and Gear et al. (1971) suggested that gastritis may be the basic disease process and ulceration secondary.

Acute gastritis may be caused by food poisoning, acute alcoholism, shock, certain drugs, acute illnesses, and uremia. Symptoms include anorexia, nausea, vomiting, diffuse epigastric discomfort, and fever. Treatment is supportive since acute gastritis heals spontaneously when the irritant is removed. Usually no food is given orally in the early acute phase.

The cause of chronic gastritis is unknown, but it occurs in association with stomach cancer, gastric ulcer, pernicious anemia, duodenogastric reflux, sprue, diabetes mellitus, chronic iron deficiency, chronic use of aspirin, and normal aging (Wintrobe et al., 1974, p. 1452). It may often occur without symptoms. Peroral biopsy can be used to establish a histological basis for diagnosis of chronic gastritis. Gastroscopic appearance and severity of clinical symptoms do not always correlate with histological findings (Samloff, 1965).

Acid output in gastric juice appears to be decreased in chronic gastritis. However, it is possible that damage to the gastric mucosal barrier has allowed back diffusion of HCl from the stomach into the mucosal cells after it has been secreted into the stomach. This loss of already secreted acid may account for the apparent lack of HCl when measured by usual methods. Alteration of the gastric mucosal barrier may play an important role in the development of chronic gastritis, as it does in peptic ulcer. If this is the case, the rational management of chronic gastritis should be based on neutralization or marked reduction of gastric acid output, as in gastric or duodenal ulcer (Ivey, 1974). Treatment may thus include use of antacids; avoidance of irritants that may damage the mucosal barrier, such as alcohol, caffeine, black pepper, and aspirin; and frequent, small feedings.

REFERENCES

1. Adibi, S. A. 1976. Intestinal phase of protein assimilation in man. *Am. J. Clin. Nutr.*, **29:** 205.

2. American Dietetic Association. 1971. Position paper on bland diet in the treatment of chronic duodenal ulcer disease. *J. Am. Dietet. Assoc.,* **59:** 244.

3. Anonymous. 1976. Taste is more than a matter of taste. *Med. World News,* July 12, p. 54.

4. Babka, J. C. and D. O. Castell. 1973. On the genesis of heartburn. *Am. J. Dig. Dis.,* **18:** 391.

5. Beeson, P. B. and W. McDermott (Eds.). 1975. Textbook of Medicine, vol. II, 14th ed. Philadelphia: Saunders.

6. Behm, V., D. R. King, and G. Murchie. 1974. Nutritional care of the patient following gastric surgery. *Dietet. Currents* (Ross Laboratories), **1** (No. 2): 1.

7. Berkowitz, D. 1964. Blood lipid responses to feedings of a polyunsaturated fat nutritional preparation and milk-cream mixture. *Am. J. Clin. Nutr.,* **15:** 218.

8. Bevan, G. 1975. The medical therapy of peptic ulcer. *Postgrad. Med. J.,* **51** (Supplement 5): 14.

9. Biggar, B. L., M. N. Lewis, and R. M. Zollinger. 1960. Nutrition following gastric resection. II. One to seven years after surgery. *J. Am. Dietet. Assoc.,* **37:** 344.

10. Brady, J. V. 1958. Ulcers in "executive monkeys". *Sci. Am.,* **199** (No. 4): 95.

11. Buckler, K. G. 1967. Effect of gastric surgery upon gastric emptying in cases of peptic ulceration. *Gut,* 8: 137.

12. Caron, H. S. and H. P. Roth. 1972. Popular beliefs about the peptic ulcer diet. *J. Am. Dietet. Assoc.,* **60:** 306.

13. Caron, H. S. and H. P. Roth. 1971. Objective assessment of cooperation with an ulcer diet: Relation to antacid intake and to assigned physician. *Am. J. Med. Sci.,* **261** (Feb.): 61.

14. Carson, J. S. and A. Gormican. 1976. Disease-medication relationships in altered taste sensitivity. *J. Am. Dietet. Assoc.,* **68:** 550.

15. Cayer, D. and J. M. Ruffin. 1964. Experiences with a polyunsaturated fat nutritional preparation in the dietary management of patients with peptic ulcer. *Am. J. Clin. Nutr.,* **15:** 227.

16. Castell, D. O. 1975. Diet and the lower esophageal sphincter. *Am. J. Clin. Nutr.,* **28:** 1296.

17. Cleator, I. G. M., J. L. Stoller, F. R. C. Johnstone, I. B. Holubitsky, and R. C. Harrison. 1972. Comparison between the effect of pentagastrin and Histalog on gastric acid secretion. *Am. J. Dig. Dis.,* **17:** 713.

18. Cobb, J. S., S. Bank, I. N. Marks, and J. H. Louw. 1971. Gastric emptying after vagotomy and pyloroplasty. *Am. J. Dig. Dis.,* **16:** 207.

19. Cohen, S. and G. H. Booth, Jr. 1975. Gastric acid secretion and lower-esophageal-sphincter pressure in response to coffee and caffeine. *N. Eng. J. Med.,* **293:** 897.

20. Cooke, A. R. 1976. The role of the mucosal barrier in drug-induced gastric ulceration and erosions. *Am. J. Dig. Dis.,* **21:** 155.

21. Cox, A. G., M. R. Bond, D. A. Podmore, and D. P. Rose. 1964. Aspects of nutrition after vagotomy and gastrojejunostomy. *Brit. Med. J.,* **5381:** 465.

22. Crane, R. K. 1969. A perspective of digestive-absorptive function. *Am. J. Clin. Nutr.,* **22:** 242.

23. Davenport, H. W. 1975. The gastric mucosal barrier. *Mayo Clin. Proc.,* **50:** 507.

24. Davenport, H. W. 1972. Why the stomach does not digest itself. *Sci. Am.,* **226** (No. 1): 86.

25. Debas, H. T. 1977. Regulation of gastric acid secretion. *Fed. Proc.,* **36:** 1933.

26. Dennish, G. W. and D. O. Castell. 1972. Caffeine and the lower esophageal sphincter. *Am. J. Dig. Dis.,* **17:** 993.

27. Desnuelle, P. and P. Lavary. 1963. Specificities of lipases. *J. Lip. Res.,* **4:** 369.

28. Desor, J. A. and O. Maller. 1975. Taste correlates of disease states: Cystic fibrosis. *J. Ped.*, **87:** 93.

29. Dodsworth, J. M. and J. E. Fischer. 1974. Surgical therapy of chronic peptic ulcer. *Surg. Clin. No. Am.*, **54:** 529.

30. Doll, R., P. Friedlander, and F. Pygott. 1956. Dietetic treatment of peptic ulcer. *Lancet*, **1:** 5.

31. Dragstedt, L. R. 1963. A guide for the surgical treatment of peptic ulcer. *Am. J. Surg.*, **105:** 239.

32. Eddy, R. L. 1971. Metabolic bone disease after gastrectomy. *Am. J. Med.* **50:** 442.

33. Fiddian-Green, R. G., I. N. Marks, S. Bank, and J. H. Louw. 1976a. Maximum acid output and risk of peptic ulcer. *Lancet*, **2:** 1367.

34. Fiddian-Green, R. G., I. N. Marks, S. Bank, and J. H. Louw. 1976b. Maximum acid output and position of peptic ulcers. *Lancet*, **2:** 1370.

35. Foltz, E. L. 1964. Neurophysiological mechanisms in production of gastrointestinal ulcers. *J. Am. Med. Assoc.*, **187:** 413.

36. Gear, M. W. L., S. C. Truelove, and R. Whitehead. 1971. Gastric ulcer and gastritis. *Gut*, **12:** 639.

37. George, J. D. 1968. Gastric acidity and motility. *Am. J. Dig. Dis.*, **13:** 376.

38. Gillespie, I. E. 1968. The surgical treatment of peptic ulcer. *Postgrad. Med. J.*, **44:** 608.

39. Goodhart, R. S. and M. E. Shils (Eds.). 1973. *Modern Nutrition in Health and Disease*, 5th ed. Philadelphia: Lea and Febiger.

40. Greenall, M. J., P. J. Lyndon, J. C. Goligher, and D. Johnston. 1975. Long term effect of highly selective vagotomy on basal and maximal acid output in man. *Gastroent.*, **68:** 1421.

41. Guyton, A. C. 1971. *Textbook of Medical Physiology*, 4th ed. Philadelphia: Saunders.

42. Hambidge, K. M., C. Hambidge, M. Jacobs, and J. D. Baum. 1972. Low levels of zinc in hair, anorexia, poor growth, and hypogeusia in children. *Ped. Res.*, **6:** 868.

43. Hambidge, K. M. and A. Silverman. 1973. Pica with rapid improvement after dietary zinc supplementation. *Arch. Dis. Child.*, **48:** 567.

44. Harkins, R. W. and H. P. Sarett. 1968. Medium-chain triglycerides. *J. Am. Med. Assoc.*, **203:** 272.

45. Hartroft, W. S. 1964. The incidence of coronary artery disease in patients treated with the Sippy diet. *Am. J. Clin. Nutr.*, **15:** 205.

46. Henkin, R. I. 1967. The role of taste in disease and nutrition. *Borden's Rev. Nutr. Res.*, **28** (No. 4): 71.

47. Henkin, R. I., P. J. Schechter, and C. F. T. Mattern. 1971. Idiopathic hypogeusia and dysgeusia, hyposmia, and dysosmia. *J. Am. Med. Assoc.*, **223:** 914.

48. Hiatt, G. A. and R. F. Wells. 1974. Clinical physiology review: Gastrin. *Am. J. Gastroent.*, **62:** 59.

49. Hines, J. D., A. V. Hoffbrand, and D. L. Mollin. 1967. The hematologic complications following partial gastrectomy. *Am. J. Med.*, **43:** 555.

50. Hogan, W. J., S. R. Viegas de Andrade, and D. H. Winship. 1972. Ethanol-induced acute esophageal motor dysfunction. *J. Appl. Physiol.*, **32:** 755.

51. Holt, P. R. 1972. The roles of bile acids during the process of normal fat and cholesterol absorption. *Arch. Intern. Med.*, **130:** 574.

52. Hussey, H. H. 1974. Zinc in taste and smell deviations. (Editorial.) *J. Am. Med. Assoc.*, **228:** 1669.

53. Ingelfinger, F. J. 1973. How to swallow, and belch and cope with heartburn. *Nutr. Today*, **8** (No. 1): 4.

54. Ingelfinger, F. J. 1967. Gastrointestinal absorption. *Nutr. Today,* **2** (Mar.): 2.

55. Ippoliti, A. F., V. Maxwell, and J. I. Isenberg. 1976. The effect of various forms of milk on gastric-acid secretion. *Ann. Int. Med.,* **84:** 286.

56. Isenberg, J. I. 1975. Peptic ulcer disease. *Postgrad. Med.,* **57:** 163.

57. Isselbacher, K. J. 1967. Biochemical aspects of lipid malabsorption. *Fed. Proc.,* **26:** 1420.

58. Isselbacher, K. J. 1966. Biochemical aspects of fat absorption. *Gastroent.,* **50:** 78.

59. Isselbacher, K. J. 1965. Metabolism and transport of lipid by intestinal mucosa. *Fed. Proc.,* **24:** 16.

60. Ivey, K. J. 1974. Gastritis. *Med. Clin. No. Am.,* **58:** 1289.

61. Ivey, K. J. 1973. What's new in chronic gastritis? *Med. J. Aust.,* **2:** 857.

62. Ivey, K. J., L. DenBesten, and J. A. Clifton. 1970. Effect of bile salts on ionic movement across the human gastric mucosa. *Gastroent.,* **59:** 683.

63. Jacobs, E. and J. Pringot. 1973. Gastric ulcers due to the intake of potassium chloride. *Am. J. Dig. Dis.,* **18:** 289.

64. Kaplan, B. M., M. A. Spellberg, M. M. Norton, and R. Pick. 1965. Effect on serum cholesterol of a corn oil and skim milk mixture in peptic ulcer patients. *Am. J. Med. Sci.,* **250:** 621.

65. Katz, D. and C. S. Pitchumoni. 1973. Management of hiatal hernia-esophagitis complex in the elderly. *Geriatrics,* **28** (No. 10): 84.

66. Katz, J. 1973. Gastrointestinal hormones. *Med. Clin. No. Am.,* **57:** 893.

67. Kennedy, T. 1974. The vagus and the consequences of vagotomy. *Med. Clin. No. Am.,* **58:** 1231.

68. Kotrba, C. and C. F. Code. 1969. Gastric acid secretory responses to some purified foods and to additions of sucrose or olive oil. *Am. J. Dig. Dis.,* **14:** 1.

69. Laureta, H. C., C. Chou, and E. C. Texter, Jr. 1964. An appraisal of the management of peptic ulcer including comparative studies of the value of a polyunsaturated fat nutritional preparation in the management of gastric hypersecretion. *Am. J. Clin. Nutr.,* **15:** 211.

70. Lewis, M. N., J. King, J. H. Quaele, and R. M. Zollinger. 1958. Nutrition following gastric resection. I. The immediate postoperative period. *J. Am. Dietet. Assoc.,* **34:** 1195.

71. McConnell, R. J., C. E. Menendez, F. R. Smith, R. I. Henkin, and R. S. Rivlin. 1975. Defects of taste and smell in patients with hypothyroidism. *Am. J. Med.,* **59:** 354.

72. McHardy, G., R. C. Judice, and H. E. Cradic. 1964. Effect of polyunsaturated fat diet on serum lipids of hypercholesteremic patients with peptic ulcer. *Am. J. Clin. Nutr.,* **15:** 229.

73. Makhlouf, G. M., A. L. Blum, and E. W. Moore. 1970. Undissociated acidity of human gastric juice. *Gastroent.,* **58:** 345.

74. Mansbach, C. M., II. 1976. Conditions affecting the biosynthesis of lipids in the small intestine. *Am. J. Clin. Nutr.,* **29:** 295.

75. Menguy, R. 1964. Current concepts of the etiology of duodenal ulcer. *Am. J. Dig. Dis.,* **9:** 199.

76. Newcomer, A. D. 1973. Digestion and absorption of protein. *Mayo Clin. Proc.,* **58:** 624.

77. Olsen, W. A. 1974. Carbohydrate absorption. *Med. Clin. No. Am.,* **58:** 1387.

78. Phillips, S. F. 1972. Pathophysiology of gastritis: Recent concepts and clinical significance. *So. Med. J.,* **65:** 1187.

79. Pittman, A. C. and F. W. Robinson. 1962. Dietary management of the "dumping" syndrome. *J. Am. Dietet. Assoc.,* **40:** 108.

80. Ross, J. R. 1971. Postgastrectomy syndromes and their management. *Surg. Clin. No. Am.,* **51**: 615.

81. Saint-Hilaire, S., M. K. Lavers, J. Kennedy, and C. F. Code. 1960. Gastric acid secretory value of different foods. *Gastroent.,* **39**: 1.

82. Samloff, I. M. 1965. Gastritis: Pathology and diagnosis. *Am. J. Gastroent.,* **44**: 437.

83. Schneider, M. A., V. DeLuca, Jr., and S. J. Gray. 1956. The effect of spice ingestion upon the stomach. *Am. J. Gastroent.,* **26**: 722.

84. Shafer, R. B. and G. R. Onstad. 1975. Measurement of fat absorption utilizing [131]iodine-triolein and nonabsorbable radioactive markers. *Am. J. Med. Sci.,* **269**: 327.

85. Shafer, R. B., D. Ripley, W. R. Swaim, K. Mahmud, A. Doscherholmen. 1973. Hematologic alterations following partial gastrectomy. *Am. J. Med. Sci.,* **266**: 240.

86. Shultz, K. T., F. A. Neelon, L. B. Nilsen, and H. E. Lebovitz. 1971. Mechanism of postgastrectomy hypoglycemia. *Arch. Intern. Med.,* **128**: 240.

87. Sun, D. C. H., S. H. Roth, C. S. Mitchell, and D. W. Englund. 1974. Upper gastrointestinal disease in rheumatoid arthritis. *Am. J. Dig. Dis.,* **19**: 405.

88. Tovey, F. I. and M. Tunstall. 1975. Duodenal ulcer in black populations in Africa south of the Sahara. *Gut,* **16**: 564.

89. Trier, J. S. 1976. Morphology of the gastric mucosa in patients with ulcer diseases. *Am. J. Dig. Dis.,* **21**: 138.

90. Weinstein, L., R. E. Olson, T. B. Van Itallie, E. Caso, D. Johnson, and F. J. Ingelfinger. 1961. Diet as related to gastrointestinal function. *J. Am. Med. Assoc.,* **176**: 935.

91. Weiss, J. M. 1972. Psychological factors in stress and disease. *Sci. Am.,* **226** (No. 6): 104.

92. Welsh, J. D. 1977. Diet therapy of peptic ulcer disease. *Gastroent.,* **72**: 740.

93. Willis, M. T. and R. W. Postlewait. 1962. Dietary problems after gastric resection. *J. Am. Dietet. Assoc.,* **40**: 111.

94. Wintrobe, M. M., G. W. Thorn, R. D. Adams, E. Braunwald, K. J. Isselbacher, and R. G. Petersdorf (Eds.). 1974. *Harrison's Principles of Internal Medicine,* 7th ed. New York: McGraw-Hill.

95. Wollaeger, E. E. 1973. Role of the ileum in fat absorption. *Mayo Clin. Proc.,* **48**: 836.

96. Woodward, E. R. 1975. Sliding esophageal hiatal hernia and reflux peptic esophagitis. *Mayo Clin. Proc.,* **50**: 523.

97. Wright, L. E. and D. O. Castell. 1975. The adverse effect of chocolate on lower esophageal sphincter pressure. *Am. J. Dig. Dis.,* **20**: 703.

98. Yodfat, Y. 1972. A population study of peptic ulcer. *Israel J. Med. Sci.,* **8**: 1680.

STUDY GUIDE

Familiarity with normal digestive-absorptive processes is important to an understanding of pathological conditions affecting the GI tract.

1. List the major components of saliva, gastric juice, intestinal juice, pancreatic juice, and bile.

2. Describe the mechanisms for stimulating and inhibiting the flow of saliva, gastric juice (HCl in particular), pancreatic juice, and bile, including the effects of various GI hormones.

3. Discuss several factors that may be involved in the normal resistance of the stomach to the

corrosive action of gastric juice and describe possible relationships between this barrier and back-diffusion of H^+.

4. Describe the microscopic anatomy of intestinal mucosa and relate this to the general processes involved in normal digestion-absorption of proteins, carbohydrates, LCT, MCT, NaCl, and water.

Procedures that are valuable in diagnosis of GI disease include (1) radiography, (2) endoscopy, (3) secretory studies, (4) absorptive studies, and (5) peroral biopsy.

5. Give examples of each of the procedures listed above and discuss their usefulness in diagnosing diseases of the upper GI tract.

Lack of teeth, poorly fitting dentures, and inability to move the jaw affect normal chewing ability and may lead to inadequate food intake.

6. Explain possible relationships among chewing ability, nutritional status, and apparent digestive abnormalities.

7. Make and explain appropriate recommendations concerning food intake for patients with chewing problems.

Nutrient deficiencies may produce oral lesions.

8. For each of the following clinical signs, suggest possible nutrient deficiencies and treatment: magenta tongue; swollen, red, fissured tongue with hypertrophied fungiform papillae; cheilosis; angular stomatitis; hemorrhagic interdental papillae.

Abnormalities of taste and smell may be produced by a variety of factors and can markedly influence food intake.

9. Describe several factors that may influence taste sensitivity and discuss why this type of information is valuable to the dietitian.

Swallowing is initiated voluntarily but is concluded by involuntary mechanisms that may sometimes fail to function normally.

10. Describe the normal sequences involved in swallowing.

11. What is achalasia and how may it be treated?

Gastroesophageal reflux and symptomatic hiatal hernia share similar symptoms and dietary treatment.

12. Explain the significance of findings that the following decrease LES pressure in humans: fatty meals, whole milk, chocolate, and alcohol.

13. A patient complains of heartburn. Explain a possible cause and make recommendations for treatment.

14. Describe a hiatal hernia, the symptoms that may accompany it, and give dietary suggestions that may help alleviate the symptoms. Explain the rationale behind these suggestions.

The etiology of peptic ulcer is unknown but several factors have been suggested as possible contributors to its development.

15. Explain possible influences of each of the following on the development and maintenance of peptic ulcer and its symptoms.
    (a) Excessive secretion of gastric acid
    (b) Delayed emptying of the stomach
    (c) Excessive use of caffeine, coffee, alcohol, and cigarettes
    (d) Ingestion of drugs, particularly aspirin
    (e) Psychological and emotional stress
    (f) Genetic influences

Peptic ulcer is treated medically with antacids, anticholinergic drugs, and diet.

16. Discuss the rationale for use of antacids in treatment of peptic ulcer and list advantages and disadvantages for each of several compounds.

17. Evaluate the traditional bland diet in terms of its proven ability to:
    (a) Inhibit gastric acid secretion
    (b) Neutralize gastric acidity
    (c) Decrease gastric motor activity
    (d) Aid healing of ulcer
    (e) Control stomach distention
    (f) Avoid mechanical and chemical irritation to gastric mucosa

18. Discuss and explain the role of milk in the treatment of peptic ulcer, including both advantages and disadvantages of its use.

19. Recommend and explain an effective approach to the nutritional care of a patient with active peptic ulcer disease.

20. Make dietary recommendations for a patient with active peptic ulcer who has been advised to slowly reduce obesity.

Complications of peptic ulcer include hemorrhage, obstruction, and perforation.

21. Describe the basic problem in each of the complications listed above and indicate the general type of treatment usually given.

Surgical treatment may be recommended when medical treatment of peptic ulcer is not effective.

22. Describe the general procedure followed in (1) subtotal gastrectomy, (2) antrectomy, and (3) vagotomy with drainage procedure.

23. Describe the triad that characterizes Zollinger-Ellison syndrome and indicate the usual treatment for this disorder.

Certain nutritional problems may be produced as a result of surgical procedures for the treatment of peptic ulcer disease.

24. Discuss and explain why optimal nutritional care during both the immediate and long-term postoperative period is extremely important for the patient with gastric resection.

25. Recommend appropriate nutritional care for a postgastrectomy patient while hospitalized and give suggestions for counseling at discharge, explaining the rationale for dietary suggestions.

26. Explain possible reasons for development and suggested treatments of the following conditions that may occur after gastric resection:
    (a) Hypoglycemia
    (b) Underweight
    (c) Anemia
    (d) Osteomalacia
    (e) Diarrhea

The prognosis in peptic ulcer is usually good for the immediate attack but less favorable for the long range.

27. Explain why the above statement is usually true.

Concepts of gastritis have changed as progress has been made in characterizing this disorder.

28. Describe possible causes of acute gastritis.

29. Discuss possible relationships between chronic gastritis and gastric ulcer and similarities in medical treatment.

13

Intestinal Disorders

Because the small intestine is the site of absorption for food nutrients, disorders of this organ are often reflected in an altered nutritional status of the body. A vicious circle may develop since malabsorption itself, with an accompanying lack of available nutrients, contributes to continuing degeneration of cells in the intestinal mucosa.

Approximately half of the United States population has digestive complaints. At least 25 percent of older patients experience constipation, with the major contributing factors being insufficient bulk in the diet to stimulate peristalsis, abuse of laxatives, decreased fluid intake, decreased muscle tone, poor dentition, and medications. Diverticulosis is a common problem in Western Society, experienced by 40 percent of those 70 years of age and older. A high residue diet may protect against this disorder (Berman and Kirsner, 1972). Trends in the incidence of digestive disease show a declining frequency of gastric and duodenal ulcers and an increasing incidence of cancer of the colon and pancreas (Almy et al., 1975).

There is still much to be learned about the relationships between diet and intestinal disorders, in terms of both prevention and treatment. Much reliance has been placed on traditional and ritualistic diets in treatment. As new research findings clarify underlying physiological processes, diet therapy in intestinal disease is becoming more rational. This chapter first discusses the general malabsorption syndrome and then specific intestinal disorders, many of them involving malabsorption, with dietary implications for each.

13.1 Malabsorption Syndrome

Malabsorption may be defined as any disorder with impaired absorption of fat, carbohydrate, protein, vitamins, minerals, electrolytes, and/or water. It is an abnormal physiologic state, developing as a consequence of and in association with a wide variety of diseases, affecting principally but not exclusively the small intestine. There are many causes of malabsorption that reflect the intricate and complex digestive and absorptive mechanisms in humans and their vulnerability to a wide variety of pathologic processes (Kirsner, 1969). A classification of malabsorption causes is given in Table 13.1.

Severe protein malnutrition was shown by Mayoral et al. (1967) to produce a clinically, biochemically, and histologically definable, mild-to-moderate malabsorption syndrome in adult humans. The abnormalities

Table 13.1 CLASSIFICATION OF MALABSORPTION SYNDROMES*

Intraluminal factors	Changes in intestinal wall
Decrease in effective intestinal length	Mucosal epithelial cell
Resection of stomach or small bowel	Celiac disease of childhood
Intestinal fistulization	Gluten-induced enteropathy
Hypermotility (hyperthyroidism, enterotoxins)	Tropical sprue
Decreased digestive activity	Disaccharidase deficiency
Pancreatic juice	Radiation enteritis
Pancreatitis	Drug-induced (nitrogen mustard,
Carcinoma of pancreas	6-mercaptopurine)
Pancreatectomy	Triglyceride esterifying enzyme deficiency
Cystic fibrosis	Ground substance
Bile	Lymphoma, leukemia
Hepatitis	Regional enteritis
Cirrhosis	Tuberculosis
Biliary obstruction (bile duct, stone stricture, pancreas)	Carcinoma, sarcoma
Inadequate resorption of bile salts	**Abnormalities in blood or lymphatic channels**
Changes in intestinal microorganism population	Blood
Blind loop	Arterial or venous insufficiency (arteriosclerosis, thrombosis)
Small intestinal diverticula	Congestive heart failure
Intestinal stasis	Lymphatics
Visceral neuropathy (diabetes mellitus)	Intestinal lymphangiectasia
Primary neurologic diseases	Lymphatic obstruction
Partial obstruction	**Indeterminate**
Oral antibiotics (neomycin)	Zollinger-Ellison syndrome
Intestinal parasites	Abetalipoproteinemia
Acute infectious diarrhea (viral, bacterial)	Protein-losing enteropathy
Gastric achlorhydria	Pernicious anemia
	Hyperthyroidism
	Hypoparathyroidism
	Hemochromatosis
	Kwashiorkor
	Adrenal-pituitary insufficiency

* Adapted from Johnson, 1965.

regressed to normal with protein repletion alone. When protein malnutrition was associated with severe hookworm disease, iron deficiency anemia, or both, the concomitant presence of these conditions did not influence the course of regression of the malabsorptive state to normal with protein treatment. Severe malabsorption of all substances studied (nitrogen, fat, vitamin A, glucose, D-xylose, and vitamin B_{12}) was found in 32 children with protein-calorie malnutrition that were observed on admission to the hospital and throughout recovery. With nutritional recovery, malabsorption decreased in the following sequence: absorption of nitrogen, D-xylose, and vitamin A improved soon after therapeutic diets were initiated; fat and vitamin B_{12} absorption recovered more slowly (Viteri et al., 1973).

An example of malabsorption of a single nutrient is pernicious anemia, where lack of intrinsic factor from the stomach interferes with the absorption of vitamin B_{12} in the ileum. Most cases of intestinal malabsorption, however, involve more than one mechanism and more than one nutrient. Even when the basic cause may involve only long-chain triglyceride (LCT) digestion or absorption, secondary confusion and congestion in the intestine may interfere to some degree with the normal digestion-absorption of other nutrients such as sugars and amino acids. In abetalipoproteinemia the mucosal cells cannot synthesize beta lipoproteins and thus no chylomicrons are made to transport LCT into the lacteals. Fat builds up in mucosal cells and steatorrhea (abnormal excretion of fat in the stools) results. Other fat soluble nutrients are present with the fat in the lumen of the intestine and are not well absorbed. Decreased vitamin D absorption influences calcium absorption. Calcium and iron, as well as other metals, may form soaps with the fatty acids in the intestine and become less available for absorption. Disaccharidases and peptide hydrolases at the brush borders of the microvilli may less effectively hydrolyze disaccharides and peptides (Ingelfinger, 1968).

Malabsorption syndrome presents similar clinical signs and symptoms regardless of the basic cause. These include:

1. Steatorrhea, with stools that are fat-filled, light, frothy, greasy, floating, and foul-smelling.
2. Abdominal pain and cramping from gas and erratic intestinal motility.
3. Signs of protein malnutrition from long-term amino acid malabsorption, including decreased plasma protein levels, edema, and eventually osteoporosis resulting from lack of protein for bone matrix formation.
4. Bleeding tendencies due to lack of vitamin K absorption.
5. Anemia caused by inadequate absorption of vitamin B_{12}, folacin, and/or iron.
6. Hypocalcemia from malabsorption of vitamin D coupled with increased loss of calcium soaps in the stools.
7. A variety of deficiency symptoms from failure to absorb water-soluble vitamins.

8. Diarrhea resulting from increased amounts of unabsorbed sugars in the intestinal lumen which cause an osmotic shift of fluid into the gut, thus producing fluid and electrolyte loss from the body. Fermentation of disaccharides by bacteria in the colon and lower small intestine may produce acetic and lactic acids which also contribute to the irritation and diarrhea.

9. Weight loss, weakness, pallor, and starvation in spite of an apparently adequate food intake.

In dealing with a patient suspected of having malabsorption, Escovitz and Rubin (1973) suggested that the clinician should (1) establish the presence of a malabsorption syndrome by suitable testing; (2) assess the nutritional deficiencies present; (3) diagnose the specific disorder responsible for the malabsorption; (4) institute specific and supportive therapy; and (5) follow the patient closely to be sure that his or her response to therapy and clinical course are satisfactory, since a poor response to treatment often indicates an erroneous diagnosis. Therapy must be directed toward the specific cause in order to be effective.

13.2 Gluten Sensitive Enteropathy or Celiac Disease

Many names have been applied to this disorder, including celiac disease, nontropical sprue, celiac sprue, sprue syndrome, idiopathic sprue, idiopathic steatorrhea, primary malabsorption, gluten-induced enteropathy, and gluten sensitive enteropathy. Of these names, only gluten-induced or gluten sensitive enteropathy characterizes both the etiological and functional abnormalities found in affected patients. Gluten sensitive enteropathy (GSE) is a disease of the small intestine, affecting primarily the proximal portion, and it occurs in both children and adults. It is characterized by pathological changes in the jejunal mucosa and malabsorption of a variety of dietary components. Both these abnormalities improve upon removal of gluten from the diet and can recur on its reintroduction (Katz and Falchuk, 1975; Kowlessar, 1972).

History

Samuel Gee in 1888 was the first to clearly describe the celiac syndrome (Anderson, 1959). Since then many others have attempted to find an effective treatment for it and to delineate the cause. Because the feces in patients with celiac disease usually contained large amounts of fat and undigested starch granules, these patients were given diets low in both fat and starch. In 1938 Haas pointed out the poor correlation between steatorrhea and fat intake in celiac disease and suggested that the steatorrhea was connected with carbohydrate metabolism. In 1949 Sheldon showed that the severity of the steatorrhea was significantly less when a starch-free (flour-free) diet was used (Weijers and Van de Kamer, 1965). A monumental contribution in the history of dietary treatment for celiac disease was made by Dicke and Weijers in 1950 when, as students in the Netherlands, they presented theses to substantiate the observation that wheat flour in the diet of patients with celiac disease aggravated the condition. In 1953 Dicke et al. reported their findings of a deleterious effect by wheat in celiac disease and recovery when diets free of wheat and rye cereals were given. They later showed that the gluten of these cereals, particularly the gliadin fraction, was responsible for the toxic effect (Van de Kamer et al., 1953). Although possible reasons for the damaging effect of gluten on the intestinal mucosa have since been suggested by a number of researchers, the exact mechanism is not known.

Incidence

It is difficult to determine true incidence of GSE because overt symptoms are not always present and diagnosis not always complete. GSE appears to be more common in certain European countries than in the United States. This may be due to a larger intake of gluten by people in Europe or to the way in which wheat is refined in the United States (Katz and Falchuk, 1975). The incidence in England is 1 in 3,000 and may be similar in the United States. Kowlessar and Phillips (1970) observed a preponderance of females over males by a ratio of 4 to 1, but other workers have found the disorder to be evenly distributed between the sexes. GSE appears to be confined largely to whites but has been reported in East Indians. Very rarely is it found in Negroes.

A familial tendency has been observed in the incidence of GSE, with inheritance probably as a Mendelian dominant gene with incomplete penetrance. In family studies where small bowel biopsy has been performed, 5 to 10 percent of asymptomatic relatives have been found to have the disease. A good screening test for GSE is not available, although Carswell and Ferguson (1972) suggested that measurement of food antibodies in blood serum, possibly occurring because the food proteins penetrate the damaged mucosa, may have nonspecific value in screening.

Signs, Symptoms, and Pathology

The classical clinical features of GSE in children are chronic diarrhea, weight loss, failure to thrive, enlarged abdomen, muscle wasting, anorexia, and crampy abdominal pain with distention (Fig. 13.1). Symptoms in adults are similar except for the effect on growth. The diarrhea consists of frequent, foul-smelling stools, varying from watery to loose to semisolid, but with a low specific gravity allowing them to float. Malabsorption of fat results in loss of kilocalories in the stools and contributes to loss of weight. A variety of protein, vitamin, and mineral deficiency symptoms usually occurs. Although the intraluminal digestion of proteins is usually normal in GSE, delayed absorption of amino acids and peptides may occur and thus interfere with protein synthesis in the body. The hypoproteinemia seen in many cases may be partially due to protein weeping from the damaged mucosa. Hypoproteinemia can lead to peripheral edema (Kowlessar and Phillips, 1970).

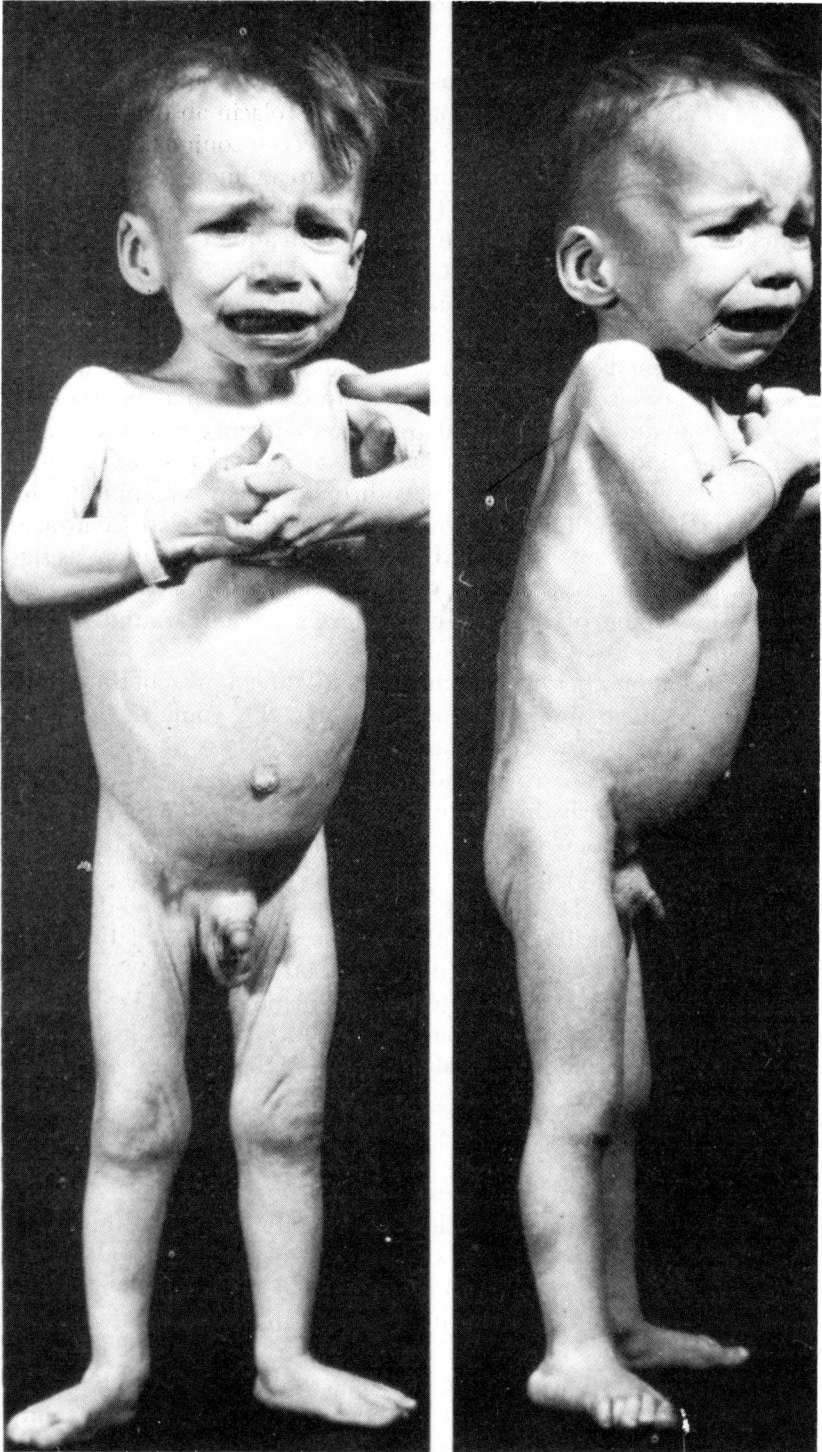

Fig. 13.1 Characteristic profile of a child with gluten sensitive enteropathy. Note typical facies, "pot" belly, muscle wasting (especially proximal limbs and buttocks.) (From A. J. Katz, Z. M. Falchuk, and H. Shwachman, "The Co-Existence of Cystic Fibrosis and Celiac Disease, *Pediatrics*, **57**:715, 1976; by permission of the authors and the American Academy of Pediatrics.)

Anemia may result from malabsorption of folacin, vitamin B_{12}, and/or iron. Baker et al. (1964) reported that defective folacin absorption in GSE was associated with an intestinal enzymatic defect in conjugating synthetic folic acid and in deconjugating natural folates to a glutamyl state favoring intestinal absorption. Melvin et al. (1970), measuring calcium absorption and endogenous calcium loss in nine patients with adult GSE using balance and isotopic techniques, reported that negative calcium balance was due to an excessive excretion of endogenous fecal calcium and that true absorption of dietary calcium was normal. Seven of the nine patients had histological signs of osteomalacia and all nine had low plasma vitamin D levels. Tetany, diffuse bone pain, and susceptibility to fractures may be secondary to loss of calcium and vitamin D malabsorption. Easy bruising, ecchymosis, bleeding gums, and bleeding from or into various organs are results of vitamin K malabsorption and hypoprothrombinemia. Vitamin B_6 deficiency was reported by Reinken et al. (1976) in children with acute GSE. Depression of plasma zinc levels and lowered taste discrimination, as signs of zinc deficiency, were observed by Solomons et al. (1976) in adult patients with GSE. Depression of plasma copper levels was also found in these patients, suggesting trace element malabsorption.

A substantial number of patients with GSE do not present the classical clinical features of the disorder. They may show only vomiting, acute watery diarrhea, chronic iron deficiency anemia, weakness, depression, and short stature in children (Brown and Lillibridge, 1975).

GSE affects primarily the mucosa of the small intestine without involving the submucosa, muscularis, and serosa. Normal mucosal epithelial cells are columnar with basally oriented nuclei. Cells in the crypts between villi normally carry on active DNA and RNA synthesis but lack a well-developed brush border, disaccharidase enzymes, and other evidence of full differentiation. As these cells migrate up the villi in 3 to 5 days, they acquire the characteristics of mature enterocytes. As the microvillus brush border develops and receives its full complement of enzymes, the cells lose their ability to replicate. Normal epithelial cells are sloughed off at the tip of the villi as new cells take their place (Fig. 13.2).

In GSE the migration rate of cells from the crypt to tip of the villus is shortened to 1 to 2 days (Katz and Falchuk, 1975). The villous structure disappears and the epithelium presents a flat surface (Fig. 13.3) when viewed under a light microscope. With an electron microscope, the surface epithelial cells are shown to be strikingly abnormal, with irregular apical surfaces, broken brush borders, and microvilli that are broad, short, and in clusters. Rubin (1971) reported that crypt cells in patients with GSE are identical to normal intestinal crypt cells, although the mucosal cells at the surface of the villi are abnormal. He has suggested that the villous atrophy in this disease may result because the epithelial cells are damaged as soon as they migrate from the crypt to the surface of the villi, and their life span is thus shortened. The shortened life span of the cells is not compensated for by an increased rate of cell replication in the elongated crypts. Normal

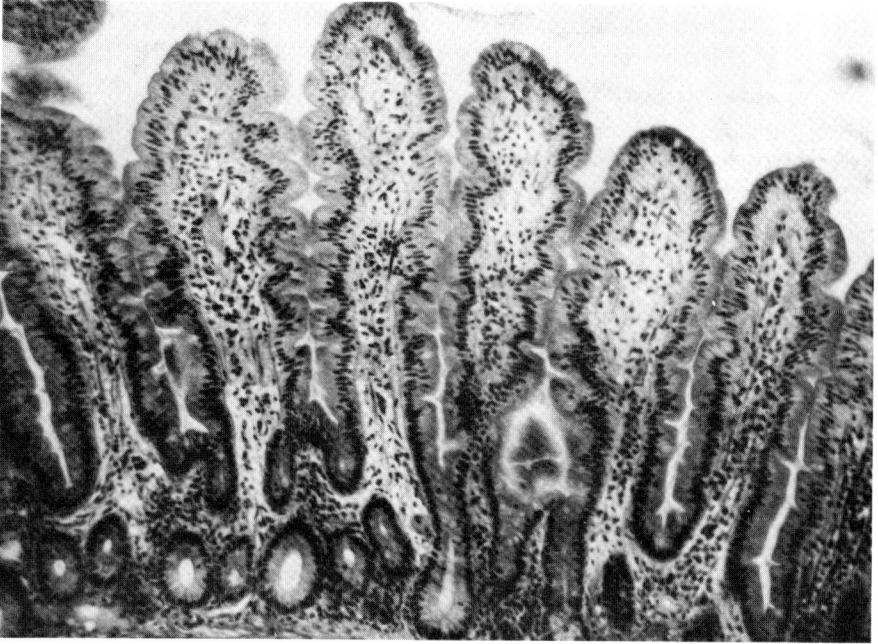

Fig. 13.2 The normal jejunal mucosa. The epithelial cells are columnar and their nuclei are basally oriented. The villus height-to-crypt-depth ratio is 4 : 1. There are plasma cells and lymphocytes in the lamina propria (× 180). (From A. J. Katz and Z. M. Falchuk, "Current Concepts in Gluten Sensitive Enteropathy, *Pediatric Clinics of North America*, **22**: 767, 1975; by permission of the authors and W. B. Saunders Company.)

absorption cannot occur through the abnormal intestinal mucosa that is characteristic of GSE. There is variability in the degree of malabsorption seen in patients with this disorder, however, that probably results from differences in both the severity and the extent of the intestinal lesions.

Pathogenesis

Two major mechanisms have been postulated to explain the damaging effect of gluten on the intestinal mucosa, although additional research data are required to prove either one. The first postulate is that GSE is due to an inborn error of metabolism with an enzyme deficiency resulting in the accumulation of undigested toxic gluten peptides that subsequently damage the mucosa. The second proposes that an abnormality in the immune system is responsible for the damage.

The harmful factor in gluten is the gliadin fraction (the 70 percent alcohol-soluble portion of gluten). Enzymatic digestion of gliadin by pepsin and crude pancreatic enzymes fails to destroy its toxicity. Ultrafiltrates and dialysates of peptic and crude pancreatic enzyme digests of gliadin or gluten also retain their toxicity. However, total acid hydrolysis, deamidation with 1 N HCl for 45 minutes, crude papain, and crude hog intestinal peptidases render both gluten and its enzymatically derived peptides non-

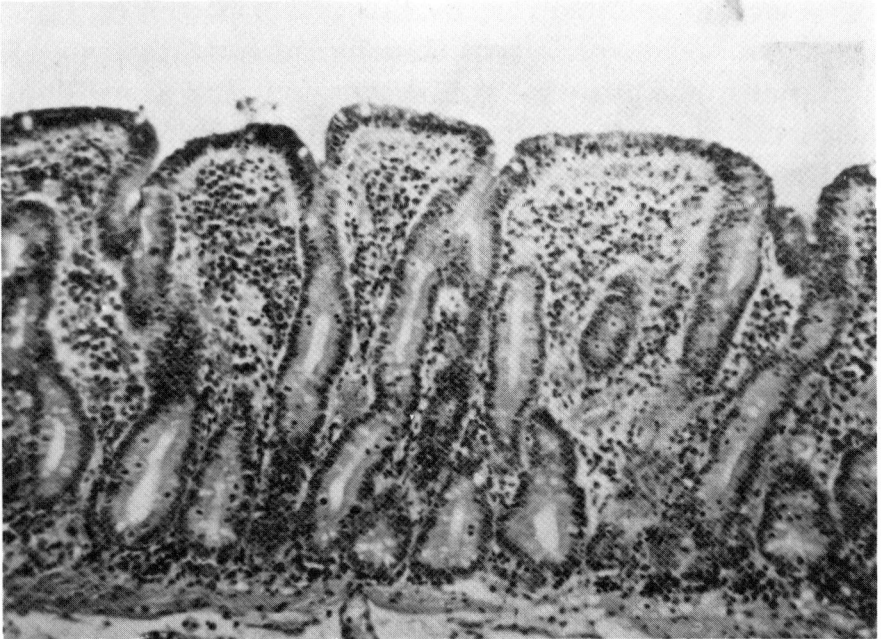

Fig. 13.3 The gluten sensitive enteropathy mucosa. The epithelial cells are cuboidal and their nuclei are not basally oriented. There are increased numbers of mitoses in the crypts, and the villi are flat. There are increased inflammatory cells present in the lamina (× 180). (From A. J. Katz and Z. M. Falchuk, "Current Concepts in Gluten Sensitive Enteropathy, *Pediatric Clinics of North America*, **22**:767, 1975; by permission of the authors and W. B. Saunders Company.)

toxic. A water eluate of material from the ultrafiltrate of a peptic, tryptic, crude pancreatic enzyme digest of gliadin was shown to contain peptides that were toxic when given to patients with GSE but nontoxic to control subjects. Apparently the normal intestinal mucosa can break down these peptides without difficulty but the mucosa of patients with GSE cannot. A primary mucosal enzyme deficiency is suggested by these data, but no specific enzymes have been isolated from normal mucosa and shown to be absent from the mucosa of individuals with GSE (Kowlessar and Phillips, 1970). Also, enzyme deficiencies have only been demonstrated in patients with active disease in whom epithelial cell function is abnormal and not always in patients with the disease in remission (Katz and Falchuk, 1975). Berg et al. (1970) were unable to demonstrate a specific deficiency of any particular dipeptidase activity in 18 subjects with the flat intestinal mucosa pattern seen in celiac disease. They concluded that the decrease of intestinal disaccharidases and dipeptidases found in celiac disease may be secondary to primary damage of the mucosa. This conclusion does not exclude the possibility that the disease is based on a lack of some intestinal peptidase not assayed in this study. The enzyme deficiency hypothesis of pathogenesis in GSE remains alive but unproved.

The theory that GSE is related to an immunologic mechanism is based on observations such as the following: (1) a high proportion of patients with

GSE have antibodies in serum to gluten or gliadin, although they also have antibodies to other food proteins such as those from milk and egg; (2) precipitins have been demonstrated in intestinal secretions of GSE patients against a peptic-tryptic digest of gluten; and (3) some patients with active disease respond promptly with clinical improvement after the administration of antiinflammatory glucocorticoids (Katz et al., 1976).

The intestinal mucosa of patients with GSE has been shown to respond to oral gluten with the production of specific antigluten antibody, whereas subjects without GSE did not respond in this fashion (Falchuk and Strober, 1974; Katz and Falchuk, 1975). Although this offers evidence that the local mucosal immunologic system is stimulated during the development of active GSE, it does not answer the question as to whether the immunologic events demonstrated represent the primary defect in GSE or a secondary phenomenon. Neither does this clarify whether or not the low-molecular-weight peptides that have previously been isolated and studied are producing the immune effect, and if so, by what mechanism (Kowlessar, 1972).

Diagnosis

The diagnosis of GSE is usually made on the basis of (1) the demonstration of impaired intestinal absorption; (2) the finding of characteristic histological changes in the duodenojejunal mucosa; and (3) the definite clinical response to withdrawal of dietary gluten (Anderson et al., 1972). Since all patients with GSE do not present the same clinical picture, interpretation of findings by the clinician is important in diagnosis.

Measurement of fat absorption will demonstrate impaired intestinal absorption in patients with possible GSE. However, steatorrhea is not always present and other tests, such as xylose absorption, or indications of folate and iron deficiency resulting from malabsorption should also be considered.

The peroral biopsy is very important in diagnosing GSE. However, abnormal intestinal mucosal changes are not specific for GSE and must be interpreted in line with other findings. The appearance of the intestine is the result of a reaction by the mucosa to a number of toxic influences. A therapeutic test of dietary gluten removal is usually not satisfactorily substituted for a peroral biopsy. The peroral biopsy gives confirmation to the diagnosis that is important in long-term care as response to a gluten-free diet is noted. Anderson et al. (1972) noted that GSE is occurring earlier now in infants than in the 1950s, probably because of the increasingly common practice of introducing solid foods, which may be derived from wheat cereal, into the diet in early infancy.

Dietary Management

No therapy in addition to dietary treatment is usually necessary in GSE. A gluten-free diet often brings dramatic results, with improvement in mood and appetite in 3 to 5 days, followed by weight gain in about 1 week.

Abnormal stools may take several weeks and abdominal distention even longer to disappear. In the absence of such a response, the diagnosis may be seriously reconsidered, as long as the clinician can be reasonably sure that a rigid gluten-free diet is being followed (Anderson et al., 1972).

Samloff et al. (1965) observed jejunal mucosal changes by serial biopsies before and after the institution of a gluten-free diet in three patients with GSE. In normal control subjects, lipid was found to be distributed as a fine haze in the superficial epithelial cells and as distinct droplets in the lamina propria. In untreated GSE, lipid droplets were limited to the superficial epithelium and to a thin band in the region of the epithelial cell basement membrane with none being found in the deeper portions of the lamina propria. Three to 5 days after the gluten-free diet was started, lipid droplets appeared in the lamina propria of GSE patients and subsequently they disappeared from the superficial epithelial cells. Fecal fat excretion gradually decreased parallel with the improvement in lipid distribution.

The response to a gluten-free diet has been related to the strictness of dietary adherence. Benson et al. (1964) reported that dietary adherence was strict in 12 adult patients with GSE and suboptimal in 14. Those in the strict group had a greater degree of improvement. Although the patients in the suboptimal group obtained a "clinical remission," the results of the more sensitive tests of intestinal absorption were likely to be abnormal. Significant clinical improvement was noted within a few days to a few weeks following introduction of a gluten-free diet. In some cases it was rapid, in others moderate, and in a few patients it was delayed or atypical. Most of the atypical responses could be explained by dietary violations.

The gluten-free diet is planned to avoid the cereal grains wheat, rye, oats, and barley. Although there is still some controversy as to the harmful effects of the proteins in oats and barley, they are generally excluded from the diet for individuals with GSE. Greif and Longenecker (1974) reported a similar effect of oats and wheat gluten challenges for four adults and two children with GSE, as measured by the xylose absorption test. It is the gluten of wheat flour that is responsible for the excellent breadmaking properties of this grain. As the flour proteins, gliadin and glutenin, are hydrated and the resulting dough is kneaded, they develop into the extensible and elastic substance called gluten. Rice, corn, and soybean flours, which may be substituted in a gluten-free diet, do not have this gluten-developing property and produce breads that are lower in volume and more crumbly in texture than are breads made from wheat flour. A number of gluten-free bread recipes have been published, however, and may be made at home as well as on a commercial basis (Johnson and Penfield, 1976; Nishita et al., 1976; Kulp et al., 1974; Smith, 1971; Sorensen, 1970; McGreer, 1967). The recipes use wheat or rice starch with methyl cellulose, guar gum, xanthan gum, or similar substances as stabilizers to substitute for the missing gluten.

Foods commonly allowed and those disallowed on a gluten-free diet are listed in Table 13.2. The individual following a gluten-free diet must

Table 13.2 A GLUTEN-FREE DIET

Foods Allowed	Foods Not Allowed
Beef, lamb, pork, veal, fish, or poultry prepared with allowed foods	Breaded meat or fish; creamed meat products thickened with wheat flour; luncheon meats, sausage, frankfurters, bologna; commercial ground beef with cereal fillers; croquettes
Cheese	Processed cheese products unless known to be wheat-free; cheese sauces
Milk, as tolerated	Malted milk; commercial chocolate milk
Eggs	Egg dishes thickened with wheat flour
Fruits	
Vegetables prepared plain or creamed with allowed flours	Creamed or escalloped vegetables if thickened with wheat flour or topped with bread crumbs
Bread and cereal products made from arrowroot, cornmeal, wheat starch, soybean, rice, potato, or gluten-free wheat flour only; tapioca; sago; cereals made from corn or rice; gluten-free bread; cornstarch; gluten-free rice wafers	Whole wheat, white, or gluten flours; bread, biscuits, rolls, muffins; crackers, pretzels, corn chips, and other snack foods; rusks, zweiback; rye krisp; doughnuts, pancakes, waffles, or any product made from wheat, rye, barley, or oat grains; bran or bran cereals, farina, grapenuts, oatmeal, shredded or puffed wheat, buckwheat, pablum, or other cereals made from wheat, rye, barley, or oat grains; prepared flour mixes; macaroni, noodles, spaghetti, and other alimentary pastes
Soups made with allowed foods, thickened with cream, cornstarch, potato, soybean, or rice flour; clear broth without any cereal additives	Soups containing commercially prepared noodles, macaroni, or spaghetti; soup mixes and bases; bouillon cubes
Fats—butter; margarine; cream; corn, peanut, safflower, or cottonseed oil; meat or poultry fat; mayonnaise; olives; nuts; peanut butter; olive oil	Commercial salad dressings
Desserts—cornstarch, tapioca, or rice pudding; custard; bavarian cream; gelatin; homemade ice cream; meringues; fruit; cakes, cookies, pastries, and desserts made with cornmeal, cornstarch, potato, rice, or soya flours or gluten-free wheat starch	Commercial ice cream with cereal additives; cakes, pastries, cookies, and puddings unless prepared with allowed flours; ice cream cones
Sweets—white, brown, or maple sugars; honey; molasses; sorghum; syrups; jellies; jams; preserves; marmalade; marshmallows	Candies of unknown composition
Beverages—milk, as tolerated; carbonated beverages; coffee; tea; pure cocoa; fruit juices	Postum; instant coffee; malted drinks; Ovaltine; ale and beer; fruit punch powders
Miscellaneous Gravies and sauces thickened with rice or potato flours, gluten-free wheat starch, or cornstarch; plain pickles; relishes; pure spices; pure flavorings; baking chocolate	Sauces and seasonings made with disallowed cereal products; commercial meat sauces; prepared mustard; soysauce; horseradish

learn to read carefully all food labels and avoid both gluten and its derivatives. Malt, prepared from sprouted grain, and brewer's yeast, grown on cereal mixtures, may cause difficulty and thus any malt-flavored food should be avoided. Brewer's yeast may sometimes be found in such prepared foods as root beer and cream cheese dip. Beer and ale contain gluten derivatives, although distilled liquors do not. The individual on a gluten-free diet must know what he or she is eating. Foods without listed ingredients and unknown recipes must be checked further before being used.

Intestinal disaccharidase deficiencies have been reported in GSE (Lifshitz et al., 1965). However, patients with known mucosal abnormalities from any cause might be expected to have abnormal disaccharidase activity and the deficiency in GSE is possibly secondary to other mucosal changes. A lactose-free diet has been recommended by some workers, at least for the first few weeks of therapy, in children with GSE (Katz and Falchuk, 1975). Disaccharidase deficiency appears to decrease as patients respond to a gluten-free diet, without dietary restriction of disaccharides, although lactase activity continues to be less than that of normal control subjects in many cases (McNicholl et al., 1976). Persistently low lactase levels may be an indication of regular ingestion of gluten, either overtly or inadvertently, or it may be related in some way to an inherited defect.

A diet that is nutritionally well balanced, with adequate protein, vitamins, and minerals, is essential for patients with GSE. This is especially true if substantial weight loss occurred before the diagnosis was made. Appropriate replacement therapy should be made for specific deficiencies, such as iron, folacin, vitamin D, vitamin K, and calcium.

Prognosis and Follow-Up Studies

A number of investigators have followed patients with GSE over a period of years after diagnosis and the initiation of a gluten-free diet. McNicholl et al. (1976) studied 40 children who had been receiving gluten-free diets for a mean of 6 years (3.7 to 11.8). Control subjects were normal siblings of children with celiac disease. Body weight was of almost normal distribution with 17 of 36 children at or over the 50th percentile, whereas at initial diagnosis only three of 32 whose weights were recorded were above the 25th percentile and none was above the 50th. Height was also of almost normal distribution after treatment. Mucosal morphology was regarded as normal in 16 and showed minimal or slight changes in 20. Long-term treatment was generally effective. These 40 children were then fed normal diets to determine whether they were still gluten sensitive. Thirty-six of them reverted to a characteristic state of mucosal damage in a mean of 15.4 months (4 to 35), thus confirming persistent gluten sensitivity. The other four children still had normal appearance of the mucosa after 2.6 and 5.4 years, two of them showing a gradual reduction in mucosal enzyme levels, which may indicate latent GSE.

Hamilton and McNeill (1972) studied 23 children with proven celiac disease 3.8 ± 1.0 years after initiation of dietary therapy. They challenged these children, while they were hospitalized, with a constant dose of wheat gluten for 6 days. Twelve of the 23 children had no deleterious effects after the 6 days on gluten and also had normal duodenal biopsies. They were discharged from the hospital and allowed a slice of bread or its equivalent in flour each day while being followed over a period of time. Three of the 12 children developed significant symptoms after 1 to 6 months and showed mucosal abnormalities at that time. In eight of nine asymptomatic patients, duodenal biopsy 1 year later showed typical lesions of GSE. In the other child, the biopsy findings were equivocal, but symptoms developed after 15 months on gluten, at which time a mucosal lesion was found. These authors concluded that long-term diet therapy is necessary for all cases of GSE diagnosed in childhood.

Young and Pringle (1971) reported that 20 children who remained on a gluten-free diet for periods of 8 to 19 years gained weight, grew normally, and had no complications. However, 24 children who did not, developed suboptimal growth and chronic ill health and were prone to diarrheal attacks, iron deficiency, and megaloblastic anemia. They recommended a life-long gluten-free diet for patients with GSE. Visakorpi et al. (1970) pointed out that a considerable number of patients with GSE develop a clinically "silent" state after the initial treatment. Even though overt symptoms are lacking, intestinal biopsies show that gluten intolerance is permanent. Similar conclusions were drawn by Ruffin et al. (1964). Celiac disease or GSE carries with it an increased risk of malignancy of the gastrointestinal tract, both in the form of tumors of lymphoid tissue and as carcinoma. McCrae et al. (1975) sought information on 130 cases of GSE that had been lost to follow-up after the diagnosis. Most of these patients were unaware of the need for continuing treatment and had returned to a normal diet with only a few instances of reported symptoms. Since it has been suggested that effective treatment, particularly a gluten-free diet, for GSE may lessen the risk of malignancy, it is important to know that many cases of GSE can continue undetected and perhaps undetectable unless a jejunal biopsy is performed. The size of the population at risk in this respect is not known but is thought to be large. Diagnosis and then life-long treatment of GSE with a gluten-free diet is important in all cases. Many individuals with GSE are apparently unable to maintain dietary treatment over a long period of time without continuing dietary advice and counseling (McCrae et al., 1975).

13.3 Tropical Sprue

A syndrome of unknown etiology characterized by intestinal malabsorption, chronic diarrhea, and multiple nutritional disorders was recognized in India and other areas of the Far East many centuries ago. Several different names have been given to this disorder over the years, but gradually the term *tropical sprue* has gained prominence. This disease continues to occur predominantly in India and Ceylon but also in Puerto Rico. It is found sporadically in the United States and other parts of the world except Africa, where it is extremely rare. The disease is characteristic of the white race (Mayer, 1966).

Soldiers and civilians from temperate climates who visit or live in some parts of the tropics may develop tropical sprue. A study of Peace Corps volunteers in Pakistan showed that close association with the native population makes the visitor more susceptible to development of this disorder than are foreigners to the tropics who remain relatively isolated from the natives. Symptoms can begin soon after arrival in the tropics or later, even following return to a northern climate. Davis (1970) reported a case of tropical sprue in a healthy, white 17-year-old New York high school junior who spent 2 months as an exchange student with a Hindu family in western India. Food eaten with the family was vegetarian, with eggplant, rice, and other Indian dishes supplemented occasionally by eggs and daily by water buffalo milk of unknown purity. Once a week he went to a restaurant where he ate chicken and other items. He did not like the food and ate as little as possible, gradually losing weight. Severe diarrhea occurred shortly before his return to the United States and persisted. A jejunal biopsy showed moderate shortening and broadening of the villi with an increase in inflammatory cell infiltration in the lamina propria. Although not specific, the changes were compatible with the diagnosis of tropical sprue. He was treated with oral doses of folic acid (5 mg per day) and tetracycline (250 mg twice daily) for several months. No vitamin B_{12} supplement was given since a Schilling test had been normal. His diarrhea subsided, fatigue lessened, and weight increased with treatment.

The typical clinical picture of tropical sprue includes glossitis, anorexia, flatulent indigestion, diarrhea, steatorrhea, hyperchromic macrocytic anemia, weight loss, and development of several nutritional deficiencies as a result of the malabsorption syndrome. All these clinical phenomena may not be present, however, and the disease must be distinguished from other conditions with malabsorption syndromes (Mayer, 1966; Ghitis et al., 1967). Biopsy of the small intestine aids in diagnosis. Wheby et al. (1971), from studies in Puerto Rico, have concluded that the ileum and jejunum are usually equally affected with lesions in tropical sprue. Malabsorption has been shown to include amino acids (Klipstein and Corcino, 1975). Jejunal lactase activity was shown by Desai et al. (1967) to be significantly lower in Indian patients with tropical sprue than in control subjects, although the Indian controls had lower lactase levels than those usually reported in western populations. Treatment with tetracycline caused a rise in disaccharidase activity in some patients. Circulating antibodies to gliadin were not found in patients with tropical sprue by Menendez-Corrada and Belaval (1968).

Although the cause of tropical sprue is still unknown, the best treatment appears to be a nutritionally complete diet, beginning with a high-protein, high-vitamin, low-fat modification, folic acid supplements (15 mg per day intramuscularly at the beginning, followed by an oral maintenance dose of 5 mg per day), a water-soluble vitamin K supplement, and antibiotic treatment. Vitamin B_{12} supplements may be necessary. The lesions in the mouth should heal rapidly, intestinal lesions and symptoms gradually improve, and the anemia should respond to treatment (Mayer, 1966). In mild cases, recovery is usually complete. However, Rickles et al. (1972), in a study of long-term follow-up on antibiotic-treated tropical sprue in Puerto Rico, reported a high rate of either relapse or recurrence of intestinal abnormalities after cessation of treatment.

13.4   Disaccharidase Deficiencies

A number of small intestinal disaccharidases, localized in the brush border, have been identified in the human. Four or five different maltases have been found, some with the ability to act only on maltose and others having isomaltase and sucrase activity as well. One or two lactases and two sucrases have also been reported. In inherited disaccharidase deficiencies the enzyme defect often seems to be multiple. Isomaltase (hydrolyzes alpha-1,6 linkage) and sucrase (invertase) activities are usually absent simultaneously, in spite of the fact that these two activities are exerted by two or three different enzymes. Lactose intolerance also may be a two-enzyme defect. In humans enzyme activity increases from the proximal to the distal duodenum with peak activity occurring in the jejunum or proximal ileum. Levels of disaccharidases are low in the distal ileum and there is no appreciable activity in the stomach or colon. Hydrolysis of lactose in the adult occurs at a slower rate than does that of maltose or sucrose (Welsh, 1970; Dahlqvist, 1966).

Classification

Disaccharidase deficiency may be either primary or secondary. Primary deficiencies are often congenital although late onset lactase deficiency that is probably under genetic control occurs in older children and adults. Congenital deficiencies are characterized by the complete absence of enzyme activity but with normal intestinal morphology. They have been described for both lactase and sucrase-isomaltase.

Secondary lactase deficiency appears to be common and may be associated with GSE, regional enteritis, irritable colon, duodenal ulcer, ulcerative colitis, cystic fibrosis, and viral hepatitis. This association, however, may occur because of the high incidence of primary late onset lactase deficiency in older children and adults, with the presence of lactase deficiency in these disease states being a coincidental rather than a secondary finding. In mucosal damage, the activity of all of the disaccharidases may be decreased but lactase seems to be most sensitive to injury and the slowest to recover (Lebenthal, 1975). A classification of disaccharide intolerance suggested by Bayless and Huang (1969) is given in Table 13.3.

Table 13.3 CLASSIFICATION OF DISACCHARIDE INTOLERANCE*

I. **Lactose intolerance**
A. Congenital physiologic lactase deficiency in premature infants
B. Congenital lactase deficiency, presumably genetically determined
C. Acquired lactase deficiency, in older children and adults, probably genetically determined
D. Acquired, secondary to diffuse mucosal damage and part of generalized disaccharidase deficiency
    1. Mucosal damage (celiac disease, tropical sprue, intestinal lymphangiectasis, and so on)
    2. Acute gastroenteritis (especially infants)
    3. Kwashiorkor
    4. Neomycin administration
    5. *Giardia lamblia* infestation
    6. Postbowel surgery in infants (presumed mucosal damage)
E. Acquired, secondary to alteration in intestinal transit
    1. Small bowel resection
    2. Postgastrectomy or pyloroplasty (may unmask a preexisting deficiency)
    3. Lactose intolerance without lactase deficiency
F. Suggested disease associations
    1. Ulcerative colitis
    2. Regional enteritis
    3. Irritable colon syndrome
    4. Osteoporosis
II. **Sucrose intolerance**
A. Congenital, sucrase-isomaltase deficiencies, genetically determined
B. Seemingly acquired sucrose intolerance in adults, sucrase-isomaltase deficiency, presumably also genetically determined and similar to the congenital deficiencies
C. Acquired, secondary to diffuse mucosal damage

---

* Bayless and Huang, 1969.

Pathogenesis of Gastrointestinal Symptoms in Carbohydrate Malabsorption

Retention of undigested disaccharides in the intestine increases the osmotic load of the intraluminal contents and causes an excess quantity of fluid to be drawn into the intestine in order to dilute the sugar concentration. This increases the motility of the intestine and contributes to the development of abdominal cramps and bloating, as well as diarrhea. In addition, undigested sugars are fermented by bacteria, producing lactic and other acids. Normally the stools contain no more than 30 to 40 mg lactic acid, but in disaccharidase-deficient subjects 1000 mg or more may be produced. The excess acid may act as an irritant to the bowel, thus increasing the severity of diarrhea. Carbon dioxide and hydrogen gas are additional products of bacterial action in the intestine that contribute to distention and abdominal discomfort (Lebenthal, 1975).

Diagnosis

The classic picture of disaccharidase deficiency in infants is persistent diarrhea, abdominal distention, vomiting, and failure to thrive, all of which disappear on removal of the malabsorbed disaccharide from the diet. However, the symptoms may be variable and are influenced by the age at which sugars are introduced into the diet, the quantity of sugar ingested, and the degree of enzyme deficiency. The older child and adult with late onset lactose intolerance may have only crampy pain without diarrhea on ingestion of milk. These individuals may be unaware of the association between this symptom and the ingestion of milk or may simply assume that milk has this effect on everyone (Lebenthal, 1975).

Disaccharide tolerance tests are usually used to establish a diagnosis of deficiency. The patient must be free of diarrhea before a test can be performed. Therefore, the suspected disaccharide should be eliminated from the diet for several days prior to the test. The test is performed in the morning when the patient is fasting. For infants and children, the test sugar solution is usually given in the amount of 2 g sugar per kg body weight or 50 g per sq m body surface. For adults, the amount is 50 to 100 g. Blood samples for glucose determination are drawn before the sugar is given and at 20 or 30 minute intervals during the next 2 hours. The stools should be collected for several hours, their consistency observed, pH measured, and content of disaccharide and lactic acid measured. Normally, the administration of maltose, isomaltose, sucrose, or lactose causes a marked blood sugar peak that is more than 30 or 50 mg/100 ml above the fasting level, the pH of the stools is unaltered, and no sugar or lactic acid is excreted in the feces. If the patient is intolerant to the tested sugar, the blood glucose curve will be comparatively flat (Fig. 13.4). Abdominal pain, diarrhea, or both are likely to be present, stools will contain disaccharide, and the lactic acid, formed by bacterial fermentation, will produce a low pH. Giving the same quantity of monosaccharide as a control test should result in a normal blood glucose rise with no abdominal symptoms. Peroral biopsy of intestinal mucosa can provide samples of tissue for assay of disaccharidase activity to confirm the diagnosis of disaccharidase deficiency (Dahlqvist, 1966).

Sucrase-Isomaltase Deficiency

Primary sucrase-isomaltase deficiency is inherited as an autosomal recessive trait. It is relatively rare in most populations but more than 150 cases have been presented in the literature. Symptoms begin with introduction of sucrose into the diet. Starch appears to play a less important role in the pathogenesis since the condition can be effectively managed on a low-sucrose or sucrose-free diet. Isomaltose makes up only a small percentage of the total linkages in the starch molecule and it is usually not necessary to limit starch intake. Some commercial cow's-milk formulas for infants, all soy-milk formulas, and many therapeutic formulas contain sucrose. If a sucrose-containing formula is not used from birth, sucrose and isomaltose are usually added to the diet in increasing amounts after 4 weeks of age in the form of juices, puréed fruits, vegetables, cereals, breads, and prepared foods. Intermittent, rather than constant, diarrhea in these patients may be explained by the variation in sucrose content of the diet from day to day. Patients with sucrase-isomaltase deficiency have shown no increased ability

(a) Normal

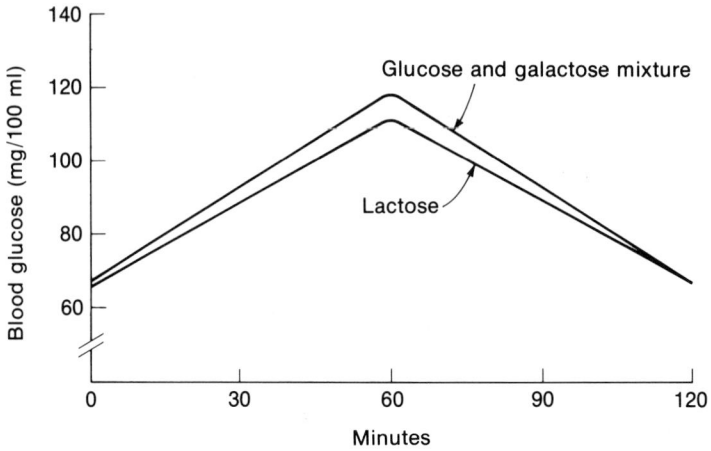

(b) Lactose intolerance

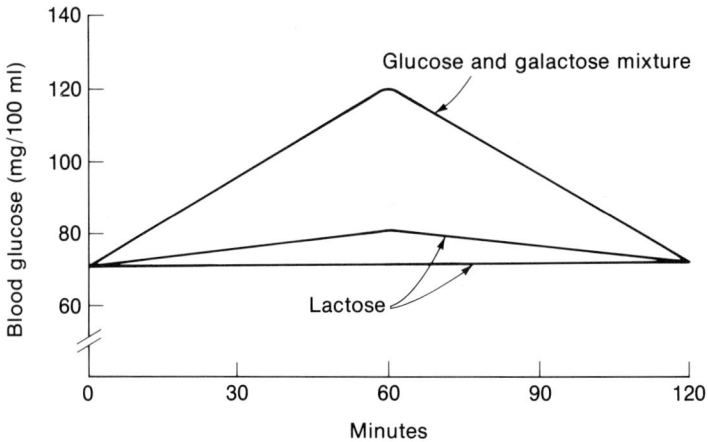

Fig. 13.4 (a) Normal blood glucose levels or (b) low blood glucose levels, indicating varying degrees of lactose intolerance, with oral administration of 50 g of lactose.

to tolerate usual amounts of sucrose in their diets as they grow older and thus dietary treatment should continue throughout life (Ament et al., 1973).

Ament et al. (1973) reported on seven cases of sucrase-isomaltase deficiency that were diagnosed in four families. The patients became free of symptoms within 24 hours when placed on sucrose-free diets. After a week of observation they were allowed to add fruits and vegetables which contained up to 2 percent sucrose (Table 13.4).

Lactose Intolerance

Primary congenital lactase deficiency is probably rare. Lactose-containing products must be eliminated from the diet and nonmilk formulas used for

Table 13.4 COMMON FOODS* CONTAINING 2 PERCENT OR LESS SUCROSE†

Food	Less than 1% Sucrose	Less than 2% but greater than 1% Sucrose
Fruits and fruit juices	Gooseberries	Boysenberries
	Loganberries	Cherries, bing
	Blackberries (dewberries)	Figs
	Cranberries	Grapes, Tokay or Thompson seedless
	Currants, black or red	Guava
	Lemons	Lime juice
	Rhubarb	Pears
	Pomegranates	Raspberries
	Tomatoes	Strawberries
	Tomato juice	
Vegetables	Bamboo shoots	Beans, lima
	Beans, snap, string, green	Carrots
	Cabbage	Rutabagas
	Cauliflower	Squash, golden, crookneck
	Celery	Beans, mung (bean sprouts)
	Corn	Peas, cow (black-eyed peas)
	Cucumber	
	Eggplant	
	Lettuce	
	Potatoes, white	
	Pumpkin	
	Radishes	
	Squash, Hubbard, butternut	
Grains, cereals, nuts, sweetening agents	Cornmeal	Wheat flour
	Puffed rice	Whole grain cereals and crackers which use whole wheat (such as puffed wheat, Nabisco Triscuits)
	Rice, brown or white	
	Wheat flour, patent	Honey
	Macaroni	Kraft dressings (Green Goddess, herb, garlic, and Golden Caesar)
	Spaghetti	
	Kraft mayonnaise	
	Kraft salad bowl mayonnaise	Pecans

* All foods, whether fresh, frozen, or canned, prepared without the addition of cane sugar (sucrose, invert sugar).
† Ament et al., 1973.

infants with this disorder. The lactase deficiency will be life-long. In markedly premature infants, a transient lactase deficiency may be present.

In 1965 several investigators at the Johns Hopkins School of Medicine gave lactose to American blacks and whites, none of whom had had GI complaints. They found that about 70 percent of the blacks were intolerant to lactose, whereas only 6 to 15 percent of the whites showed clinical symptoms from lactose ingestion. This was an unexpected finding and suggested there might be significant differences among ethnic groups in the ability to handle lactose (Kretchmer, 1972). Many reports since that time have extended these findings. Huang and Bayless (1968) reported that 19 of 20 healthy Oriental adults living in the United States developed abdominal cramps and diarrhea after ingesting an amount of lactose equivalent to that in 1 quart of milk, and 14 reported similar symptoms after 1 to 2 glasses of milk. Only two of 20 Caucasians tested at the same time were intolerant to milk and lactose. Lactose tolerance tests were performed on 32 healthy Jewish adults living in western Canada by Leichter (1971) with the finding that 68.8 percent of these subjects were lactose intolerant on the basis of a maximal blood glucose rise of less than 20 mg/100 ml after a lactose challenge. The lactose intolerance of this group was similar to that of a group of Jews living in Israel. A group of 38 healthy adults of Slavic origin living in western Canada showed an intolerance level of 23.9 percent (Leichter, 1972). Flat blood glucose curves in response to a lactose load were reported in 76 of 90 (84 percent) impoverished Peruvian Mestizo children ranging in age from 10 months to 17 years (Paige et al., 1972b). Signs of intolerance increased with age and 73 percent of the children below 3 years had normal tests, with a sharp drop in tolerance developing thereafter. More than 80 percent of Alaskan Eskimos and Indians were found to be intolerant of lactose (Duncan and Scott, 1972). A high proportion of Zambian Africans had hypolactasia, although a high concentration of the enzyme was found at birth in this population (Cook et al., 1973). Sowers and Winterfeldt (1975) found 47 percent of 17 nonrelated Mexican Americans to be lactose intolerant. Their additional findings of intolerance in two successive generations of three families and in both sexes of the families adds support to the suggestion that lactose intolerance has a genetic basis without sex predilection.

From the preceding data it is apparent that 60 to 90 percent of noncaucasian peoples have low lactase levels after early childhood, whereas only 5 to 15 percent of Caucasians fall in this category. It has not been clearly shown if this is solely a genetic phenomenon or if there is some influence due to adaptation as a result of customary milk drinking (Jones and Latham, 1974).

Because of widespread lactose intolerance, the role of milk in the diet of older children and adults has been questioned. Paige et al. (1972a) performed lactose tolerance tests on a random sample of Baltimore elementary school children who were categorized as either milk drinkers or nonmilk drinkers on the basis of observation during the school lunch period. Twenty percent of the Negro children and 10 percent of the white children were nonmilk drinkers. An association was demonstrated in the Negro nonmilk drinkers between poor milk consumption, lactose induced symptoms, and lactose malabsorption. It was also found that many of the Negro children who showed lactose intolerance on testing were consuming some milk. At a later time, Paige et al. (1975a) determined that 48 of 89 (54 percent) black elementary school children showed a flat lactose tolerance curve on testing. Twenty-eight of these 48 children (58 percent) were defined as nonmilk drinkers. These investigators concluded that some lactose intolerant children may have sufficient levels of lactase to hydrolyze the lactose in moderate amounts of milk, even though they are deficient in lactase.

Nandi and Parham (1972) did not find a correlation between milk consumption as adults and lactose intolerance in two groups of university students, 20 Oriental and 20 Caucasian. Stephenson and Latham (1974) found that the number and severity of abdominal symptoms were significantly higher in 16 lactose intolerant adults than in 19 lactose tolerant individuals after consumption of similar quantities of lactose or milk. However, the lactose intolerant subjects were able to consume nutritionally useful quantities of milk without undue symptoms developing. Garza and Scrimshaw (1976) found that none of a group of 69 black and 30 white children 4 to 9 years of age was intolerant to 240 ml of milk, although a high proportion of the black children, particularly those 6 or more years of age, were lactose intolerant on the standard tolerance test. It is important to point out that the test doses of lactose used in the standard tolerance tests are equivalent to consuming 1 quart of milk or more at one time. Smaller amounts of milk, such as 1 cup, may be tolerated by many individuals with lactase deficiency of varying degrees. It has been generally concluded that, provided milk is introduced into the diet gradually, there are no significant difficulties attending the consumption of supplementary amounts of skim milk for groups of school children and pregnant or lactating women throughout the world (Woodruff, 1976; Food and Nutrition Board, 1972). The Committee on Nutrition, American Academy of Pediatrics (1974) has stated that cow's milk is a valuable substitute for human milk in infancy and a useful food for older infants and children, although the amount of milk that should be consumed by them cannot be stated with convincing accuracy. They felt that the available evidence is insufficient to warrant discouraging programs for increasing the supply and consumption of milk in developing countries where childhood malnutrition is widespread.

A lactose-free or low-lactose diet should be consumed when lactose definitely cannot be tolerated. Since lactose is "milk sugar," this means that milk and products containing milk must be restricted. Milk contributes a number of valuable nutrients to the diet and dairy products are the major source of dietary calcium for populations in the United States, contributing 76 percent. Approximately 43 percent of the riboflavin and 23 percent of the protein available for dietary consumption in the United States come from dairy products (National Dairy Council, 1971). Fermented dairy products, particularly cultured buttermilk and yogurt, may be well tolerated by lactase deficient individuals. Much of the lactose in these products is hydrolyzed by the bacterial cultures used in their processing. It is also possible that the bacteria added in the process of culturing these products may continue to produce lactase in the intestinal tract after ingestion. Gallagher et al. (1974) reported that three lactase deficient patients tolerated fermented dairy products without adverse symptoms whereas nonfermented dairy products caused moderate to severe symptoms. Cheese may also be used by lactose intolerant individuals to supply good quality protein and calcium without lactose.

Lactose-reduced milk has been produced by treatment with lactase before processing. Several investigators have shown that milk with 50 to 90 percent less lactose than is usually contained in milk may be consumed by many patients with lactose intolerance with few adverse effects (Payne-Bose et al., 1977; Jones et al., 1976; Turner et al., 1976; Paige et al., 1975b). A lactase preparation is also available and may be given with meals. Kobayashi et al. (1975) demonstrated that intestinal absorption of calcium and magnesium was reduced in normal infants on a lactose-free milk formula and enhanced in infants who were fed a proprietary milk formula and given a lactase preparation in addition (mixed with the formula 10 minutes before feeding). Further study in this regard with lactose intolerant infants may be warranted.

13.5 Inflammatory Bowel Disease

There are two major types of chronic nonspecific inflammatory bowel disease. One is regional ileitis, regional enteritis, or Crohn's disease, a chronic granulomatous disease involving lesions chiefly in the ileum and jejunum. The bowel wall is thickened, rigid, and inflamed, and commonly has fistulas between adherent intestinal loops, between the ileum and colon, and/or between the ileum and other organs. The symptoms include abdominal pain, which is frequently worse after eating, and persistent diarrhea. Appetite declines and considerable weight loss may occur. A similar kind of granulomatous disease may affect the colon, with similar symptoms, and has been called Crohn's disease of the colon.

The second type of inflammatory bowel disease is ulcerative colitis. This disorder causes an abnormal, inflamed colonic mucosa that is edematous and hyperemic. The mucosa becomes so fragile that it bleeds easily and it has a characteristic histologic appearance. The rectum is usually extensively involved and the disease carries a greater than usual risk of developing carcinoma of the large bowel. The symptoms include abdominal pain, diarrhea, and rectal bleeding but may vary greatly in severity. Most patients have remissions and exacerbations. Severe attacks of persistent diarrhea are accompanied by fever, tachycardia, anorexia, and weight loss.

The causes of these diseases are unknown and treatment is symptomatic and empirical. Surgical treatment is usually reserved for complications such as obstruction, perforation, bleeding, or fistulation. Weight loss and nutritional deprivation is common in both types of disease, particularly in severe cases. Most patients with acute disease are anorectic and often afraid to eat because of associated symptoms. When they do consume food, persistent diarrhea limits the absorption of essential nutrients. Therefore, they often suffer from subacute starvation and break down body tissues to supply nitrogen and energy nutrients. Providing nutritional support for these patients is extremely important although often difficult to accomplish Rocchio and Randall, 1974).

There have been many suggestions of a relationship between the onset of ulcerative colitis and abnormalities in the personality structure of the patients and their ways of coping with life stresses. McMahon et al. (1973) found significant personality differences between patients with inflammatory bowel disease and their healthy siblings. The patients had a psychological fixation short of autonomy, while their siblings went through normal identity crises and emerged as more independent, mature individuals. However, about half of the patients with ulcerative colitis appear to be normal in their psychologic behavior, having maintained strong interpersonal relations and having shown success in educational pursuits, trade, or profession.

Incidence

Inflammatory bowel diseases are worldwide and occur among all races. In the United States the exact incidence is unknown but regional enteritis appears to be about one-third as common as ulcerative colitis, with an annual incidence of 2 to 3 per 100,000. The incidence of ulcerative colitis appears to be increasing in the United States (Wintrobe et al., 1974, p. 1477). Mendeloff et al. (1966) found the incidence of ulcerative colitis among Jews to be 4.5 times that among non-Jews, and regional enteritis among Jews was 9 times that among non-Jews. The diseases may occur at any age but the peak incidence is between 15 and 35 years.

Nutritional Care

The objectives of medical treatment for inflammatory bowel disease are to (1) minimize mortality and invalidism, (2) avoid complications, and (3) enable the patient to adjust to the disease, but treatment is not generally curative. Rest and administration of drugs, particularly corticosteroids, are prescribed during active periods of the disease. Maintaining nutritional status at as optimal a level as possible plays a useful role in helping the patient adapt to the stress of the disease. Nutritional care must be individualized since the problems vary with the stage and severity of the disorder. In acute stages the patient may not be able to take food orally and parenteral feeding is a possible alternative. Defined-formula diets have also been recommended under certain conditions. At most stages of the disease, however, the patient needs to be encouraged to eat a nutritionally balanced diet composed of foods that he or she is able to tolerate. When diarrhea is profuse, some restriction of dietary fiber or indigestible residue is advisable. The low-residue diet has traditionally been recommended in inflammatory bowel disease but may be unpalatable for some patients. It is more important that a patient consumes energy, protein, and other essential nutrients in whatever form he can tolerate than that he follows a prescribed low-residue diet. Milk has commonly been implicated in exacerbations of the disease (Citrin, 1964). Lactase deficiency was found by Cady et al. (1967) in 46 percent of 32 male patients with ulcerative colitis. Tandon et al. (1971) reported that 23.5 percent of 51 non-Jewish patients with ulcerative colitis had lactose intolerance as indicated by lactose tolerance tests, whereas 84.2 percent of 19 Jewish patients had lactose intolerance. In general, milk does not need to be restricted unless it is not tolerated on an individual basis. Circulating antibodies to milk proteins were low in 51 patients tested by Jewell and Truelove (1972), suggesting that milk allergy is not a factor in the etiology of ulcerative colitis.

Favorable results have been reported from the use of a fat-reduced diet for patients with ileal dysfunction both under metabolic ward conditions and during continued treatment outside the hospital (Andersson, 1974). It was suggested that the daily fat intake should be limited to not more than 50 g. In spite of a reduction of energy with this diet, nine of 10 patients did not lose weight, and several increased their total body potassium, indicating an increase in lean body mass. Fat absorption studies indicated that steatorrhea and azotorrhea were marked with butter or glyceryl monostearate but decreased when dietary fat was either cottonseed oil or glyceryl monolinoleate. MCT were most effective in lowering fecal fat excretion, however.

Gerson and Cohen (1976) reported that absorption of folic acid was normal in five patients with regional enteritis. They suggested that the folic acid deficiency common in this disorder is largely caused by malnutrition rather than malabsorption.

Defined-Formula Diets
Defined-formula diets are discussed in Sec. 10.3. Some of these products available commercially contain MCT along with amino acids or protein hydrolysates and simple sugars. When patients with inflammatory bowel disease are unable to tolerate regular foods, they may be able to absorb sugars and amino acids if these substances are infused slowly and continuously. The use of defined-formula diets can provide enough kilocalories and amino acid nitrogen to maintain positive nitrogen and caloric balance and thus avert the effects of starvation. Positive balance usually can be maintained in women by providing 2500 to 3000 kcal with 20 g nitrogen per day and in men by giving 3000 to 4000 kcal with 27 g nitrogen (Rocchio and Randall, 1974).

The formula diet is usually fed through a small nasogastric tube. During the first 3 to 5 days both the rate and concentration are gradually increased. Diarrhea, high gastric residue, or elevated blood sugar with glycosuria are signs that the intake has become excessive and the rate of administration should be reduced. Patients must be weighed daily and fluid retention evaluated. Intake and output should be recorded accurately and urine tested for glucose four times a day (Rocchio and Randall, 1974). Rocchio et al. (1974) reviewed a series of 40 patients with inflammatory bowel disease who had been given a defined-formula diet. Nitrogen balance studies in 14 cases and body composition studies in seven cases showed a marked anabolic response followed by nutritional improvement despite extensive GI disease. Bounous et al. (1974) reported that, with use of a semihydrolyzed elemental diet for 22 patients with intestinal disease, the improved nutritional status was sometimes accompanied by healing of local intestinal lesions. In severely debilitated, cachectic patients, however, the defined-formula diet was administered in association with intravenous alimentation.

Parenteral Feeding

Total parenteral nutrition (TPN) is discussed in Sec. 10.4. Reilly et al. (1976), from a review of patient records at the Massachusetts General Hospital, reported that surgery was avoided in approximately 70 percent of the patients with Crohn's disease who received TPN after the usual medical treatment had failed. Patients with Crohn's disease of the colon had a less favorable prognosis and 43 percent of these patients underwent surgery. Parenteral feeding did not appear to affect the course of ulcerative colitis, as almost all patients in this group were eventually treated by colectomy (removal of the colon). Anderson and Boyce (1973) reported that TPN for 30 days brought definite improvement marked by weight gain, diminished pain, decreased diarrhea, and increased serum albumin in eight patients with advanced regional enteritis, characterized by multiple areas of involvement, previous surgery, and failure on medical therapy. However, clinical remission was transient in seven of the eight patients. The authors concluded that although TPN could not be considered a primary form of treatment, it may be useful in patients with regional enteritis in order to restore nutrition, induce remission, and prepare a debilitated patient for surgery.

Medium-Chain Triglycerides (MCT)

MCT are prepared from coconut oil by a hydrolysis, molecular distillation, and reesterification process. The final product is a liquid fat with a melting point below 0°C, made up entirely of saturated fatty acids of chain lengths ranging from C6 to C10. A typical MCT preparation contains 80 percent C8, 17 percent C10, and 1 to 2 percent of either C6 or C12. Its energy yield is approximately 8.2 to 8.4 kcal per g (Hashim, 1967). The difference in digestion and absorption between MCT and LCT is discussed in Sec. 12.1. They appear to be most useful in the dietary treatment of malabsorptive diseases that are characterized by decreased pancreatic lipase or bile acid output; congenital malformation of the small intestine; intestinal lymphatic drainage problems; blind-loop syndromes; and resection of the small intestine (Hashim, 1967; Holt et al., 1965). They may be useful in selected cases of inflammatory bowel disease.

MCT oil may be used in food preparation in place of vegetable oil or other fats. The simplest ways to introduce MCT in food preparation are in salad dressings, blenderized with skim milk or fruit juices, and in sautéed foods. It has also been used to make cookies, bread, pancakes, French toast, muffins, popovers, pie crusts, pilaf, a modified form of ice cream, and various casserole mixtures (Schizas et al., 1967; Bowman, 1973; Howard and Morse, 1973).

Low-Residue Diets

In mild attacks of inflammatory bowel disease, most patients require only rest at home and a nutritious diet that is usually low in indigestible fiber or residue. There is no evidence that severe dietary restrictions contribute significantly to the long-term management, but it is usually wise to restrict bulk, particularly raw fruits and vegetables, nuts, and whole grains, at the time of active disease. Indigestible residue in the intestinal tract may increase transit time and contribute to the maintenance of existing diarrhea. As the disease subsides, a regular diet may be resumed, as tolerated. Vitamin supplementation is reasonable for poorly nourished patients. A severe attack is a medical emergency with the presence of dehydration, fever, weight loss, severe diarrhea, anemia, hypoalbuminemia, and signs of malnutrition, and requires hospitalization. Patients are temporarily managed without food or fluids by mouth and parenteral feeding may be useful at this time (Grand and Homer, 1975).

In the 1920s Hosoi, Alvarez, and Mann performed studies on dogs, with the lower ileum attached to the rectum, in which they measured the residue resulting from the feeding of large quantities of a single food. They concluded that gelatin, hard-cooked eggs, cottage cheese, and meats had low residues, whereas raw egg white, banana, potato, lard, butter, apple, prune, and milk were high-residue foods. Although the application of this research to human dietetics is not clear, milk was considered for many years to be a high-residue food and was restricted in a low-residue diet. In human subjects with ileotomies it has been found that 600 ml of milk per day, taken in place of 600 ml of water and added to an otherwise palatable and balanced diet, did not increase the volume of ileal effluent. Milk has not emerged as a high residue food for humans on the basis of several reported fecal studies (Weinstein et al., 1961), and should not be eliminated from a low-residue diet for reasons of residue. As previously discussed, milk may not be well tolerated by patients with inflammatory bowel disease because of lactase deficiency.

The usual low-residue diet is a modified-fiber diet. Foods high in indigestible fiber are restricted. When additional information on the fiber content of foods becomes available, the fiber content of low-residue diets may be estimated more accurately than is now possible. Foods to be avoided and those that may be included in a moderately low residue (fiber-modified) diet are listed in Table 13.5.

Nutritional Implications of Surgical Treatment

When medical management of regional enteritis has failed, surgery may be indicated. It may involve a bypass procedure, in which the fecal stream is diverted by dividing the ileum and anastomosing the undiseased portion to

Table 13.5 A MODERATELY LOW-RESIDUE (FIBER-MODIFIED) DIET

Foods Allowed	Foods not Allowed
Tender meat, fish, fowl	Meats with tough connective tissue
Cooked eggs	
All types of milk and dairy products	
All types of fats	
Refined bread and cereal products	Whole grain cereal products and bran
Tender, cooked vegetables and juices	Raw vegetables
Ripe bananas and cooked or canned fruits and juices, without skins or seeds	Raw fruits, except ripe banana
Desserts prepared from allowed foods	
Tea, coffee, carbonated beverages, and seasonings, as tolerated	
	Nuts, seeds, hulls, and fibrous skins on any food

the side of the transverse colon, or it may involve a resection of the small bowel to remove the diseased portion. Recurrence is similar in bypass or resection (Wheelock, 1974).

When more than two-thirds of the small intestine is removed from the adult patient, severe metabolic disturbances and a state of undernutrition are often observed with weight loss, muscle wasting, diarrhea, and malabsorption, and is called the short-bowel syndrome. Patients with this syndrome are capable of absorbing glucose and most water-soluble vitamins relatively efficiently. Amino acid absorption improves with time. However, fats are poorly tolerated and absorption may remain permanently impaired. There is a decrease in the bile salt pool and in the absorption of vitamin B_{12} with loss of the terminal ileum. Bowel motility often increases, as does gastric acid secretion. If nutritional support can be given by parenteral means for several weeks or months postoperatively, the remaining intestine will adapt by increasing villus size and efficiency of cellular metabolic activity.

Nutritional management following massive small-bowel resection has been divided into three stages by Richmond and Curreri (1974). During the first stage, TPN is used and there is no oral intake of fluids or food. Patients must be closely monitored to maintain electrolyte balance and provide sufficient nitrogen and energy nutrients. This stage may last 2 to 3 months in some cases, but cautious trial of oral isotonic fluids may be attempted after 3 to 4 weeks if 20 to 30 percent of the small bowel has been left intact. The second stage of management may begin once a successful trial with oral isotonic fluid has been completed and a gradual transition to an oral nutritional program is made. Extreme patience on the part of the dietitian and physician is necessary during this stage in implementing a progressive dietary program that can be tolerated by the patient. Appetite seldom returns until the rate and volume of parenteral fluids are substantially reduced, but both parenteral and oral routes must be used for a time in order to maintain adequate nutrition. Richmond and Curreri prefer to begin GI feedings by using extremely diluted solutions of simple defined-formula diets given through a nasogastric feeding tube at a constant rate by pump. Intake may be adjusted gradually to include commercial formulas containing polypeptides and small carbohydrate polymers. These compounds are less hyperosmolar than are amino acids and simple sugars. Finally, trials of fat administration may be attempted, probably using MCT at first. Within 3 to 6 months following massive bowel resection, it is usually possible to provide total daily caloric requirements orally. Thereafter, in the third stage, the diet can be varied to include most foodstuffs, as tolerated on an individual basis. Trial of new foods should be recorded in a dietary diary so that a pattern of tolerance can be identified. Richmond and Curreri suggested that patients avoid alcohol, extremely spicy foods, excessive coffee, milk products and other foods with high fat content during the first year. Thereafter, cautious ingestion of these foods may be attempted.

The usual surgical procedure for complications of ulcerative colitis and Crohn's disease of the colon involves removal of the colon and creation of an ileostomy by bringing the end of the ileum to the surface of the abdomen. External collection devices are available that permit the post-operative patient to carry on normal life activities. A continent ileotomy, providing a reservoir from a segment of terminal ileum that is split and folded back on itself, has been employed in some cases (Handelsman and Fishbein, 1976). Colectomy can cure ulcerative colitis and postsurgical metabolic problems do not usually occur.

Bone and Sorensen (1974) followed all ileostomy patients that were alive in 1971 after total proctocolectomy performed at the university hospitals in Aarhus, Denmark. One patient had formed stools, but all the others had watery to semisolid bowel movements, depending on their diets. Half of the patients reported a continual flow of bowel contents throughout the day, whereas in the others there was more or less a tendency to periodicity. As a rule, voluminous intestinal material appeared in the ileostomy bag 1 to 2 hours after meals, with nothing appearing in between. Several patients were able to keep the bag empty in the forenoon and afternoon by avoiding food and drink between meals. Most of the ileostomy patients emptied their bags four to eight times in 24 hours, partly depending on diet. Hill et al. (1975) reported that the mean weight of ileostomy fluid for 24 hours on a calculated normal diet was 570 ± 275 g for 10 ileostomy patients. This weight fell to 441 ± 194 g with substitution of a defined-formula diet for normal foods. The mean water content of the ileostomy fluid rose slightly with the formula diet. However, the consumption of an additional 2 liters of water resulted in no change in the water content of the ileal effluent. The study suggested that when a patient consumes a formula diet as the sole nutritional source for a period of time, bland, clear fluids will not increase the volume of fistula fluid. In general, foods with moderately low residue may be most appropriate for persons with ileostomies, but individualization to determine patient tolerance is extremely important.

13.6   Diverticulosis and Diverticulitis

Multiple herniations of the mucosa and submucosa of the colon through the circular muscle layer are referred to as diverticulosis (Fig. 13.5). The mucosal and submucosal layers are surrounded by a circular muscle that forms a complete tube. The colon's longitudinal muscle layer, which is on the outside of the circular muscle, does not completely cover the colon surface but is gathered into three areas, called *taenia,* between which the wall of the colon is thinner. The colonic wall is further weakened at certain points between the longitudinal muscles where blood vessels pierce the circular muscle layer. Diverticula tend to form in these weakened areas as the mucosa and submucosa are pushed by increased intraluminal pressure through the tunnels made by blood vessels. In large diverticula, feces may not be expelled and may harden into faecoliths within the diverticula. Diverticula commonly occur in two rows on each side of the colon (Painter, 1974; Shapiro, 1974).

Diverticulitis is a complication of diverticulosis, usually defined as a micro- or macroperforation of a diverticulum, with localized abdominal pain and fever. For many years diverticulosis was thought to be a symptomless condition and all symptoms that occurred were attributed to diverticulitis. However, it is now generally accepted that diverticulosis may periodically produce symptoms such as marked local abdominal tenderness or pain with exacerbation after eating. Patients with attacks or symptoms

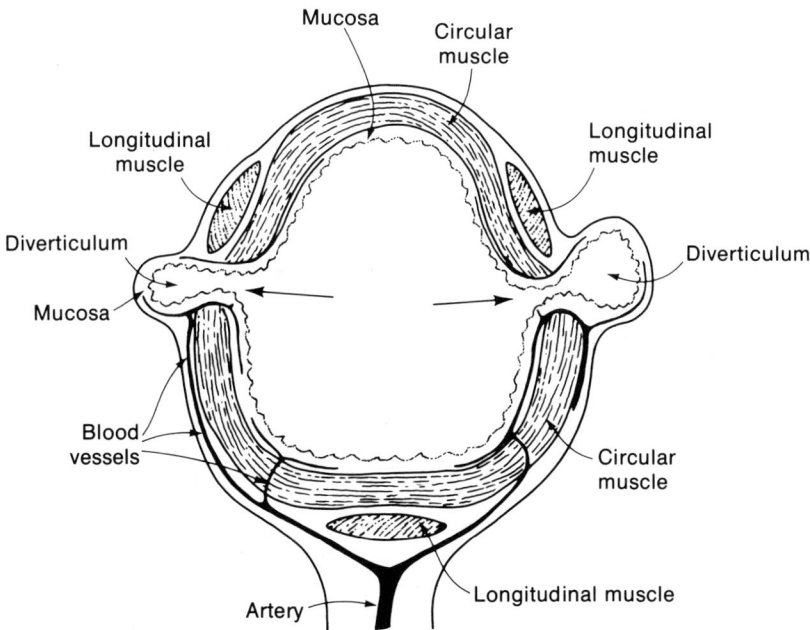

Fig. 13.5 Herniation of mucosa through the circular muscle of the colon produces diverticula (shown in cross section of colon).

due to diverticulosis do not usually have fever and the white blood count is not elevated. Treatment of diverticulitis includes giving nothing by mouth, along with continuous nasogastric suction if signs of obstruction are present or if the patient is nauseated; appropriate intravenous fluid; and broad-spectrum antibiotics. Surgery is indicated if the perforation has caused generalized peritonitis, persisting intestinal obstruction, the development of a fistula, or if medical therapy fails (Beeson and McDermott, 1975, pp. 1196 and 1278–1279).

Pathogenesis and Etiology of Diverticulosis

Diverticular disease of the colon has dramatically increased in the western world since 1900, when it was rarely found. It now affects 45 percent of Australian colons and 35 percent of British ones over the age of 60, with a similar incidence in the United States and France (Painter, 1974). The disease is rare in Africa, Thailand, India, and Iran. Diverticular disease is now increasing in Japan. It is more prevalent among Japanese who have been born and reared in Hawaii where they have consumed a westernized diet than it is among Japanese citizens living in Japan (Painter and Burkitt, 1975).

Dietary factors, particularly the amount of fiber, have been implicated in the etiology of diverticulosis and in an explanation for the relatively recent marked increase of this disorder in westernized countries. A decrease in dietary fiber, with concurrent decrease in stool weights and intestinal transit times, has occurred over the past 75 years with western-type diets of refined foods. The consistency of stools is firmer with less fiber in the diet (Burkitt and Painter, 1975). Payler (1973) reported that the average intestinal transit time in English school boys was reduced from 64.5 to 45.9 hours and average daily stool weights increased from 135 to 163 g after the replacement of white by wholemeal bread and the addition of 2 dessert-spoonsful of bran to the daily diet. Africans on unrefined carbohydrate foods had intestinal transit times of approximately 14 hours, while school teachers on an intermediate fiber diet had times of 20 hours, and university medical students on more refined carbohydrate foods had 28 hours (Burkitt and Painter, 1975). Intestinal transit time (using carmine as a marker) averaged about 9.5 hours in rural South African Negro children 9 to 12 years of age when ingesting a mean of 10 g crude fiber per day in their usual diets (Walker, 1975).

The explanation for pathogenesis of diverticular disease has been related to changing pressures in the colon, which can be measured with the use of water-filled, open-ended tubes placed in various positions in the colon. Circular muscles of the colon normally contract in segments (Fig. 13.6) to form rings in order to move or halt the content of the colon, allowing absorption of water and avoiding diarrhea. Pressure is produced within a segment between contracting rings. The greater the degree of segmentation, the greater the intracolonic pressures. If the colon is wide and filled with indigestible material, it is less likely to contract its lumen by

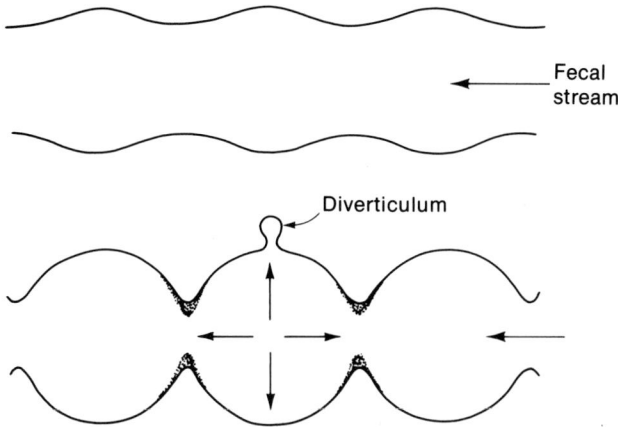

Fig. 13.6 Hypersegmentation of the colon may increase intraluminal colonic pressure within a segment, resulting in development of a diverticulum.

segmentation than is a narrow unfilled colon. Fecal material that is hard in consistency requires greater muscle contraction in order to move it along the intestinal tract than do feces of a soft consistency, with greater pressure being produced in the colon by the more powerful contractions. Intracolonic pressure, localized in a segment of the colon, may be great enough to force the mucosa and submucosa through the circular muscle at the weak points of the wall where blood vessels have pierced the muscle, thus producing diverticula (Fig. 13.5) (Burkitt and Painter, 1975; Painter, 1974). With less dietary fiber, producing less indigestible residue in the colon, hypersegmentation and intraluminal pressure is theoretically increased, thus increasing the likelihood of diverticular disease.

Dietary Treatment of Diverticulosis

For many years a low-residue diet was standard treatment for diverticular disease. However, with the explanation of pathogenesis as hypersegmentation of the colon, treatment with a high-residue diet appeared to be more logical since it would provide greater indigestible bulk so that hypersegmentation would be less likely to occur. The softer stool consistency associated with a high-residue diet would also require less powerful muscle contractions to control the movement of the fecal mass. No evidence is available to support the use of the traditional low-residue diet in the management of diverticular disease (Plumley and Francis, 1973). In fact, ingestion of low-residue diets for 2 years has been shown to lead to formation of diverticula in rats. In rabbits on low-residue diets, raised intracolonic pressures have been noted (Hodgson, 1974).

Painter et al. (1972) treated 70 patients with symptomatic diverticular disease without organic stenosis over a 4-year period by giving increasing amounts of wheat bran until the patients did not have to strain to defecate. Most patients needed 2 teaspoonsful (12 to 14 g) of bran three times a day but some required several tablespoonsful a day. At least 39 of the subjects suffered from flatulence when the bran treatment was initially started, but this disappeared within 3 weeks. Each of the patients complained of more than one pretreatment symptom, including nausea, heartburn, flatulence, distention, abdominal pain, and constipation. The patients were also asked to use 100 percent whole wheat bread, fresh fruits, and vegetables and to stop adding refined sugar to their drinks. These dietary changes, along with the addition of bran, relieved or abolished 88.6 percent of the symptoms of uncomplicated diverticular disease. Plumley and Francis (1973) in the United Kingdom developed a high-fiber bran crispbread as an acceptable way for patients to consume large amounts of bran. The basic recipe called for 52 percent wheat gluten, 7 percent wheat flour, and 41 percent wheat bran, to which were added calcium carbonate (commensurate with phytic acid content) and salt. The crispbread contained 4 percent crude fiber, determined by the standard method of hydrolysis with dilute acid and alkali. Forty-eight people with diverticular disease ate six slices of crispbread per day over a 6-month to 3-year period. Of the total 98 presenting symptoms, 73 percent were satisfactorily controlled by the addition of the crispbread to the diet.

Wheat bran may be the preferable source of bulk for patients with diverticular disease, although scientific proof for this is not available. Goldstein (1972) has advised avoidance of *excess* quantities of raw fruits and vegetables for patients with diverticular disease because of the likely mild laxative effect. Fresh fruits and vegetables are also often expensive. Goldstein has further recommended avoidance of excessive quantities of spices, such as pepper, because these substances appear to increase bowel irritability, although no scientific proof for this assertion can be cited. Additional data on the mechanisms of wheat bran or other high fiber foods in relieving symptoms of diverticulosis are desirable. Published clinical studies are still preliminary and often not well controlled (Connell, 1976). The amount and type of bran required to decrease intestinal transit time has not been clarified (Wyman et al., 1976; Kirwan et al., 1974).

It has been postulated that the so-called spastic colon, which has been classified as one type of irritable bowel syndrome, may be a forerunner of diverticular disease as similar colonic pressures and other abnormalities have been reported in these two disorders (Goldstein, 1972; Boy et al., 1976). It has therefore been suggested that high-fiber diets may be helpful in *prevention* of diverticular disease although proof for this suggestion is not yet available. Lyford et al. (1975) did not find a clearcut beneficial effect of bran on irritable bowel syndrome for a group of 27 patients.

13.7   Dietary Fiber

Terminology concerned with fiber is imprecise at the present time. An exact definition for dietary fiber has not been agreed upon but probably includes the nondigestible plant carbohydrates (cellulose, hemicelluloses, and pectin) and lignin, a nondigestible noncarbohydrate substance found in woody materials. Data on fiber appearing in food composition tables are chiefly "crude fiber," which is determined in the laboratory by sample treatment with dilute acid and extraction with alkali. Crude fiber is mainly cellulose with some lignin. About 85 percent of the hemicellulose and 50 to 90 percent of lignin is lost in the acid-alkaline measurement procedure. A neutral-detergent method of measuring fiber leaves lignin, cellulose, and hemicellulose but pectin is lost. Few data on foods are available using this method (Van Soest and Robertson, 1977). Some values for indigestible residue of foods determined by an enzymatic method have been published (Hellendorn, 1975 and 1976).

Table 13.6   CRUDE FIBER IN FOODS*

Food	Measure	Weight (g)	Crude Fiber (g)	Kcal
Almonds, whole, shelled	$\frac{1}{4}$ cup	36	0.9	195
Apple, fresh, whole	1 ($2\frac{1}{2}''$ diam.)	115	1.2	61
Apricots, canned, light syrup	4 halves, 2 tbs juice	100	0.4	66
Asparagus, cooked, cut	$\frac{1}{2}$ cup	72	0.5	15
Banana, fresh, sliced	$\frac{1}{2}$ cup	75	0.4	64
Beans, kidney, cooked	$\frac{1}{2}$ cup	93	1.4	109
Beans, snap, boiled	$\frac{1}{2}$ cup	63	0.6	15
Beef	Any quantity		0.0	
Bran, Kellogg's, All-Bran	$\frac{1}{2}$ cup	28	2.4	64
Bran flakes, 40%, Kellogg's	$\frac{3}{4}$ cup	28	1.1	97
Bread, white	1 slice	27	0.05	74
Bread, whole wheat	1 slice	25	0.4	61
Broccoli, fresh, boiled	$\frac{1}{2}$ cup	78	0.8	20
Carrot, raw	1 ($1\frac{1}{8}''$ diam., 7" long)	81	0.8	30
Corn flakes	1 cup	28	0.2	112
Crackers, graham	4 ($2\frac{1}{2}''$ square)	28	0.3	108
Egg	Any quantity		0.0	
Farina, regular, cooked	$\frac{3}{4}$ cup	183	Trace	76
Grapefruit juice, canned, unsweetened	$\frac{1}{2}$ cup	118	Trace	51
Lettuce, iceberg, leaves, chopped	1 cup	56	0.3	8
Macroni, elbow, cooked tender (14–20 min)	$\frac{1}{2}$ cup	70	0.07	78
Oatmeal, cooked	$\frac{1}{2}$ cup	120	0.2	66
Orange, fresh, navel	1 ($2\frac{3}{8}''$ diam.)	131	0.7	45
Peas, green, frozen, boiled	$\frac{1}{2}$ cup	84	1.6	57
Peanuts, shelled	2 tbs	18	0.4	104
Pineapple, raw, diced	$\frac{1}{2}$ cup	78	0.3	40
Raisins, uncooked, not packed	$\frac{1}{4}$ cup	73	0.7	105
Soybeans, mature, cooked	$\frac{1}{2}$ cup	90	1.3	117
Spinich, leaves, cooked	$\frac{1}{2}$ cup	90	0.5	20
Wheat, cracked, cooked	$\frac{1}{2}$ cup	123	0.4	55

* Watt and Merrill, 1963.

Although data on crude fiber are not very meaningful in a physiologic sense, they are all that is now generally available to use in estimating fiber intake (Bing, 1976; Trowell, 1976). Table 13.6 lists crude fiber content of selected foods.

The usual intake of crude fiber has not been satisfactorily estimated. There has been a decline in the consumption of whole wheat flour and cereals in the United States from 160 lb per capita in 1900 to less than 100 lb in 1970. Consumption of fresh fruits and vegetables has also declined from 250 lb per capita in 1940 to under 180 lb in 1970. However, the consumption of processed fruits and vegetables has increased in the same period from 65 lb to almost 110 lb per person, giving a minimum net decrease in fruits and vegetables of 25 lb per person. Therefore, it is esti-mated that fiber intake from fruits and vegetables has declined by about 20 percent and fiber from cereal products has decreased by as much as 50 percent thus far during the twentieth century (Scala, 1974). Trowell (1972) and Robertson (1972) reported from dietary surveys that the average indi-vidual in Great Britain consumed 4 to 8 g fiber daily. Hardinge et al. (1958) have shown that a group of American vegetarians consumed 8 to 11 g fiber per day. South African Negro schoolchildren were estimated to consume 10 g fiber daily (Walker, 1975), whereas rural African tribesmen have been reported to consume 15 to 20 g fiber per day. Dorfman et al. (1976) used recall diet histories in seven subjects with no disease and 14 with colon disease to estimate fiber intake. They found a mean intake of 3.5 g with a range of 1.6 to 11 g daily. No statistical differences in intake were found between patients with or without colon disease in this small sample.

13.8   Cancer of the Large Bowel

In western populations, cancer causes 10 to 21 percent of total deaths. Of these, 15 to 20 percent are due to colon cancer. Thus colon cancer accounts for 2 to 4 percent of all deaths. In the United States, the disease is responsi-ble for 37,000 deaths annually. Colon cancer is either unknown or very rare in primitive and developing populations. There is an average of six cases per year among a million or more blacks in Johannesburg, whereas in a South African white population of the same size and age structure, about 95 cases could be expected. Mortality is slightly lower in blacks than whites in the United States. Japanese immigrants to Hawaii and the United States have a higher mortality from colonic cancer than do their compatriots in Japan. Colon cancer is slightly more common in men than women (Walker, 1976; Walker and Burkitt, 1976).

The major cause of colon cancer appears to be environmental, with diet being one of the most important factors. The carcinogens involved may be either ingested or of endogenous origin. Several hypotheses concerning the relationships between diet and cancer of the colon have been suggested although there are few research data to clearly establish the role of diet in development of the cancer. The hypotheses include: (1) national intakes of protein, particularly animal protein, are correlated with colon cancer mortality rates and suggest that the level of dietary protein may be of significance; (2) increased fat intake is a major associated factor and probably a chief etiological cause; (3) colon cancer may be a sequelae of increased intake of sugar or other refined carbohydrates; and (4) depletion of fiber is the primary predisposing factor for colon cancer (Walker, 1976; Howell, 1975). The hypotheses involving protein, fat, and sugar intake are supported wholly or in part from close associations between national intakes of the particular food components and mortality rates from cancer of the colon. These types of studies are limited by the reliability of data both on nutrient intake and on mortality. In addition, they do not show a cause and effect relationship but may serve as guides for further research (Walker and Burkitt, 1976).

A study of Japanese migrants to Hawaii (Berg et al., 1975) attempted to show food items that differentiated between patients with bowel cancer and hospital controls matched for age, sex, and race. Although total use of meat differentiated cases from controls, with cases using a greater amount of meat, the relative risks associated with chicken and some sources of pork were not significant. The meat item with the highest relative risk (in terms of above versus below average use) was beef. Fish, eggs, and dairy products did not yield differences between cases and controls. Howell (1975) submitted data from international food consumption patterns (from FAO) as well as surveys of food consumption in the United States (from USDA) to factor analysis and found that her data supported the findings of the case-control study in regard to meat consumption, particularly beef. From information reviewed by Howell, there was little basis for rejecting any of the dietary hypotheses that have been suggested with respect to colorectal cancer.

Various laboratory studies have suggested that fecal bile acids and total neutral sterols may be involved in the development of colon cancer. Concentration of these substances was found to be higher in the feces of British subjects than in Ugandan adults, populations that are prone and nonprone, respectively, to colon cancer. These compounds were also found to be more concentrated in the feces of colon cancer patients as compared with controls. Decreasing dietary fat decreased the concentration of fecal bile acids and neutral sterols. A high-fat diet (40 percent of kcal) with 15 g per day of fiber produced decreases in fecal bile acid concentration when compared with diets lower in fiber. Raising the fiber intake had a greater effect than reducing fat intake on decreasing fecal sterols. Since addition of fiber to the diet usually increases the total volume of feces voided, the *concentration* of bile acids and neutral steroids may be decreased, although the *total amount* excreted may be unchanged or even increased since fiber binds bile acids in varying amounts. The binding is apparently influenced by several factors, including the type of fiber (Eastwood and Mowbray, 1976; Cummings et al., 1976). Dietary fiber has the ability to bind not only bile acids and potentially toxic substances but also other nutrients in the intestine. Phytic acid, which is an indigestible component of cereal fibrous material, may bind mineral elements, including calcium, magnesium, and zinc (Reinhold et al., 1976; Leveille, 1975). This should be kept in mind when considering large increases in dietary fiber.

The pattern and type of microflora in the intestine has been reported by some investigators to differ in colon cancer patients from that of non-cancer patients. However, no consistently significant differences between cancer prone and nonprone populations have been found by other re-searchers (Walker, 1976). It has been suggested that bile acids and sterols may be degraded by intestinal bacteria to yield pre-, co-, or actual carcino-gens and that diets with little indigestible residue, that remains in the bowel for comparatively long periods of time, may allow greater contact between the carcinogens and the bowel mucosa, thus increasing the likelihood that cancer will develop. Decreasing fat intake or increasing fiber intake may decrease the concentration of these potentially noxious materials by de-creasing the concentration of sterols from which they are formed. In addi-tion, increasing fiber intake may decrease contact in the bowel by increasing transit time of the larger volume of feces (Walker and Burkitt, 1976).

It may be difficult to suggest widespread dietary changes for the pre-vention of colon cancer that will be acceptable. Kahaner et al. (1976) found that six subjects consuming 3 oz daily of a high fiber bran breakfast food changed their eating behavior during the 3-week experimental period. They decreased their intake of eggs, butter, and breakfast meats since they chose to eat the major portion of the bran during breakfast. They increased milk and fruit intake since these foods made the bran more palatable. Five subjects added the supplement to between meal snacks and thus increased their daily caloric intake. Not withstanding the knowledge that increased fiber content may have beneficial effects, none of the subjects continued eating the high-fiber food after the experimental period was concluded. It would appear that a worthwhile increase in intake of fiber-containing foods is unlikely to occur for the general population unless bran is added com-mercially to widely consumed breakfast foods or other products. Further-more, the minimal dietary change that will bring beneficial results in the prevention of colon cancer is not known (Walker, 1976). Perhaps research concerned with education and motivation of individuals and groups, along with additional data on physiologic and biochemical effects of diet on cancer, will bring some answers to the many questions that yet remain unanswered.

13.9   Constipation and Diarrhea

Approximately 500 ml of chyme pass through the ileocecal valve of the normal adult each day. As this residue is slowly passed along the colon by the kneading and churning movement of segmentation, fluid is absorbed. Net forward velocity is normally about 5 cm per hour and ingestion of food doubles this rate. The sigmoid reservoir of the colon collects the formed residue. When the rectum fills and becomes sufficiently distended, centers in the sacral part of the spinal cord facilitate a defecation reflex. The willful act of defecation is a complex, coordinated, learned habit. Voluntary inhibition of this act and ignoring the impulse returns the stool to the sigmoid and descending colon (Benson, 1975).

Constipation is defined as the condition resulting from insufficient frequency of defecation, deficient quantity of stool, or production of abnormally hard and dry stools (Benson, 1975). Diarrhea may be defined as an increase in the frequency, volume, or fluidity of stools (Phillips, 1975). In both cases these definitions are related to the usual habit of each individual, the number and volume of bowel movements considered to be normal varying from one person to another and in different cultures. In the United States, a normal person may have as many as two or three formed stools per day or as few as three per week, as long as they are soft and comfortable movements. The African Bantu may consider himself constipated if he does not have three or four bowel movements every day (Ackerman, 1972).

Benson (1975) classified the causes of simple chronic constipation as:

1. Imagined. The patient assumes that a daily bowel movement is absolutely essential for health.
2. Rectal. Elimination is delayed though stool consistency is normal. Habits are poor. Breakfast stimulates the gastrocolic reflex and this stimulation is lost for non-breakfast eaters. If the reflex urge is not heeded, for many reasons involving social and job pressures, the individual gradually becomes insensitive to it.
3. Colonic. Delay in the passage of residue through the colon leads to a dry, hard stool that is difficult to eliminate. Several organic, mechanical, or metabolic conditions may contribute to this. Probably the most common nonorganic cause is inadequate dietary residue and water intake. In the elderly patient, decreased appetite, inadequate dentition, distaste for vegetables, and reduced funds for food purchases may all conspire to provide low-residue diets that do not stimulate the rectosigmoid by distention. Drugs may also cause colonic constipation, including opiates, anticholinergic agents, ganglionic blockers used to treat hypertension, nonabsorbable antacids, antidepressants, sedatives, and antiparkinsonism agents. These all tend to harden the stool, impair responsiveness to rectal distention, reduce segmentation by the colon, and disrupt the complex, learned behavior of elimination.
4. Constipation in children. Parental concern with toilet training is often excessive and emotional upsets precede many attacks of constipation in children. The child may use delayed defecation as an attention-getting device. In some cases, the toilet seat is simply too high to permit adequate squatting.

Generalized symptoms accompanying chronic constipation may include dull headache, lassitude, anorexia, low-back pain, weakness, giddiness, bloating, and lower abdominal discomfort. The laxative habit often becomes established when purgatives fail to clear up the symptoms. A vicious circle may develop with laxatives and enemas being used constantly in order to produce a bowel movement. This contributes to development of the irritable-colon syndrome, where a spastic, tender, cordlike left colon causes alternating constipation and diarrhea (Benson, 1975).

Any organic or metabolic causes of constipation should be determined and treated by dealing with the basic cause. Education of the patient with bad habits of hygiene should include an explanation of the gastrocolic reflex. Mistaken notions of the patient about constipation, foods, and laxatives should be dispelled. Results come slowly and the patient should be advised to expect this as new habits are being formed. A regular morning routine should be encouraged, with breakfast included. Hot water and lemon juice, taken on arising, may serve to initiate the gastrocolic reflex (Benson, 1975).

The dietary residue should be increased, particularly in the elderly, for treatment of colonic constipation. This may come from cooked or canned fruits and vegetables, raw fruits and vegetables (if tolerated), whole grain breads and cereals, and added bran (2 to 3 tsp three times a day). Bran may cause flatulence initially but this usually disappears within a few weeks. In some individuals, the lactose from milk may loosen the stool, especially in blacks and others who have lactase deficiency. The amount of dietary residue that will be effective in relieving constipation is not known and undoubtedly depends on the individual patient. Five to six servings of fruits and vegetables daily, along with four to six servings of whole grain bread or cereals should be sufficient.

Laxatives, in general, should be immediately discontinued with the high-fiber diet. Certain patients, however, may temporarily require mild stimulation from laxatives, under supervision of a physician, as adaptation to additional dietary residue and improved health habits occurs. Physical activity will also be helpful in maintaining regularity of bowel function.

The colon normally absorbs daily approximately 2.5 liters water, 400 meq Na^+, and 560 meq Cl^- into the general circulation, while it secretes about 45 meq K^+ and 260 meq HCO_3^- into the lumen. Bile acid is absorbed to some extent from the colon in the enterohepatic circulation. Natural fiber in the stool holds water by adsorption and traps water in the interstices of the fiber. It also adsorbs bile acids. Failure to absorb sufficient water from the stool allows it to move forward and stimulate the receptor areas of the rectosigmoid, resulting in urgency to defecate and diarrhea. The segmenting activity of the colon is decreased in a diarrheal state (Connell, 1974).

Osmotic diarrhea occurs when an excessive concentration of small water soluble molecules remains in the bowel lumen. Lactase deficiency may produce this type of diarrhea. Secretory diarrhea occurs when the mucosa of the bowel is stimulated to secrete a fluid similar to extracellular fluid. This may occur as a result of bacterial toxins, formation of dihydroxy bile acids, fatty acids and hydroxy fatty acids, and some hormones. Exudative diarrhea results from the outpouring of serum proteins, blood, or mucus from sites of inflammatory, ulcerative, and infiltrative diseases. Common causes of acute diarrhea include gastroenteritis, bacterial infections, parasitic infestations, and drugs. Treatment of acute diarrhea considers the cause but is also aimed at fluid and electrolyte replacement. Oral replacement of body fluid with glucose-saline solutions provides a simple, effective remedy (Phillips, 1975). Hirschhorn and Denny (1975) suggested the use of an oral glucose-electrolyte solution containing, in mmol per liter, 81 Na^+, 18 K^+, 71 Cl^-, 28 HCO_3^-, and 139 glucose for children throughout the world with acute diarrhea. Bicarbonate should be deleted if vomiting is also present. This correction of fluid volume depletion and acidosis often permits children to take food by mouth very early in treatment and thus overcome the nutritional deficits produced by diarrhea. Sherman et al. (1975) treated infants with severe diarrhea in the early stages with an oral defined-formula diet.

Chronic diarrhea often accompanies diverse intestinal disorders, including GSE, inflammatory bowel disease, colon cancer, and disaccharidase deficiencies. The underlying cause should be treated whenever possible. Functional diarrhea may occur without apparent cause. Motility patterns of the colon are abnormal in some patients and pain may be correlated with high peaks of intraluminal pressure (Phillips, 1975). The irritable bowel syndrome, an apparent functional disorder, may be responsible for intermittent diarrhea. Treatment of functional diarrheas includes reassurance and explanation for the patient. If specific foods are suspected as exacerbating agents, they should be avoided. An increase in dietary fiber may be helpful. An effort should be made, on an individual basis, to correct any nutritional deficiencies that are often associated with chronic diarrhea (Gardner, 1962).

REFERENCES

1. Ackerman, L. V. 1972. Some thoughts on food and cancer. *Nutr. Today,* **7** (Jan.-Feb.): 2.

2. Almy, T. P., A. I. Mendeloff, D. Rice, A. Lilienfeld, H. Klarman, R. Rawson, and W. R. Cunnick. 1975. Prevalence and significance of digestive disease. *Gastroent.,* **68** (Part 2): 1351.

3. Ament, M. E., D. R. Perera, and L. J. Esther. 1973. Sucrase-isomaltase deficiency—a frequently misdiagnosed disease. *J. Ped.,* **83:** 721.

4. American Academy of Pediatrics, Committee on Nutrition. 1974. Should milk drinking by children be discouraged? *Pediatrics,* **53:** 576.

5. Anderson, C. M., M. Gracey, and V. Burke. 1972. Coeliac disease. *Arch. Dis. Child.,* **47:** 292.

6. Anderson, D. L. and H. W. Boyce, Jr. 1973. Use of parenteral nutrition in treatment of advanced regional enteritis. *Am. J. Dig. Dis.,* **18** (New Series): 633.

7. Anderson, D. M. 1959. History of celiac disease. *J. Am. Dietet. Assoc.,* **35:** 1158.

8. Andersson, H. 1974. Fat-reduced diet in the symptomatic treatment of patients with ileopathy. *Nutr. and Met.,* **17:** 102.

9. Baker, H., O. Frank, and H. Sobotka. 1964. Mechanisms of folic acid deficiency in nontropical sprue. *J. Am. Med. Assoc.,* **187:** 119.

10. Bayless, T. M. and S. Huang. 1969. Inadequate intestinal digestion of lactose. *Am. J. Clin. Nutr.,* **22:** 250.

11. Beeson, P. B. and W. McDermott (Eds.) 1975. *Textbook of Medicine,* vol. II, 14th ed. Philadelphia: Saunders.

12. Benson, G. D., O. D. Kowlessar, and M. H. Sleisenger. 1964. Adult celiac disease with emphasis upon response to the gluten-free diet. *Medicine,* **43:** 1.

13. Benson, J. A., Jr. 1975. Simple chronic constipation. *Postgrad. Med.,* **57:** 55.

14. Berg, N. O., A. Dahlqvist, T. Lindberg, and Å. Nordén. 1970. Intestinal dipeptidases and disaccharidases in celiac disease in adults. *Gastroent.,* **59:** 575.

15. Berg, J. W., W. Haenszel, and S. S. Devesa. 1975. Epidemiology of gastrointestinal cancer. In *Seventh National Cancer Conference Proceedings.* Philadelphia: Lippincott.

16. Berman, P. M. and J. B. Kirsner. 1972. The aging gut. 2. Diseases of the colon, pancreas, liver, and gallbladder, functional bowel disease, and iatrogenic disease. *Geriatrics,* **27** (No. 4): 117.

17. Bing, F. C. 1976. Dietary fiber—in historical perspective. *J. Am. Dietet. Assoc.,* **69:** 498.

18. Bone, J. and F. H. Sorensen. 1974. Life with a conventional ileostomy. *Dis. Colon Rectum,* **17:** 194.

19. Bounous, G., G. Devroede, H. Haddad, R. Beaudry, B. J. Perey, and L. Lejeune. 1974. Use of an elemental diet for intestinal disorders and for the critically ill. *Dis. Colon Rectum,* **17:** 157.

20. Bowman, F. 1973. MCT cookies, cakes, and quick breads: quality and acceptability. *J. Am. Dietet. Assoc.,* **62:** 180.

21. Boy, J. A. E., M. A. Eastwood, W. D. Mitchell, J. L. Pritchard, and A. N. Smith. 1976. Fecal characteristics contrasted in the irritable bowel syndrome and diverticular disease. *Am. J. Clin. Nutr.,* **29:** 1480.

22. Brown, M. R. and C. B. Lillibridge. 1975. When to think of celiac disease. *Clin. Ped.,* **14** (No. 1): 76.

23. Burkitt, D. and N. Painter. 1975. Gastrointestinal transit times; stool weights and consistency; intraluminal pressures. In *Refined Carbohydrate Foods and Disease,* D. P. Burkitt and H. C. Trowell (Eds.). New York: Academic Press.

24. Cady, A. B., J. B. Rhodes, A. Littman, and R. K. Crane. 1967. Significance of lactase deficit in ulcerative colitis. *J. Lab. Clin. Med.,* **70:** 279.

25. Carswell, F. and A. Ferguson. 1972. Food antibodies in serum—a screening test for coeliac disease. *Arch. Dis. Child.,* **47:** 594.

26. Citrin, Y. 1964. Milk and ulcerative colitis. *Arch. Int. Med.,* **113:** 519.

27. Connell, A. M. 1976. Natural fiber and bowel dysfunction. *Am. J. Clin. Nutr.,* **29:** 1427.

28. Connell, A. M. 1974. Clinical aspects of motility. *Med. Clin. No. Am.,* **58:** 1201.

29. Cook, G. C., N. Asp, and A. Dahlqvist. 1973. Lactose absorption kinetics in Zambian African subjects. *Brit. J. Nutr.,* **30:** 519.

30. Cummings, J. H., M. J. Hill, D. J. A. Jenkins, J. R. Pearson, and H. S. Wiggins. 1976. Changes in fecal composition and colonic function due to cereal fiber. *Am. J. Clin. Nutr.,* **29:** 1468.

31. Dahlqvist, A. 1966. Disaccharide intolerance. *J. Am. Med. Assoc.,* **195:** 225.

32. Davis, J. S. 1970. Tropical sprue in upstate New York. *J. Am. Med. Assoc.,* **213:** 735.

33. Desai, H. G., A. V. Chitre, D. V. Parekh, and K. N. Jeejeebhoy. 1967. Intestinal disaccharidases in tropical sprue. *Gastroent.,* **53:** 375.

34. Dicke, W. K., H. A. Weijers, and J. H. Van de Kamer. 1953. Coeliac disease. 2. The presence in wheat of a factor having a deleterious effect in cases of coeliac disease. *Acta Paediat.,* **42:** 34.

35. Dorfman, S. H., M. Ali, and M. H. Floch. 1976. Low fiber content of Connecticut diets. *Am. J. Clin. Nutr.,* **29:** 87.

36. Duncan, I. W. and E. M. Scott. 1972. Lactose intolerance in Alaskan Indians and Eskimos. *Am. J. Clin. Nutr.,* **25:** 867.

37. Eastwood, M. and L. Mowbray. 1976. The binding of the components of mixed micelle to dietary fiber. *Am. J. Clin. Nutr.,* **29:** 1461.

38. Escovitz, G. H. and W. Rubin. 1973. The malabsorption syndrome. *Med. Clin. No. Am.,* **57:** 907.

39. Falchuk, Z. M. and W. Strober. 1974. Gluten-sensitive enteropathy: Synthesis of anti-gliadin antibody *in vitro. Gut,* **15:** 947.

40. Food and Nutrition Board-National Research Council. 1972. Background information on lactose and milk intolerance. *Nutr. Rev.,* **30:** 175.

41. Gallagher, C. R., A. L. Molleson, and J. H. Caldwell. 1974. Lactose intolerance and fermented dairy products. *J. Am. Dietet. Assoc.,* **65:** 418.

42. Gardner, F. H. 1962. Nutritional management of chronic diarrhea in adults. *J. Am. Med. Assoc.,* **180:** 147.

43. Garza, C. and N. S. Scrimshaw. 1976. Relationship of lactose intolerance to milk intolerance in young children. *Am. J. Clin. Nutr.,* **29:** 192.

44. Gerson, C. D. and N. Cohen. 1976. Folic acid absorption in regional enteritis. *Am. J. Clin. Nutr.,* **29:** 182.

45. Ghitis, J., K. Tripathy, and G. Mayoral. 1967. Malabsorption in the tropics. 2. Tropical sprue versus primary protein malnutrition: vitamin B_{12} and folic acid studies. *Am. J. Clin. Nutr.,* **20:** 1206.

46. Goldstein, F. 1972. Diet and colonic disease. *J. Am. Dietet. Assoc.,* **60:** 499.

47. Grand, R. J. and D. R. Homer. 1975. Approaches to inflammatory bowel disease in childhood and adolescence. *Ped. Clin. No. Am.,* **22:** 835.

48. Greif, M. B. and J. B. Longenecker. 1974. Determination of the sensitivity to oats in celiac patients. (Reported at American Dietetic Association Annual Meeting, Philadelphia.)

49. Hamilton, J. R. and L. K. McNeill. 1972. Childhood celiac disease: Response of treated patients to a small uniform daily dose of wheat gluten. *J. Ped.,* **81:** 885.

50. Handelsman, J. C. and R. H. Fishbein. 1976. Permanent ileostomy without external appliance: Kock internal reservoir (pouch) operation. *Johns Hopkins Med. J.,* **138:** 161.

51. Hardinge, M. G., A. C. Chambers, H. Crooks, and F. T. Stare. 1958. Nutritional studies of vegetarians. III. Dietary levels of fiber. *Am. J. Clin. Nutr.,* **6:** 523.

52. Hashim, S. A. 1967. Medium-chain triglycerides—Clinical and metabolic aspects. *J. Am. Dietet. Assoc.,* **51:** 221.

53. Hellendoorn, E. W. 1976. Beneficial physiologic action of beans. *J. Am. Dietet. Assoc.,* **69:** 249.

54. Hellendoorn, E. W. 1975. Enzymatic determination of the indigestible residue (dietary fibre) content of human food. *J. Sci. Food Agric.,* **26:** 1461.

55. Hill, G. L., W. S. J. Mair, J. P. Edwards, D. B. Morgan, and J. C. Goligher. 1975. Effect

of a chemically defined liquid elemental diet on composition and volume of ileal fistual drainage. *Gastroent.,* **68** (Part I): 676.

56. Hirschhorn, N. and K. M. Denny. 1975. Oral glucose-electrolyte therapy for diarrhea: A means to maintain or improve nutrition? *Am. J. Clin. Nutr.,* **28:** 189.

57. Hodgson, J. 1974. Diverticular disease. *Am. J. Gastroent.,* **62:** 116.

58. Holt, P. R., S. A. Hashim, and T. B. Van Itallie. 1965. Treatment of malabsorption syndrome and exudative enteropathy with synthetic medium chain triglycerides. *Am. J. Gastroent.,* **43:** 549.

59. Hosoi, K., W. C. Alvarez, and F. C. Mann. 1928. Intestinal absorption: Search for low residue diet. *A.M.A. Arch. Intern. Med.,* **41:** 112.

60. Howard, B. D. and E. H. Morse. 1973. Muffins and pastry made with medium-chain triglyceride oil. *J. Am. Dietet. Assoc.,* **62:** 51.

61. Howell, M. A. 1975. Diet as an etiological factor in the development of cancers of the colon and rectum. *J. Chron. Dis.,* **28:** 67.

62. Huang, S. and T. M. Bayless. 1968. Milk and lactose intolerance in healthy Orientals. *Science,* **160:** 83.

63. Ingelfinger, F. J. 1968. For want of an enzyme. *Nutr. Today,* **3** (No. 3): 2.

64. Jewell, D. P. and S. C. Truelove. 1972. Circulating antibodies to cow's milk proteins in ulcerative colitis. *Gut,* **13:** 796.

65. Johnson, C. F. 1965. Malabsorption syndromes. *Postgrad. Med.,* **37:** 667.

66. Johnson, J. J. and M. P. Penfield. 1976. A home-baked, yeast-leavened, low-protein bread. *J. Am. Dietet. Assoc.,* **69:** 653.

67. Jones, D. V. and M. C. Latham. 1974. Lactose intolerance in young children and their parents. *Am. J. Clin. Nutr.,* **27:** 547.

68. Jones, D. V., M. C. Latham, F. V. Kosikowski, and G. Woodward. 1976. Symptom response to lactose-reduced milk in lactose-intolerant adults. *Am. J. Clin. Nutr.,* **29:** 633.

69. Kahaner, N., H. Fuchs, and M. H. Floch. 1976. The effect of dietary fiber supplementation in man. I. Modification of eating habits. *Am. J. Clin. Nutr.,* **29:** 1437.

70. Katz, A. J., Z. M. Falchuk, W. Strober, and H. Schwachman. 1976. Gluten-sensitive enteropathy: Inhibition by cortisol of the effect of gluten protein *in vitro. N. Eng. J. Med.,* **295:** 131.

71. Katz, A. J. and Z. M. Falchuk. 1975. Current concepts in gluten sensitive enteropathy (celiac sprue). *Ped. Clin. No. Am.,* **22:** 767.

72. Kirsner, J. B. 1969. Clinical observations on malabsorption. *Med. Clin. No. Am.,* **53:** 1169.

73. Kirwan, W. O., A. N. Smith, A. A. McConnell, W. D. Mitchell, and M. A. Eastwood. 1974. Action of different bran preparations on colonic function. *Brit. Med. J.,* **4:** 187.

74. Klipstein, F. A. and J. J. Corcino. 1975. Malabsorption of essential amino acids in tropical sprue. *Gastroent.,* **68:** 239.

75. Kobayashi, A., S. Kawai, Y. Ohbe, and Y. Nagashima. 1975. Effects of dietary lactose and a lactase preparation on the intestinal absorption of calcium and magnesium in normal infants. *Am. J. Clin. Nutr.,* **28:** 681.

76. Kowlessar, O. D. 1972. Dietary gluten sensitivity updated. *J. Am. Dietet. Assoc.,* **60:** 475.

77. Kowlessar, O. D. and L. D. Phillips. 1970. Celiac disease. *Med. Clin. No. Am.,* **54:** 647.

78. Kretchmer, N. 1972. Lactose and lactase. *Sci. Am.,* **227** (Oct.): 71.

79. Kulp, K., F. N. Hepburn, and T. A. Lehmann. 1974. Preparation of bread without gluten. *Bakers Dig.,* **48** (June): 34.

80. Lebenthal, E. 1975. Small intestinal disaccharidase deficiencies. *Ped. Clin. No. Am.*, **20**: 757.

81. Leichter, J. 1972. Lactose tolerance in a slavic population. *Am. J. Dig. Dis.*, **17** (New Series): 73.

82. Leichter, J. 1971. Lactose tolerance in a Jewish population. *Am. J. Dig. Dis.*, **16** (New Series): 1123.

83. Leveille, G. A. 1975. The importance of dietary fiber in food. *Bakers Dig.*, **49** (Apr.): 34.

84. Lifshitz, F., A. P. Klotz, and G. H. Holman. 1965. Intestinal disaccharidase deficiencies in gluten-sensitive enteropathy. *Am. J. Dig. Dis.*, **10** (New Series): 47.

85. Lyford, C., J. Fischer, B. Buess, R. Rhodes, and J. B. Rhodes. 1975. Controlled clinical trial of bran in irritable bowel syndrome. *Clin. Res.*, **23**: 253A.

86. Mayer, J. 1966. Tropical malnutrition. 2. Sprue and kwashiorkor. *Postgrad. Med.*, **39** (No. 4): A-111.

87. Mayoral, L. G., K. Tripathy, F. T. García, S. Klahr, O. Bolãnos, and J. Ghitis. 1967. Malabsorption in the tropics: A second look. I. The role of protein malnutrition. *Am. J. Clin. Nutr.*, **20**: 866.

88. Melvin, K. E. W., G. W. Hepner, P. Bordier, G. Neale, and G. F. Joplin. 1970. Calcium metabolism and bone pathology in adult coeliac disease. *Qtr. J. Med.*, 39 (New Series, No. 153): 83.

89. Mendeloff, A. I., M. Monk, C. I. Siegel, and A. Lilienfeld. 1966. Some epidemiological features of ulcerative colitis and regional enteritis. *Gastroent.*, **51**: 748.

90. Menéndez-Corrada, R. and M. E. Belaval. 1968. Gluten antibodies and tropical sprue. *Am. J. Dig. Dis.*, **13** (New Series): 987.

91. McCrae, W. M., M. A. Eastwood, M. R. Martin, and W. Sircus. 1975. Neglected coeliac disease. *Lancet*, **1**: 187.

92. McGreer, R. H. 1967. A gluten-free wheat product made with cellulose gum. *J. Am. Dietet. Assoc.*, **51**: 534.

93. McMahon, A. W., P. Schmitt, J. F. Patterson, and E. Rothman. 1973. Personality differences between inflammatory bowel disease patients and their health siblings. *Psychosom. Med.*, **35** (No. 2): 91.

94. McNicholl, B., B. Egan-Mitchell, F. Stevens, R. Keane, S. Baker, C. F. McCarthy, and P. F. Fottrell. 1976. Mucosal recovery in treated childhood celiac disease (gluten-sensitive enteropathy). *J. Ped.*, **89**: 418.

95. Nandi, M. A. and E. S. Parham. 1972. Milk drinking by the lactose intolerant. *J. Am. Dietet. Assoc.*, **61**: 258.

96. National Dairy Council. 1971. Lactose intolerance. *Dairy Council Dig.*, **42** (No. 6): 31.

97. Nishita, K. D., R. L. Roberts, M. M. Bean, and B. M. Kennedy. 1976. Development of a yeast-leavened rice-bread formula. *Cer. Chem.*, **53**: 626.

98. Paige, D. M., T. M. Bayless, and W. S. Dellinger, Jr. 1975a. Relationship of milk consumption to blood glucose rise in lactose intolerant individuals. *Am. J. Clin. Nutr.*, **28**: 677.

99. Paige, D. M., T. M. Bayless, S. Huang, and R. Wexler. 1975b. Lactose hydrolyzed milk. *Am. J. Clin. Nutr.*, **28**: 818.

100. Paige, D. M., T. M. Bayless, and G. G. Graham. 1972a. Milk programs: Helpful or harmful to Negro children? *Am. J. Pub. Health*, **62**: 1486.

101. Paige, D. M., E. Leonardo, A. Cordano, J. Nakashima, B. Adrianzen T., and G. G. Graham. 1972b. Lactose intolerance in Peruvian children: effect of age and early nutrition. *Am. J. Clin. Nutr.*, **25**: 297.

102. Painter, N. S. 1974. The high fibre diet in the treatment of diverticular disease of the colon. *Postgrad. Med. J.,* **50:** 629.

103. Painter, N. S., A. Z. Almeida, and K. W. Colebourne. 1972. Unprocessed bran in treatment of diverticular disease of the colon. *Brit. Med. J.,* **2:** 137.

104. Painter, N. and D. Burkitt. 1975. Diverticular disease of the colon. In *Refined Carbohydrate Foods and Disease,* D. P. Burkitt and H. C. Trowell (Eds.). New York: Academic Press.

105. Payler, D. K. 1973. Food fibre and bowel behaviour. Letter. *Lancet,* **1:** 1394.

106. Payne-Bose, D., J. D. Welsh, H. L. Gearhart, and R. D. Morrison. 1977. Milk and lactose-hydrolyzed milk. *Am. J. Clin. Nutr.,* **30:** 695.

107. Phillips, S. F. 1975. Diarrhea. *Postgrad. Med.,* **57:** 65.

108. Plumley, P. F. and B. Francis. 1973. Dietary management of diverticular disease. *J. Am. Dietet. Assoc.,* **63:** 527.

109. Reilly, J., J. A. Ryan, W. Strole, and J. E. Fischer. 1976. Hyperalimentation in inflammatory bowel disease. *Am. J. Surg.,* **131:** 192.

110. Reinhold, J. G., B. Faradji, P. Abadi, and F. Ismail-Beigi. 1976. Decreased absorption of calcium, magnesium, zinc and phosphorus by humans due to increased fiber and phosphorus consumption as wheat bread. *J. Nutr.* **106:** 493.

111. Reinken, L., H. Zieglauer, and H. Berger. 1976. Vitamin B_6 nutriture of children with acute celiac disease, celiac disease in remission, and of children with normal duodenal mucosa. *Am. J. Clin. Nutr.,* **29:** 750.

112. Richmond, D. and P. W. Curreri. 1974. Nutritional management following massive small bowel resection. *Dietet. Currents* (Ross Laboratories), **1** (No. 4): 1.

113. Rickles, F. R., F. A. Klipstein, J. Tomasini, J. J. Corcino, and N. Maldonado. 1972. Long-term follow-up of antibiotic-treated tropical sprue. *Ann. Int. Med.,* **76:** 203.

114. Robertson, J. 1972. Change in the fiber content of the British diet. *Nature,* **238:** 290.

115. Rocchio, M. A., J. M. Cha, and K. F. Haas. 1974. Use of chemically defined diets in the management of patients with acute inflammatory bowel disease. *Am. J. Surg.,* **127:** 469.

116. Rocchio, M. A. and H. T. Randall. 1974. Nutrition in inflammatory disease of the bowel. *Intake: Perspectives in Clinical Nutrition* (Eaton Laboratories), No. 7.

117. Rubin, W. 1971. Celiac disease. *Am. J. Clin. Nutr.,* **24:** 91.

118. Ruffin, J. M., S. M. Kurtz, J. L. Borland, Jr., C. R. W. Bain, and W. M. Roufail. 1964. Gluten-free diet for nontropical sprue. *J. Am. Med. Assoc.,* **188:** 42.

119. Samloff, I. M., J. S. Davis, and E. A. Schenk. 1965. A clinical and histochemical study of celiac disease before and during a gluten-free diet. *Gastroent.,* **48:** 155.

120. Scala, J. 1974. Fiber. *Food Technol.,* **28** (No. 1): 34.

121. Schizas, A. A., J. A. Cremen, E. Larson, and R. O'Brien. 1967. Medium-chain triglycerides—Use in food preparation. *J. Am. Dietet. Assoc.,* **51:** 228.

122. Shapiro, J. L. 1974. Diverticular disease of the colon. *So. Med. J.,* **67:** 710.

123. Sherman, J. O., C. A. Hamly, and A. K. Khachadurian. 1975. Use of an oral elemental diet in infants with severe intractable diarrhea. *J. Ped.,* **86:** 518.

124. Smith, E. B. 1971. Gluten-free breads for patients with uremia. *J. Am. Dietet. Assoc.,* **59:** 572.

125. Solomons, N. W., I. H. Rosenberg, and H. H. Sandstead. 1976. Zinc nutrition in celiac sprue. *Am. J. Clin. Nutr.,* **29:** 371.

126. Sorensen, M. K. 1970. A yeast-leavened, low-protein, low-electrolyte bread. *J. Am. Dietet. Assoc.,* **56:** 521.

127. Sowers, M. F. and E. Winterfeldt. 1975. Lactose intolerance among Mexican Americans. *Am. J. Clin. Nutr.*, **28**: 704.

128. Stephenson, L. S. and M. C. Latham. 1974. Lactose intolerance and milk consumption: the relation of tolerance to symptoms. *Am. J. Clin. Nutr.*, **27**: 296.

129. Tandon, R., H. Mandell, H. M. Spiro, and W. R. Thayer, Jr. 1971. Lactose intolerance in Jewish patients with ulcerative colitis. *Am. J. Dig. Dis.*, **16** (New Series): 845.

130. Trowell, H. 1976. Definition of dietary fiber and hypotheses that it is a protective factor in certain diseases. *Am. J. Clin. Nutr.*, **29**: 417.

131. Trowell, H. C. 1972. Ischemic heart disease and dietary fiber. *Am. J. Clin. Nutr.*, **25**: 926.

132. Turner, S. J., T. Daly, J. A. Hourigan, A. G. Rand, and W. R. Thayer, Jr. 1976. Utilization of a low-lactose milk. *Am. J. Clin. Nutr.*, **29**: 739.

133. Van de Kamer, J. H., H. A. Weijers, and W. K. Dicke. 1953. Coeliac disease. 4. An investigation into the injurious constituents of wheat in connection with their action on patients with coeliac disease. *Acta Paediat.*, **42**: 223.

134. Van Soest, P. J. and J. B. Robertson. 1977. What is fibre and fibre in food? *Nutr. Rev.*, **35** (No. 3): 12.

135. Visakorpi, J. K., P. Kuitunen, and E. Savilahti. 1970. Frequency and nature of relapses in children suffering from the malabsorption syndrome with gluten intolerance. *Acta Paediat. Scand.*, **59**: 481.

136. Viteri, F. E., J. M. Flores, J. Alvarado, and M. Béhar. 1973. Intestinal malabsorption in malnourished children before and during recovery. *Am. J. Dig. Dis.*, **18**: 201.

137. Walker, A. R. P. 1976. Colon cancer and diet, with special reference to intakes of fat and fiber. *Am. J. Clin. Nutr.*, **29**: 1417.

138. Walker, A. R. P. 1975. Effect of high crude fiber intake on transit time and the absorption of nutrients in South African Negro schoolchildren. *Am. J. Clin. Nutr.*, **28**: 1161.

139. Walker, A. R. P. and D. P. Burkitt. 1976. Colonic cancer—hypotheses of causation, dietary prophylaxis, and future research. *Dig. Dis.*, **21**: 910.

140. Watt, B. K. and A. L. Merrill. 1963. *Composition of Foods*. U.S. Department of Agriculture.

141. Weijers, H. A. and J. H. Van de Kamer. 1965. Some considerations of celiac disease. *Am. J. Clin. Nutr.*, **17**: 51.

142. Weinstein, L., R. E. Olson, T. B. Van Itallie, E. Caso, D. Johnson, and F. J. Ingelfinger. 1961. Diet as related to gastrointestinal function. *J. Am. Med. Assoc.*, **176**: 935.

143. Welsh, J. D. 1970. Isolated lactase deficiency in humans: Report on 100 patients. *Medicine*, **49**: 257.

144. Wheby, M. S., V. L. Swanson, and T. M. Bayless. 1971. Comparison of ileal and jejunal biopsies in tropical sprue. *Am. J. Clin. Nutr.*, **24**: 117.

145. Wheelock, F. C., Jr. 1974. Surgical management of regional ileitis, ulcerative colitis, and granulomatous colitis. *Surg. Clin. No. Am.*, **54**: 675.

146. Wintrobe, M. M., G. W. Thorn, R. D. Adams, E. Braunwald, K. J. Isselbacher, and R. G. Petersdorf (Eds.). 1974. *Harrison's Principles of Internal Medicine*, 7th ed. New York: McGraw-Hill.

147. Woodruff, C. W. 1976. Milk intolerances. *Nutr. Rev.*, **34**: 33.

148. Wyman, J. B., K. W. Heaton, A. P. Manning, and A. C. B. Wicks. 1976. The effect on intestinal transit and the feces of raw and cooked bran in different doses. *Am. J. Clin. Nutr.*, **29**: 1474.

149. Young, W. F. and E. M. Pringle. 1971. 110 children with coeliac disease, 1950–1969. *Arch. Dis. Child.*, **46**: 421.

CLIENT REFERENCES

Gluten Sensitive Enteropathy

1. *Celiac Disease.* Recipes for Parents and Patients. 1968. Toronto, Canada: The Hospital for Sick Children.

2. French, A. B. *Low Gluten Diet with Tested Recipes.* Ann Arbor, Mich.: University Hospital.

3. Sheedy, C. B. and N. Keifetz. 1969. *Cooking for Your Celiac Child.* New York: Dial Press.

4. Wood, M. N. 1967. *Gourmet Food on a Wheat-Free Diet.* Springfield, Ill.: Charles C. Thomas.

High Fiber Diets

5. Ewald, E. B. 1973. *Recipes for a Small Planet.* New York: Ballantine Books.

6. Johnson, G. Whole foods for high-fiber cooking. American Digestive Disease Society, 7720 Wisconsin Avenue, Suite 217, Washington, D.C. 20014.

7. Kraus, B. 1975. *The Barbara Krause Guide to Fiber in Foods.* New York: New American Library.

STUDY GUIDE

Malabsorption is associated with a variety of causes or diseases.

1. List several abnormal conditions in which malabsorption usually occurs and explain the probable cause in each case.

2. Explain the usual clinical signs and symptoms that occur in patients with extensive malabsorption from any cause.

3. Describe and explain several tests that might demonstrate the presence of malabsorption syndrome in a patient.

The cause of gluten sensitive enteropathy (GSE) is not known but several hypotheses have been advanced to explain its pathogenesis.

4. Cite research findings that seem to support the "lack of enzyme" hypothesis to explain GSE and discuss their limitations.

5. Describe an immunologic hypothesis to explain the cause of GSE and discuss pros and cons for this hypothesis.

The intestinal mucosa undergoes extensive structural change in GSE, leading to abnormal function.

6. Explain relationships between abnormalities in intestinal mucosal structure and the classical clinical features of GSE.

7. Be able to recognize, from microphotographs, normal intestinal mucosa and mucosa typical of a patient with GSE.

Several tests may be used in the diagnosis of GSE.

8. For fat balance, D-xylose absorption, lactose tolerance test, and peroral biopsy, describe and explain expected results in a patient who will be diagnosed to have GSE.

A gluten-free diet is the primary treatment for GSE.

9. Explain why a gluten-free diet should be effective in treating GSE.

10. Recommend an approach to counseling a patient with newly diagnosed GSE and explain why this approach is likely to be effective.

11. Describe the usual time course for improvement of clinical and of histological signs after beginning dietary treatment for a patient with GSE.

12. Explain why the usual recommendation to GSE patients is for lifelong adherence to a gluten-free diet.

13. Adapt a gluten-free diet so that it will be satisfactory for a patient with GSE and secondary lactase deficiency.

Tropical sprue is a disease of uncertain etiology with symptoms similar to those of GSE.

14. Describe and explain a treatment program that is usually effective in treatment of tropical sprue.

Various disaccharidase deficiencies produce similar symptoms.

15. Outline and explain a probable mechanism for development of abdominal symptoms with any disaccharidase deficiency.

16. Distinguish between primary and secondary disaccharidase deficiency and give examples of each.

Although primary sucrase-isomaltase deficiency is relatively rare, a number of cases have been reported in the literature.

17. Give nutritional counseling to the mother of an infant with sucrase-isomaltase deficiency and explain the prognosis for this condition.

18. Describe and explain the results of a sucrose tolerance test in this case.

Lactose intolerance is widespread and particularly prevalent among some ethnic groups.

19. Describe the types of studies that have lead to the conclusion that lactose intolerance occurs predominantly among non-Caucasian peoples and discuss implications for feeding programs throughout the world.

20. Give instructions for diet, emphasizing particular precautions that should be followed, to patients with severe lactase deficiency; to those with mild lactose intolerance.

Two types of nonspecific inflammatory bowel disease are regional enteritis or Crohn's disease and ulcerative colitis.

21. Explain common clinical signs and symptoms of regional enteritis and of ulcerative colitis and discuss nutritional implications.

22. Give appropriate dietary and nutritional suggestions for patients with inflammatory bowel disease in both the mild active and inactive stages of the disease, explaining rationale for the suggestions.

23. Describe the general types of surgical procedures that may be used for patients with regional enteritis and with ulcerative colitis when medical treatment has been unsuccessful.

24. Give recommendations for nutritional management when a patient has undergone massive small bowel resection and explain the rationale behind the treatment.

Dietary factors have been implicated in the etiology and treatment of diverticular disease of the colon.

25. Describe and explain a hypothesis for development of diverticula in the colon involving intraluminal pressures and relate it to dietary fiber.

26. Justify the use of high-fiber diets in the treatment and possible prevention of diverticular disease of the colon.

Dietary fiber is of great physiologic interest but laboratory measurement is difficult.

27. Distinguish among dietary fiber, crude fiber, and neutral-detergent fiber in terms of components and measurement techniques.

28. From available data, estimate ranges of usual crude fiber intake for populations in the western world and in developing countries.

Several hypotheses link diet with incidence of colon cancer.

29. Describe four hypotheses that suggest a relationship between diet and cancer of the colon and discuss research evidence for each.

Chronic constipation is present when defecation is insufficiently frequent or stools are hard and dry.

30. Describe several causes of simple chronic constipation and suggest possible treatments, particularly dietary, in each case.

31. Estimate the total amount of crude fiber in a meal pattern that might be suggested for a patient with chronic colonic constipation.

Diarrhea is characterized by an increase in the frequency, volume, or fluidity of stools and may be acute or chronic.

32. Describe major physiological effects of diarrhea, list some common causes of acute diarrhea, and suggest appropriate general nutritional therapy.

33. Suggest appropriate nutritional care for patients with chronic functional diarrhea, such as the irritable bowel syndrome.

14

Pancreatitis and Gallbladder Disease

Pancreatitis often occurs in association with biliary tract disease. Secretion of pancreatic digestive juice and bile shares a common channel in the final stage of emptying into the duodenum. The potential for reflux of these juices into either the pancreatic or bile ducts is always present. Other factors undoubtedly contribute to the relationships that have been noted between pancreatitis and diseases of the biliary tract.

This chapter reviews normal pancreatic physiology and discusses pancreatitis. Gallbladder disease is also discussed, as well as dietary implications for both abnormalities.

14.1 Pancreatitis

Normal Pancreatic Physiology

The pancreas functions both as an endocrine and an exocrine gland. It is composed, therefore, of two major types of secreting tissue. (1) The cells of the acini secrete digestive enzymes, which combine with water and electrolytes secreted by the epithelial and centro-acinous cells of interspersed ducts before reaching the duodenum. (2) The islets of Langerhans, having no means for emptying their secretions externally, secrete insulin and glucagon directly into the blood stream. The pancreas secretes approximately 2000 ml of pancreatic juice daily through its system of ducts which culminate in the major duct of Wirsung. This duct then joins the common bile duct, forming the hepatopancreatic ampulla of Vater as it opens into the duodenum (Fig. 14.1). The sphincter of Oddi controls the opening.

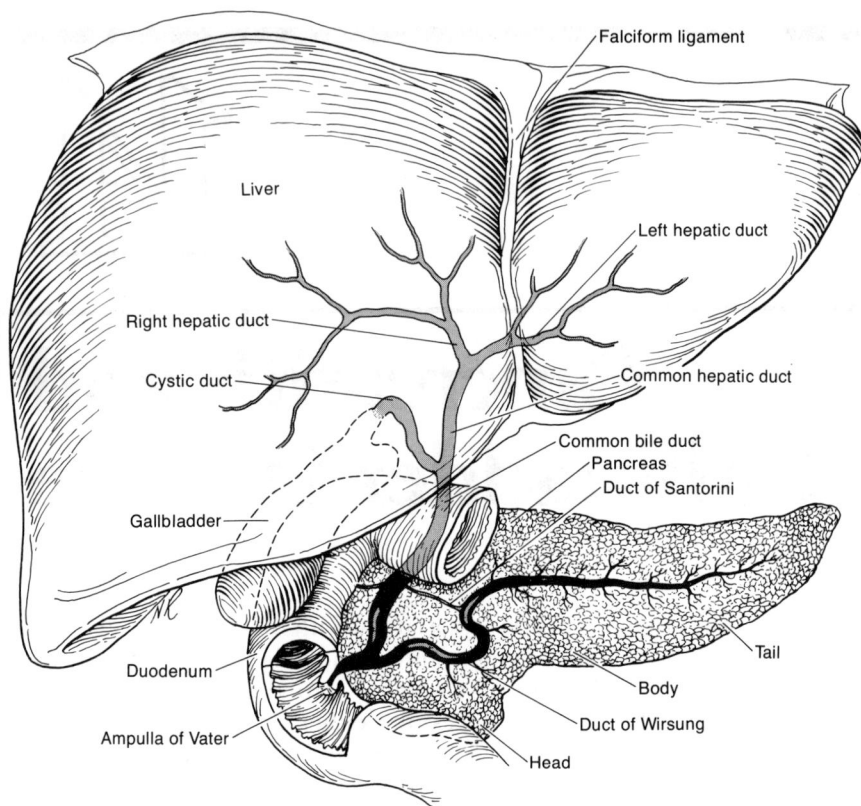

Fig. 14.1 The pancreas in relation to the liver, gallbladder, and duodenum. (From Gerard J. Tortora and Nicholas P. Anagnostakos, *Principles of Anatomy and Physiology*, 2d ed., New York: Harper & Row, 1978; by permission of the publisher.)

The exocrine secretions of the pancreas are under complex neurohumoral control. Parasympathetic impulses are transmitted along the vagus nerve to the pancreas during the cephalic and gastric phases of stomach digestion, stimulating primarily enzyme production. The enzymes are temporarily stored in the acini and released in greater quantity when the secretion of watery fluid is more strongly stimulated by the gastrointestinal (GI) hormone secretin (Guyton, 1971). Secretin is produced by intestinal mucosal cells in response to the delivery of acid from the stomach. The presence in the duodenum of amino acids and peptides as products of protein digestion is the primary stimulus for secretion of cholecystokinin-pancreozymin (CCK) by mucosal cells. The presence of fat also stimulates hormone secretion. These hormones reach the pancreas via the blood stream. Secretin causes pancreatic secretion of large quantities of fluid containing a high concentration of HCO_3^- (pH 7.5 to 8.5), while CCK stimulates enzyme secretion. Gastrin also has some stimulatory effect on pancreatic secretion.

At the cellular level, the control of pancreatic secretion probably involves receptor sites that release adenyl cyclase and activate intracellular cyclic AMP. There may be activation of an ATPase in the water and electrolyte secreting cells with the released energy being used for active extrusion from the cells of Na^+ as well as HCO_3^-. Control of enzyme secretion is exerted by change in the rate of synthesis and the rate at which the inactive enzyme (zymogen) granules are extruded from the cell. Apparently secretion of enzymes occurs first in response to stimulation of the cell, and when the cells are depleted of enzymes to a critical level, enzyme synthesis increases (Brooks, 1973).

The major portion of ingested food is digested by enzymes secreted by the pancreas; thus a pancreatic abnormality that substantially decreases its output of enzymes may have a marked effect on the digestive process. The proteolytic enzymes of the pancreas are the endopeptidases (trypsin, chymotrypsin, and elastase) that attack the peptide bonds on the inside of a protein or peptide molecule and the exopeptidases (carboxypeptidases A and B) that hydrolyze the terminal peptide bonds. Proteolytic enzymes are synthesized and secreted in their inactive forms as zymogens or proenzymes and are activated in the duodenum. The duodenal enzyme, enterokinase, activates trypsinogen. Trypsin in turn activates the other pancreatic enzymes. Enterokinase is localized at the brush border of the duodenal mucosa and is thought to be released by the action of bile salts. Since the proteolytic enzymes of pancreatic juice are powerful hydrolyzing agents, the pancreas must be protected from autodigestion. This normally occurs by (1) secretion of proteinases in an inactive form, (2) separating the zymogens from other cell proteins in granules that are surrounded by membranes, and (3) providing some enzyme inhibitors in pancreatic tissue. Substances that inhibit the action of trypsin have also been isolated from soybean, lima bean, and other species of beans and have been found to be polypeptides that form complexes with trypsin. They are inactivated by usual cooking procedures (Beck, 1973).

Lipase with the ability to attack the hydrophobic esters of long-chain fatty acids and glycerol is present in the pancreatic granules and is secreted in an active form. It requires a water-fat interface for its action, however, since it has both a hydrophylic and a hydrophobic part. Phospholipase A is secreted as an inactive proenzyme that is activated in the duodenum by the proteolytic enzymes and, after activation, catalyzes the conversion of lecithin to lysolecithin and fatty acid. Phospholipase A has been implicated in the production of acute pancreatitis, and it has been suggested that the transformation of lecithin to lysolecithin in the pancreas causes membrane damage leading to necrosis of pancreatic cells. Cholesterol esterase is also packaged by the pancreas in the secretory granules (Beck, 1973).

Pancreatic alpha-amylase is present in the secretory granules in an active form. It attacks the 1-4-alpha-junctions of the amylose and amylopectin fractions of starch, yielding maltose, maltotriose, and small branched alpha-dextrins. These compounds are hydrolyzed to glucose by maltase and isomaltase at the brush border of the mucosa. Other pancreatic enzymes include ribonuclease, deoxyribonuclease, and collagenase (Beck, 1973).

Etiology and Pathogenesis

Pancreatitis is a recurrent, continuous, and sometimes relentless disease involving inflammation of pancreatic tissue, edema, death of cells, and sometimes hemorrhage. Acute pancreatitis refers to an acute clinicopathologic entity which may or may not reoccur. The essential lesion is necrosis (death) of the acinous cells. Activated enzymes produced by these cells escape into the interstitial tissues with resulting edema, vascular engorgement and inflammation. With superimposed infection, abscesses can form in the pancreas. Resolution of the inflammatory process may occur with accompanying fibrosis and calcification of the pancreatic tissues, which may persist in more severe forms of the disease (Beeson and McDermott, 1975, p. 1245).

After two or three attacks of acute pancreatitis, the designation "relapsing pancreatitis" may be applicable. Each attack increases the destruction of pancreatic tissue. A common clinical form of chronic pancreatitis is chronic relapsing pancreatitis. The parenchyma of the organ, subjected to cycles of necrosis, edema, and calcification, are gradually and extensively replaced by fibrotic tissue with the disappearance of acinous and islet tissue. Since the disease process is frequently more severe in the head of the pancreas, and the islet cells are concentrated in the body and tail, disturbances in carbohydrate metabolism due to lack of insulin appear relatively late in the course of this disease (Beeson and McDermott, 1975, p. 1250). In many cases the acute disease does not progress to chronic pancreatitis and in some patients the characteristics of the chronic disease may be present at the time of the first attack.

A number of factors have been proposed to explain the etiology of pancreatitis, but three influences appear to account for 90 to 95 percent of all cases. These are (1) the presence of biliary tract disease, (2) alcoholism, and (3) idiopathic processes with exact etiology unknown. The association between pancreatitis and biliary tract or gallbladder disease has not been completely clarified, but mechanical factors have been suggested. It is possible that the ampulla of Vater is blocked by a gallstone, thus obstructing the secretion of pancreatic juice and bile through the common duct and allowing injury to the tissues of the pancreas from the released enzymes. Reflux into the pancreatic duct of unconjugated bile salts and lysolecithin, produced in the duodenum by the action of bacteria, is another possible mechanism to explain the association between gallbladder disease and acute pancreatitis.

A suggestion as to the mechanism for the effect of alcohol consumption in large quantities on the development of pancreatitis is that alcohol stimulates gastrin release, and excessive HCl secretion in the stomach, which causes increased secretin and CCK secretion and, thereby, augmented pancreatic juices. At the same time, a direct effect of ethanol may increase the resistance of the sphincter of Oddi, causing elevated intrapancreatic ductal pressure. It is also possible that bile may reflux into the pancreatic duct during vomiting and retching that often accompany excess alcohol consumption. Although proof is not available in humans, direct toxic effects of alcohol on the pancreas are suggested by animal studies. The pancreatitis associated with alcoholism is almost always of the chronic type. It has been suggested that obstruction of small ducts in the pancreas by proteinaceous material, that may be characteristic of some forms of chronic pancreatitis, may be related in some way to alcoholism. Protein malnutrition accompanies alcoholism in many cases and may have some influence on the development of pancreatitis. Even though the precise effects of alcoholism on pancreatitis have not been clarified, abstinence from alcohol seems to have a favorable effect on the natural history of the disease (Baum and Iber, 1973).

A number of miscellaneous causes of acute pancreatitis include hyperlipoproteinemias I and V, diabetic ketoacidosis, malnutrition, uremia, hypercalcemic states, infection, trauma, pancreatic cancer, and various drugs such as glucocorticoids, isoniazid, salicylates, and indomethacin (Beeson and McDermott, 1975, pp. 1244–1245; Howorth, 1973).

Clinical Features

Pain in the upper abdomen is the prime symptom in many cases of acute pancreatitis and is characterized as steady, severe, and gnawing. Other symptoms include nausea, vomiting, fever, tachycardia, abdominal distention, and leukocytosis. Levels of serum calcium, potassium, and sodium are lowered. Robertson et al. (1976) studied the pathogenesis of the hypocalcemia in nine patients with acute pancreatitis and concluded that relative parathyroid insufficiency may account for it. Another explanation is that calcium is sequestered in damaged fatty tissue surrounding the pancreas. Release of lipase causes hydrolysis of triglycerides in this tissue and the liberated fatty acids form calcium soaps.

Serum amylase is generally regarded as the single most important practical diagnostic test in acute pancreatitis. It will be elevated within 24 to 48 hours after onset of the disease, probably the result of transperitoneal absorption of the enzyme from the pancreas (Salt and Schenker, 1976). Serum lipase usually rises in parallel with amylase activity but amylase can be more easily and rapidly measured in the laboratory.

In the early stages of chronic pancreatitis the outstanding feature is recurrent attacks of severe abdominal pain. Later stages are characterized by metabolic disturbances, such as diabetes, steatorrhea, and azotorrhea, with concomitant weight loss. Between attacks the patient may be free of symptoms except for abdominal distention and fullness. With progression of the disease, intervals between attacks become shorter (Beeson and McDermott, 1975, p. 1250).

Dietary Treatment

The major nutritional consequence of pancreatic exocrine insufficiency is loss of fat and nitrogen in the stool. Starch digestion and assimilation is not as much affected because amylase is also produced in the duodenum and the salivary glands. Deficiency symptoms from lack of fat-soluble vitamins are rarely evident in patients with chronic pancreatitis, whereas they are often apparent in other cases of malabsorption syndrome. Fat-soluble vitamins are often well absorbed in spite of steatorrhea—probably because they depend more on bile salts for absorption than they do on pancreatic lipase—food intake is reasonably normal, and no mucosal defect interferes with absorption (Taubin and Spiro, 1973). A number of patients with pancreatic insufficiency show a defect in absorption of vitamin B_{12}, although only a small percentage of them have megaloblastic anemia. The defect is improved with administration of bicarbonate or pancreatic extract or both and involves binding of vitamin B_{12} in the intestinal lumen with unidentified nonintrinsic factor substances (Bernstein and Herbert, 1973).

Diabetes occurs in approximately 25 percent of all patients with chronic pancreatitis. This frequency increases to 75 percent when pancreatic calcification is present. However, diabetic ketoacidosis, microangiopathy, and nephropathy are rare in patients with pancreatitis. The diabetes is usually mild but in some cases may require insulin, particularly to prevent large losses of glucose in the urine and consequent weight loss. Oral hypoglycemic agents may be tried before insulin is given (Bank et al., 1975; Taubin and Spiro, 1973). Joffe et al. (1973) studied the fat tolerance of nine patients with chronic pancreatitis complicated by secondary diabetes. They found not only decreased absorption of dietary fat but also impaired removal of chylomicron triglyceride from the plasma as a consequence of the lack of insulin. Severe episodes of hypoglycemia may occur in patients with chronic pancreatitis who are taking insulin because of erratic absorption of energy nutrients. Restriction of dietary carbohydrate only adds to this problem and is not warranted in these diabetic patients. In pancreatectomy for carcinoma of the pancreas no endogenous insulin will be available and these patients require exogenous insulin (Taubin and Spiro, 1973).

Pancreatic enzymes are available for replacement of insufficient secretion. High concentrations must be given in order to be effective since lipase can be inactivated by either pepsin or HCl in the stomach and trypsin is inactivated to some degree when both pepsin and acid are present. Gastric aspiration studies showed that 60 percent of lipase activity and 40 percent of trypsin activity disappeared before the food materials left the stomach. This partial inactivation by gastric juice may explain the variable responses to the use of pancreatic extracts. Available enzyme preparations include (1) pancreatin, an alcoholic extract of porcine pancreas standardized for its ability to digest starch and casein *in vitro*, but without standardization of its lipase activity, and (2) pancrealipase, a lipase-enriched mixture of enzymes extracted from whole hog pancreas. Trade names for pancreatin include Ilozyme, Panteric, and Viokase, while a trade name for pancrealipase is

Cotazyme. There is controversy concerning the optimal frequency of administration for pancreatic enzymes (Taubin and Spiro, 1973).

Although pancreatic replacement therapy is the primary treatment for pancreatic steatorrhea, altering the dietary fat intake may bring additional benefits and allow normal weight maintenance for a patient with chronic pancreatitis. When the amount of protein or fat is increased in the diet, the same fraction is absorbed as before. Even though the total amount of fat or protein lost in the feces will increase when larger amounts are eaten, the amounts absorbed will also increase. Too much dietary fat, however, may not only increase diarrhea but also act as a strong stimulant to pancreatic secretion. Experimental pancreatitis is more damaging in animals fed a high-fat diet. There must be a balance between the desire to give more kilocalories to maintain body weight and the adverse effects of a high-fat diet. Taubin and Spiro (1973) suggested that the total caloric intake should generally be between 3000 and 6000 kcal, providing 100 to 150 g protein and 400 g or more of carbohydrate. Concomitant with pancreatic enzyme replacement, fat intake should begin with 50 g daily and gradually be increased to 200 g or until steatorrhea becomes clinically apparent.

Patients with acute and complicated pancreatitis may not be able to eat. In addition, stimulation of pancreatic secretion is undesirable when the pancreas is inflamed and edematous. Total parenteral feeding may be used for these patients in order to maintain a reasonably good nutritional status during the illness. Defined-formula diets containing amino acids, glucose or sucrose, and electrolytes have been used when seriously ill patients with pancreatitis can take something orally but cannot tolerate normal foods. Voitk et al. (1973) used such a diet for six patients with pancreatitis who could not tolerate conventional food and found that they responded well with complete recovery in all but one case. The defined-formula diet apparently did not stimulate the pancreas and healing occurred more readily. Positive nitrogen balance was maintained. With use of normal foods during the treatment of acute pancreatitis, it is appropriate to try small meals, as tolerated, that are low in fat, moderately high in protein, and as high in kilocalories as possible.

Medium-chain triglycerides (MCT) may be well tolerated by some patients with pancreatitis since they are hydrolyzed more readily by pancreatic lipase than are long-chain triglycerides (LCT). They may also be absorbed without hydrolysis. MCT do not delay gastric emptying, as do LCT, and may thus contribute to abdominal discomfort and diarrhea. Many patients do not find them palatable. Their role in long-term treatment of chronic pancreatitis needs further assessment (Taubin and Spiro, 1973).

In summary, dietary treatment of pancreatitis must be individualized with consideration for the stage and severity of the disease. In acute and complicated cases, total parenteral feeding or the use of defined-formula diets may be advantageous. For maintenance of an adequate nutritional state in patients with chronic pancreatitis, pancreatic enzyme replacement therapy should be used. In addition, the caloric level of the diet should be kept high enough to minimize weight loss by using a high-protein, high-carbohydrate diet with fat intake gradually adjusted from 50 g up toward 200 g, depending on the total caloric intake.

14.2 Gallbladder Disease

In nearly all cases, gallbladder disease is secondary to the development of gallstones (cholelithiasis). Since the presence of gallstones does not always produce symptoms, the exact prevalence of this disorder is not known. However, there is some indication that the frequency of gallstones in the general populations of the western world has increased in recent years (Holland and Heaton, 1972). Symptoms of gallbladder disease may occur with cholecystitis, which is an inflammation of the gallbladder in response to blockage of the cystic duct, usually with a gallstone. This does not commonly involve infection. Surgery has been the treatment of choice for gallstones that are producing symptoms of cholecystitis. However, there is controversy concerning the advisability of removing stones that are asymptomatic. With research on the processes involved in the development of gallstones and the ability to dissolve them by giving an orally administered bile acid, alternatives to surgery may become available.

Gallstone Formation

Gallstones have traditionally been classified into those containing cholesterol, those containing pigment, and mixed varieties. Chemical analysis, however, shows that stones vary in composition continuously over a wide spectrum. Pure pigment stones occur in the gallbladder in hemolytic states and cirrhosis of the liver. With few exceptions, however, gallstones contain cholesterol in amounts varying continuously from a few percent to 100 percent. In western countries, cholesterol is the predominant component, averaging 74 percent of the stone in the United States. Minor components include calcium carbonate, calcium palmitate, and calcium phosphate. Gallstones thus become chiefly a problem of cholesterol precipitation from bile (Heaton, 1975).

Liver cells secrete bile containing conjugated bile salts, various organic anions such as conjugated bilirubin, Na^+, K^+, phospholipids (mostly lecithin), and cholesterol dispersed in water. It is secreted continuously and flows from bile capillaries and ducts either directly into the duodenum or, during fasting periods, into a relaxed gallbladder, where it is stored. Within the gallbladder, the bile is modified by the active absorption of Na^+, Cl^-, and HCO_3^-, with water following passively. This results in an increase of solids from 3 to 11 percent and a reduction in pH from 7.6 to 6. The total volume of bile secreted averages 15 ml per kg per day. Secretion of CCK into the blood causes contraction of the gallbladder and relaxation of the sphincter of Oddi. Most of the bile salts entering the intestine are actively reabsorbed in the distal ileum, returned to the liver by the portal vein, and resecreted in bile. Primary bile acids, synthesized in the liver, are cholic acid and chenodeoxycholic acid. They are conjugated with either glycine or taurine and form bile salts with Na^+ or K^+. The secondary bile acids, deoxycholic acid and the relatively insoluble lithocholic acid, are formed in the colon by bacterial dehydroxylation of the cholic and chenodeoxycholic acids, respectively, that were not reabsorbed in the ileum. Deoxycholic acid is readily absorbed from the colon. Normal hepatic bile contains salts of cholic, chenodeoxycholic, deoxycholic, and lithocholic acids in concentration ratios of about $10:10:5:1$ (Wintrobe et al., 1974, pp. 1557–1558).

Cholesterol is virtually insoluble in water and is held in solution in the bile by bile acid and phospholipid, forming mixed micelles. It has been suggested that gallstones are likely to form when there is an increase in the cholesterol concentration of bile, either absolute or relative to bile acid and phospholipid. Under these conditions the bile becomes supersaturated with cholesterol, crystal precipitation occurs, and crystals aggregate to form stones of varying sizes (Ho, 1976). The reasons why bile may become supersaturated with cholesterol have not been clarified. Using radiolabeled bile acid, it was possible to show that men with gallstones had a total bile acid pool approximately half the size of control subjects. It was suggested that a reduction in the bile acid pool may be implicated in the production of a lithogenic (calculi forming) bile (Lukie and Dietschy, 1973).

Epidemiology of Gallstones

Gallstones are common in all western countries for which statistics are available. In the Framingham, Massachusetts survey, 8 percent of the population in the 30-to-62-year age group had symptoms of gallbladder disease, or after death were found to have autopsy evidence of it. In a large autopsy series done in Philadelphia and covering the period from 1920 to 1949, gallstones were found in 16.8 percent of women and 7.8 percent of men over age 20. Some groups of American Indians, particularly the Pima in Arizona, have been found to have a very high incidence of gallstones (Heaton, 1975). Bernstein et al. (1973) reported an overall occurrence rate for gallbladder disease of 15.7 percent in a group of 62,739 weight-conscious women. For each decade of life there was a statistically significant increase in the degree of obesity for women with a history of gallbladder disease as compared with women having no history of the disease. Women with a history of the disease also had more live births than women without the disease for every decade of life studied. Thus, obesity and parity were both found to be important risk factors in the development of gallbladder disease. The disease is more prevalent in women than men. Gallbladder disease is generally considered, from clinical evidence, to increase with age. However, a study by Bainton et al. (1976) of prevalence in a South Wales industrial town, using a weighted sample in order to insure adequate numbers of subjects in all age and sex categories, showed no marked increase in prevalence of gallstones with age in either sex. The overall prevalence rates were 6.2 percent for men 45 to 69 years of age and 12.1 percent for women of the same ages. Symptoms of dyspepsia said to be suggestive of gallstones were found with approximately equal frequency in those with and without gallbladder disease as determined by cholecystography for gallstones.

Gallstones have apparently become more common in western civilization since the beginning of the twentieth century. They are also being found in younger segments of the population than previously. A survey in Canada has revealed that 26 percent of cholecystectomy patients are under 35 years of age (Plant et al., 1973). In developing countries, urbanization and westernization are followed by an increase in incidence of gallstones (Heaton, 1975).

Diet and Gallstone Formation

Diet has been suggested as having an exogenous influence on bile metabolism and gallstone formation. However, clearcut influences have not been documented. A survey in an Appalachian community with an abnormally high incidence of gallbladder disease (age adjusted prevalence rate of 16.7 percent) suggested a relationship between gallstones and socioeconomic factors. It was postulated that diet might help to explain this relationship since most families in the eastern Kentucky and rural Appalachian area had excessive intakes of fats, meat, and cholesterol (Richardson et al., 1973). In certain species, particularly the prairie dog which has a bile composition similar to human bile, the feeding of cholesterol has been shown to increase the degree of supersaturation of cholesterol in gallbladder bile, resulting in cholesterol crystals and gallstones (Ho, 1976). A relationship between gallstones and serum cholesterol was not found in the Framingham study. Neither was a definite correlation found between serum cholesterol levels and the presence of gallstones in a series of 245 patients, aged 60 to 100 years, for which determinations of serum cholesterol as well as autopsy data were available (Hove and Geill, 1968).

From a review of autopsy records for subjects in an atherosclerosis prevention trial, Sturdevant et al. (1973) reported that men who ate an experimental diet (low-cholesterol, low-saturated fat, high-polyunsaturated fat, high-plant sterol) were more likely to have gallstones than were those who ate a standard American diet. It has been suggested that polyunsaturated fatty acids may increase the excretion of cholesterol into bile as serum levels are decreased. This may change the balance of cholesterol and bile salts and contribute to gallstone formation. The gallstone threat in the atherosclerosis prevention trial would seem less serious than the threat of coronary heart disease in highly susceptible persons. Other findings that suggest a relationship between the oversecretion of cholesterol by the liver into the bile and production of a supersaturated bile include: (1) the increased cholesterol output in bile of women with gallstones and supersaturated bile, as compared with control subjects, when directly measured over a 24-hour period, although the test subjects were all obese and the controls nonobese; (2) the increased flux of cholesterol into bile, with a resulting supersaturated bile, when the hypolipidemic drug clofibrate is given; and (3) the frequent dissolution of gallstones and undersaturation of bile with cholesterol when the bile acid chenodeoxycholic acid is fed on a regular basis (Heaton, 1975). The use of chenodeoxycholic acid to dissolve gallstones is being tested in a national cooperative gallstone study (Anonymous, 1976).

Dietary fiber may influence the secretion of cholesterol in bile by influencing the proportion in the bile of the bile salts, chenodeoxycholate and deoxycholate. Feeding chenodeoxycholate reduces cholesterol secretion and thus makes bile undersaturated while feeding deoxycholate makes the bile more saturated with cholesterol. Feeding of deoxycholate apparently causes displacement of chenodeoxycholate in the bile. Feeding bran to human subjects caused a decrease of deoxycholate in bile, possibly because of the binding of deoxycholate by fiber and reduction of its absorption in the intestinal tract (Heaton, 1975). In 1961 and 1971, Plant et al. (1973) compared incidence of gallbladder disease and gross dietary intakes for the populations of three communities with over 200,000 people in each— Windsor, Ontario, Canada: Luton, Bedfordshire, England; and Rennes, Brittany, France. Incidence of gallbladder disease doubled in the 10-year period and was six times higher in North America than in Western Europe. Prepared or processed foods seemed to be consumed more in Canada, to a lesser extent in England, and hardly at all in rural France. In addition, the authors suggested that the relative preponderance of thin people with gallbladder disease, in North America particularly, made it unlikely that diet alone could be the cause of the increased incidence. Many questions are raised by the studies that associate a refined diet with gallbladder disease. What is it about refined or processed foods that affects the disease process? Is it lack of fiber, large amounts of accompanying cholesterol and fat, or might certain chemical additives in the processed foods alter the enterohepatic circulation of bile salts or the hepatocytes themselves? Further studies are necessary before definite conclusions can be drawn as to the relationships between diet and gallstone formation.

Cholecystitis

Acute cholecystitis is a sterile inflammatory response of the gallbladder wall to blockage of the cystic duct, aided by lymphatic and venous obstruction. A gallstone is usually involved in the blockage but occasionally it may be due to other causes, such as stricture or pressure. Bacterial infection may occur secondary to the obstruction. Symptoms usually include severe right-upper-quadrant pain, nausea, vomiting, fever, and minimal jaundice. Low-grade hyperbilirubinemia and increased serum alkaline phosphatase activity are often associated findings. A radiologic procedure for diagnosis may involve the administration of a contrast material given orally. The drug is absorbed, excreted in the bile, and concentrated in the gallbladder, allowing visualization with x-ray (cholecystography). To visualize bile ducts, a contrast material may be given intravenously before x-ray (cholangio-

Table 14.1 FOODS HIGH IN FAT CONTENT THAT SHOULD BE LIMITED OR DISALLOWED ON A LOW-FAT DIET

Food Group	Foods High in Fat Content
Meat, fish, poultry	Fatty meats Products containing unremovable visible fat, as bacon, sausage, spareribs, frankfurters, luncheon meats, duck, or goose Fried meat, fish, or poultry
Milk and milk products	Whole milk Most cheeses Cream Ice cream
Bread and cereal products	Sweetrolls and quickbreads Cakes, cookies, pastry Many flour-based snack foods, especially if fried
Vegetables	Potato chips Fried potatoes and other fried vegetables
Fruits	Avocados Olives
Fats	Butter and margarine Oil and shortening Mayonnaise and salad dressings
Desserts	Those containing chocolate, nuts, cream, or other fats Doughnuts, cakes, cookies, pastries Ice cream
Sweets	Candies made with cream, chocolate, or other fats
Miscellaneous	Cream soups or chowders, unless made with skim milk or allowed whole milk Peanut butter Buttered popcorn Fried foods

graphy) (Beeson and McDermott, 1975, p. 1311; Wintrobe et al., 1974, pp. 1520 and 1563).

In 75 percent of patients, symptoms of acute cholecystitis usually disappear after 1 to 4 days with conservative management. The other 25 percent usually require immediate surgical intervention. Treatment in any case is typically cholecystectomy, but this may be done either within the first 48 hours or several weeks later after the symptoms have regressed and the patient can be prepared for surgery. Preparation for surgery in the acute case may need to include parenteral vitamin K to correct a deficiency that may occur with only a few days inadequate absorption of this nutrient in a marginally-nourished individual. An obese patient should be encouraged to lose weight before elective surgery since obesity increases the surgical risk. Repeated attacks of mild to severe acute cholecystitis merit the clinical diagnosis of chronic cholecystitis. In the chronic disease, the gallbladder mucosa and smooth muscle are partly replaced by fibrous tissue and the ability to concentrate bile is impaired. A few patients may have vague abdominal discomfort and dyspeptic symptoms thought to be due to chronic cholecystitis, but find that the symptoms do not improve after surgical removal of the gallbladder (Wintrobe et al., 1974, pp. 1563–1565).

Patients hospitalized with acute cholecystitis have often been vomiting and unable to eat before admission. This causes dehydration that can be corrected by intravenous fluids. Nasogastric suction may also be used for the acutely ill patient. In chronic cholecystitis a low-fat diet containing 40 to 60 g fat daily may give some symptomatic relief but has no effect on the course of the disease. Since the presence of fat in the duodenum stimulates the production of CCK which causes contraction of the gallbladder, high-fat diets theoretically increase discomfort. However, protein and peptides in the duodenum also affect CCK production and discomfort may result from taking almost any type of food. It has been reported that similar foods are incriminated by patients for any disease of the GI tract that causes dyspepsia. Foods high in fat content that need to be limited or disallowed on a low-fat diet are listed in Table 14.1. A typical pattern and menu for a diet containing approximately 50 g fat daily is given in Table 14.2.

Table 14.2 DIET PATTERN AND MENU FOR A LOW-FAT DIET (50 G)*

Diet Pattern		Approximate Amount of Fat (g)	Menu
Breakfast			
Fruit or fruit juice	2 servings		Grapefruit juice
Bread or cereal product	2 servings		Cracked wheat cereal
			Rye toast
Fat	1 serving	5	Margarine
Milk, 2% fat	1 cup	5	Milk, 2% fat
Coffee with sugar			Coffee with sugar
Lunch			
Lean meat, fish, poultry	2 oz	6	Chef's salad with turkey and chipped beef
Fat	2 servings	10	French dressing
Vegetable	1 serving		Carrot and celery sticks
Bread product	2 servings		Soda crackers
Fruit or fat-free dessert	1 serving		Canned apricots
Dinner			
Lean meat, fish, poultry	3 oz	9	Roast leg of veal
Potato or substitute	1 serving		Baked potato
Vegetables	1–2 servings		Boiled broccoli
Bread product	2 servings		Whole wheat bread
Fat	2 servings	10	Margarine
Fruit or fat-free dessert	1 serving		Whipped cherry gelatin with bananas
Milk, 2% fat	1 cup	5	Milk, 2% fat
Total fat		50	

* Approximately 1500 kcal.

Fat digestion appears to be unimpaired following cholecystectomy. The liver continues to produce bile but does not store it. After a fatty meal, a high initial intraluminal bile salt concentration does not appear because the meal cannot stimulate the release of stored bile. However, Simmons and Bouchier (1972) reported that lipolysis and micellar lipid concentrations were normal in 10 postcholecystectomy patients following a test meal. Bile salt concentrations in the intestine were slightly reduced in comparison to control subjects but concentrations were sufficient to insure effective lipolysis. Patients who have undergone cholecystectomy should be able to follow a diet of normal composition soon after surgery without encountering digestive difficulties.

REFERENCES

1. Anonymous. 1976. National study focuses on gallstone-dissolving drug. *Med. World News,* July 26, p. 32.

2. Bainton, D., G. T. Davies, K. T. Evans, and I. H. Gravelle. 1976. Gallbladder disease. *N. Eng. J. Med.,* **294:** 1147.

3. Bank, S., I. N. Marks, and A. I. Vinik. 1975. Clinical and hormonal aspects of pancreatic diabetes. *Am. J. Gastroent.,* **64:** 13.

4. Baum, R. and F. L. Iber. 1973. Alcohol, the pancreas, pancreatic inflammation, and pancreatic insufficiency. *Am. J. Clin. Nutr.,* **26:** 347.

5. Beck, I. T. 1973. The role of pancreatic enzymes in digestion. *Am. J. Clin. Nutr.,* **26:** 311.

6. Beeson, P. B. and W. McDermott. (Eds.) 1975. *Textbook of Medicine,* vol. II, 14th ed. Philadelphia: Saunders.

7. Bernstein, L. and V. Herbert. 1973. The role of pancreatic exocrine secretions in the absorption of vitamin B_{12} and iron. *Am. J. Clin. Nutr.,* **26:** 340.

8. Bernstein, R. A., L. H. Werner, and A. A. Rimm. 1973. Relationship of gallbladder disease to parity, obesity, and age. *Health Ser. Rep.,* **88:** 925.

9. Brooks, F. P. 1973. The neurohumoral control of pancreatic exocrine secretion. *Am. J. Clin. Nutr.,* **26:** 291.

10. Guyton, A. C. 1971. *Textbook of Medical Physiology.* Philadelphia: Saunders.

11. Heaton, K. 1975. Gallstones and cholecystitis. In *Refined Carbohydrate Foods and Disease,* D. P. Burkitt and H. C. Trowell (Eds.). New York: Academic Press.

12. Ho, K. 1976. Comparative studies on the effect of cholesterol feeding on biliary composition. *Am. J. Clin. Nutr.,* **29:** 698.

13. Holland, C. and K. W. Heaton. 1972. Increasing frequency of gall bladder operations in the Bristol clinical area. *Br. Med. J.,* **3:** 672.

14. Hove, E. and T. Geill. 1968. Serum cholesterol and incidence of gallstones. *Geriatrics,* **23** (Jan.): 114.

15. Howorth, M. B., Jr. 1973. Pancreatitis and hyperlipoproteinemia. *So. Med. J.,* **66:** 1260.

16. Joffe, B. I., L. Krut, D. Mendelson, and H. C. Seftel. 1973. Oral fat tolerance studies in chronic pancreatitis. *Am. J. Gastroent.,* **59:** 522.

17. Lukie, B. E. and J. M. Dietschy. 1973. Cholesterol gallstone formation: recent advances in pathophysiology. *Texas Med.,* **69:** 90.

18. Plant, J. C. D., I. Percy, T. Bates, J. Gastard, and Y. Hita de Nercy. 1973. Incidence of gallbladder disease in Canada, England, and France. *Lancet,* **2:** 249.

19. Richardson, J. D., F. D. Scutchfield, W. H. Proudfoot, and A. S. Benenson. 1973. Epidemiology of gallbladder disease in an Appalachian community. *Health Ser. Rep.*, **88:** 241.

20. Robertson, G. M., E. W. Moore, D. M. Switz, G. W. Sizemore, and H. L. Estep. 1976. Inadequate parathyroid response in acute pancreatitis. *N. Eng. J. Med.*, **294:** 512.

21. Salt, W. B., II and S. Schenker. 1976. Amylase—its clinical significance—a review of the literature. *Medicine,* **55:** 269.

22. Simmons, F. and I. A. D. Bouchier. 1972. Intraluminal bile salt concentrations and fat digestion after cholecystectomy. *S. Afr. Med. J.,* **46:** 2089.

23. Sturdevant, R. A. L., M. L. Pearce, and S. Dayton. 1973. Increased prevalence of cholelithiasis in men ingesting a serum cholesterol-lowering diet. *N. Eng. J. Med.*, **288:** 24.

24. Taubin, H. L. and H. M. Spiro. 1973. Nutritional aspects of chronic pancreatitis. *Am. J. Clin. Nutr.,* **26:** 367.

25. Voitk, A., R. A. Brown, V. Echave, A. H. McArdle, F. N. Gurd, and A. G. Thompson. 1973. Use of an elemental diet in the treatment of complicated pancreatitis. *Am. J. Surg.,* **125:** 223.

26. Wintrobe, M. M., G. W. Thorn, R. D. Adams, E. Braunwald, K. J. Isselbacher, and R. G. Petersdorf (Eds.). 1974. *Harrison's Principles of Internal Medicine,* 7th ed. New York: McGraw-Hill.

STUDY GUIDE

A knowledge of normal pancreatic physiology is essential to an understanding of pathological changes in pancreatitis.

1. Describe the endocrine and exocrine structure and function of the pancreas and indicate how this is changed by pancreatitis.

2. Outline the mechanisms whereby exocrine pancreatic secretions are stimulated and list the major components of the pancreatic juice.

3. Describe the usual clinical features of acute and chronic pancreatitis and explain why steatorrhea, azotorrhea, and diabetes may be features of chronic pancreatitis.

4. Explain possible relationships between pancreatitis and biliary tract disease; between pancreatitis and alcoholism.

Dietary treatment of pancreatitis is aimed at sparing the damaged pancreas while nourishing the patient adequately.

5. Suggest appropriate dietary treatment for patients with acute and with chronic pancreatitis and explain the rationale for the recommendations.

6. Justify the use of pancreatic enzyme replacement therapy for patients with pancreatitis and describe the types of products available.

7. Discuss possible advantages for use of a defined-formula diet in treatment of pancreatitis and explain its effectiveness.

8. What nutritional considerations should be given to secondary diabetes that is present in a patient with chronic pancreatitis and why?

Bile plays an essential role in the digestion-absorption of fats from the small intestine.

9. List the major components of bile, describe the enterohepatic cycle of bile salts, and explain the role of bile in normal digestion-absorption.

Gallstone formation in the gallbladder appears to be related to the state of supersaturation of cholesterol in bile.

10. Discuss the present state of knowledge that relates dietary factors to the development of gallstones.

Obstruction of bile flow by gallstones may produce inflammation and pain.

11. Explain symptoms and signs that usually accompany acute cholecystitis.

12. Give appropriate suggestions for the nutritional care and instruction of a patient hospitalized for an acute attack of cholecystitis, during and after hospitalization, when the patient is released without surgery.

13. Give useful dietary suggestions for a patient following cholecystectomy and explain the rationale behind these recommendations.

14. Write diet patterns and representative menus for diets limited to 40, 50, or 60 g fat daily.

15

Food Allergies

Individuals may experience abnormal reactions to the food they eat, the air they breathe, or the substances they touch. Not only may foreign substances produce hypersensitivity, but sensitization to autologous substances (autosensitization) may also develop. The term *allergy* was coined in the early 1900s to mean altered reactivity of the body to a foreign substance, called an antigen, on second exposure to it. Increased study of the allergic reaction, along with widespread use of the term allergy, has led to a preference among scientists for use of the term *hypersensitivity* to refer to true allergies in which a definite immunological reaction is involved.

15.1   Allergic Reactions

In investigations conducted around the beginning of the twentieth century, it was observed that injection of the antitoxins to diphtheria and other agents induced not protection but injury in some individuals. Since "phylaxis" means protection from harm, this phenomenon was called anaphylaxis or loss of protection. The reaction was later shown to be caused by a "transferable" substance in the blood. Experimental anaphylaxis has been used with laboratory animals in studying hypersensitivity and immunity. Anaphylactic shock is an overwhelming reaction of the body that may sometimes be experienced by an allergic patient. In 1921 it was shown that the skin of a normal recipient of blood serum from a sensitized donor reacted immediately on contact with the sensitizing antigen. This demonstration led to additional studies of the antibody involvement in allergy and indirectly prompted the use of skin tests in clinical allergy diagnosis (National Institute of Allergy and Infectious Diseases, 1972).

The immune system in human beings is composed of cooperating cellular and humoral components. Each plays its own role in protecting the integrity and safety of the body from invasive substances. The humoral immune system in the human is composed of five known blood serum immunoglobulins (Ig): IgG, IgM, IgA, IgD, and IgE. IgE is present in the serum in the smallest amount but has been shown to be very potent and required for an allergic reaction. The reaction, however, is also influenced by several other factors, including (1) the total number of mast cells (connective tissue cells that may elaborate granules containing histamine) and basophils (histamine-containing leukocytes) throughout the body, as well as the number in a given region; (2) the number of IgE-binding sites per basophil and mast cell; (3) the amount of histamine in each cell; (4) the processing of the allergen (antigen) in the body, which may be affected by the permeability of the skin and mucous membranes, the amount and types of enzymes able to process the antigens, the number and types of carrier proteins that turn haptens (incomplete antigens) into active antigens, and the tissue reactivity to various mediators such as histamine, bradykinin, serotonin, and SRS-A (slow-reacting substance of anaphylaxis) (Hamburger, 1976).

It is thought that the following events occur in an allergic reaction. (1) Specific antibodies of the IgE class are formed as a result of exposure to an antigen. These protein antibodies contain two combining sites on one end for binding with the antigen and a unique arrangement of amino acids at the other end of the molecule for binding to the surface membrane of tissue mast cells and blood basophils. (2) The antigen again enters the body and binds to its specific antibody which has attached itself to an IgE-binding site on a mast cell in tissues of the body or on a basophil in the blood. (3) Binding of the antigen triggers the release of histamine from the mast cell or basophil. (4) The histamine produces changes in blood vessels and nerve endings that result in blood vessel engorgement (flare) and edema (wheal). The allergic responses may be hives in the skin, sneezing in the nose, or spasms of the bronchioles in the lungs causing asthma. In the blood vessels, if the reaction is generalized, a massive dilatation can cause a precipitous fall in blood pressure, leading to shock. This entire process occurs within a few seconds to a few minutes after the antigen-antibody reaction (Hamburger, 1976). Three requisites for an allergic reaction would appear to be: (1) a susceptible or sensitized individual; (2) the presence of an allergen or sensitizing substance; and (3) an effector or shock organ.

Many antigens are proteins. Some low-molecular weight, nonprotein substances have also been involved in allergic reactions. It has been suggested that these comparatively small molecules, such as many color and flavor additives to food, may act as haptens by combining with body proteins to become complete antigens (Feingold, 1968; Lockey, 1971). It has also been suggested that an individual may be allergic to insoluble substances such as corn or wheat starch. Skin testing cannot be used to evaluate allergy to insoluble substances because an extract cannot be made to use in testing (Lietze, 1969).

Many years ago it was observed that allergy tended to be familial. Because of the complex nature of the problem, the mode of inheritance has not been determined. Not one but many of the variables involved in an antigen-antibody reaction are probably under some degree of genetic control. In addition, specific criteria for defining allergy are not uniformly applied (Hamburger, 1976).

15.2 Environmental and Food Effects on Allergy Development

The actual frequency of food allergy in early life depends on whether one demands all the criteria that are necessary to make the diagnosis sure from a scientific point of view or whether one assumes its existence on a clinical basis. The practicing physician is primarily concerned with clinical experience and often bases his or her diagnosis on criteria that are difficult to reproduce and may not withstand the exacting scrutiny needed to convert them to scientific facts (Blumstein and Richardson, 1964). According to Gerrard (1974) there are some reactions in young patients that the clinician feels may be allergic but, as he is not always certain of the allergen or even the mechanism of the response, is unable to prove his point. It is for this reason that the field of clinical allergy is not always clearcut and the incidence of true allergy not definitely known.

The question of environmental influence, including food intake, on the development of allergy in humans is controversial with some data suggesting a marked influence and other data suggesting none. Glaser and Johnstone (1953) reported that only 15 percent of children coming from allergic families and fed soy milk from birth to 6 months of age developed allergic diseases within 6 years, whereas 65 percent of sibling controls and 52 percent of nonrelated controls fed cow's milk developed allergic illnesses. The control groups were retrospectively selected, however, and proper precautions were not taken to prevent bias. Johnstone and Dutton (1966) then completed a prospective study in which 235 children chosen from allergic families were followed to 10 years of age and reported that allergy occurred in 18 percent of the group fed soy milk and in 50 percent of the controls fed cow's milk.

Brown et al. (1969) studied 427 children from a general pediatric practice for 12 to 27 months. Soy and cow's milk were used without regard to family history of allergy. Allergic reactions developed in 10.6 percent of the children given soy milk and 13.3 percent of those given cow's milk. Halpern et al. (1973) followed, for varying periods of time up to 7 years, 1753 infants fed breast, soy, or cow's milk from birth to 6 months of age.

There were 45.8 percent with an immediate family history of allergy, 15.6 percent with a remote history, and 38.6 percent with a negative history. Allergy occurred in 12.4 percent of the total group with a similar incidence in the three milk groups. The cow's-milk group showed allergy earlier than did the breast-milk group (12.6 versus 18.5 months). Allergy to soy milk occurred in 0.5 percent of the patients and to cow's milk in 1.8 percent. Feeding egg yolk before 3 weeks or after 6 months of age did not affect the development of allergy. These workers concluded that feeding breast or soy milk in place of cow's milk formulas from birth to 6 months did not affect the development of childhood allergy.

Environmental modifications in a study by Hamburger (1976) include exclusive breast feeding; delay of diphtheria, pertussis, and tetanus immunization; hypoallergenic food and clothing; and dust, contactant, and inhalant restraints. Preliminary data suggest that the expression of allergic symptoms in infants is influenced by the environment, although serum IgE levels are unaffected. Elevated serum IgE levels in humans appear to be associated with allergic diseases in those with the genetic predisposition to maintain such elevated levels of serum IgE.

15.3   Testing for Allergy

The history is of great value in diagnosing food allergy. Many patients, especially children, will experience fairly clearcut reactions to foods, and the patient or his parents can often make an association between certain symptoms and food ingestion. The reactions that are generally labeled as allergic include asthma, hay fever or rhinitis, hives, and some types of eczema. A wide range of other symptoms sometimes may be considered to have an allergic origin and include abdominal pain, headache, fatigue, and diarrhea (Grogan, 1969).

Skin testing is used in an attempt to identify specific allergens. Crude aqueous extracts of foods, pollen, dust, animal dander, insects, and other substances, commercially available in varying concentrations, are applied to a skin scratch or given by intradermal injection. Positive reactions appear within 15 to 20 minutes and are characterized by wheal and erythema formation and local pruritus (Wintrobe et al., 1974, p. 370). Since many false positive reactions occur, skin tests alone cannot produce a positive diagnosis of food allergy. It is usually preferable to diagnose food allergies by use of histories and possible elimination diets. The number and type of skin tests performed should be guided by the patient's history. The testing results may be of some assistance to the clinician when using an elimination diet or when adding suspected foods back to the diet (Grogan, 1969).

Diet testing in a patient suspected of having food allergy may take several forms. A simple elimination diet removes only one or two foods that are suspected of causing allergy. Egg, milk products, and cereal grains are some of the most common food allergens although they are difficult to avoid because they are present in various forms in many prepared foods. Food labels must be carefully read in order to eliminate these substances from the diet. Extra precaution should be taken to eliminate all the related foods when a specific food group is in question (Grogan, 1969).

A number of extensive elimination test diets and recipes have been described by Rowe (1972). Many of these are limited to a few hypoallergic foods that must be followed rigidly. If improvement of symptoms is observed on a major elimination diet, single food-family groups can be added slowly after periods of about 10 days. If symptoms reoccur after the addition of a single food, it is probable that this food is a cause of the allergic reaction and must be eliminated from the diet. If no improvement of allergic symptoms is observed after the use of elimination diets, it is probable that the allergy is not of food origin. The foods included in elimination test diets are those considered least likely to produce allergic reactions. Grogan (1969) suggested the following as a useful hypoallergic test diet: a milk substitute; rice cereal; apples and pears; carrots and sweet potatoes; lamb.

The foods to be used on Rowe's (1972) cereal-free elimination diet are:

Tapioca (pearl or minute)	Apricots
White potatoes	Grapefruit
Sweet potatoes or yams	Lemon
Soybean potato bread	Peaches
Lima bean potato bread	Pineapples
Soy milk (Mull-Soy) (free of corn glucose)	Prunes
	Pears
Lamb	Cane or beet sugar
Chicken, fryers, roosters, and capon (no hens)	Salt
	Sesame oil (not Chinese)
Bacon	Soybean oil
Liver (lamb)	Margarine (without milk solids or corn oil)
Peas	
Spinach	Gelatin (Knox)
Squash	White vinegar
String beans	Vanilla extract
Tomatoes	Lemon extract
Artichokes	Cornstarch-free baking powder
Asparagus	Baking soda
Carrots	Cream of tarter
Lettuce	Maple syrup or syrup made with cane sugar flavored with maple
Lima beans	

The fruits used on the diet may be fresh or canned with cane or beet sugar (no corn sugar, glucose).

A detailed daily food diary with a record of the degree of symptoms may be helpful when a patient is experiencing sporadic reactions. This approach is especially valuable in investigating persistent urticaria (Grogan, 1969). Provocative diets may occasionally be used in diagnosing food allergy. A food that is suspected of causing allergy is deliberately added to the diet and the patient observed for symptoms. If previous reactions have been anaphylactic, this procedure should be done in a physician's office. At least three separate diet provocations have been suggested before eliminating a major food from the diet for a prolonged period of time (Grogan, 1969).

Sensitivity to cow's milk may be difficult to document for several reasons. There are individual variations in intestinal absorption of ingested proteins, a multiplicity of antigens in milk, differing antibody responses following ingestion of milk, variations in specific organ responses to antigen-antibody interaction, and variations in the time required for clinical sensitivity to be recognized following milk ingestion (Heiner et al., 1964). Goldman et al. (1963) confirmed the diagnosis of milk allergy in 89 children by oral challenge with milk and/or purified milk proteins. Every one of 45 patients challenged with the amounts of the purified milk proteins (casein, alpha lactalbumin, beta lactoglobulin, and bovine serum albumin (BSA)) found in 100 ml skim milk had an allergic reaction to one or more of the proteins. The frequencies of reactions in this case were casein, 57 percent; BSA, 51 percent; beta lactoglobulin, 66 percent; and alpha lactalbumin, 54 percent.

15.4   Treatment

The only logical treatment for food allergy is elimination and avoidance of the specific food allergen for an extended period. Food allergy is often transient and may disappear after avoidance of the incriminated foods for several weeks or months. Thus, important basic foods to which an individual is allergic might be carefully reintroduced into the diet at 6-month or yearly intervals to test for continuing allergy. When foods are completely cooked they may be less likely to be allergenic. Many possible antigens may be present in any food, and identification of the specific one producing an allergic reaction is difficult. Cow's milk has been shown, through gel diffusion techniques, to contain more than 20 different antigens capable of eliciting precipitins in some humans who regularly ingest it (Heiner et al., 1964).

Milk is a major food in the diets of infants and young children and requires careful replacement if this becomes necessary. Its substitute should contain protein, fat, and carbohydrate in amounts approximately equal to that of human milk, along with adequate amounts of minerals and vitamins. In circumstances where commercially prepared milk substitutes are not available, formulas containing a mixture of fructose, olive oil, and rice combined with a high-quality protein such as egg yolk may be used. Cow's-milk substitutes usually available on the market include (1) meat-base formulas such as Lambase and (2) soy milk preparations. A number of soy milk formulas are made. Some of them have no added vitamins and require supplementation (Freier and Kletter, 1970). A careful reading of labels on products used for milk allergic patients is necessary. Rowe (1972) does not advise the use of Nutramigen, which is a preparation of enzymatically hydrolyzed casein with added corn oil, sugar, starch, minerals, and vitamins, since it contains traces of casein. With available substitutes for cow's milk, attempts at desensitization for infants with milk allergy are not usually necessary. Goat's milk may be tolerated by some children who cannot handle cow's milk, but often this is not true because antigens in the two milks are similar. Milk allergy usually disappears spontaneously within 1 to 2 years.

A child with several major food allergies, such as wheat, milk, and eggs, may have serious nutritional problems. The diet must be planned carefully so that individual nutritional requirements are adequately met. The diet is usually monotonous and often low in kilocalories. Essential fatty acids may be deficient if the mother has not been instructed to add an oil to the diet. Nutritional deficiencies can produce anorexia, further complicating adequate intake. If diarrhea is present, absorption of dietary nutrients may be limited. Multivitamin supplements are usually not recommended for children with allergy. Rather, crystalline synthetic vitamins are added one at a time or at most three together. Some children may be allergic to the nonvitamin materials that are included in a multivitamin preparation (Feeney, 1969).

A knowledge of food sources and related botanical food groups is important in managing a patient with food allergy. A food allergen such as corn is found in many hidden sources. Baking powders usually contain cornstarch as an inert ingredient, and monosodium glutamate may be derived from corn. Many vegetable gums are used in processed foods and may be factors in allergic response. They are often present in jellied candies, chewing gums, processed cheese foods, and whipped toppings. When eggs must be eliminated from the diet so must custards, certain puddings, some ice creams and candies, cakes, muffins, egg noodles, mayonnaise, and Ovaltine. Some breads and pretzels are glazed with an egg mix (Feeney, 1969). A number of commercial products are available for use by patients with food allergies, and food technologists are expanding the variety of these types of food in the market (Bowman et al., 1973). Recipe books designed for use by people with food allergies have been published (Wood, 1967). With careful counseling and planning, nutritionally adequate and esthetically acceptable diets may be provided for individuals with food allergies while eliminating the allergenic foods.

REFERENCES

1. Blumstein, G. I. and F. M. Richardson. 1964. Food allergy in first year of life. *Med. Sci.,* Oct., p. 88.

2. Bowman, F., W. Dilsaver, and I. Lorenz. 1973. Rationale for baking wheat-, gluten-, egg-, and milk-free products. *Bakers Dig., 47* (Apr.): 15.

3. Brown, E. B., B. M. Josephson, H. S. Levine, and M. Rosen. 1969. A prospective study of allergy in a pediatric population. *Am. J. Dis. Child., 117:* 693.

4. Feeney, M. C. 1969. Nutritional and dietary management of food allergy in children. *Am. J. Clin. Nutr., 22:* 103.

5. Feingold, B. F. 1968. Recognition of food additives as a cause of symptoms of allergy. *Ann. Allergy, 26:* 309.

6. Freier, S. and B. Kletter. 1970. Milk allergy in infants and young children. *Clin. Ped., 9:* 449.

7. Gerrard, J. W. 1974. Allergy in infancy. *Ped. Annals, 3:* 9.

8. Glaser, J. and D. E. Johnstone. 1953. Prophylaxis of allergic disease in newborn. *J. Am. Med. Assoc., 153:* 620.

9. Goldman, A. S., D. W. Anderson, Jr., W. A. Sellers, S. Saperstein, W. T. Kniker, and S. R. Halpern. 1963. Milk allergy. 1. Oral challenge with milk and isolated milk proteins in allergic children. *Pediatrics, 32:* 425.

10. Grogan, F. T., Jr. 1969. Food allergy in children after infancy. *Ped. Clin. No. Am., 16:* 217.

11. Halpern, S. R., W. A. Sellars, R. B. Johnson, D. W. Anderson, S. Saperstein, and J. S. Reisch. 1973. Development of childhood allergy in infants fed breast, soy, or cow milk. *J. Allergy Clin. Immun., 51:* 139.

12. Hamburger, R. N. 1976. Allergy and the immune system. *Am. Scientist, 64:* 157.

13. Heiner, D. C., J. F. Wilson, and M. E. Lahey. 1964. Sensitivity to cow's milk. *J. Am. Med. Assoc., 189:* 563.

14. Johnstone, D. E. and A. M. Dutton. 1966. Dietary prophylaxis of allergic disease in children. *N. Eng. J. Med., 274:* 715.

15. Lietze, A. 1969. The role of particulate insoluble substances in food allergy. III. Heat labile antibody to wheat starch in sera of wheat sensitive patients. *Ann. Allergy, 27:* 9.

16. Lockey, S. D., Sr. 1971. Reactions to hidden agents in foods, beverages and drugs. *Ann. Allergy, 29:* 461.

17. National Institute of Allergy and Infectious Diseases. 1972. Allergy research. DHEW Publication No. (NIH) 72–281.

18. Rowe, A. H. 1972. *Food Allergy.* Springfield, Ill.: Charles C. Thomas.

19. Wintrobe, M. M., G. W. Thorn, R. D. Adams, E. Braunwald, K. J. Isselbacher, and R. G. Petersdorf (Eds.). 1974. *Harrison's Principles of Internal Medicine,* 7th ed. New York: McGraw-Hill.

20. Wood, M. N. 1967. *Gourmet Food on a Wheat-Free Diet.* Springfield, Ill.: Charles C. Thomas.

CLIENT REFERENCES

1. Allergy Recipes. 1969. The American Dietetic Association, 430 North Michigan Avenue, Chicago, Ill. 60611.

2. Baking for People with Food Allergies. U.S. Department of Agriculture Home and Garden Bulletin No. 147. U.S. Government Printing Office, Washington, D.C. 20402.

3. Good Housekeeping's 125 Great Recipes for Allergy Diets. 1967. Good Housekeeping Bureau.

4. Little, B. 1968. *Recipes for Allergics.* New York: Vantage Press.

5. Sainsbury, I. S. 1974. *The Milk-Free and Milk-Free, Egg-free Cookbook.* Springfield, Ill.: Charles C. Thomas.

6. Shattuck, R. R. 1974. *Creative Cookery Without Wheat, Milk and Eggs.* New York: A. S. Barnes.

7. Wood, M. N. 1967. *Gourmet Food on a Wheat-Free Diet.* Springfield, Ill.: Charles C. Thomas.

8. Wood, M. N. 1972. *Delicious and Easy Rice Flour Recipes.* Springfield, Ill.: Charles C. Thomas.

STUDY GUIDE

Allergies represent abnormal reactions to the food one eats, the air one breathes, or substances one touches.

1. Describe what occurs theoretically in the body as an allergic reaction is precipitated, including roles of antigens, antibodies, haptens, and histamine. What is the significance of IgE in allergic reactions?

2. Describe signs of allergic reactions involving the skin; the respiratory tract; the gastrointestinal tract.

3. What is meant by anaphylactic shock?

4. What types of substances may act as allergens for the human. Give examples.

It has been suggested that hypoallergenic environmental controls may delay or prevent the development of allergy in susceptible individuals.

5. Describe and discuss the significance of some of the controversial data concerning effects of early feeding on the development of allergies.

Various tests or procedures may be used as aids in the diagnosis of allergies.

6. Outline the major steps involved and the limitations in the use of each of the following procedures for diagnosis of food allergies: histories; skin tests; elimination test diets; provocative diets; food diaries.

7. Suggest an appropriate use for Rowe's cereal-free elimination diet, giving examples of patients that may profit from it.

The logical treatment for food allergy is elimination of the specific food allergen for an extended period of time.

8. Describe the feeding problems created for an infant with milk allergy and suggest feasible solutions to these problems.

9. List several specific substances in milk that may be responsible for the allergic reaction in a milk-sensitive individual.

10. Evaluate the probable long-term prognosis for a child with food allergy.

Great care must be used in planning menus for a diagnosed allergy patient who is sensitive to several common foods that may be present in hidden forms in the diet.

11. Give appropriate dietary suggestions to a patient who is allergic to several common foods, including milk, wheat, and egg, and explain the rationale for your suggestions.

UNIT 5

Metabolic Abnormalities

16

Diabetes Mellitus - Development and Diagnosis

A few decades ago diabetes mellitus was defined quite simply as a disease of metabolism characterized by hyperglycemia and glycosuria resulting from the inability of the cell to utilize glucose. As time has elapsed since the discovery of insulin and its use in the treatment of diabetes, the great complexity of this disease has become more apparent. It is now commonly defined not only in terms of high blood glucose values and spilling of sugar in the urine, but also in terms of metabolic abnormalities in fat and protein metabolism and disorders in the structure and function of blood vessels. The principal early symptoms are usually related to the metabolic abnormalities and later developments involve complications with blood vessels such as retinopathy, nephrosclerosis, and atherosclerosis.

This chapter presents several factors apparently involved in the etiology and pathogenesis of diabetes mellitus. It includes a discussion of insulin and glucagon as well as interrelationships between obesity and diabetes. Treatment and complications of diabetes are discussed in Chap. 17.

16.1 Types of Diabetes Mellitus

Diabetes may result from various causes, including destruction of pancreatic islet cells from chronic inflammation or surgical removal, disorders of other endocrine glands, and administration of drugs such as corticosteroids or estrogen-progesterone combinations. A possible role of viruses in the development of diabetes has been suggested (Steinke and Taylor, 1974). However, the most commonly accepted etiology for diabetes mellitus is genetic or hereditary. Diabetes with a hereditary tendency may also be called primary or idiopathic (Wintrobe et al., 1974, pp. 533–534).

Genetic diabetes is subdivided into two general types with differing characteristics and problems of management—maturity-onset and juvenile-onset diabetes. Maturity- or adult-onset diabetes is relatively mild and associated with a moderately obese state. Individuals developing this type of disease usually do so after the age of 35 to 40 years, although it has been reported in children and adolescents (Fajans et al., 1976). It is characterized by resistance to the development of ketosis except under unusual stress. The onset of the disease is gradual and symptoms are often minimal. However, degenerative complications involving the vascular system are common. Insulin is secreted although in insufficient amount or delayed in time so that glucose is not adequately removed from the blood. Hyperinsulinemia, especially in the obese patient, has been frequently reported (Felig, 1971; Jackson et al., 1972).

Juvenile- or growth-onset diabetes is usually comparatively severe and often difficult to keep under good control with ketosis developing readily. The onset is usually during childhood or adolescence but it sometimes occurs in an adult, usually a nonobese adult. A child with diabetes is likely to maintain the severe ketosis-prone disease during adulthood. A sudden onset with accompanying weight loss is characteristic. Blood insulin is undetectable within a few years after the disease is diagnosed and exogenous insulin must be given. Wide variations in blood sugar are often present and management of diet, insulin, and exercise is difficult. Chronic degenerative changes in the vascular system appear to be related to the duration of the disease.

Approximately 80 percent of individuals with diabetes are of the mild, maturity-onset type and are obese. About 10 percent have a mild, stable form of the disorder but are nonobese adults. About 5 percent are children with a moderately severe and ketosis-prone form of the disease, and the remaining 5 percent are adults having a severe juvenile-type disease (Lilly, 1973, p. 2).

16.2 Prevalence

The actual number of individuals in the United States with diabetes mellitus is not known but 4.4 million cases have been estimated (U.S. Public Health Service, 1969). About 1.6 million of these do not know that they have the disease; they are undiagnosed.

Incidence of diabetes increases with age. The rate of diagnosed diabetes among individuals who are less than 25 years of age is 1.6 per 1000 noninstitutional population, and for persons between 25 and 44 years it is 8.0 per 1000. The rate for those between 45 and 54 years of age is 20.0 per 1000. Between ages 65 and 74 the rate reaches a peak of 64.4 and drops to 57.9 per 1000 for persons 75 years of age or older (U.S. Public Health Service, 1969).

A mail survey by Gorwitz et al. (1976) of 1,720,212 enrolled Michigan school-age children identified 2816 children with diabetes mellitus, a ratio of 1 case per 611 or 1.6 per 1000. The number of diabetic children increased with advancing age up to a maximum at 14 to 15 years. At that point the rate was approximately 1 per 450. In this study, rates were higher for females than males and for whites than nonwhites. The overall national diabetes diagnosis rate presented by the U.S. Public Health Service (1969) was slightly higher for women than for men by 1966 fiscal year figures, being 12.9 per 1000 for males and 16.1 for females.

The incidence of diabetes is increasing in the United States. Several factors may contribute to this increase. (1) Diabetes is more prevalent in the older age groups and the aging population is increasing in number. (2) The life expectancy of the treated diabetic is increasing. (3) Children with diabetes are living to maturity and bearing children of their own with excellent chances for survival of the newborn infants. (4) The potential for diabetes is being increased as intermarriage of families with diabetes continues. (5) Obesity is prevalent and may contribute to the development of diabetes in predisposed individuals.

16.3   Nutrition and the Development of Diabetes

Diabetes is a universal disease that is found in persons from all nations of the world. However, some nations have a lesser incidence of the disease than others. It has been noted that this disease is found more commonly in portions of the world where there is an abundance of available food and less commonly in agriculturally depressed areas. In any nation, diabetes is more common in times of prosperity than in times of famine and war.

In the 1930s and 1940s Himsworth published papers on diet and the incidence of diabetes. He first suggested that the consumption of large amounts of carbohydrate was related to an increased incidence of diabetes. Later, however, he wrote that changes in prevalence of and mortality from diabetes in a population more closely paralleled the consumption of fat. This seemed a paradox because "the consumption of fat has no deleterious influence on sugar tolerance. . . ." Many years later, Yudkin (1964) reported that, in a comparison of 41 countries, fat intake increased generally as sugar intake increased. This is probably because many foods that contain sugar also contain fat, e.g., cakes, candies, chocolates, pastries, and ice creams. There are exceptions, of course. Meats contain fat without sugar and sugar may be added to beverages without fat. National consumption figures were used in Yudkin's study and these relationships may not always hold on an individual basis. However, Yudkin proposed that sugar was more likely a direct causative agent for diabetes than was fat.

Cohen (1972) reported that diabetes increased significantly among Yemenite and Kurdish Jews after they had lived in Israel for more than 25 years, in comparison to the very low incidence of diabetes among new immigrants from the same areas. Dietary studies revealed that one of the major differences in food consumption was a substantial increase in sucrose intake by the older settlers. Almost no sucrose had been consumed in Yemen. An association between the increased sucrose consumption and increased incidence of diabetes is suggested.

West and Kalbfleisch (1971) studied 12 age-matched populations in 11 countries (many in Central and South America). They found a positive association between prevalence of diabetes and dietary intake of fat and of sugar and a negative association between prevalence of diabetes and total carbohydrate consumption. However, they thought that these relationships might be partly or completely incidental because of certain inconsistencies in the data. Increased prevalence of diabetes also correlated well with elevated serum cholesterol levels. The most impressive and consistent association in these studies was between prevalence of diabetes and fatness (weight in relation to height).

All researchers have not found significant relationships between sugar or fat intake and prevalence of diabetes. However, it is difficult to get reliable dietary data on age-matched populations, and failure to show a significant relationship, particularly in a small study, does not necessarily prove that this relationship does not exist in the population as a whole. Kahn et al. (1971) were involved in a collaborative study between Israel and the National Heart and Lung Institute in the United States. This was basically a heart disease study on 10,000 men that covered a 2-year period, but these same data were used to look at factors related to diabetes incidence. Diabetes developed in 131 individuals during the study. No significant associations were found between diabetes incidence and intake of total carbohydrate, sugar, saturated fatty acids, animal protein, or total kilocalories. An association was found between diabetes incidence and height/weight ratio or obesity, with more diabetes occurring among those with lower height/weight ratios. The researchers suggested that it is beneficial for an individual to metabolize most of the energy nutrients consumed rather than store a significant part of these substances as fat.

Populations characterized by leanness have a very low incidence of diabetes whether they consume chiefly carbohydrates or fats. The Masai in Africa eat only about 20 percent of their kilocalories as carbohydrate with a diet of meat, milk, and blood. The Zulus, on the other hand, traditionally eat about 85 percent of their kilocalories as carbohydrate. However, both groups are lean and virtually free of diabetes. Many American Indian tribes have a very high incidence of diabetes along with a high incidence of obesity. The Athabaskan Indians in Alaska, living on a high-fat, low-carbohydrate diet, have a low incidence of both diabetes and obesity. When diabetes does occur in populations with little obesity, it is usually mild and with few accompanying signs of atherosclerosis (Albrink and Davidson, 1971).

O'Sullivan and Mahan (1965), in an Oxford, Massachusetts study that continued over a 17-year period, found no relationship between body weight and blood sugar levels in the general study population of more than 3,000 subjects. However, the rate of development of diabetes in overweight subjects with blood sugar levels of 140 mg/100 ml or more was much greater than that of normal weight individuals with the same blood sugar levels. It was suggested that obesity may not be a direct cause but may increase the risk of developing diabetes when a tendency toward the disease is present. That is, obesity, as an important environmental factor, may uncover an inherited tendency toward diabetes.

Since there are probably many factors involved in the development of diabetes, including genetics, relationships between dietary intake and incidence of the disease are not simple and clearcut. There *may* be a positive influence on the incidence of diabetes by high sucrose consumption but more definitive research is necessary to clarify whether or not this is a real effect. Obesity is apparently associated with diabetes but must be interrelated with other influences as well.

16.4   Insulin

In 1869, while still a medical student, Langerhans described islets in the structure of the pancreas. These are now known to contain at least two major types of cells, the *alpha* and *beta* cells, which differ in their morphology and staining characteristics. The beta cells secrete the hormone, insulin, and the alpha cells secrete glucagon. Delta cells that secrete other hormones are also present. Characteristic granules are found in each type of cell. Fig. 16.1 shows the histology of the pancreas.

Insulin was discovered in 1921 by two researchers in Toronto, Canada. Banting was a surgeon established in private practice when he became interested in research on pancreatic extracts. He left his practice to work without salary in a university laboratory in order to confirm some of his theories. Best was a student of biochemistry with an interest in medicine, later completing both science and medical degrees. These researchers produced pancreatic extracts with the ability to lower the blood sugar of depancreatized dogs. After the discovery of insulin, one of the first problems was to find a method of increasing the yield of pancreatic extracts because the demand for the life-saving substance was enormous. This, then, became a challenge for industrial technology (Groen, 1972).

Synthesis and Secretion of Insulin

Insulin is the first protein for which the amino acid sequence was established (Sanger, 1959). For this monumental accomplishment, Sanger re-

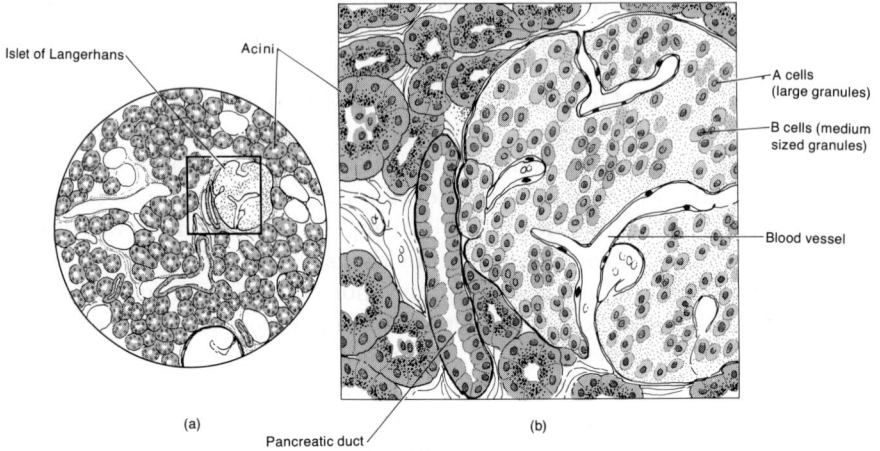

Fig. 16.1 Histology of the pancreas. (*a*) View of two islets of Langerhans (cells that produce hormones) and several acini (cells that produce digestive enzymes). (*b*) Enlarged aspect of a portion of an islet of Langerhans and several acini. (From Gerard J. Tortora, *Principles of Human Anatomy,* New York: Harper & Row, 1977; by permission of the publisher.)

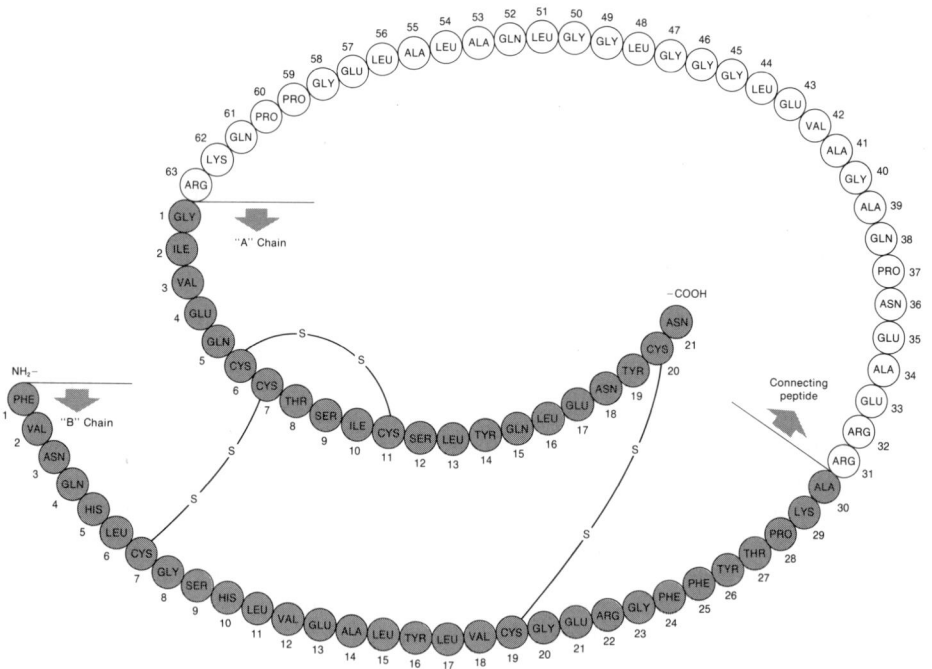

Fig. 16.2 The primary structure of porcine proinsulin. The sequence of procine proinsulin is represented by the amino acids in the darker circles. The sequence of the connecting peptide is depicted by the amino acids in the open circles. (From R. E. Chance, "Amino Acid Sequences of proinsulins and Intermediates," *Diabetes,* **21** (Supplement 2):461, 1972; by permission of Eli Lilly and Company.)

ceived a Nobel prize. Insulin was also the first protein to be synthesized (Katsoyannis, 1966). Its synthesis is not yet possible on a commercial basis, however, and the available insulins are usually extracted from beef or pork pancreas.

The biosynthesis of insulin in beta cells of the islets of Langerhans involves first the production of a precursor molecule called proinsulin. Proinsulin is a polypeptide that includes both the A and B chains of insulin within its amino acid sequence. A connecting peptide (C-peptide) joins the two chains. The amino acid sequence of porcine proinsulin is shown in Fig. 16.2. The conversion of proinsulin to insulin requires the hydrolysis of the connecting peptide from the proinsulin molecule. Proinsulin has little biologic activity and accounts for only 5 to 15 percent of the total insulin in blood (Felig, 1971).

A model of the biologic events in formation, storage, and release of insulin in beta cells of the rat pancreas has been proposed by Lacy (1972). In this model (Fig. 16.3) the intracellular metabolism of glucose acts as a signal for proinsulin synthesis to begin without the endoplasmic reticulum of the cell. The proinsulin formed is then transferred to the Golgi complex by way of microvescular carriers where it is made into beta granules. Enzymatic conversion of proinsulin to insulin by peptidases probably occurs here. Mature beta granules are released from the Golgi complex and are enclosed by smooth membranous sacs. Some of the beta granules are ap-

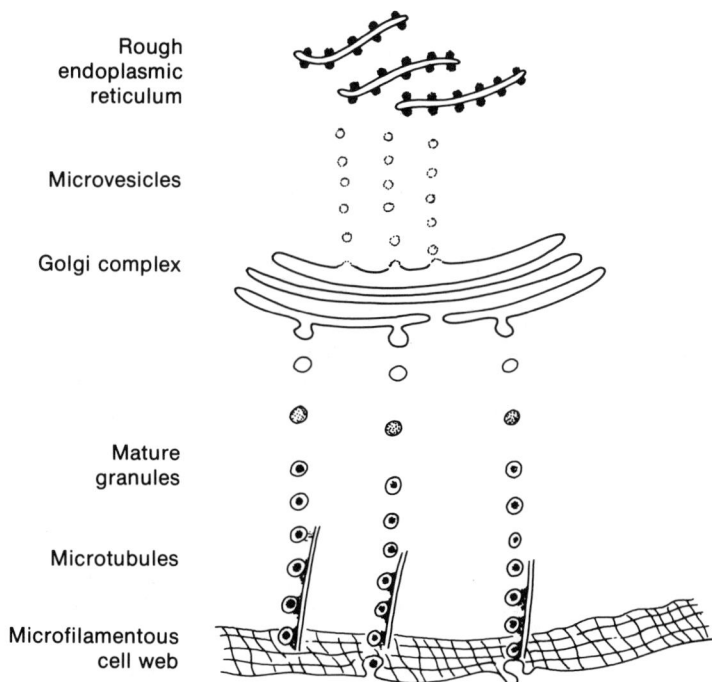

Fig. 16.3 Beta granule formation and secretion from beta cells in the islets of Langerhans.

parently microcrystals of zinc and insulin. After release from the Golgi complex, the beta granules either remain free in the cytoplasm or become attached to a microtubular system close to the cell membrane. Glucose metabolism initiates the entrance of calcium into the cell which triggers a change in the physical conformation of the microtubules. They contract to displace the beta granules to the cell surface. The membranous sacs encasing the granules fuse with the plasma membrane, and the granules may be released by the process of emiocytosis (from the Greek *emesis* or vomiting) at specific locations on the plasma membrane. This leaves tiny cytoplasmic projections between the sites of release of beta granules. A microfilamentous cell web just beneath the cell membrane may control the access of the granules to the membrane and their extrusion (Malaisse, 1973).

Some parts of the proposed model of insulin secretion are firmly established while others require further testing. The formation of proinsulin in the endoplasmic reticulum and the formation of beta granules in the Golgi complex are documented (Steiner et al., 1974). It has been confirmed that calcium plays a role in insulin release from the beta cell, possibly by influencing the microtubular-microfilamentous web system (Malaisse, 1972; Sharp et al., 1975). It is not yet clear whether glucose must enter the beta cell and be metabolized in order to exert its effect on insulin release or if glucose releases insulin by interacting with a glucoreceptor within the cell membrane (Cerasi, 1975). Whether the production of cyclic AMP through the action of adenylate cyclase is involved as an intermediary process in the glucose stimulation of insulin release has not been firmly established but has been strongly suggested as a possible mechanism (Cerasi, 1975; Malaisse, 1972; Sharp et al., 1975).

Glucose is the most important substance that stimulates insulin secretion. The response of the beta cell to a sudden increase in blood glucose occurs in two phases as illustrated in Fig. 16.4. There is an initial rapid release of insulin from an easily mobilized pool, followed by a second more gradual release from a more slowly responsive pool plus newly synthesized insulin and small amounts of proinsulin (Felig, 1971).

When glucose is taken orally, higher levels of blood insulin are observed than when glucose is given intravenously, attributed to the release of upper gastrointestinal (GI) hormones. The hormones stimulate insulin secretion immediately, preparing the system for absorption of glucose. One of the hormones secreted has been called "gut glucagon" because its polypeptide structure and immunological characteristics resemble pancreatic glucagon. However, gut glucagon does not have the gluconeogenic and glycogenolytic properties of pancreatic glucagon. Secretin, gastrin, and cholecystokinin-pancreozymin (CCK) have also been shown to stimulate insulin release. In addition, CCK stimulates glucagon secretion by pancreatic alpha cells (Raptis et al., 1972; Chisholm et al., 1969).

Amino acids are capable of stimulating insulin secretion, although there are individual differences in their capacities. Other substances that stimulate insulin secretion include pancreatic glucagon, the sulfonylurea

Biphasic Insulin Response to Glucose

Phase I: Rapid Release

Stimuli
- Glucose
- Amino acids
- Sulfonylureas
- Glucagon
- GI hormones

Content: Stored, preformed insulin

Phase II: Delayed Release

Stimulus: Glucose

Content
- Preformed insulin
- Newly synthesized insulin
- Proinsulin

Time (minutes)

Stimulus

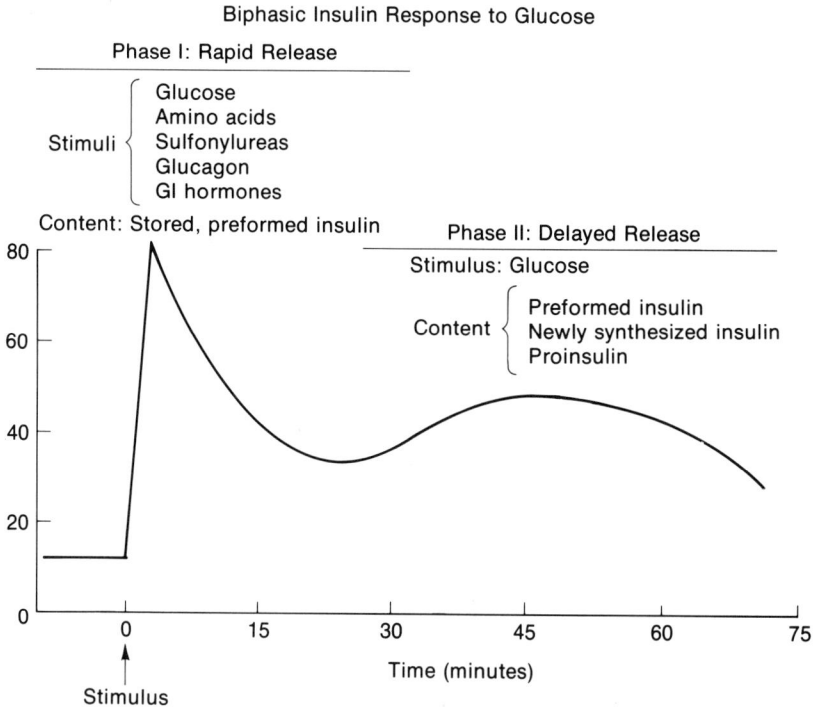

Fig. 16.4 Biphasic insulin secretory response following glucose administration. The initial rapid phase consists of stored, preformed insulin released from a rapidly mobilizable pool of beta-cell granules and can be elicited by a variety of stimuli as well as glucose. The delayed secondary response is observed with glucose only and consists of newly synthesized insulin and small amounts of proinsulin in addition to secretion of preformed, stored insulin. (From Philip Felig, "Pathophysiology of Diabetes Mellitus, *Medical Clinics of North America,* **55:** 823, 1971; by permission of the author and W. B. Saunders Company.)

drugs, and theophylline. Epinephrine is a potent inhibitor of insulin secretion (Felig, 1971).

Metabolic Effects of Insulin

Insulin is directly involved in some phases of the metabolism of fat and protein as well as carbohydrate. Under experimental conditions insulin can be shown to influence fat and protein metabolism in the absence of, and independent of, its action on glucose. However, in physiological systems these effects are well integrated so that insulin's primary role is to encourage conservation and storage of all the metabolic fuels (Felig, 1971).

Many tissues require insulin for the transport of glucose across cell membranes but some do not. Cells requiring insulin include striated muscle, adipocytes, mammary gland, anterior pituitary, lens of the eye, and aorta. On the other hand, cells in the liver, kidney tubule, intestinal mucosa, lymph nodes, nerves and brain, and erythrocytes do not require insulin for glucose transport.

Liver.   Although liver cells do not require insulin for the entry of glucose, it is necessary for normal metabolism. The liver receives glucose directly from the GI tract through the portal vein and disposes of approximately 70 percent of any oral glucose load. It continuously releases glucose throughout a 24-hour period at the rate of 2 to 3.5 mg per kg body weight per minute (200 to 350 g per day) as a result of its capacity for glycogenolysis and gluconeogenesis. Insulin is secreted directly into the portal system and the liver removes 50 to 80 percent of the hormone reaching it. Insulin acts on the liver to both encourage glucose uptake and suppress glucose production and release. It apparently does this by influencing the activity of various cellular enzymes. Insulin probably acts in the liver to enhance the activity of glucokinase, which catalyzes the phosphorylation of glucose to glucose-6-phosphate. It stimulates glycogen synthetase and also promotes inactivation of phosphorylase, which releases glucose from glycogen. The levels of certain key enzymes in gluconeogenesis are suppressed and controlled by insulin. The overall effect is net liver glucose storage. In addition, insulin encourages fatty acid synthesis from glucose, esterification of these fatty acids with glycerol, and release of the triglycerides into the blood as very low density (pre-beta) lipoproteins. Hydrolysis of liver proteins to amino acids is reduced by insulin (Felig, 1971).

Muscle.   In muscle tissue insulin increases glucose transport across cell membranes with phosphorylation of glucose occurring in the process. It stimulates the transport of amino acids into the cells and acts on ribosomes to stimulate protein synthesis. It also appears to affect glycogen synthetase and encourages glycogen storage. The products of muscle glycogenolysis enter glycolysis since muscle lacks the enzyme glucose-6-phosphatase and free glucose cannot be released from stored glycogen. Glucose utilization by muscle tissue is increased during exercise but this augmented utilization is not insulin-dependent. It accounts for the frequent decrease in insulin requirements of the insulin-treated diabetic during exercise and the tendency toward hypoglycemia at this time.

Adipose Tissue.   Insulin is necessary for the transport of glucose across cell membranes in adipose tissue with rapid phosphorylation of the sugar. Glucose is further metabolized to (1) yield two-carbon fragments that participate in fatty acid synthesis, or (2) produce alpha-glycero-phosphate that is esterified with the fatty acids to yield triglycerides. Once glucose has entered the adipocyte, these additional metabolic events are indirect effects of the action of insulin. Insulin directly affects fat metabolism by stimulating the enzyme lipoprotein lipase and thus encourages the entrance of fatty acids into adipocytes as they are released from the hydrolysis of circulating chylomicrons and pre-beta lipoproteins. In addition, it directly inhibits a lipase within the fat cell. Thus, fat storage is encouraged by the action of insulin. The antilipolytic effect of insulin occurs at insulin concentrations less than those necessary to effect glucose transport (Felig, 1971).

The effects of insulin on carbohydrate, fat, and protein metabolism are all directed toward the building up of tissue stores. Insulin is a "fattening" hormone since fat synthesis is encouraged while lipolysis is inhibited. Glucose uptake, with a concomitant decrease in blood glucose, is encouraged and the glucose directed toward storage as glycogen. A decrease in the amount of new glucose formed by gluconeogenesis is also evident as a decreased output of amino acids from muscle limits the substrate available to the liver for this purpose (Fig. 16.5).

Several suggestions have been offered as to how insulin acts at the molecular level in achieving its many integrated effects. It has been proposed that the hormone acts by initiating a disturbance at the cell membrane as it attaches to a specific receptor site and then transmits information through the cell by various intracellular messenger molecules. Cyclic AMP has been suggested as a potential messenger. Ions, such as K^+, Ca^{++}, and Mg^{++}, have also been proposed as possible messengers. A messenger may act on a biochemical reaction that is shared by various metabolic processes and switch this key reaction in either an anabolic or a catabolic direction (Fain and Rosenberg, 1972; Krahl, 1972; Levine, 1972; Park et al., 1972; Weber, 1972).

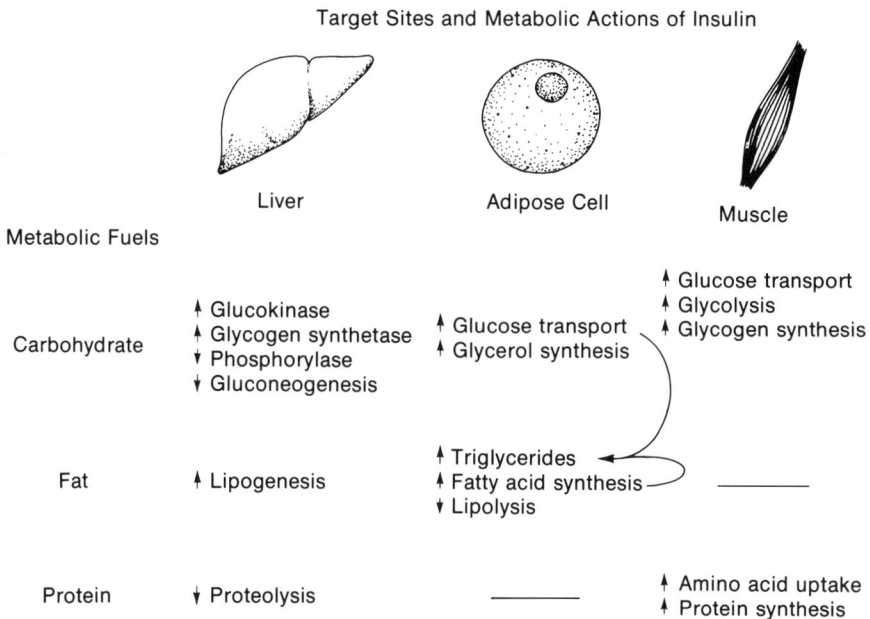

Fig. 16.5 Target sites and metabolic action of insulin. The diverse effects of insulin on the major metabolic fuels tend to reinforce each other. (From Philip Felig, "Pathophysiology of Diabetes Mellitus, *Medical Clinics of North America*, **55**: 825, 1971; by permission of the author and W. B. Saunders Company.)

Measurement and Standardization of Insulin

The first standard for insulin potency was based on the hypoglycemic effect of the insulin on rabbits. As insulin extracts became more purified with improved manufacturing processes, however, a uniform standard was adopted that was based on absolute weight of insulin prepared from a recrystallized composite sample. The first standard of insulin contained approximately 8 units per mg but by 1972 the standard was 24 units per mg (Lilly, 1973, pp. 44–45).

Insulin is available in various concentrations, such as 40 units per ml, 100 units per ml, etc. To minimize the possibility of confusion and error on the part of the person with diabetes as he or she injects insulin, the American Diabetes Association, the U.S. Food and Drug Administration, and insulin manufacturers in Canada and the United States agreed in 1971 that only one concentration of insulin should be routinely used. The accepted concentration is 100 units per ml or U-100. A transition is being made toward the exclusive use of U-100 insulin in the routine treatment of diabetes (Lilly, 1973, pp. 46–47).

Insulin is present in blood serum in very small quantities and has been difficult to measure accurately. Several serum insulin assay methods have been reported (Batchelor, 1967) and each method has its own particular problems. Biologic assay methods have included use of (1) rat epididymal fat pad, (2) rat diaphragm muscle, and (3) a radioimmunologic technique.

Radioimmunoassay is the most commonly used assay method for insulin and is based on the reaction between insulin antibodies at very low concentration and insulin-[131]I. The quantity of *labeled* antigen-antibody complex is decreased by the addition of *unlabeled* insulin. After the antigen-antibody reaction has occurred, the insulin-antibody complex can be separated from the free insulin in the mixture by electrophoresis and the ratio of *labeled* Bound/Free (B/F) insulin determined. Ratios of B/F labeled insulin from serum samples are compared with a standard curve produced with known quantities of insulin. The radioimmunoassay is the most sensitive and specific method for blood insulin assay. Normal values for fasting plasma immunoreactive insulin (IRI) are 10–30 μU per ml. Blood insulin levels normally rise postprandially and have been reported to range from 20 to 300 μU per ml when measured as IRI (Batchelor, 1967). The exact state of insulin in the blood remains to be elucidated. It may exist not only as a single molecule but also as a dimer, trimer, or large polymer (Ogawa, 1969).

Glucagon and Insulin

Glucagon is a polypeptide that is produced by the alpha cells of the islets of Langerhans in the pancreas. It has powerful gluconeogenic and glycogenolytic effects on the liver, thus promoting hepatic glucose production, opposing the effect of insulin that encourages glucose uptake and storage in body tissues. The relative concentration of these two hormones, glucagon and insulin, has the capability of controlling the moment-to-moment balance of glucose across the liver in accordance with energy needs of the body (Unger and Orci, 1977). Insulin-induced hypoglycemia is associated with a rise in glucagon concentration measured in the pancreaticoduodenal vein (Ohneda et al., 1969). Glucagon is a hormone of "glucose need." Dietary carbohydrate restriction lowers fasting serum insulin and raises fasting glucagon levels in normal human subjects (Unger, 1972).

It has been suggested that diabetes mellitus is a bihormonal disease characterized by a deficiency of endogenous insulin and abnormal regulation of endogenous glucagon. Reynolds et al. (1977) found that unstable diabetics failed to decrease glucagon secretion during hyperglycemia and also failed to increase glucagon secretion during hypoglycemia. Stable diabetics demonstrated some ability to increase glucagon secretion during hypoglycemia and consequently showed less wide blood glucose fluctuations.

Sherwin et al. (1976) challenged the importance of glucagon in diabetes and suggested that the action of glucagon is dependent on coexistent insulin deficiency. However, from a review of the role of glucagon in diabetes, Unger and Orci (1977) concluded that there is a hypersecretion of glucagon by the alpha cells in severe diabetes and glucagon is a factor in the development of endogenous hyperglycemia and ketoacidosis.

A peptide called somatostatin that is produced by the hypothalamus is an inhibitor of glucagon release by the alpha cells, but it also inhibits insulin secretion and growth hormone release. In early studies it was shown that postprandial hyperglycemia could be controlled in some diabetic patients receiving insulin when glucagon release was depressed by giving somatostatin. However, additional studies (Felig et al., 1976) have shown that the decline in blood sugar following somatostatin administration persists for only 60 to 120 minutes. The improvement in postprandial hyperglycemia produced by somatostatin is apparently the result of an inhibitory effect of this peptide on carbohydrate absorption in the GI tract rather than an effect on enhancement of carbohydrate disposal.

16.5 Pathophysiology

Diabetes mellitus in humans is a complex disease and relationships between intermediary metabolic abnormalities and vascular changes have not been clarified. However, lack of insulin, on either an absolute or relative basis, characterizes the diabetic syndrome.

In juvenile-onset diabetes insulin deficiency is usually very severe. After the disease is well established there is often no extractable pancreatic insulin and no measurable insulin in the circulating blood. The individual with juvenile-onset diabetes is dependent on exogenous insulin for survival. However, in at least one-third of juvenile diabetics there is a period of temporary remission, sometimes called the "honeymoon period," that usually occurs within 3 months after the onset of the disease. The remission may last from several days to months but rarely exceeds a year, and glucose tolerance may be normal during this time (Wintrobe et al., 1974, p. 535).

Maturity- or adult-onset diabetes develops more slowly than does the juvenile-onset disease. Some insulin is produced by the maturity-onset diabetic but pancreatic beta cell secretory responses have been altered so that a subnormal amount of insulin is available to body tissues.

While some patients exhibit classic juvenile-onset diabetes and other show characteristic maturity-onset diabetes, some patients develop a diabetes that has characteristics of both types. It should be emphasized that comments about each particular type of diabetes are generalizations.

In both types of diabetes, insulin lack produces the classic sign of hyperglycemia which is usually associated with excretion of sugar in the urine (glycosuria). Metabolic changes that are observed in diabetes reflect the degree of insulin deficiency. When little or no insulin is secreted, as in juvenile-onset diabetes, metabolism in the fasting as well as the fed state is markedly affected (Fig. 16.6). Because there is decreased uptake and oxidation of glucose in muscle tissue, there is loss of muscle glycogen and failure to synthesize more. There is also release of amino acids, particularly alanine (Felig et al., 1970), to supply the liver with a substrate for gluconeogenesis. In adipose tissue there is decreased fatty acid uptake and increased lipolysis, probably because of the lack of insulin to stimulate lipoprotein lipase and inhibit lipase activities. Serum fatty acid concentration is thus elevated in the diabetic state and this may further decrease glucose utilization in body tissues (Hales, 1966). Decreased glucose uptake by adipose tissue causes lack of alpha-glycerophosphate and fatty acid for triglyceride synthesis. The liver receives many of the fatty acids released by adipose tissue and metabolizes part of them to produce ketone bodies (beta-hydroxybutyric acid and acetoacetic acid) (Fig. 16.7). The liver normally produces small amounts of ketones that are metabolized in extrahepatic tissues such as muscle. In the severe diabetic state, however, an excess of ketones results from a diminished utilization of acetyl CoA for fatty acid synthesis or tricarboxylic acid (TCA) cycle metabolism and a decreased rate of ketone uptake by muscle tissue. Beta-hydroxybutyric acid and acetoacetic acid are generally present in a ratio of 3 : 1. They rapidly dissociate as they are released into the blood stream, causing an increase in hydrogen ion concentration and a fall in serum bicarbonate. Acetone is formed by nonenzymatic decarboxylation of acetoacetic acid and also circulates in the blood. It does not contribute hydrogen ion to lower the blood pH but is responsible for a fruity odor on the breath of a diabetic in acidosis (Felig, 1974). Ketones are excreted in the urine (ketonuria). Since they are strong acids, the kidney must combine them with fixed base for excretion, leading to loss of sodium and potassium from the body.

The liver responds to persistent insulin lack with increased gluconeogenesis, utilizing as substrate amino acids from muscle. Glycogenolysis is enhanced, glucose phosphorylation decreased, and little or

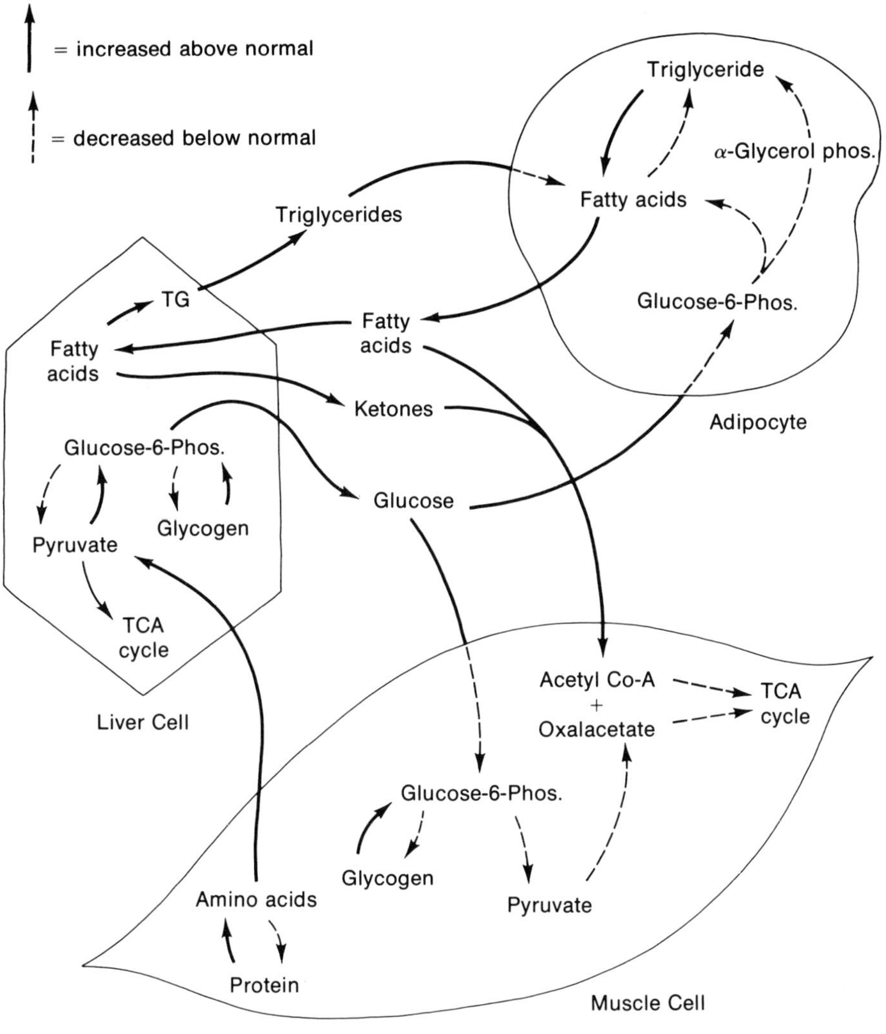

Fig. 16.6 Metabolic abnormalities in diabetes mellitus.

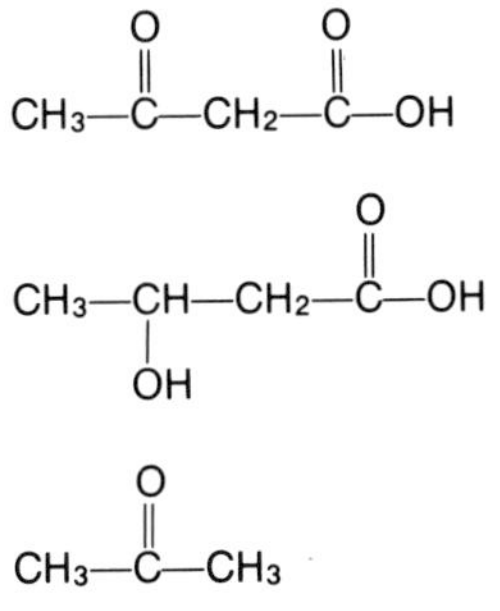

Acetoacetic acid

Beta-hydroxybutyric acid

Acetone

Fig. 16.7 Ketone bodies.

no new glycogen synthesized in the liver as a result of insulin deficiency. There is an excess of glucose in the system resulting from both underutilization by tissues and overproduction by the liver. A sorbitol pathway operates in the metabolism of excess glucose (Fig. 16.8). In this pathway glucose is not phosphorylated but is directly reduced by aldose reductase to the sugar alcohol, sorbitol. The further conversion of sorbitol to fructose may occur with the action of the enzyme sorbitol dehydrogenase. Sorbitol penetrates cell membranes poorly and, once formed, may be trapped intracellularly. Presence of large amounts of sorbitol in nerve cells and in the lens of the eye has been suggested as a factor in the development of some diabetic-related neuropathies and cataract formation (Wintrobe et al., 1974, p. 537).

The net result of metabolic changes in severe juvenile-onset diabetes is marked hyperglycemia which causes an osmotic diuresis with loss of water, glucose, and electrolytes. With the high glucose concentration in extracellular fluid, water is drawn from cells in order to maintain isotonicity. Hyperlipidemia, negative nitrogen balance, depleted fat stores, weight loss, general dehydration, and ketoacidosis are major features of the uncontrolled severe diabetic state characterized by marked insulin deficiency.

When some insulin is secreted, metabolic abnormalities are less pronounced. In mild maturity-onset diabetes, the failure of the beta cell to secrete insulin may be apparent only when it is called upon to produce insulin in response to a glucose load. Secretion may be adequate to maintain normal fasting blood sugar values. A moderate insulin deficiency, however, does not allow maintenance of normal fasting blood sugar nor adequate handling of usual oral carbohydrate intakes. The symptoms of hyperglycemia and glycosuria develop. Ketosis is not usually present in maturity-onset diabetes except during periods of unusual stress. Patients with this type of diabetes appear to be ketosis-resistant. Apparently the insulin that is produced is sufficient to prevent excessive lipolysis of adipose tissue and to allow utilization of sufficient glucose to control ketone balance in the body.

Conflicting data have been reported regarding patterns of insulin secretion in mild maturity-onset diabetes. In some studies, glucose-induced insulin secretion was found to be greater than normal in subjects with mild

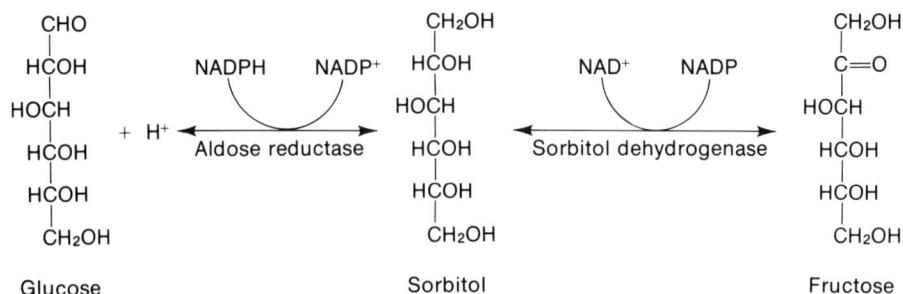

$$
\begin{array}{ccccc}
\text{CHO} & & & \text{CH}_2\text{OH} & \\
| & & & | & \\
\text{HCOH} & \text{NADPH} \quad \text{NADP}^+ & \text{HCOH} & \text{NAD}^+ \quad \text{NADP} & \text{CH}_2\text{OH} \\
| & & | & & | \\
\text{HOCH} & + \text{H}^+ & \text{HOCH} & & \text{C}=\text{O} \\
| & \xleftarrow{\qquad\qquad} & | & \xleftarrow{\qquad\qquad} & | \\
\text{HCOH} & \text{Aldose reductase} & \text{HCOH} & \text{Sorbitol dehydrogenase} & \text{HOCH} \\
| & & | & & | \\
\text{HCOH} & & \text{HCOH} & & \text{HCOH} \\
| & & | & & | \\
\text{CH}_2\text{OH} & & \text{CH}_2\text{OH} & & \text{HCOH} \\
& & & & | \\
& & & & \text{CH}_2\text{OH} \\
\text{Glucose} & & \text{Sorbitol} & & \text{Fructose}
\end{array}
$$

Fig. 16.8 The sorbitol pathway.

diabetes although it was less than normal in those with more severe diabetes (Chiles and Tzagournis, 1970; Johansen, 1972). Impaired insulin output even in the early stages of mild maturity-onset diabetes has been reported by others (Fujita et al., 1975). In maturity-onset diabetes, the impaired response of insulin secretion to a glucose load appears to occur primarily during the initial rapid-release phase (see Fig. 16.4). There is a delay in insulin secretion at this stage, allowing an abnormally high blood glucose level to develop relatively quickly. Then an excessive secretion of insulin apparently occurs, in response to the abnormally high blood glucose level, during the second phase. Excessive secretion of insulin may eventually lead to hypoglycemia after 4 to 5 hours. As the disease progresses, insulin secretion decreases and hypoglycemia is less likely to occur (Wintrobe et al., 1974, p. 535). Although the concept of delayed insulin secretion in mild maturity-onset diabetes is generally accepted, a few researchers have not found delayed secretion in diabetic subjects as compared to normal controls (Fujita et al., 1975; Felig, 1971; Jackson et al., 1972). Further research should help to clarify the reported differences.

16.6   Obesity and Diabetes

Some degree of glucose intolerance is commonly associated with the obese state, an incidence of 50 to 75 percent having been reported, depending on age (Smith and Levine, 1964). Conversely, approximately 80 percent of all diabetics are obese. The relationships between obesity and diabetes are not clarified, but it is obviously important to try to understand something about the puzzle inherent in the closeness of these two conditions.

Numerous studies have reported that markedly obese people have abnormally high levels of immunoreactive insulin (IRI) circulating in the blood when compared with normal weight control subjects. Some researchers have found a significant positive correlation between basal serum insulin and body weight (Bierman et al., 1968; Rosselin et al., 1971), although other workers have not found the correlation to be significant (Stephan et al., 1972). When an oral glucose challenge is given to obese subjects, they often show an insulin response that is increased above normal, and the serum levels may remain high for a relatively long period of time (Karam et al., 1963). The hyperinsulinism of obesity appears to be due to hypersecretion rather than to impaired clearance (Nikkila and Taskinen, 1971). Hyperinsulinism of obese subjects has been shown to return to normal on weight reduction (Kalkhoff et al., 1971), and normal subjects have developed hyperinsulinism after they have been made obese by forced feeding (Sims et al., 1971), suggesting that insulin hypersecretion is a consequence of the obesity rather than a cause.

A cause of hyperinsulinism in obesity has been thought to be a compensating mechanism by the pancreatic beta cell in response to decreased insulin sensitivity or resistance to the action of insulin in peripheral tissues.

Obese subjects often have elevated blood glucose levels during a glucose tolerance test even in the presence of hyperinsulinism (Rabinowitz and Zierler, 1962). As beta cells produce additional insulin to compensate for tissue resistance, hyperplasia (increase in cell number) of the islet cells may result. Salans et al. (1968) reported a decreased response to insulin of enlarged adipose tissue cells from obese subjects. The insulin resistance of large adipocytes may be due to an intracellular defect in glucose metabolism (Olefsky, 1976). However, Davidson (1972) was not able to demonstrate insulin insensitivity in abdominal adipose tissue from obese humans.

Grey and Kipnis (1971) suggested that the hyperinsulinemia of obesity may be a result, at least in part, of dietary factors rather than being produced exclusively as a consequence of cell insulin resistance. They fed isocaloric high-carbohydrate (62 percent) and low-carbohydrate (25 percent) diets to obese subjects during two successive 3-week periods. The high-carbohydrate diet produced higher serum insulin levels than did the low-carbohydrate diet, even with some weight loss by subjects in this study. Drenick et al. (1972) also suggested that excessive food intake stimulates hyperinsulinism in obese individuals, at least initially, and peripheral tissue resistance may be secondary to the chronic overproduction of insulin. Flatt (1972) postulated that an elevation of serum-free fatty acids in the obese individual, because of the large adipose tissue mass in the body, is the primary cause of elevated blood glucose and insulin levels because the increased free fatty acids depress the uptake of glucose by tissues.

Diabetes complicates even further the relationships between obesity and hyperinsulinism. Bompiani and Laudicina (1972) found apparent hyperinsulinism in both obese diabetics and obese nondiabetics. However, the pattern of insulin secretion after stimuli such as glucose differed markedly between simple obesity and diabetic obesity, with the first phase of insulin secretion being delayed in the diabetics. The percent of serum insulin increase over the basal insulin level was used as an indication of the magnitude of the beta cell response and was similar in nonobese control subjects and obese nondiabetics. The response was significantly lower in obese diabetics. Hyperinsulinism was relative and not absolute in the obese diabetic since it coexisted with a diminished beta cell response. Obese and nonobese diabetics apparently have in common the decreased insulin secretion capacity that is not shared by obese nondiabetics.

Associations between obesity and diabetes mellitus in populations from various countries have been reported on several occasions. The overall prevalence of adult-onset diabetes in a community appears to be largely determined by the prevalence of obesity in that population. In spite of these obvious associations, the nature of the relationship remains speculative. It has been suggested that, in obese individuals, the necessity of producing excessive quantities of insulin over a long period of time eventually results in exhaustion of the pancreas if they are genetically predisposed to diabetes. This is an attractive hypothesis but is not supported by data at the present. It is generally accepted, however, that caloric restriction and weight loss play important roles in the treatment of obese diabetic patients since improvement in clinical symptoms usually accompanies weight loss (Smith and Levine, 1964).

16.7 Etiology

It is generally agreed that genetic factors are important in the etiology of diabetes mellitus for most patients although the actual mechanisms of inheritance are not clear (Tattersall and Fajans, 1975). The familial nature of this disease was first reported by Morton in 1696 when he described a family with four diabetic siblings (Harris, 1950).

Autosomal recessive inheritance has been a favored hypothesis for the transmission of diabetes. Under this hypothesis all of the offspring of conjugal diabetics should inherit a predisposition to diabetes and, assuming full penetrance, all should develop the disease. Observed risks have been shown to be much lower than this (Frias and Rosenbloom, 1973).

A multifactorial mode of inheritance for diabetes has also been suggested. This claims that an additive effect of several genes at a number of loci determine the predisposition to diabetes.

Studies on twins have provided evidence for the hereditary nature of diabetes. Identical twins (monozygotic) are identical genetically. Fraternal (dizygotic) twins are no more alike genetically than are siblings. The rate of similarity (concordance) of identical twins has been compared to that of fraternal twins to give an indication of the relative effects of heredity and environment on the development of diabetes. White (1965) reported concordance to be 48 percent among identical twins but only 2 percent among fraternal twins studied. Tattersall and Pyke (1972) found 65 of 96 pairs (68 percent) of identical twins to be concordant for diabetes. However, of the 59 pairs in which the index twin developed diabetes *before* the age of 40, 31 (53 percent) were concordant and among the 37 pairs in which the index twin was diagnosed *after* the age of 40, all but 3 pairs (92 percent) were concordant. They also noted that half of the concordant twins were of the maturity-onset type, but almost all of the discordant twins were juvenile-onset diabetics. Further studies by Tattersall and Fajans (1975) suggested two different types of inheritance for the disease. In the families of maturity-onset patients, there was a diabetic parent 85 percent of the time, direct vertical transmission of the disease through three generations in 46 percent of the families, latent diabetes in 53 percent of the siblings tested, and the diabetic phenotype in the families was consistent with most affected individuals having the maturity-onset type of disease. These findings are compatible with an autosomal dominant mode of inheritance.

In the families of juvenile-onset diabetics, however, only 11 percent of the subjects had a diabetic parent, three generation inheritance was found in only 6 percent of the families, and only 11 percent of the tested siblings were diabetic. These differences suggest a need for careful definition of the phenotype of diabetes when the genetics of a population is analyzed.

Sound genetic counseling of patients concerning diabetes is difficult. However, counseling all diabetic patients on the basis of one mode of inheritance is incorrect (Zonana and Rimoin, 1976).

It has been suggested that juvenile-onset diabetes may be due to destruction of pancreatic beta cells by viruses. The lines of evidence supporting this hypothesis of the etiology of diabetes include studies by British workers of the seasonal incidence, more frequent in fall and winter, of juvenile-onset, insulin-requiring diabetes and an apparent relationship to elevated antibodies to Coxsackie virus Group B, Type 4. Viruses have also been isolated that produce a specific lesion in the pancreatic islets of mice. However, no such virus has yet been cultured from human tissues nor excreted by newly diagnosed diabetic patients (Steinke and Taylor, 1974).

Spontaneous diabetes syndromes have been observed in laboratory animals, such as sand rats (Schmidt-Nielsen et al., 1964), that had previously become habituated to semidesert vegetation, which is low in carbohydrate and high in fiber, and subsequently were fed ad libitum high-carbohydrate laboratory chow. The diabetic syndrome is frequently accompanied by obesity. A hypothesis has been proposed by Trowell (1975) that dietary fiber-depleted starchy foods are conducive to the development of diabetes in susceptible human genotypes.

Some evidence has suggested that insulin-dependent diabetes is an autoimmune disease resulting from production of antibodies against pancreatic beta cells (Huang and Maclaren, 1976). This hypothesis requires further exploration.

16.8 Stages in the Development of Diabetes

Diabetes apparently develops over a period of time or in stages. This is especially true of the maturity-onset, noninsulin-dependent types of disease. Individuals with a strong predisposition to develop diabetes, including healthy monozygotic twin siblings of diabetics and children of diabetic parents, have been considered to be prediabetics. All these potential diabetics, however, do not eventually develop diabetes and the firm diagnosis of prediabetes, or diabetes premellitus, as the first stage in the development of diabetes can only be made retrospectively after the patient has developed frank diabetes. It has been generally thought that no detectable metabolic disorders are present in prediabetes but Cerasi et al. (1972) reported decreased sensitivity of the beta cells to glucose in prediabetic subjects. They have suggested that the prediabetic state is characterized by normal glucose tolerance but decreased insulin secretion after glucose stimulation (Cerasi and Luft, 1972). Siperstein has questioned the concept that the beta cell is the primary site of diabetes development and has reported thickening of capillary basement membranes from muscle tissue of prediabetics (off-

Table 16.1 STAGES OF DIABETES MELLITUS

	FBS*	OGTT†	CGTT‡
Prediabetes	Normal	Normal	Normal
Chemical diabetes	Normal	↓ tolerance	May show ↓ tolerance when GTT normal
Clinical or overt diabetes	↑	↓ tolerance but test not usually necessary	Not necessary

* Fasting blood sugar.
† Oral glucose tolerance test.
‡ Cortisone glucose tolerance test.

spring of two diabetic parents). However, Williamson has attributed Siperstein's findings to a progressive age-related thickening of the basement membrane (Beeson and McDermott, 1975, pp. 1603–1604). The prediabetic state cannot be diagnosed in clinical practice and remains in the realm of the researcher.

The next stage of development for diabetes is chemical diabetes. The patient at this stage is asymptomatic but shows some degree of glucose intolerance on testing. Fasting blood sugar is usually normal but a glucose tolerance test (GTT) is abnormal. Serum insulin levels may be increased at this stage, especially in the maturity-onset type of disease. The stage of chemical diabetes has sometimes been divided into a subclinical stage, in which the standard GTT is normal but a cortisone-GTT is abnormal, and a latent stage, in which the standard GTT is abnormal and fasting blood sugar may be either normal or slightly increased. The cortisone-GTT requires the administration of cortisone acetate approximately 8½ and 2 hours before a GTT is given (Fajans, 1963). The administration of cortisone, which is glucogenic, produces an added stress that may unmask a slight insulin secreting deficiency not apparent on a standard GTT.

When fasting blood glucose levels are consistently abnormal, clinical or overt diabetes is diagnosed. At this stage the body has not been able to compensate for insulin secretion deficiencies and glucose intolerance is readily apparent. A GTT is not necessary at this stage. The stages of diabetes are summarized in Table 16.1.

16.9   Diagnosis

A case of diabetes becomes known only when diagnosed by a physician. Screening of large population groups has been practiced in recent years as an aid to the physician in detecting diabetes and encouraging treatment. By screening apparently healthy subjects, those who *probably* have the disease can be separated from those who *probably do not.* Both blood and urine tests for glucose have been used in screening but blood tests have greater validity and reproducibility.

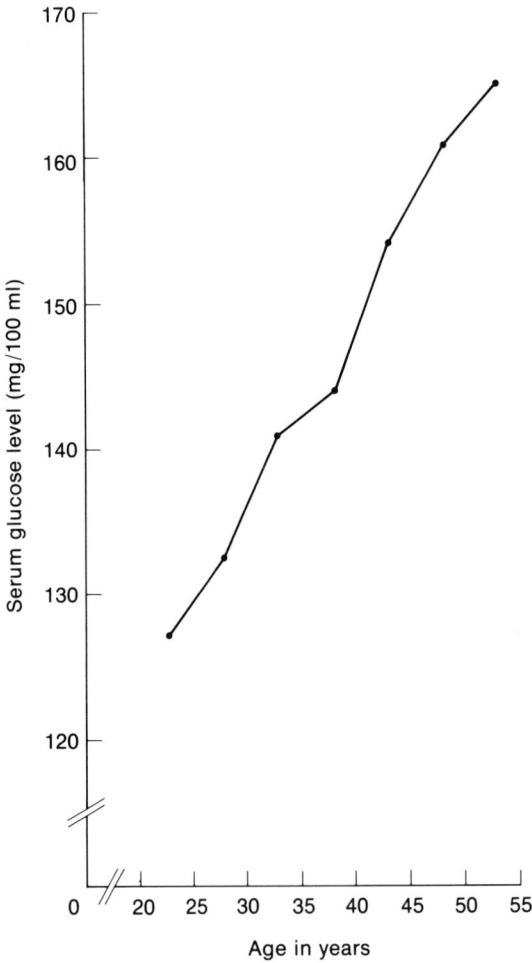

Fig. 16.9 Mean 1-hour serum glucose level by age. (From Nancy Phillips and Thomas Duffy, "Effect of Age, Hours Since Last Food, Time of Day, and Ketonuria on 1-Hour Glucose Tolerance," Health Services Reports, 87, **649**: 650, 1972.)

Glucose Tolerance Testing

The major sign for diagnosis of diabetes is demonstration of the inability to handle glucose, called glucose intolerance. Blood glucose values, both fasting and postprandial, may be measured. Whereas it is generally agreed that a 1-hour postprandial blood glucose value of 200 mg/100 ml or higher indicates diabetes, there is considerable discussion as to whether abnormality begins at 160, 170, or 180 mg/100 ml (Wintrobe et al., 1974, p. 538). West (1975) conducted an informal survey of the diagnostic criteria employed by 20 physicians with a special interest in diabetes and found a considerable range in the criteria used as plasma glucose values were interpreted, to the degree that disparities would result in major differences in the rates of "diabetes." The American Diabetes Association has released a guide to physicians for designing and interpreting GTTs (American Diabetes Association, 1974).

The upper limits for normalcy in blood glucose values increase with age. Phillips and Duffy (1972) reported that serum glucose levels of nondiabetic women increased linearly with age at the rate of 1.3 mg/100 ml per year (Fig. 16.9). Sandberg et al. (1973) suggested that release of growth hormone in older individuals is not adequately inhibited by the ingestion of glucose and, therefore, produces a state of insulin insensitivity with a resulting increase in blood glucose concentration. Williamson et al. (1971) adjusted values from normal oral GTTs upward by 10 mg/100 ml per decade over 40 years of age. There are also circadian variations in blood glucose levels of normal subjects, with lower values in the morning and higher values at 6 P.M. and midnight (Aparicio et al., 1974). If a subject has not been consuming a diet containing 250 to 300 g carbohydrate for at least 3 days before a standard oral GTT is given, a decreased glucose tolerance may be observed. Physical inactivity decreases glucose tolerance and a patient undergoing prolonged bed rest may give false positive results.

The usual procedure for a standard oral GTT includes first determining the level of fasting blood glucose, then giving a glucose solution to drink within 5 minutes (about 100 g glucose), and measuring blood glucose at $\frac{1}{2}$-, 1-, 2-, and 3-hour intervals. In some cases a 5-hour GTT may be desirable to check for postprandial hypoglycemia that may develop as a result of delayed insulin secretion in the early stages of maturity-onset diabetes. Urine samples are also tested for the presence of sugar (glycosuria). Upper-normal values obtained with venous blood measured by the autoanalyzer method are shown in Fig. 16.10 and may be: fasting, 100 mg/100 ml; $\frac{1}{2}$ hour (or peak value), 170 mg; 1 hour, 170 mg; 2 hours, 120 mg; and 3 hours, 110 mg/100 ml (Wintrobe et al., 1974, p. 539). Capillary blood glucose levels will be higher than venous blood levels; plasma or serum levels will be higher than whole blood. Several methods of analysis

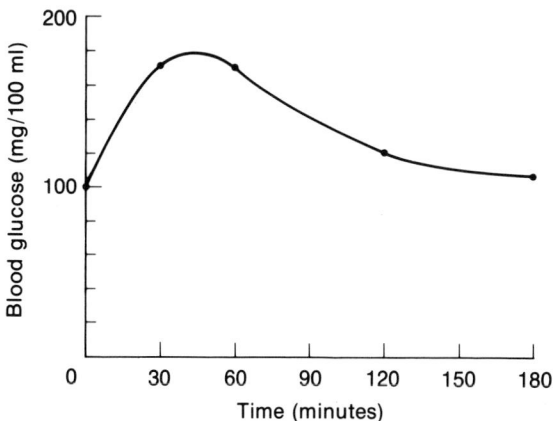

Fig. 16.10 Upper-normal blood glucose levels in oral glucose tolerance test (venous blood measured in autoanalyzer).

may be used for blood glucose. The only method that measures glucose per se uses glucose oxidase. Other methods, such as Nelson-Somogyi and Folin-Wu, measure all reducing substances.

An intravenous GTT may be desirable when intestinal absorption is abnormal. Olefsky et al. (1973) found a high incidence of diagnostic disagreement when the results of oral and intravenous GTTs were compared, however.

Clinical Signs

Juvenile-onset diabetes characteristically presents with symptoms of polyphagia, polyuria, polydipsia, weight loss, lassitude, and irritability. If the condition remains undiagnosed, nausea, vomiting, dehydration, acidosis, stupor, coma, and finally death will result. This progression may be rapid, especially in small children, or it may continue over a period of weeks to months. Unnoticed hyperglycemia and glucosuria may be brought to the attention of a physician by superimposed infection or stress.

Maturity-onset diabetes has a less stormy beginning and frequently symptoms are minimal or absent. Sometimes the patient consults a physician because of the vascular problems or a wound that does not heal. Glucose intolerance will be apparent on testing.

REFERENCES

1. Albrink, M. J. and P. C. Davidson. 1971. Dietary therapy and prophylaxis of vascular disease in diabetics. *Med. Clin. No. Am.,* **55:** 877.

2. American Diabetes Association. 1974. Educational Pamphlet on Detection and Diagnosis of Diabetes: Plasma glucose procedures.

3. Aparicio, N. J., F. E. Puchulu, J. J. Gagliardino, M. Ruiz, J. M. Llorens, J. Ruiz, A. Lamas, and R. DeMiguel. 1974. Circadian variation of the blood glucose, plasma insulin, and human growth hormone levels in response to an oral glucose load in normal subjects. *Diabetes,* **23:** 132.

4. Batchelor, B. R. 1967. Insulin-like activity. *Diabetes,* **16:** 418.

5. Beeson, P. B. and W. McDermott (Eds.). 1975. *Textbook of Medicine,* vol. II, 14th ed. Philadelphia: Saunders.

6. Bierman, E. L., J. D. Bagdade, and D. Porte, Jr. 1968. Obesity and diabetes: The odd couple. *Am. J. Clin. Nutr.,* **21:** 1434.

7. Bompiani, G. D. and E. Laudicina. 1972. Obesity and diabetes. *Israel J. Med. Sci.,* **8:** 823.

8. Cerasi, E. 1975. Mechanisms of glucose stimulated insulin secretion in health and in diabetes: Some re-evaluations and proposals. *Diabetologia,* **11:** 1.

9. Cerasi, E. and R. Luft. 1972. The prediabetic state, its nature and consequences—A look toward the future. *Diabetes,* **21** (Supplement 2): 685.

10. Cerasi, E., R. Luft, and S. Efendic. 1972. Decreased sensitivity of the pancreatic beta cells to glucose in prediabetic and diabetic subjects. *Diabetes,* **21:** 224.

11. Chiles, R. and M. Tzagournis. 1970. Excessive serum insulin response to oral glucose in obesity and mild diabetes. *Diabetes,* **19:** 458.

12. Chisholm, D. J., J. D. Young, and L. Lazarus. 1969. The gastrointestinal stimulus to insulin release. I. Secretin. *J. Clin. Investig.,* **48:** 1453.

13. Cohen, A. M. 1972. Environmental aspects of diabetes. *Israel J. Med. Sci.,* **8:** 358.

14. Davidson, M. B. 1972. Effect of obesity on insulin sensitivity of human adipose tissue. *Diabetes,* **21:** 6.

15. Drenick, E. J., A. S. Brickman, and E. M. Gold. 1972. Dissociation of the obesity-hyperinsulinism relationship following dietary restriction and hyperalimentation. *Am. J. Clin. Nutr.,* **25:** 746.

16. Fain, J. N. and L. Rosenberg. 1972. Antilipolytic action of insulin on fat cells. *Diabetes,* **21** (Supplement 2): 414.

17. Fajans, S. S. 1963. Cortisone-glucose tolerance test. *J. Am. Med. Assoc.,* **186:** 279.

18. Fajans, S. S., J. C. Floyd, Jr., R. B. Tattersall, J. R. Williamson, S. Pek, and C. I. Taylor. 1976. The various faces of diabetes in the young. *Arch. Int. Med.,* **136:** 194.

19. Felig, P. 1971. Pathophysiology of diabetes mellitus. *Med. Clinics No. Am.,* **55:** 821.

20. Felig, P. 1974. Diabetic ketoacidosis. *N. Eng. J. Med.,* **290:** 1360.

21. Felig, P., T. Pozefsky, E. Marliss, and G. F. Cahill, Jr. 1970. Alanine: Key role in gluconeogenesis. *Science,* **167:** 1003.

22. Felig, P., J. Wahren, R. Sherwin, and R. Hendler. 1976. Insulin, glucagon, and somatostatin in normal physiology and diabetes mellitus. *Diabetes,* **25:** 1091.

23. Flatt, J. 1972. Role of the increased adipose tissue mass in the apparent insulin insensitivity of obesity. *Am. J. Clin. Nutr.,* **25:** 1189.

24. Frias, J. L. and A. L. Rosenbloom. 1973. The genetics of diabetes. *Metabolism,* **22:** 355.

25. Fujita, Y., A. L. Herron, Jr., and H. S. Seltzer. 1975. Confirmation of impaired early insulin response to glycemic stimulus in nonobese mild diabetics. *Diabetes,* **24:** 17.

26. Gorwitz, K., G. G. Howen, and T. Thompson. 1976. Prevalence of diabetes in Michigan school-age children. *Diabetes,* **25:** 122.

27. Grey, N. and D. M. Kipnis. 1971. Effect of diet composition on the hyperinsulinemia of obesity. *N. Eng. J. Med.,* **285:** 827.

28. Groen, J. J. 1972. Discovery of insulin told as a human story. *Israel J. Med. Sci.,* **8:** 476.

29. Hales, C. N. 1966. The glucose-fatty acid cycle and the aetiology of diabetes. *Proc. Nutr. Soc.,* **25:** 61.

30. Harris, H. 1950. The familial distribution of diabetes mellitus: A study of the relatives of 1241 diabetic propositi. *Ann. Eugen.,* **15:** 95.

31. Himsworth, H. P. 1935–1936. Diet and the incidence of diabetes mellitus. *Clin. Sci.,* **2:** 117.

32. Himsworth, H. P. 1949. The syndrome of diabetes mellitus and its causes. *Lancet,* **1:** 465.

33. Huang, S. and N. K. Maclaren. 1976. Insulin-dependent diabetes: A disease of autoaggression. *Science,* **192:** 64.

34. Jackson, W. P. U., W. Van Miegham, and P. Keller. 1972. Insulin excess as the initial lesion in diabetes. *Lancet,* **1:** 1040.

35. Johansen, K. 1972. Normal initial plasma insulin response in mild diabetes. *Metabolism,* **21:** 1177.

36. Kahn, H. A., J. B. Herman, J. H. Medalie, H. N. Neufeld, E. Riss, and U. Goldbourt. 1971. Factors related to diabetes incidence: A multivariate analysis of two years and observation on 10,000 men. *J. Chron. Dis.,* **23:** 617.

37. Kalkhoff, R. K., H. J. Kim, J. Cerletty, and C. A. Ferrou. 1971. Metabolic effects of weight loss in obese subjects. *Diabetes,* **20:** 83.

38. Karam, J. H., G. M. Grodsky, and P. H. Forsham. 1963. Excessive insulin response to glucose in obese subjects as measured by immunochemical assay. *Diabetes,* **12:** 197.

39. Katsoyannis, P. G. 1966. Synthesis of insulin. *Science,* **154:** 1509.

40. Krahl, M. E. 1972. Insulin action at the molecular level. *Diabetes,* **21** (Supplement 2): 695.

41. Lacy, P. E. 1972. The secretion of insulin. *Diabetes,* 21 (Supplement 2): 510.

42. Levine, R. 1972. Action of insulin: An attempt at a summary. *Diabetes* 21 (Supplement 2): 454.

43. Lilly Research Laboratories. 1973. Diabetes Mellitus, 7th ed. Indianapolis, Ind.: Eli Lilly and Company.

44. Malaisse, W. J. 1972. Role of calcium in insulin secretion. *Israel J. Med. Sci.,* **8:** 244.

45. Malaisse, W. J. 1973. Insulin secretion: Multifactorial regulation for a single process of release. *Diabetologia,* **9:** 167.

46. Nikkila, E. A. and M. Taskinen. 1971. The insulin secretion rate in obesity. *Postgrad. Med. J.,* Supplement, p. 412.

47. Ogawa, 'S. 1969. Insulin in blood. *N.Y. State J. Med.,* **69:** 1201.

48. Ohneda, A., E. Aguilar-Parada, A. M. Eisentraut, and R. H. Unger. 1969. Control of pancreatic glucagon secretion by glucose. *Diabetes,* **18:** 1.

49. Olefsky, J. M. 1976. The insulin receptor: Its role in insulin resistance of obesity and diabetes. *Diabetes,* **25:** 1154.

50. Olefsky, J. M., J. W. Farquhar, and G. M. Reaven. 1973. Do the oral and intravenous glucose tolerance tests provide similar diagnositc information in patients with chemical diabetes mellitus? *Diabetes,* **22:** 202.

51. O'Sullivan, J. B. and C. M. Mahan. 1965. Blood sugar levels, glycosuria, and body weight related to development of diabetes mellitus. *J. Am. Med. Assoc.,* **194:** 587.

52. Park, C. R., S. B. Lewis, and J. H. Exton. 1972. Relationship of some hepatic actions of insulin to the intracellular level of cyclic adenylate. *Diabetes,* **21** (Supplement 2): 439.

53. Phillips, N. and T. Duffy. 1972. Effect of age, hours since last food, time of day, and ketonuria on 1-hour glucose tolerance. *Health Ser. Repts.,* **87:** 649.

54. Rabinowitz, D. and K. L. Zierler. 1962. Forearm metabolism in obesity and its response to intra-arterial insulin. Characterization of insulin resistance and evidence for adaptive hyperinsulinism. *J. Clin. Invest.,* **41:** 2173.

55. Raptis, S., K. E. Schroder, G. Rothenbuchner, and E. F. Pfeiffer. 1972. Effect of the gastrointestinal hormones, secretin and cholecystokinin-pancreozymin, on insulin and glucagon release in healthy and diabetic subjects. *Israel J. Med. Sci.,* **8:** 769.

56. Reynolds, C., G. D. Molnar, D. L. Horwitz, A. H. Rubenstein, W. F. Taylor, and N. Jiang. 1977. Abnormalities of endogenous glucagon and insulin in unstable diabetes. *Diabetes,* **26:** 36.

57. Rosselin, G. E., J. R. Claude, E. P. Eschwege, E. Patois, J. M. Warnet, and J. L. Richard. 1971. Diabetes survey. Plasma insulin during 0–2 hour oral glucose tolerance test systematically carried out in a professional group. *Diabetologia,* **7:** 34.

58. Salans, L. B., J. L. Knittle, and J. Hirsch. 1968. The role of adipose cell size and adipose tissue insulin sensitivity in the carbohydrate intolerance of human obesity. *J. Clin. Invest.,* **47:** 153.

59. Sandberg, H., N. Yoshimine, S. Maeda, D. Symons, and J. Zavodnick. 1973. Effects of an oral glucose load on serum immunoreactive insulin, free fatty acid, growth hormone and blood sugar levels in young and elderly subjects. *J. Am. Ger. Soc.,* **21:** 433.

60. Sanger, F. 1959. Chemistry of insulin. *Science,* **129:** 1340.

61. Schmidt-Nielsen, K., H. B. Haines, and D. B. Hackel. 1964. Diabetes mellitus in the sand rat induced by standard laboratory diets. *Science,* **143:** 689.

62. Sharp, G. W. G., C. Wollheim, W. A. Muller, A. Gutzeit, P. A. Trueheart, B. Blondel, L. Orci, and A. E. Renold. 1975. Studies on the mechanism of insulin release. *Fed. Proc.,* **34:** 1537.

63. Sherwin, R. S., M. Fisher, R. Hendler, and P. Felig. 1976. Hyperglucagonemia and blood glucose regulation in normal, obese and diabetic subjects. *N. Eng. J. Med.,* **294:** 455.

64. Sims, E. A. H., E. S. Horton, and L. B. Salans. 1971. Inducible metabolic abnormalities during development of obesity. *Ann. Rev. Med.,* **22:** 235.

65. Smith, M. and R. Levine. 1964. Obesity and diabetes. *Med. Clinics No. Am.,* **48:** 1387.

66. Steiner, D. F., W. Kemmler, H. S. Tager, and J. D. Peterson. 1974. Proteolytic processing in the biosynthesis of insulin and other proteins. *Fed. Proc.,* **33:** 2105.

67. Steinke, J. and K. W. Taylor. 1974. Viruses and the etiology of diabetes. *Diabetes,* **23:** 631.

68. Stephan, F., P. Reville, R. Thierry, and J. L. Schlienger. 1972. Correlations between plasma insulin and body weight in obesity, anorexia nervosa and diabetes mellitus. *Diabetologia,* **8:** 196.

69. Tattersall, R. B. and S. S. Fajans. 1975. A difference between the inheritance of classical juvenile-onset and maturity-onset type diabetes of young people. *Diabetes,* **24:** 44.

70. Tattersall, R. B. and D. A. Pyke. 1972. Diabetes in identical twins. *Lancet,* **2:** 1120.

71. Trowell, H. C. 1975. Dietary-fiber hypothesis of the etiology of diabetes mellitus. *Diabetes,* **24:** 762.

72. U.S. Department of Health, Education and Welfare, Public Health Service. 1969. *Diabetes Source Book.* PHS, DHEW Publication: No. 1168.

73. Unger, R. H. 1972. Insulin/glucagon ratio. *Israel J. Med. Sci.,* **8:** 252.

74. Unger, R. H. and L. Orci. 1977. Role of glucagon in diabetes. *Arch. Int. Med.,* **137:** 482.

75. Weber, G. 1972. Integrative action of insulin at the molecular level. *Israel J. Med. Sci.,* **8:** 325.

76. West, K. M. 1975. Substantial differences in the diagnostic criteria used by diabetes experts. *Diabetes,* **24:** 641.

77. West, K. M. and J. M. Kalbfleisch. 1971. Influence of nutritional factors on prevalence of diabetes. *Diabetes,* **20:** 99.

78. White, P. 1965. The inheritance of diabetes. *Med. Clinics No. Am.,* **49:** 857.

79. Williamson, J. R., N. J. Vogler, and C. Kilo. 1971. Microvascular disease in diabetes. *Med. Clinics No. Am.,* **55:** 847.

80. Wintrobe, M. M., G. W. Thorn, R. D. Adams, E. Braunwald, K. J. Isselbacher, and R. G. Petersdorf (Eds.). 1974. *Harrison's Principles of Internal Medicine,* 7th ed. New York: McGraw-Hill.

81. Yudkin, J. 1964. Dietary fat and dietary sugar in relation to ischaemic heart disease and diabetes. *Lancet,* **2:** 4.

82. Zonana, J. and D. L. Rimoin. 1976. Inheritance of diabetes mellitus. *N. Eng. J. Med.,* **295:** 603.

STUDY GUIDE

There are two major types of diabetes mellitus.

1. Identify differences and similarities between juvenile-onset and adult-onset diabetes

Diabetes, particularly the maturity-onset disease, develops through several stages.

2. Outline the major characteristics of prediabetes, chemical diabetes, and overt or clinical diabetes.

3. Explain how a possible prediabetic individual might be identified.

Several factors have been suggested in the etiology of diabetes mellitus.

4. Evaluate the evidence for several proposed mechanisms for inheritance of diabetes.

5. Discuss the possible role of viruses and of fiber in etiology of diabetes.

Insulin has both direct and indirect effects on body metabolism.

6. Describe a proposed theory for insulin secretion by pancreatic beta cells and distinguish between proinsulin and insulin.

7. Describe two phases of insulin secretion in the body and explain how this pattern may be altered in many maturity-onset diabetics.

8. List types of cells that require and those that do not require insulin for the transport of glucose across cell membranes.

9. Describe probable effects of insulin on metabolism in muscle cells, adipose cells, and liver cells, and explain pathological changes that occur in diabetes, both mild and severe.

10. Relate the classical symptoms of polyphagia, polydipsia, and polyuria in severe diabetes to the metabolic abnormalities described in (9).

11. Discuss possible relationships between insulin and glucagon in nondiabetic and diabetic individuals.

Methods are available for measuring blood insulin levels.

12. Explain the general principles involved in the measurement of serum insulin by radioimmunoassay.

13. Compare with normal weight nondiabetics the usual levels of fasting blood insulin for obese nondiabetics, normal weight juvenile-onset diabetics, and obese maturity-onset diabetics.

A relationship is apparent, but unexplained, between obesity and diabetes.

14. Give possible explanations for hyperinsulinism in the obese.

15. Discuss possible interrelationships between obesity and diabetes.

A glucose tolerance test (GTT) is often used in the diagnosis of diabetes mellitus.

16. Describe the usual procedure involved in an oral GTT and identify abnormal patterns of blood glucose in the test.

17. Explain differences in procedure and expected results between a standard oral GTT and a cortisone-GTT and suggest when each of these tests might be useful.

18. Outline clinical and laboratory data that are useful in diagnosis of juvenile-onset and adult-onset diabetes.

17

Diabetes Mellitus – Treatment and Complications

Diet therapy is a major component of treatment for any type of diabetes mellitus and is the *fundamental* element of therapy in most cases of maturity-onset disease (West, 1973). Diet is balanced with appropriately prescribed hypoglycemic medication (insulin or oral agents) and exercise.

The Committee on Food and Nutrition of the American Diabetes Association presented a special report in 1971 on the principles of nutrition and dietary recommendations for patients with diabetes mellitus. They emphasized the importance of (1) controlling caloric intake to achieve ideal weight; (2) spacing food intake regularly in relation to insulin injection and physical activity; (3) adjusting proportions and types of carbohydrate and fat to the extent permitted by the present state of research knowledge; and (4) individualizing treatment to meet specific patient needs.

This chapter emphasizes dietary treatment in relation to type of diabetes and use of hypoglycemic agents. Complications of diabetes are also discussed.

17.1 Correction of Obesity

Weight reduction is of primary importance in treatment of the obese maturity-onset diabetic. With reduction to normal body weight, glucose intolerance and hyperinsulinemia often return to normal. It is usually not easy for an obese diabetic to consistently follow a low-kilocalorie diet. Strong motivation is essential. The long-term success rate for obese individuals who have been advised to lose weight for medical reasons is generally reported to be poor. A real appreciation by dietitians, physicians, and patients of the profoundly beneficial effects of weight reduction for obese maturity-onset diabetics may increase the vigor and skill that is applied to programs aimed at the correction of obesity (West, 1973).

It is not clarified completely as to whether obesity associated with diabetes is influenced by genetic makeup and deranged metabolism of the disease itself or is due simply to an excessive intake of kilocalories. Feldman et al. (1969) reported that fat was distributed on the body differently in diabetics than in nondiabetics, especially in females, with a greater proportion of fat on the trunk for those with diabetes—a more masculine characteristic. They suggested that this may be due to a disturbance of male/female hormone balance. In any case, the correction of obesity must be accomplished through caloric restriction. The type of diet used for weight reduction may be similar to that used in the nondiabetic obese patient. Low-kilocalorie diets are discussed in Sec. 5.6. Bistrian et al. (1976) reported successful weight reduction in seven insulin-requiring, adult-onset diabetics who were markedly obese by use of a protein-sparing modified fast. The only food given was lean beef or equivalent animal protein to supply 0.8 to 1.0 g protein per kg ideal body weight per day. Insulin was discontinued after 0 to 19 days. Modified fasting for weight reduction is discussed in Sec. 5.2.

The dietitian should continually search for innovative approaches to obese patients with diabetes, either individually or in groups, so that their personal motivation to achieve normal weight through consumption of a nutritious low-kilocalorie diet is maintained at a high level. The importance of this effort was emphasized by the Committee on Food and Nutrition of the American Diabetes Association (1971) in a statement that "the single most important objective in dietary treatment of diabetic patients is control of total caloric intake to attain ideal body weight." Although the advantages of weight reduction in the obese maturity-onset diabetic are apparent on a short-term basis, more research is needed to determine the long-term effects on vascular changes, morbidity, and mortality.

17.2 Composition of the Diet

The goals of diet therapy for patients with diabetes are to control hyperglycemia and glycosuria and also to reduce the known risk factors associated with atherosclerosis, to which the diabetic is predisposed, particularly in the United States (Committee on Food and Nutrition, 1971; Weinsier et al., 1974a). Although the optimum proportions of dietary carbohydrate and fat to achieve these goals are not well established, some data have been reported and will be discussed.

Dietary Fat Modification and Hyperlipidemia

In the late 1920s, early 1930s, and even later, some clinicians proposed high-carbohydrate and relatively low-fat diets for individuals with diabetes (Himsworth, 1935–1936 and 1949), although these suggestions were not generally accepted. There was concern even then about possible relationships among high-fat diets, atherosclerosis, and premature coronary heart disease (CHD) in patients with diabetes.

Serum triglycerides, nonesterified fatty acids, and possibly cholesterol are increased in poorly controlled diabetes. These increased blood lipid levels may persist in some diabetic patients in spite of reasonably good control of hyperglycemia. It is important to know whether the hyperlipidemia noted in a diabetic patient is due to poor control of the disease state or to other causes. This can only be determined by careful testing.

Obesity per se has been shown by Sailer et al. (1966) to be related to an increase in plasma triglycerides and this effect may be increased in an obese individual with diabetes. Diabetics seem to respond to dietary treatment of hyperlipidemias in much the same way as do nondiabetics, however, as long as reasonable control of hyperglycemia is maintained (Schroepfer et al., 1960). Dietary treatment of hyperlipidemia is discussed in Sec. 20.4.

Stone and Connor (1963) gave to a group of diabetic subjects a diet restricted to 100 mg cholesterol daily, with 20 percent of kilocalories as fat (slightly increased in polyunsaturates) and 64 percent carbohydrate. Diabetic control was good or excellent in most of the patients, serum cholesterol levels were reduced, and serum triglycerides did not increase with the elevated carbohydrate. One young man in the experimental group was taking over 500 g carbohydrate daily without any increase in insulin requirements. Bierman and Hamlin (1961) fed to diabetic subjects a formula diet containing 15 percent protein, 85 percent carbohydrate, and no fat and found that this caused hypertriglyceridemia in a number of cases. Stone and Connor suggested that approximately 20 percent fat may prevent the increase in serum triglycerides that has been reported with diets very low in fat.

Albrink (1971) stressed the importance of dietary treatment for any lipid abnormalities found in diabetic patients. There must be a careful measurement of blood lipids, however, in order to determine the need for and most appropriate type of diet therapy. She has suggested that serum lipids should be measured 2 to 3 months after any acute illness, when the eating pattern is usual, when weight has been steady for at least 2 weeks, and when no alcohol has been taken for at least 24 hours. Testing should be repeated two or three times at weekly intervals, after which classification of hyperlipoproteinemia can be made and an appropriate diet prescribed. In cases of severe diabetes with hyperlipoproteinemia, correction of obesity by caloric restriction is very important, just as it is in the milder type of diabetes that is noninsulin-dependent. It is expected that successful dietary treatment of hyperlipoproteinemias in diabetic patients will decrease their risk of developing premature CHD. More research is needed to determine if this will actually occur, however.

Kinsell (1962) made a case a number of years ago for the routine use of diets high in polyunsaturated fat for diabetics. However, the Committee on Food and Nutrition of the American Diabetes Association (1971) felt that because of "uncertainties regarding the long-term effects of the ingestion of large quantities of unsaturated fat . . . . possible additional benefits to be gained by this dietary modification were not sufficient to warrant inclusion as a general recommendation for diabetics at the present time."

Dietary Carbohydrate and Glucose Tolerance

Before the discovery of insulin in 1921, extreme dietary carbohydrate and kilocalorie restrictions were essential for diabetic patients. There were realistically no alternatives. After insulin therapy became available, a somewhat more liberal allowance of dietary carbohydrate was commonly made but there was still considerable carbohydrate restriction in comparison to usual consumption by the nondiabetic population. Traditionally, 150 to 200 g carbohydrate per day have been recommended for diabetics. Some reported data suggest advantages for a higher level of dietary carbohydrate.

Brunzell et al. (1971) reported improved glucose tolerance with 85 percent carbohydrate, 15 percent protein, and fat-free formula diets given seven normal and five mild diabetic subjects. The carbohydrate was either dextrose or dextrimaltose. Some of the subjects developed elevated serum triglyceride levels on the high carbohydrate intake. In an extension of this study, Brunzell et al. (1974) reported that glucose tolerance was improved, as indicated by a 22 mg/100 ml decrease in fasting plasma glucose, on the high-carbohydrate diet in diabetics who were treated with insulin or oral hypoglycemic agents. This diet given before treatment with hypoglycemic medication did not improve glucose tolerance, however, and glucosuria was actually increased by the high-carbohydrate intake in this case. Weinsier et al. (1974a) found diabetic control and insulin secretory capacity to be maintained in mild and moderately severe diabetic outpatients on 60 percent carbohydrate, 25 percent fat diets for 20 weeks. Kiehm et al. (1976) fed a 75 percent carbohydrate diet of regular foods, containing 15 g crude fiber, to 13 diabetic subjects. After 2 weeks on the diet, glucose tolerance was improved to the extent that the five subjects on sulfonylureas were able to discontinue this medication and insulin was decreased or discontinued in five subjects. Insulin requirements and fasting plasma glucose values were not changed in three men requiring 40 to 55 units of insulin. Anderson (1977) reported that glucose tolerance was slightly improved by a 75 percent carbohydrate diet fed for a week to men with chemical diabetes. More research is needed to clarify the effects of high-carbohydrate diets on glucose tolerance in diabetics, but apparently a relatively high proportion of carbohydrate in the diet of a treated diabetic does not decrease glucose tolerance.

Ernest et al. (1965) followed nine diabetic patients on a carbohydrate-rich, fat-poor diet for $1\frac{1}{2}$ to $2\frac{1}{2}$ years to determine if the diet would normalize some of the vascular changes that were occurring, particularly retinopathy. They found a decrease in hard exudates in the retina, but proliferative lesions tended to progress regardless of the high-carbohydrate diet.

The Committee on Food and Nutrition of the American Diabetes Association (1971) suggested that there is probably no need to restrict the proportion of carbohydrate within the allowed kilocalories. The usual 45 percent of kilocalories or even somewhat higher levels might be used. Hypertriglyceridemia should be monitored on an individual basis for those susceptible to this condition. With the possible use of relatively high carbohydrate diets, primarily from complex carbohydrates such as starch, dietary patterns may be adapted to individual needs and desires.

17.3   Chromium and Diabetes

In 1959 Schwarz and Mertz reported impaired glucose tolerance in rats raised on purified diets that could be prevented by trivalent chromium. A syndrome resembling moderately severe diabetes mellitus that occurred in chromium-deficient rats could be rapidly reversed by feeding chromium. Chromium (III) is evidently a cofactor with insulin in affecting the uptake of glucose at the cellular level (National Research Council, 1974a).

Evidence for a chromium deficiency in humans is based partly on the impairment of oral or intravenous glucose tolerance that is improved by increased chromium intake (World Health Organization, 1973). The causes of glucose intolerance are many and deficiency of chromium may be one contributing factor in some individuals. Small numbers of diabetic patients have been studied to determine their response to chromium supplementation. In a few subjects, an improvement in glucose tolerance has been noted, whereas in others there has been no improvement (Glinsmann et al., 1966; Schroeder, 1968; Sherman et al., 1968). A readily absorbable form of chromium is not available and limits the study of chromium nutrition in humans. Absorbable chromium in foods is evidently present in the form of a complex called the glucose tolerance factor (GTF). This factor has been isolated in the laboratory but is not available for dietary supplementation.

The concentration of chromium in human hair samples has been measured as a possible indication of body chromium status. Hambidge et al. (1968) found that the mean level of chromium in the hair of 19 children with juvenile-onset diabetes was significantly lower than that of 33 normal children. Benjanuvatra and Bennion (1975) found significantly lower concentrations of chromium in the hair of Thai diabetics with maturity-onset diabetes as compared with nondiabetics of similar age and sex. Morgan (1972) found mean liver chromium to be significantly decreased in elderly diabetic subjects in comparison to a control group.

Relationships among chromium, glucose intolerance, and diabetes are not clear. Certainly chromium deficiency does not appear to be a major cause of diabetes. However, there are chromium-responsive forms of impaired glucose tolerance and this element is essential for effective insulin action in the body.

17.4 Diet Prescriptions and Patterns

A diet prescription for an individual with diabetes may specify the total kilocalories and grams of protein, fat, and carbohydrate to be consumed on a daily basis. If the individual is insulin-dependent, it may also specify the distribution of carbohydrate throughout the day.

Kilocalories
The first step in arriving at an appropriate diet prescription is determining the daily caloric need that will allow the patient with diabetes to maintain ideal body weight and, if the patient is a child, provide for growth. The National Research Council's recommended dietary allowances (1974b) for kilocalories may be used as a guide in setting tentative caloric levels. Many adult-onset diabetics are obese and allowance must be made for satisfactory weight loss. There is great variation among normal individuals in the kilocalories required to maintain body weight, and this variation is also present among individuals with diabetes. Approximate estimates of caloric need may be made, however, and then adjusted as the regimen is tried. If a patient begins to gain undesirable weight on the initial diet prescription, the prescribed kilocalories should be reduced.

In estimating a caloric prescription, basal metabolic need may be considered first with an appropriate percentage of this amount added for physical activity. Although it probably underestimates to some degree and does not make an allowance for the slightly higher basal metabolism of men as compared to women (Pike and Brown, 1975, pp. 832–833), a rough estimate of basal metabolic energy need for a 24-hour period may be made by assuming that 1 kcal is used per kg ideal body weight per hour, or 24 kcal × ideal body weight in kg. This may be adjusted immediately by adding 100 to 300 kcal if the person is young, tall, and male or subtracting a similar amount if the person is elderly, short, and female. As an example, an estimate of basal metabolic energy need for a 24-year-old female secretary whose ideal weight is 58 kg (128 lb) would be 58 × 24 = 1392 kcal.

If the patient does light activity, 30 percent of the basal kilocalories may be added to the estimate for basal energy need. If the activity level is moderate or heavy, 50 to 75 percent of basal kilocalories may be added. For the 24-year-old secretary whose activity level is light, $0.30 \times 1392 = 418$ and $1392 + 418 = 1810$ estimated total kilocalories needed daily.

An alternate procedure for estimating caloric need is to use the following figures, which include estimates for basal metabolism:

Activity Level	Kcal/kg Ideal Wt	Kcal/lb Ideal Wt
Very light	25	11.4
Light	30	13.6
Moderate	35	15.9
Heavy	40	18.2

Using these figures, the 24-year-old secretary with light activity would require approximately 1740 kcal daily to maintain her ideal body weight.

Persons of larger body size require proportionately more energy per unit of time for physical activities than do smaller persons and slightly higher basal energy needs also accompany larger size. Weight may be used as a basis for adapting energy allowances for differences in body size as long as the individuals are not appreciably over- or underweight (National Research Council, 1974b). Ideal body weights are used in the estimation of total energy need but it should be realized that an overweight diabetic may be using additional energy to move his larger body unless he compensates by decreased activity.

Protein

Fifteen to 20 percent of total kilocalories are often derived from protein in a diabetic diet although the usual intake of protein for nondiabetics in the United States is 10 to 15 percent. For the 24-year-old secretary, requiring 1810 kcal, 15 to 20 percent of total kcal as protein calories is

$$0.15 \times 1810 \text{ kcal} = 272 \text{ kcal} \qquad \text{to} \qquad 0.20 \times 1810 \text{ kcal} = 362 \text{ kcal}$$

$$\frac{272 \text{ kcal}}{4 \text{ kcal/g protein}} = 68 \text{ g protein} \qquad \text{to} \qquad \frac{362 \text{ kcal}}{4 \text{ kcal/g protein}} = 91 \text{ g protein}$$

An alternative approach to determining protein need for the individual with diabetes is to allow 1 to $1\frac{1}{2}$ g protein per kg ideal body weight ($\frac{1}{2}$ to $\frac{2}{3}$ g/lb). Using these figures, the secretary might be given

$$1.0 \times 58 \text{ kg} = 58 \text{ g protein} \qquad \text{to} \qquad 1.5 \times 58 \text{ kg} = 87 \text{ g protein}$$

The decision for actual protein prescription should be made on an individual basis, considering physical condition and personal preferences.

Carbohydrate and Fat

Percentage of kilocalories from carbohydrate may be 40 to 60 percent. Research suggesting that a liberal intake of carbohydrate may be permitted for a diabetic is reviewed in Sec. 17.2. Increasing the level of carbohydrate in the diet allows a corresponding decrease in fat. Hyperlipoproteinemias should be treated on an individual basis with appropriate adjustment in the proportions of fat and carbohydrate.

If the 24-year-old secretary is given 50 percent of the total kilocalories as carbohydrate, she will have

$$0.50 \times 1810 \text{ kcal} = \frac{905 \text{ kcal}}{4 \text{ kcal/g Cho}}$$

$$= 226 \text{ g carbohydrate}$$

If she were receiving 68 g protein ($68 \times 4 = 272$ kcal) and 905 kcal from carbohydrate, she would have $272 + 905 = 1177$ kcal from protein and carbohydrate. Therefore, $1810 - 1177 = 633$ kcal would be available from fat. This would allow

$$\frac{633 \text{ kcal}}{9 \text{ kcal/g fat}} = 70 \text{ g fat}$$

For convenience, figures for protein, fat, and carbohydrate are often rounded off to the nearest multiple of 5. Therefore, a possible diet prescription for the 24-year-old secretary is 70 P, 70 F, and 225 Cho with 1810 kcal.

Distribution of Kilocalories

For any diabetic, kilocalories should be spread throughout the day in order to allow the body to metabolize energy nutrients at a reasonable rate without periods of overload. For the insulin-dependent diabetic it is especially important to distribute kilocalories, and particularly carbohydrate calories, so that they will be available for insulin activity (see Table 17.4). For intermediate-acting insulins taken in the morning, a snack is usually given in the afternoon or at bedtime, depending on the individual's schedule and lateness of the dinner hour. Distribution of carbohydrate and kilocalories might be 2/7, 2/7, 2/7, and 1/7 for breakfast, lunch, dinner, and bedtime feeding, respectively. For labile insulin-dependent diabetics, particularly children, additional snacks are desirable and distribution may be 2/10, 2/10, 1/10, 3/10, and 1/10, allowing for a mid-afternoon and a bedtime snack, or it may be 2/10, 1/10, 2/10, 1/10, 3/10, and 1/10, with snacks given in the mid-morning, mid-afternoon, and evening. A stable maturity-onset diabetic who is noninsulin-dependent may distribute his kilocalories approximately in thirds.

If the 24-year-old secretary is taking an intermediate-acting insulin, her carbohydrate distribution might be 65, 65, 65, and 30 or it might be 60, 60, 65, and 40 with some protein and fat being included in each meal and snack so that the total kilocalories are distributed in a similar manner to the carbohydrate.

Calculation of Diet Patterns Using Exchange Lists

The system of exchanges discussed in Sec. 2.2 was originally developed by a joint committee of the American Dietetic Association, the American Diabetes Association, and the Diabetes Branch of the United States Public Health Service in response to a need for standardization and simplification of diets for patients with diabetes (Caso, 1950). The lists have been revised and updated in order to provide flexibility in their use for nutrition counseling.

Before a diet pattern is planned, information must be gathered on the patient's usual food practices, physical activities, and living conditions. The diet pattern is fitted to the individual and, therefore, the individual must be involved in its development. Data that will be helpful in this process may be collected from the medical record, interviews with the patient and/or the patient's family, and discussions with other health professionals. Knowledge about the individual's daily schedule on weekends as well as weekdays, patterns of physical exercise, cultural and religious influences on eating patterns, economic status, usual food preparation procedures, meals eaten away from home, personal food likes and dislikes, and type of insulin or oral hypoglycemic agent prescribed is important in the development of an appropriate diet pattern. Interviews with the patient will allow the dietitian to assess the patient's present state of knowledge concerning diet and diabetes and his or her probable learning capability and interest. Clues as to what might help motivate the patient in following the diet pattern may also come from interviews.

In assigning specific amounts from each exchange list for the patient, the clinician should begin with milk, vegetables, and fruits. A patient should be encouraged to include at least 2 cups of milk in the diet pattern each day unless there is a particular reason why milk should be eliminated. If milk fat is not appropriate in a diet, skim milk or buttermilk may be used. Choices from the vegetable list should be encouraged in liberal amounts to provide vitamins, minerals, and fiber in the diet. The patient should also be instructed on good sources of vitamin A and ascorbic acid. Desserts for the diabetic patient will usually be fruit, and since most listed servings of fruits are limited in amount (10 g carbohydrate), several daily fruit exchanges may be appropriate. If the amount of simple sugar in the diet is to be restricted, fruits may need to be limited to some degree.

After an estimated number of milk, vegetable, and fruit exchanges has been determined, a subtotal of carbohydrate included in them should be made, as indicated in Table 17.1 for the diet of the 24-year-old secretary. The only remaining exchange list that contains carbohydrate is the bread group. The remainder of the carbohydrate in the diet prescription may then be divided by 15 to determine the number of bread exchanges to be included. Bread supplies complex carbohydrate in the form of starch. With relatively high carbohydrate diets and an emphasis on complex carbohydrate, bread and starchy vegetables will find a prominent place in the diet pattern.

The next step in development of the diet pattern is to subtotal the amount of protein included thus far. All the remaining protein will come from meat exchanges and, therefore, this figure may be divided by seven to

Table 17.1 TOTAL DAILY DIET PATTERN* FOR 1800-KCAL DIET OF 24-YEAR-OLD SECRETARY

Exchange List	Number of Exchanges	Protein (g)	Fat (g)	Carbohydrate (g)	Energy (kcal)
Milk, skim	2	16		24	160
Vegetable	3	6		15	75
Fruit	5			50	200
Subtotal				**89**	
Bread	9	18		135	630
Subtotal		**40**			
Meat	5	35	15		275
Subtotal			**15**		
Fat	11		55		495
Total		75	70	224	1835

* Diet prescription: P 70, F 70, Cho 225, kcal 1800 (Cho distribution 60, 60, 65, 40).

Table 17.2 DIET PATTERN IN MEALS FOR 1800-KCAL DIET OF 24-YEAR-OLD SECRETARY

Meal	Exchanges Type	Number	Protein (g)	Fat (g)	Carbohydrate (g)	Energy (kcal)
Morning	Milk	1	8		12	80
	Fruit	2			20	80
	Bread	2	4		30	140
	Fat	4		20		180
	Meat	1	7	3		55
Total			19	23	62	535
Noon	Meat	2	14	6		110
	Vegetable	1	2		5	25
	Bread	3	6		45	210
	Fat	1		5		45
	Fruit	1			10	40
Total			22	11	60	430
Evening	Meat	2	14	6		110
	Vegetable	2	4		10	50
	Bread	3	6		45	210
	Fat	3		15		135
	Fruit	1			10	40
Total			24	21	65	545
Bedtime	Milk	1	8		12	80
	Bread	1	2		15	70
	Fat	3		15		135
	Fruit	1			10	40
Total			10	15	37	325
Daily Total			75	70	224	1835

Table 17.3 MENUS FOR 1800-KCAL DIET OF 24-YEAR-OLD SECRETARY

Meal	Exchanges Type	Exchanges Number	Food	Amount
Breakfast	Milk, whole	1	Whole milk	1 cup
	Fruit	2	Orange slices	2 small oranges
	Bread	1	Cornflakes	$\frac{3}{4}$ cup
	Bread	1	Whole wheat toast	1 slice
	Fat	1	Margarine	1 tsp
	Meat, med.-fat	1	Soft cooked egg	1
Lunch			Sandwich with:	
	Meat	2	Sliced turkey	2 oz
	Vegetable	As desired	Lettuce	As desired
	Bread	2	Whole wheat bread	2 slices
	Fat	1	Mayonnaise	1 tsp
	Vegetable	1	Celery and carrot sticks	$\frac{1}{2}$ cup
	Fruit	1	Fresh fig	1
	Bread	1	Graham crackers	2 squares
Dinner	Meat	2	Baked halibut	2 oz
	Vegetable	1	Green peas	$\frac{1}{2}$ cup
		1	Cauliflower	$\frac{1}{2}$ cup
	Bread	1	Baked potato	1 small
		2	Rye bread	2 slices
	Fat	3	Margarine	3 tsp
	Fruit	1	Fresh applesauce, artificially sweetened	$\frac{1}{2}$ cup
Bedtime	Milk, whole	1	Whole milk	1 cup
	Bread	1	Soda crackers	3
	Fat	1	Margarine	1 tsp
	Fruit	1	Fresh grapes	12

determine the number of meat choices to be included. The amount of fat in the pattern may then be subtotaled and the remaining grams of fat divided by five to determine the number of fat exchanges. This completes the diet pattern on a daily basis.

The daily total diet pattern must then be divided into meals and snacks with the carbohydrate distributed as indicated in the prescription. Division into meals is illustrated for the 24-year-old secretary in Table 17.2 and illustrative menus are shown in Table 17.3. Combinations of choices from the exchange lists may be put together in various recipes. Cookbooks that consider exchange lists are available (Little and Thorup, 1972).

17.5 Type of Dietary Carbohydrate and Blood Glucose Levels

It has been generally supposed that dietary monosaccharides and oligosaccharides are absorbed more rapidly from the digestive tract than are polysaccharides and that they thus produce a greater degree of hyperglycemia in the diabetic. However, varying data have been reported. Some studies have suggested that consumption of cooked starch and glucose have similar effects on blood glucose (Althausen and Uyeyama, 1954; Nugent and Millhon, 1958). Crapo et al. (1976) reported that, in normal subjects, 50 g glucose and 100 g sucrose produced similar blood glucose response curves but the sucrose elicited a 20 percent greater plasma insulin response. They also found that carbohydrates given in meals produced lower plasma glucose responses than the same carbohydrates given alone, although insulin responses were similar. Blood glucose and insulin responses to cooked potato were somewhat less than to a glucose drink, and the responses to cooked rice were significantly lower than to either cooked potato or glucose drink. Further research is needed in diabetic subjects to clarify these effects.

Lenner (1976a and b) found that breakfasts with the highest percentage of oligosaccharides caused the smallest increase in blood glucose level in adult diabetic subjects on isocaloric breakfasts with 45 percent of kilocalories from carbohydrate. The breakfasts containing 95 percent of total carbohydrate as starch or 70 percent as starch and 25 percent as lactose produced, approximately 1 hour after consumption, the greatest elevation in blood glucose. With five insulin-treated diabetics, the initial blood glucose level was of greater importance than the kind of carbohydrate consumed in determining the blood glucose rise after breakfast. Lenner concluded that postprandial blood glucose reaches higher levels because of the consumption of carbohydrates such as starch, that are built up of glucose units only, than because of sucrose, which on hydrolysis gives rise to both glucose and fructose. The differences in blood glucose response due to type of carbohydrate did not seem to remain when the proportion of total carbohydrate was changed to as high as 70 percent or as low as 35 percent of kilocalories. Oligosaccharide-rich meals created a greater tendency toward hypoglycemia, satiety was decreased, and hunger developed sooner than with polysaccharide-rich meals. Overfeeding and resultant weight gain are potential risks in this case and diabetic diets with relatively high proportions of the total carbohydrate as polysaccharides may be justified on these grounds alone.

Lenner (1976b) found no significant differences among sucrose, fructose, and sorbitol-containing meals in regard to the effect on blood glucose or on glucosuria with nine adult diabetics. Specially sweetened foods, containing sorbitol or fructose, apparently offer no advantages to the diabetic and may be expensive.

17.6   Alcohol and Diabetes

Ethanol has a number of effects that make planning for its use important for a person with diabetes. Alcohol causes hypoglycemia in fasting glycogen-depleted subjects because gluconeogenesis is inhibited while alcohol is being metabolized by liver cells. Friedenberg et al. (1971) reported that alcohol primed the islets of Langerhans and increased insulin secretion in mildly diabetic patients. However, Nikkila and Taskinen (1975) found no increase in insulin response of more severe diabetics with administration of ethanol. Walsh and O'Sullivan (1974) reported no deterioration in control of diabetes over a 24-hour period when 20 diabetic patients were given moderate amounts of alcohol. Two of the subjects in this study developed hypoglycemia, although it was not certain that alcohol was a causal factor since insufficient data were collected. They suggested that diabetic patients (in an attempt to compensate for the extra caloric load) should *not* reduce their normal intake of food immediately before drinking. Alcohol consumed on a regular basis must be included in considering the total caloric intake if weight gain is to be avoided. It is contraindicated when hyperlipoproteinemia characterized by elevated serum triglycerides is present.

Although alcohol intake is not to be *recommended* for diabetic patients, if moderate use of alcohol has become a well-ingrained habit that the patient will continue after diabetes is diagnosed, the most appropriate use of alcohol in a normal kilocalorie diet pattern should be outlined for the patient. Small amounts of alcoholic beverages of low-carbohydrate content are probably best substituted for fat exchanges in the diet pattern. On low-kilocalorie diets, alcohol should not be used because the calories from alcohol are not accompanied by essential nutrients and it will be difficult to meet the patient's nutritional requirements on a limited number of kilocalories. Each gram of ethanol metabolized by the body yields approximately 7 kilocalories.

17.7 Education for Diabetes

An understanding by the patient of the basic nature of diabetes mellitus and its management is essential if he or she is to be successfully treated over a lifetime. The disease also affects other members of the patient's family since the family's living pattern may have to be adjusted to accommodate some of the diabetic's needs. This is especially true with juvenile-onset diabetes, which is often labile and present in a child who is still dependent on parents for supervision and support.

Success has been limited over the past 50 years in various efforts to educate the patient with diabetes. Collier and Etzwiler (1971) surveyed diabetes knowledge among juvenile diabetics and their parents and found failure to recognize symptoms associated with the development of acidosis, confusion on insulin units, deficient knowledge on testing urine for acetone, and generally poor understanding and comprehension of dietary items. The failures in diabetes education must be shared by all members of the health care team.

Results from a national health survey in 1964–1965 indicated that nearly one-fourth of the persons with diabetes in the United States had not been given a diet for their diabetes (Holland, 1968). Another fourth of the representative diabetic population did not follow the diet they had been given. Of the 53 percent who said they followed a diet, further evaluation of their apparent understanding of Food Exchange lists indicated that only about 25 percent of them could be considered to have "good knowledge" of their diets (Stulb, 1968).

West (1973) cites the following factors as important deterrents to successful diet therapy:

1. The recommended diet prescription may lack relevance to the patient's preferences and may not fit her cultural, sociologic, or economic status.
2. An insulin-dependent patient may find frequent feedings and balancing of exercise and carbohydrate inconvenient and unappealing.
3. The patient and her family may misunderstand the general goals and priorities and/or the specifics of diet therapy.
4. The physician, dietitian, or nurse may have a poor understanding of principles and methods of diet therapy.
5. The patient education system may be defective because of (*a*) limitations of professional enthusiasm and acumen; (*b*) limited teaching manpower; (*c*) lack of economic incentives for professionals and institutions to teach patients; (*d*) lack of systematic patient education efforts among health care professionals; or (*e*) underestimation of deficiencies in patients' understanding.

Although West (1973) emphasizes much that is wrong with diet counseling for diabetes, he acknowledges that there are exceptions to this failure and that some physicians and dietitians are highly skilled in both the formulation and execution of diet therapy for their diabetic patients. There is great potential for success with diet in treating diabetes with effective learning that is translated into changed behavior (Ohlson, 1968). The effectiveness of diet therapy in the control of diabetes has been demonstrated. Weinsier et al. (1974b) described a successful multifaceted educational program that includes (1) small, group-oriented learning; (2) frequent intervals of follow-up; (3) feedback on laboratory data; (4) individualization of diet prescriptions; and (5) family involvement.

17.8 Diabetes and Exercise

Muscular exercise has a blood-sugar-lowering effect in both normal and diabetic subjects (Sanders et al., 1964). Exercise energy metabolism of trained patients with well-regulated diabetes was shown by Pruett and Maehlum (1973) to be similar to that of nondiabetic subjects. Klachko et al.

(1972) monitored blood sugar changes continuously in diabetic and nondiabetic individuals participating in standardized walking exercises. Blood glucose concentrations for normal subjects resumed or slightly exceeded preexercise levels within 1 hour after the exercise period. In diabetic subjects, the continuous blood glucose tracings resumed the preexercise slopes but at a lower level than with nondiabetics.

The blood-sugar-lowering effect of exercise must be considered in planning for control in insulin-dependent diabetes. The increased glucose disappearance rate with exercise seems to be independent of insulin action and, therefore, decreases the insulin requirement. Insulin-dependent diabetic children with erratic exercise habits may have difficulty balancing dietary intake and insulin dosage to avoid hypoglycemic reactions. *Regular* exercise is an important part of a successful regimen for both adult and child diabetics.

17.9   Hypoglycemic Agents

Types of Insulin
Since insulin is a protein hormone that will be digested by proteolytic enzymes if given orally, it must be given parenterally, usually subcutaneously. A purified form of crystalline zinc-insulin in clear solution, called regular insulin, acts rapidly and is usually administered $\frac{1}{2}$ to 1 hour before a meal. When insulin is mixed with a properly buffered solution containing protamine (a basic protein) and zinc, an insulin preparation is produced with poor solubility that is slowly absorbed after injection and is available to the body over a 24- to 30-hour period. Peak activity occurs at 16 to 20 hours.

At the Hagedorn laboratories in Copenhagen, an intermediate acting insulin was developed by carefully controlling the ratio of protamine and insulin so that it approached stoichiometric proportion and the crystals that formed left behind no protamine or insulin. The insulin was named NPH, with N indicating a neutral pH, P showing the use of protamine, and H referring to Hagedorn, its discoverer. NPH insulin has some of the advantages of regular insulin and also eliminates some of the disadvantages of protamine zinc insulin. It acts over 18 to 24 hours with peak activity at 8 to 14 hours. Globin insulin is made by combining insulin with globin, a basic protein. It acts over 12 to 18 hours with peak activity at 6 to 8 hours.

When the concentration of zinc is increased to 10 times the amount required for production of regular insulin, along with a change in the buffer system, an insoluble zinc-insulin preparation can be produced without the addition of a protein. The action can be further controlled by using it in either a crystalline or amorphous (microcrystalline) form. The amorphous form is more quickly absorbed and faster acting. Ultralente is the long acting crystalline form, Semilente the fast acting amorphous form, and Lente a mixture of approximately 70 percent Ultralente and 30 percent Semilente insulins. Table 17.4 summarizes the action of various types

Table 17.4 TYPES OF INSULIN AND THEIR ACTION TIMES WHEN GIVEN SUBCUTANEOUSLY*

| | | Action (hours) | | |
| | Speed of | | | Total |
Type	Action	Onset	Peak	Duration
Regular crystalline (neutral)	Rapid	$\frac{1}{2}$	1–2	5–10
Semilente	Rapid	1	3–4	10–16
Globin	Intermediate	2	6–8	12–18
NPH	Intermediate	2	8–14	18–24
Lente	Intermediate	2	8–14	18–24
Protamine zinc	Slow	6	16–20	24–30
Ultralente	Slow	6	18–29	30–36

* Owen et al., 1976.

of insulin. Insulin preparations are generally available in concentrations of 40, 80, and 100 units per ml. Standardized use of U-100 insulin (100 units per ml) is recommended. Dietary carbohydrate must be distributed on a daily basis to cover the periods of peak insulin activity in order to avoid hypoglycemic reactions.

Oral Hypoglycemic Agents

The first hypoglycemic agent that could be taken orally was Synthalin, a guanidine derivative studied extensively during the 1930s, but its use was abandoned within a few years because of hepatic and renal toxicity (Colwell, 1976). Several sulfonylurea compounds, investigated in the 1950s, are now used in the treatment of maturity-onset diabetes, in spite of controversy concerning their safety generated as a result of reports in 1970 from the University Group Diabetes Program (UGDP). Chemical structures for tolbutamide, tolazamide, acetohexamide, and chlorpropamide are shown in Fig. 17.1. A biguanide derivative, phenformin, has also been marketed as an oral hypoglycemic agent, although recently banned by the U.S. Food and Drug Administration.

The sulfonylureas evidently exert their primary hypoglycemic effect by stimulating pancreatic insulin secretion. However, extrapancreatic effects may also be present (Colwell, 1976). Hecht et al. (1973) studied the effect of chronic chlorpropamide treatment on insulin secretion in response to intravenous glucose and found that early insulin release generally improved, although subsequent insulin release was unaffected by the chlorpropamide treatment. However, they did not find a significant relationship between this change in early insulin secretion and the observed decrease in fasting blood glucose (hypoglycemic effect). A dissociation between the insulin-releasing and hypoglycemic effects has also been demonstrated for tolbutamide (Feldman and Lebovitz, 1969).

The time of action varies among the sulfonylureas. Tolbutamide is short-acting, covering 6 to 10 hours. It is metabolized in the liver to inactive compounds that are excreted by the kidneys. Acetohexamide and tolazamide are intermediate-acting compounds, acting over a 10 to 16-hour period. They are also metabolized in the liver but are changed to other hypoglycemic compounds in the process. Chlorpropamide acts over 40 to 72 hours (Colwell, 1976). Patients using oral hypoglycemic agents should space their meals, although hypoglycemic reactions do not commonly occur.

A clinical trial to determine the effect of hypoglycemic agents on vascular complications of diabetes, in comparison with the use of insulin or diet alone, was conducted over an 8- to 10-year period by a group of 12 university-affiliated treatment centers or clinics. A common study protocol was established for the collection of comparable data, which were sent to a coordinating center for analysis. About 200 patients in each of five treatment groups were given diet and, respectively, placebo, a standard dose of tolbutamide, a standard dose of insulin, a variable dose of insulin, or a standard dose of phenformin. The mortality figures from this study after 8½ years are summarized in Table 17.5 (UGDP, 1970; Goldner et al., 1971).

The major conclusions from the UGDP study were that the combination of diet and either tolbutamide or phenformin is no more effective than diet alone in prolonging life and that diet and either tolbutamide or phenformin may be less effective than diet alone, or diet and insulin, with regard to cardiovascular mortality. The collaborators in the study emphasized a need for reevaluation of the management of patients with adult-onset dia-

Sulfonylureas

	Generic Name	Trade Name
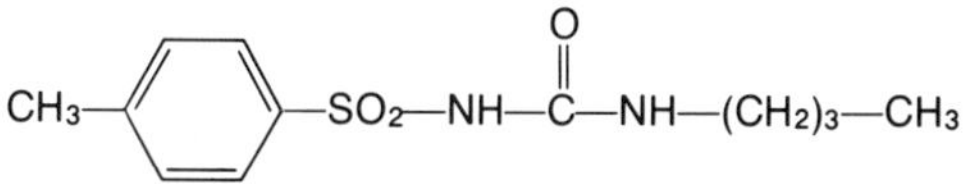	Tolbutamide	Orinase
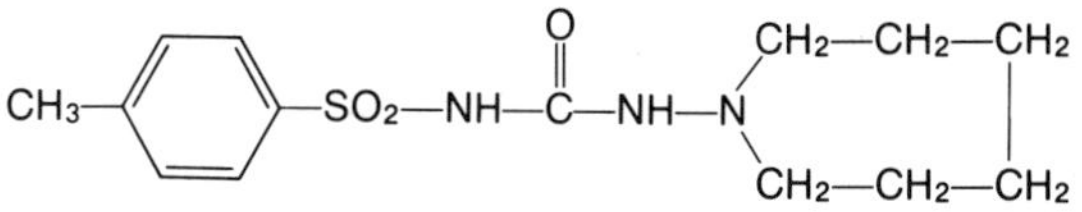	Tolazamide	Tolinase
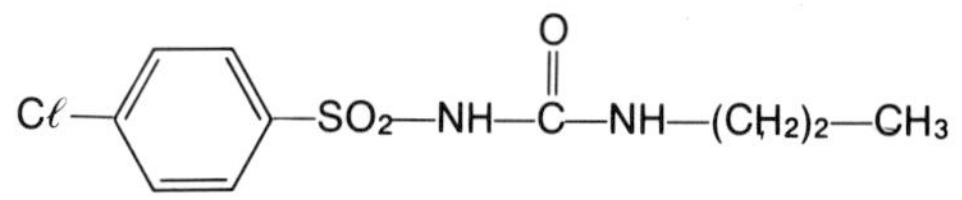	Chlorpropamide	Diabinese
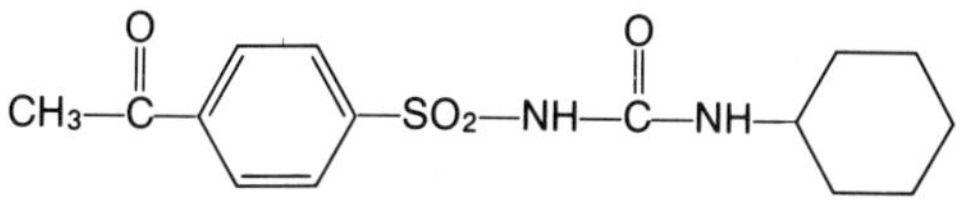	Acetohexamide	Dymelor

Fig. 17.1 Chemical structures for oral hypoglycemic agents.

Table 17.5 SUMMARY OF UGDP STUDY MORTALITY DATA*

Treatment	Number at Risk of Death	Cardiovascular-related Deaths	Total Deaths
Placebo	205	10	21
Tolbutamide	204	26	30
Insulin, standard dose	210	13	20
Insulin, variable dose	204	12	18
Phenformin		26	31

* UGDP, 1970.

betes who are not insulin-dependent. They suggested greater attention to diet and a more cautious approach to the use of oral hypoglycemic agents than had been used in the past (Goldner et al., 1971).

The UGDP study has been criticized on the basis of apparent defects in the design and execution of the study, as well as in the analysis and interpretation of data (Seltzer, 1972). The study has been assessed by a committee of the Biometric Society, however, and the probability that oral hypoglycemic agents cause premature deaths from cardiovascular disease remains valid (Shen and Bressler, 1977). It cannot be dismissed on the basis of other available evidence.

Colwell (1976) suggested that, whenever possible, control of diabetes with diet alone should be attempted. Particular emphasis should be placed on education for weight reduction. If the dietary regimen alone is unsuccessful, the physician may prescribe oral sulfonylurea compounds selectively. Insulin should be used if glucose and lipid levels are not adequately controlled by the sulfonylurea therapy.

17.10 Management of Diabetes and Complications

The availability of insulin brought about a dramatic change in the prognosis for juvenile-type, ketosis-prone diabetics. Their expected life span has been greatly lengthened and they can be kept in an excellent nutritional state with proper management. Enough exogenous insulin should be supplied, in relation to a nutritionally balanced diet, to regulate the metabolism of glucose, lipid, and protein in the body. The goal of management is similar in both juvenile- and adult-onset diabetes—to control hyperglycemia as well as possible. It has been suggested that excellent control of blood glucose levels will reduce the incidence and severity of complications of diabetes mellitus but results from controlled clinical studies to test this hypothesis are variable (Rossini, 1976; Anderson, 1975; Schmitt, 1975). The American Diabetes Association (Cahill et al., 1976) has issued a policy statement to publicize their belief that "the weight of evidence, particularly that accumulated in the past five years, strongly supports the concept that the microvascular complications of diabetes are decreased by reduction of blood glucose concentrations." They assert that the goals of therapy, therefore, should include a strong effort to maintain blood glucose levels as close to normal as possible. Acute or short-term complications of diabetes include ketoacidosis in the juvenile-onset diabetic, hyperosmolar coma in the maturity-onset diabetic, hypoglycemic reactions, susceptibility to infection, and delayed wound healing. Chronic or long-term complications include neuropathy, nephropathy, retinopathy, cataract formation, and premature arteriosclerotic heart disease.

Good control of blood glucose levels is difficult, at best, in stable diabetics and may not be possible in unstable diabetics. Service et al. (1970) found the mean amplitude of glycemic excursion (MAGE) for blood glucose during a 48-hour period to be small for normal subjects (range, 22 to 60 mg/100 ml), larger for stable diabetic subjects (67 to 82 mg/100 ml), and largest for unstable diabetics (119 to 200 mg/100 ml). With continuous intravenous infusion of insulin for seven diabetic subjects, Slama et al. (1974) found MAGE to range from 30 to 147 mg/100 ml with a mean of 71.

Ketoacidosis and Coma

Failure of glucose utilization by body tissues, excess hepatic glucose production, hydrolysis of glycogen, lipids, and proteins, and production of ketones occur as a result of marked insulin deficit. Ketones may accumulate in the blood in sufficient quantity to cause a fall in arterial pH to less than 7.25 or a decrease in serum bicarbonate to less than 10 meq per liter, or both, resulting in ketoacidosis (Felig, 1974). The high blood glucose levels lead to marked glucosuria as the renal threshold for glucose is surpassed and an osmotic effect produces large losses of water, sodium, and chloride with resulting dehydration of body cells and tissues. Ketones are excreted in the urine combined with sodium, potassium, and ammonium. Blood volume is decreased, affecting the heart and vascular system (Beeson and McDermott, 1975, p. 1613). Clinical symptoms and signs may include dry skin, air hunger (Kussmaul's respiration), florid face, rapid pulse, acetone breath, nausea, vomiting, abdominal pain, headache, thirst, dim vision, and coma. Urinalysis will be positive for glucose, acetone, and diacetic acid. Blood glucose is usually more than 250 mg/100 ml and CO_2 combining power less than 20 volumes percent.

Treatment involves intravenous fluid replacement, restoration of electrolyte balance, and administration of rapid-acting insulin in appropriate dosages. The patient is given fluids by mouth when he can tolerate them and will gradually be given an appropriate diet balanced with insulin.

Common causes of ketoacidosis are failure to take insulin because of illness and accompanying failure to eat, insulin resistance associated with infection, or possibly emotional stress (Beeson and McDermott, 1975, p. 1613). A previously undiagnosed diabetic may be first diagnosed in ketoacidosis.

Hyperosmolar Coma

The main features of hyperosmolar coma that may occur in ketosis-resistant, maturity-onset diabetes are severe hyperglycemia, hyperosmolarity of extracellular fluids, and profound dehydration. Although the etiology is not known in most cases, frequently it occurs after an illness that is accompanied by hyperglycemia and polyuria resulting from osmotic diuresis. With the high osmolarity of the blood and other extracellular fluids, water is extracted from the cells, including the cerebral cells. In many cases, the function of the brain cells is already compromised by vascular disease and coma results.

Treatment requires correcting the severe dehydration and hyperosmolarity by giving intravenous fluids and water orally when the patient is able to take it. The mortality rate has been reported to be high in this type of coma.

Hypoglycemic Reaction

Any patient on insulin and occasional patients on oral hypoglycemic agents are subject to hypoglycemic reactions due to lack of food in relation to the hypoglycemic agent. Unusual exercise without additional food may precipitate a hypoglycemic reaction. The first signs of a reaction usually involve mental confusion or mood change, followed by parasympathetic signs and symptoms, salivation, hunger, and increased gastric motility. There may then be sympathetic hyperactivity, with sweating, tachycardia, and anxiety. The pattern differs in various individuals, and within minutes the symptoms may progress to total unconsciousness. Urinalysis will be negative for sugar in a second-voided specimen and also negative for acetone and diacetic acid. Blood glucose will usually be 60 mg/100 ml or lower.

Patient education is very important to avoid hypoglycemic reactions. Recovery is usually rapid after giving readily available carbohydrate, such as orange juice, other sweetened beverages, or candy. If the patient is unconscious, glucagon may be given subcutaneously to elevate blood glucose and awaken the patient (Beeson and McDermott, 1975, p. 1617).

Somogyi Effect

A pattern of swings from hyper- to hypoglycemia and back has been described by Somogyi (1959). After a hypoglycemic reaction, the natural body defenses are called upon to raise the blood glucose level. These include increases in circulating catecholamines, glucagon, cortisol, and growth hormone. In addition, oral intake of carbohydrate may be excessive in an attempt to correct the hypoglycemia. The trend is then toward hyperglycemia and a larger than usual dose of insulin is required to correct the rebound. Occasionally another hypoglycemic reaction can follow and the sequence is repeated. These swings may be corrected by reducing the principal insulin injection and giving a smaller dose before the evening meal (Beeson and McDermott, p. 1617). Occasionally a hypoglycemic reaction may occur during the night without waking the patient. Natural body defenses will produce glucose which may then appear in the urine with testing the following morning. The patient may think that more insulin is required, creating a similar type of cycling.

Susceptibility to Infection

A delay in antibody formation and attainment of maximal titers has been observed in diabetic children following injection of staphylococcus toxin. It has also been shown that physiologic levels of insulin enhance the ability of cytotoxic lymphocytes to attack target cells. It has thus been suggested that insulin deficiency may make the diabetic more susceptible to infection because of a suboptimal lymphocyte responsiveness (Rossini, 1976). Increased glucose levels in tissues probably encourage growth of microorganisms, and changes in the vascular system increase the threat of infection. Skin infections are frequent in persons with diabetes, especially if they are in poor control. The feet, with a decreased supply of blood, are particularly susceptible to infection, and patients with diabetes must exercise care in protecting the feet from injury.

Delayed Wound Healing

Wounds often heal slowly and with difficulty in individuals with diabetes. Diabetic rats subjected to a midline incision that was then sutured had better wound strength when pressure was applied to open the wound if they were receiving insulin, in comparison with those not receiving insulin. The reason for the difference could not be determined, however. No significant correlations were found with the wound content of collagen, water, or albumin levels (Rossini, 1976).

Chronic Complications

Neurologic problems frequently accompany diabetes of relatively long duration and sometimes respond to reductions in elevated blood glucose. It has been suggested that perhaps an accumulation of sorbitol and fructose in peripheral nerves, probably in the Schwann cells, is related to the neuropathy. When glucose levels are elevated in body fluids and cells, the enzyme aldose reductase converts glucose to the sugar alcohol, sorbitol (see Fig. 16.8). Sorbitol is very slowly metabolized and also is not able to leave the cell, thus producing an osmotic effect and causing swelling (Rossini, 1976; Anderson, 1975 and 1976).

Microangiopathy in the kidneys and retina of diabetics was recognized many years ago and is a major complication of long-standing diabetes. A diagram of capillary ultrastructure is shown in Fig. 17.2. The capillary basement membrane in diabetes is both thickened and altered in chemical composition (McMillan, 1975). Williamson and Kilo (1977) suggested that capillary basement membrane thickening (CBMT) is a nonspecific reaction to and manifestation of abnormal vascular function and/or injury. However, it is a useful index for monitoring deleterious effects

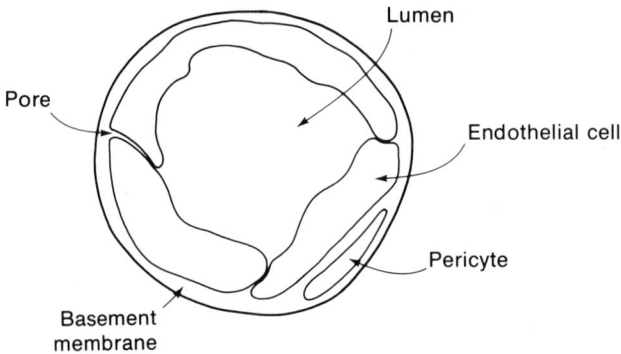

Fig. 17.2 Diagram representing a cross section of a capillary wall.

of the diabetic state. Controversy has arisen as to whether or not CBMT occurs in prediabetes and whether or not it is related to the severity and duration of diabetes. Siperstein et al. (1968) found muscle CBMT in approximately 98 percent of adult diabetic subjects tested and in 50 percent of patients who were genetically prediabetic, but they found the degree of thickening in diabetic patients to be unrelated to age, weight, severity, or duration of diabetes. Raskin et al. (1975) found muscle CBMT in only 40 percent of children with diabetes. Williamson et al. (1969 and 1971) and Kilo et al. (1972) found muscle CBMT to be related to age in both normal and diabetic subjects. Williamson and Kilo (1977) have been critical of other workers' findings of thickening in prediabetics because of methodology and failure to adjust for age and sex. They have concluded that CBMT follows rather than precedes carbohydrate intolerance and is a complication of the insulin-deficient state, although a correlation between degree of thickening and severity of carbohydrate intolerance has not been demonstrated in humans. Howard (1975) reported a significant correlation between the thickness of basement membranes and the degree and severity of spontaneous diabetic syndrome in the *Macaca nigra* monkey.

At present there is no satisfactory causal explanation for the deterioration of microcirculation in diabetes but it seems to follow sustained hyperglycemia. Neither is there satisfactory evidence that any treatment other than complete control of hyperglycemia will prevent the development of microangiopathy. Marble (1976) suggested that the development of angiopathy may be delayed and minimized by the judicious use of diet, insulin, oral hypoglycemic agents, exercise, help with emotional problems, and continuing education of the patient and his family.

Nephropathy is the most serious life-threatening complication of diabetes, with declining renal function. Typically this involves a diffuse and/or nodular glomerulosclerosis (Kimmelstiel-Wilson disease), which is characterized by CBMT in the glomerulus and accumulation of glycoprotein in the mesangial region of the glomerulus (Rossini, 1976). Also, arteriosclerosis occurs in the glomerular arterioles.

Diabetes is one of the leading causes of new blindness in the United States. One of the earliest changes in the retina is the appearance of microaneurysms. Exudates, both hard and soft, later occur. Progressive neovascularization is a major threat to vision and usually develops in eyes with extensive background retinopathy, including microaneurysms and exudates. Cataract formation may occur as a result of increased blood glucose levels and production of sorbitol and fructose in the lens of the eye by way of the sorbitol pathway. This increases the osmotic pressure and causes movement of water into the lens fibers, with the swelling resulting in myopia. If this process continues, alterations in electrolytes, amino acids, ATP, and other substrates occur, which cause precipitation of proteinaceous materials and cataracts. It is assumed that lowering blood glucose levels can inhibit this sequence of events and prevent cataract formation (Rossini, 1976).

Diabetes at all ages is associated with premature atherosclerosis. Coronary insufficiency and myocardial infarction are more common in the diabetic than in the nondiabetic. The Framingham study showed that diabetics had an increased morbidity and mortality from all cardiovascular causes (Garcia et al., 1974). Peripheral arteries are affected and gangrene of the feet caused by ischemia is more frequent in individuals with diabetes than in nondiabetics. Blood triglyceride levels are elevated in approximately one-fifth of all persons with diabetes, and 90 percent of subjects with Type IV hyperlipoproteinemia have overt diabetes or glucose intolerance. The atherosclerotic process is often out of proportion to elevated lipid levels in diabetics, however (Beeson and McDermott, 1975, p. 1610). Bennion and Grundy (1977) found both increased cholesterol synthesis and elevated plasma lipids in six adult-onset diabetics during uncontrolled hyperglycemia in comparison to that found during relative euglycemia on insulin treatment.

17.11   Testing of Urine

Frequent testing of urine for glucose shows variation at different times during the day and gives an indication of uniformity of control. The renal threshold for glucose varies from one individual to another and may change to some degree in one individual under different conditions. Urinary glucose, therefore, is not as accurate a measure as blood glucose in assessing the present status of carbohydrate metabolism in the body. However, it is more conveniently done and the patient can test urine regularly at home. If the urine is a second or double-voided sample (urine collecting in the bladder within the last 15 to 20 minutes), it should give a reasonable indication of the glucose that is being spilled from the blood into the urine.

Benedict's solution may be used to measure all reducing substances with the use of a copper reagent. This requires boiling the urine-reagent mixture. A more convenient method involves the use of reagent tablets

(Clinitest from Ames Company). Reagent strips dipped directly into a urine sample are less quantitative but offer a convenient estimate of urinary glucose (TesTape from Lilly; Clinistix from Ames Company). They utilize glucose oxidase and are thus specific for glucose. Reagent tablets and tapes are also available for the testing of urinary ketones.

17.12   Diabetes and Pregnancy

Among the metabolic changes associated with pregnancy is an increased demand by the fetus for glucose. The transplacental glucose concentration gradient is low and rapid delivery of glucose to the fetus from the mother's blood is thus facilitated. However, this lowers maternal blood glucose below usual nonpregnant levels. Increased hormone secretions, including estrogen, progesterone, cortisol, and human chorionic somatomammotropin exert a contrainsulin effect on the mother's body in order to make glucose available. If a pregnant woman has sufficient pancreatic reserve to compensate for these metabolic alterations, normal adjustments occur. In the woman with limited reserve, however, gestational diabetes results.

Gestational diabetes occurs in a pregnant woman who has previously had no signs of diabetes. Since increased risk of perinatal mortality is associated with gestational diabetes, it is important to screen for this condition so that the pregnancy may be managed more effectively. Patients with gestational diabetes have been included in the spectrum of prediabetes because of the high rate of diabetes developing in this group in succeeding years (Bates, 1974; O'Sullivan et al., 1973a).

Findings that are thought to be suggestive of gestational diabetes include family history of diabetes mellitus, weight in excess of 200 lb, unexplained fetal death, previous fetus weighing more than 9 lb, history of habitual abortion, and fetal anomalies (Bates, 1974). O'Sullivan et al. (1973b) recommended that a glucose tolerance test be given to patients with glucose levels exceeding 130 mg/100 ml whole blood on a screening test. They also suggested that screening be done on all prenatal patients 25 years of age or older.

Dietary management alone is usually sufficient to control gestational diabetes. However, some patients may require insulin. Caloric requirement is calculated on an individual basis following usual guidelines for prenatal patients. Weight gain appropriate for pregnancy should be monitored (Bates, 1974).

Pregnancy in a known diabetic is associated with an increased incidence of maternal, fetal, and neonatal complications. The mother is prone to instability in control of her disease and the newborn infant is often oversized. The pregnant diabetic and her newborn are classified as high-risk patients and optimal care should be provided (Persson, 1975).

The treatment of pregnant diabetic patients involves the same general principles as for nondiabetic pregnant women. A relatively high dietary protein level is often recommended (up to 2 g per kg body weight per day). To prevent edema and minimize hydramnios, sodium restriction and diuretics may be recommended. At least 200 g carbohydrate must be utilized to prevent ketosis (Wintrobe et al., 1974, pp. 549–550). With frequent observation, optimal insulin control, and appropriate timing of delivery, the perinatal mortality has gradually decreased in the offspring of diabetic mothers over the past few years (Persson, 1975).

17.13   Surgery in Patients with Diabetes

Surgery creates a special kind of stress for an individual with diabetes, especially when the disease is poorly controlled, yet surgery is frequently required for this population. Management of the diabetic patient during surgery will vary with the severity of the disease. A major goal is to prevent ketonuria and excessive breakdown of protein-containing tissues by providing an adequate carbohydrate intake. On the day of surgery, oral feedings are stopped and carbohydrate can be given intravenously as 5 percent or 10 percent glucose solutions. Insulin is adjusted on an individual basis, usually two-thirds of the usual dosage being given in two portions, one pre- and the other postoperatively. Glucose and insulin are given intravenously after surgery with oral liquids being taken as soon as possible. The patient resumes his usual diet as he is able to tolerate it.

17.14   Special Concerns for Diabetes in Children

In many respects the management of diabetes mellitus in children differs from that for adults. The classical signs of polyuria, polydipsia, and polyphagia are usually present initially in the child with diabetes, and he or she is often undernourished at the time of diagnosis. Since he is growing, his nutritional requirements are relatively great and must be adjusted according to his stage of growth. A child usually engages in erratic, vigorous exercise, for which he needs more food without additional insulin. Children are dependent on their parents and families and the diabetes education process must involve all of them. However, the child must eventually learn to take care of himself and his diabetes. He becomes his own diagnostician, laboratory technician, and nurse (Etzwiler, 1962). Adolescents with diabetes may have special problems from underlying anxiety and fear. Young diabetics are better able to accept the fact that they have the disease when they find that they can control it. Knowledge results in a healthy attitude (Khurana and White, 1971).

There are differences of opinion concerning the degree of dietary control that should be imposed upon children with diabetes. It has been suggested by some clinicians that the common side effects of strict dietary regimens are emotional conflicts and when a rigid diet is continued into adolescence against the patient's will, he may become resistant in other areas of diabetic care (Schmitt, 1975). Some flexibility must be included in dietary instruction and education to cover changes in activities and special needs. There does need to be reasonable consistency from day to day, however, and assurance that the diet is nutritionally balanced. Food must also be spaced appropriately to avoid hyper- or hypoglycemic periods as much as possible. Diabetic children, in general, seem to grow normally and attain adult heights that are within the range of nondiabetics.

17.15 Future Treatments for Diabetes Mellitus

A number of exciting possibilities for treating diabetes are now being studied, including transplantation of the pancreas (total or subtotal), of pancreatic islets, or of cultured beta cells. They also include the construction of an artificial pancreas (Albisser et al., 1977) or implantable device that will monitor blood glucose levels and release appropriate amounts of insulin as needed. All these procedures are for the present highly experimental and further research must be done. Research must also continue to clarify the basic causes and mechanisms of diabetes, upon which further progress in therapy depend.

REFERENCES

1. Albisser, A. M., B. S. Leibel, B. Zinman, F. T. Murray, W. Zingg, C. K. Botz, A. Denoga, and E. B. Marliss. 1977. Studies with an artificial endocrine pancreas. *Arch. Int. Med.*, **137:** 639.

2. Albrink, M. J. and P. C. Davidson. 1971. Dietary therapy and prophylaxis of vascular disease in diabetics. *Med. Clin. No. Am.*, **55:** 877.

3. Althausen, T. L. and K. Uyeyama. 1954. A new test of pancreatic function based on starch tolerance. *Ann. Int. Med.*, **41:** 563.

4. Anderson, J. W. 1977. Effect of carbohydrate restriction and high carbohydrate diets on men with chemical diabetes. *Am. J. Clin. Nutr.*, **30:** 402.

5. Anderson, J. W. 1975. Metabolic abnormalities contributing to diabetic complications. I. Glucose metabolism in insulin-insensitive pathways. *Am. J. Clin. Nutr.*, **28:** 273.

6. Anderson, J. W. 1976. Metabolic abnormalities contributing to diabetic complications. II. Peripheral nerves. *Am. J. Clin. Nutr.*, **29:** 402.

7. Bates, G. W. 1974. Management of gestational diabetes. *Postgrad. Med.*, **55:** 55.

8. Beeson, P. B. and W. McDermott (Eds.). 1975. Textbook of Medicine, vol. II, 14th ed. Philadelphia: Saunders.

9. Benjanuvatra, N. K. and M. Bennion. 1975. Hair chromium of Thai subjects with and without diabetes mellitus. *Nutr. Repts. Internat.*, **12:** 325.

10. Bennion, L. J. and S. M. Grundy. 1977. Effects of diabetes mellitus on cholesterol metabolism in man. *N. Eng. J. Med.*, **296:** 1365.

11. Bierman, E. L. and J. T. Hamlin. 1961. The hyperlipemic effects of a low-fat, high-carbohydrate diet in diabetic subjects. *Diabetes*, **10:** 432.

12. Bistrian, B. R., G. L. Blackburn, J. Flatt, J. Sizer, N. S. Scrimshaw, and M. Sherman.

1976. Nitrogen metabolism and insulin requirements in obese diabetic adults on a protein-sparing modified fast. *Diabetes,* **25:** 494.

13.   Brunzell, J. D., R. L. Lerner, W. R. Hazzard, D. Porte, Jr., and E. L. Bierman. 1971. Improved glucose tolerance with high carbohydrate feeding in mild diabetes. *N. Eng. J. Med.,* **284:** 521.

14.   Brunzell, J. D., R. L. Lerner, D. Porte, Jr., and E. L. Bierman. 1974. Effect of a fat free, high carbohydrate diet on diabetic subjects with fasting hyperglycemia. *Diabetes,* **23:** 138.

15.   Cahill, G. F., D. D. Etzwiler, and N. Freinkel. 1976. Blood glucose control in diabetes. *Diabetes,* **25:** 237.

16.   Case, E. K. 1950. Calculation of diabetic diets. *J. Am. Dietet. Assoc.,* **26:** 575.

17.   Collier, B. N. and D. D. Etzwiler. 1971. Comparative study of diabetes knowledge among juvenile diabetics and their parents. *Diabetes,* **20:** 51.

18.   Colwell, J. A. 1976. Use of oral agents in treating diabetes mellitus. *Postgrad. Med.,* **59:** 139.

19.   Committee on Food and Nutrition. 1971. Principles of nutrition and dietary recommendations for patients with diabetes mellitus. *Diabetes,* **20:** 633.

20.   Crapo, P. A., G. Reaven, and J. Olefsky. 1976. Plasma glucose and insulin responses to orally administered simple and complex carbohydrates. *Diabetes,* **25:** 741.

21.   Ernest, I., E. Linner, and A. Swanborg. 1965. Carbohydrate-rich, fat-poor diet in diabetes. *Am. J. Med.,* **39:** 594.

22.   Etzwiler, D. D. 1962. What the juvenile diabetic knows about his disease. *Pediatrics,* **29:** 135.

23.   Feldman, J. M. and H. E. Lebovitz. 1969. Biological activities of tolbutamide and its metabolites. A dissociation of insulin-releasing and hypoglycemic activity. *Diabetes,* **18:** 529.

24.   Feldman, R., A. J. Sender, and A. B. Siegelaub. 1969. Difference in diabetic and nondiabetic fat distribution patterns by skinfold measurements. *Diabetes,* **18:** 478.

25.   Felig, P. 1974. Diabetic ketoacidosis. *N. Eng. J. Med.,* **290:** 1360.

26.   Friedenberg, R., R. Metz, M. Mako, and B. Surmaczyuska. 1971. Differential plasma insulin response to glucose stimulation following ethanol priming. *Diabetes,* **20:** 397.

27.   Garcia, M. J., P. M. McNamara, T. Gordon, and W. B. Kannell. 1974. Morbidity and mortality in diabetics in the Framingham population. *Diabetes,* **23:** 105.

28.   Glinsmann, W. H., F. J. Feldman, and W. Mertz. 1966. Plasma chromium after glucose administration. *Science,* **152:** 1243.

29.   Goldner, M. G., G. L. Knatterud, and T. E. Prout. 1971. Effects of hypoglycemic agents on vascular complications in patients with adult-onset diabetes. *J. Am. Med. Assoc.,* **218:** 1400.

30.   Hambidge, K. M., D. O. Rodgerson, and D. O'Brien. 1968. Concentration of chromium in the hair of normal children and children with juvenile diabetes mellitus. *Diabetes,* **17:** 517.

31.   Hecht, A., H. Gershberg, and M. Hulse. 1973. Effect of chlorpropamide treatment on insulin secretion in diabetics: Its relationship to the hypoglycemic effect. *Metabolism,* **22:** 723.

32.   Himsworth, H. P. 1935–1936. Diet and the incidence of diabetes mellitus. *Clin. Sci.,* **2:** 117.

33.   Himsworth, H. P. 1949. The syndrome of diabetes mellitus and its causes. *Lancet,* **1:** 465.

34.   Holland, W. M. 1968. The diabetes supplement of the National Health Survey. III. The patient reports on his diet. *J. Am. Dietet. Assoc.,* **52:** 387.

35. Howard, C. F., Jr. 1975. Basement membrane thickness in muscle capillaries of normal and spontaneously diabetic *Macaca nigra. Diabetes,* **24:** 201.

36. Khurana, R. C. and P. White. 1971. Juvenile-onset diabetes. *Postgrad. Med.,* **49:** 118.

37. Kiehm, T. G., J. W. Anderson, and K. Ward. 1976. Beneficial effects of a high carbohydrate, high fiber diet on hyperglycemic diabetic men. *Am. J. Clin. Nutr.,* **29:** 895.

38. Kilo, C., N. Vogler, and J. R. Williamson. 1972. Muscle capillary basement membrane changes related to aging and to diabetes mellitus. *Diabetes,* **21:** 881.

39. Kinsell, L. W. 1962. The case for the routine use of diets high in polyunsaturated fat for diabetics. *Diabetes,* **11:** 338.

40. Klachko, D. M., T. H. Lie, E. J. Cunningham, G. R. Chase, and T. W. Burns. 1972. Blood glucose levels during walking in normal and diabetic subjects. *Diabetes,* **21:** 89.

41. Lenner, R. A. 1976a. Studies of glycemia and glucosuria in diabetics after breakfast meals of different composition. *Am. J. Clin. Nutr.,* **29:** 716.

42. Lenner, R. A. 1976b. Specially designed sweeteners and food for diabetics—a real need? *Am. J. Clin. Nutr.,* **29:** 726.

43. Little, B. and P. L. Thorup. 1972. *Recipes for Diabetics.* New York: Grosset and Dunlap.

44. Marble, A. 1976. Late complications of diabetes. A continuing challenge. *Diabetologia,* **12:** 193.

45. Morgan, J. M. 1972. Hepatic chromium content in diabetic subjects. *Metabolism,* **21:** 313.

46. McMillan, D. E. 1975. Deterioration of the microcirculation in diabetes. *Diabetes,* **24:** 944.

47. National Research Council. 1974a. *Chromium.* Washington, D.C.: National Academy of Sciences.

48. National Research Council. 1974b. *Recommended Dietary Allowances.* Washington, D.C.: National Academy of Sciences.

49. Nikkila, E. A. and M. Taskinen. 1975. Ethanol-induced alterations of glucose tolerance, postglucose hypoglycemia, and insulin secretion in normal, obese, and diabetic subjects. *Diabetes,* **24:** 933.

50. Nugent, F. A. and W. A. Millhon. 1958. Clinical evaluation of the starch tolerance test. *J. Am. Med. Assoc.,* **168:** 2260.

51. Ohlson, M. A. 1968. Suggestions for research to strengthen learning by patients. *J. Am. Dietet. Assoc.,* **52:** 401.

52. Owen, O. E., G. Boden, and C. R. Shuman. 1976. Managing insulin-dependent diabetic patients. *Postgrad. Med.,* **59:** 127.

53. O'Sullivan, J. B., D. Charles, C. M. Mahan, and R. V. Dandrow. 1973a. Gestational diabetes and perinatal mortality rate. *Am. J. Obstet. Gyn.,* **116:** 901.

54. O'Sullivan, J. B., C. M. Mahan, D. Charles, and R. V. Dandrow. 1973b. Screening criteria for high-risk gestational diabetic patients. *Am. J. Obstet. Gyn.,* **116:** 895.

55. Persson, B. 1975. Treatment of diabetic pregnancy. *Israel J. Med. Sci.,* **11:** 609.

56. Pike, R. L. and M. L. Brown. 1975. *Nutrition: An Integrated Approach,* 2nd ed. New York: Wiley.

57. Pruett, E. D. R. and S. Maehlum. 1973. Muscular exercise and metabolism in male juvenile diabetics. I. Energy metabolism during exercise. *Scand. J. Clin. Lab. Invest.,* **32:** 139.

58. Raskin, P., J. F. Marks, H. Burns, Jr., M. E. Plumer, and M. D. Siperstein. 1975. Capillary basement membrane width in diabetic children. *Am. J. Med.,* **58:** 365.

59. Rossini, A. A. 1976. Why control blood glucose levels? *Arch. Surg.,* **111:** 229.

60. Sailer, S., F. Sandhofer, and H. Braunsteiner. 1966. Overweight and triglyceride level in normal persons and patients with diabetes mellitus. *Metabolism,* **15:** 135.

61. Sanders, C. A., G. E. Levinson, W. H. Abelmann, and N. Freinkel. 1964. Effect of exercise on the peripheral utilization of glucose in man. *N. Eng. J. Med.,* **271:** 220.

62. Schmitt, B. D. 1975. An argument for the unmeasured diet in juvenile diabetes mellitus. *Clin. Ped.,* **14:** 68.

63. Schroeder, H. A. 1968. The role of chromium in mammalian nutrition. *Am. J. Clin. Nutr.,* **21:** 230.

64. Schroepfer, G. J., Jr., B. Friedrich, and F. C. Goetz. 1960. Dietary fat and serum lipids in diabetes. *N. Eng. J. Med.,* **262:** 748.

65. Schwarz, K. and W. Mertz. 1959. Chromium (III) and the glucose tolerance factor. *Arch. Biochem. Biophys.,* **85:** 292.

66. Seltzer, H. S. 1972. A summary of criticisms of the findings and conclusions of the University Group Diabetes Program (UGDP). *Diabetes,* **21:** 976.

67. Service, F. J., G. D. Molnar, J. W. Rosevear, E. Ackerman, L. C. Gatewood, and W. F. Taylor. 1970. Mean amplitude of glycemic excursions, a measure of diabetic instability. *Diabetes,* **19:** 644.

68. Shen, S. and R. Bressler. 1977. Clinical pharmacology of oral antidiabetic agents. *N. Eng. J. Med.,* **296:** 493.

69. Sherman, L., J. A. Glennon, W. J. Brech, G. H. Klomberg, and E. S. Gordon. 1968. Failure of trivalent chromium to improve hyperglycemia in diabetes mellitus. *Metabolism,* **17:** 439.

70. Siperstein, M. D., R. H. Unger, and L. L. Madison. 1968. Studies of muscle capillary basement membranes in normal subjects, diabetic, and prediabetic patients. *J. Clin. Investig.,* **47:** 1973.

71. Slama, G., M. Hautecouverture, R. Assan, and G. Tchobroutsky. 1974. One to five days of continuous intravenous insulin infusion on seven diabetic patients. *Diabetes,* **23:** 732.

72. Somogyi, M. 1959. Diabetogenic effect of hyperinsulinism. *Am. J. Med.,* **26:** 192.

73. Stone, D. B. and W. E. Connor. 1963. The prolonged effects of a low cholesterol, high carbohydrate diet upon the serum lipids in diabetic patients. *Diabetes,* **12:** 127.

74. Stulb, S. C. 1968. The diabetes supplement of the National Health Survey. IV. The patients' knowledge of the food exchanges. *J. Am. Dietet. Assoc.,* **52:** 391.

75. University Group Diabetes Program. 1970. A study of the effects of hypoglycemic agents on vascular complications in patients with adult-onset diabetes. I. Design, methods and baseline results. II. Mortality results. *Diabetes,* 19 (Supplement 2): 747.

76. Walsh, C. H. and D. J. O'Sullivan. 1974. Effect of moderate alcohol intake on control of diabetes. *Diabetes,* **23:** 440.

77. Weinsier, R. L., A. Seeman, M. G. Herrera, J. Assal, J. S. Soeldner, and R. E. Gleason. 1974a. High- and low-carbohydrate diets in diabetes mellitus. *Ann. Int. Med.,* **80:** 332.

78. Weinsier, R. L., A. Seeman, M. G. Herrera, J. J. Simmons, and M. E. Collins. 1974b. Diet therapy of diabetes. *Diabetes,* **23:** 669.

79. West, K. M. 1973. Diet therapy of diabetes: An analysis of failure. *Ann. Int. Med.,* **79:** 425.

80. Williamson, J. R. and C. Kilo. 1977. Current status of capillary basement membrane disease in diabetes mellitus. *Diabetes,* **26:** 65.

81. Williamson, J. R., N. J. Vogler, and C. Kilo. 1969. Estimation of vascular basement membrane thickness. *Diabetes,* **18:** 567.

82. Williamson, J. R., N. J. Vogler, and C. Kilo. 1971. Microvascular disease in diabetes. *Med. Clinics No. Am.,* **55:** 847.

83. Wintrobe, M. M., G. W. Thorn, R. D. Adams, E. Braunwald, K. J. Isselbacher, and R. G. Petersdorf (Eds.). 1974. *Harrison's Principles of Internal Medicine,* 7th ed. New York: McGraw-Hill.

84. World Health Organization. 1973. Trace elements in human nutrition. World Health Organization Technical Report Series No. 532.

CLIENT REFERENCES

1. Behrman, M. 1969. *A Cookbook for Diabetics.* New York: American Diabetes Association, 1 West 48th St., New York, N.Y. 10017.

2. Diabetes Forecast. American Diabetes Association publication. 1 West 48th St., New York, N.Y. 10017.

3. Donohoe, V. M. 1976. *Diabetic Cooking Made Easy,* rev'd ed. Minneapolis, Minn.: Burgess Publishing.

4. Fischer, A. E. and D. L. Horstmann. 1972. *A Handbook for the Young Diabetic,* 4th rev'd ed. New York: Intercontinental Medical Book Corp.

5. Gibbons, E. 1973. *Feast on a Diabetic Diet,* rev'd ed. New York: David McKay.

6. Gormican, A. 1971. *Controlling Diabetes with Diet.* Springfield, Ill.: Charles C. Thomas.

7. Little, B. and P. L. Thorup. 1972. *Recipes for Diabetics.* New York: Grosset and Dunlap.

8. Prater, B. M., N. J. Denton, and K. F. Oakeson. 1973. *Food and You,* 2nd rev'd ed. Salt Lake City, Utah: The Diabetes Center, 1174 East 2700 South No. 4, Salt Lake City, Utah 84106.

9. Revell, D. T. 1971. *Gourmet Recipes for Diabetics.* Springfield, Ill.: Charles C. Thomas.

10. Rosenthal, H. and J. Rosenthal. 1968. *Diabetic Care in Pictures,* 4th ed. Philadelphia: Lippincott.

11. Schmitt, G. F. 1965. *Diabetes for Diabetics.* Miami, Fla.: The Diabetes Press of America, 30 S. E. 8th St.

STUDY GUIDE

Diet is of prime importance in treating all types of diabetes and may be essentially the only treatment in maturity-onset diabetes.

1. Explain why diet is so important in the treatment of diabetes.

2. Explain and justify the following trends in the nutritional care of patients with diabetes: high carbohydrate levels; fat-modified diets; individualization of diet patterns; and emphasis on weight reduction.

3. Discuss the pros and cons of the use of alcohol in the diets of diabetic subjects and give practical suggestions for incorporating it into the diet pattern when its use is appropriate.

4. Make suggestions for planning and implementing an effective educational program for individuals with diabetes mellitus, with emphasis on nutritional aspects.

5. Explain why control of physical exercise is of importance in the management of diabetes and how it affects insulin and diet requirements.

6. Describe and explain special problems and considerations that might be encountered in the management of children with diabetes.

7. Write a diet prescription for a 21 year old man (6 ft tall, medium frame, and weighing 165 lb) who works as a mechanic, lives with his parents, and has newly diagnosed diabetes. He is taking NPH insulin. Also develop a diet pattern and sample menus for the diet prescription.

Various hypoglycemic agents are used in the treatment of diabetes mellitus.

8. List common types of insulin available and describe characteristic action.

9. List common oral hypoglycemic agents and describe characteristics of each.

10. Describe the appropriate distribution of carbohydrate and kilocalories with each type of insulin and explain the necessity for making adjustments between insulin administration and diet distribution.

11. Describe major findings of the University Group Diabetes Program and discuss the controversy over use of oral hypoglycemic agents.

Testing of urine should be a regular part of diabetic management.

12. Explain why a double-voided urine sample should be used for testing.

Short-term or acute complications may develop in a patient with diabetes.

13. Outline and explain the sequence of major biochemical changes in body metabolism leading to ketosis and diabetic acidosis and the type of treatment usually employed.

14. Explain usual reasons for the development of a hypoglycemic reaction in a person with diabetes and suggest appropriate treatment.

15. Distinguish between characteristic signs and symptoms of ketoacidosis and hypoglycemic reaction in the diabetic.

16. Describe and explain usual symptoms and treatment in nonketotic coma which may occur in adult-onset diabetes.

17. Give probable explanations for increased susceptibility to infection in diabetic patients.

The individual with diabetes is susceptible to chronic complications of the disease.

18. Describe the chief characteristics of each of the following conditions as they are likely to develop with long-standing diabetes: atherosclerosis of large blood vessels and CHD; capillary basement membrane abnormalities; nephropathy; retinopathy; and neuropathy.

19. Discuss possible relationships between "normalization" or lack of "normalization" of blood glucose and development of complications in the individual with diabetes and explain why there is controversy on this.

Pregnancy may bring special problems for the known diabetic and may unmask previously undiagnosed diabetes in other women.

20. Make and justify appropriate suggestions for the nutritional care of a patient with gestational diabetes; with previously diagnosed diabetes.

Surgery produces a special stress for the patient with diabetes mellitus.

21. Describe usual procedures for the management of a diabetic surgical patient.

18

Liver Disorders and Alcohol Metabolism

The liver is a master organ that is intimately involved in the metabolism of protein, fat, and carbohydrate. It plays a central role in the handling of nutrients for the body since most ingested substances go directly from the intestine to the liver via the portal venous system. There are thus many nutritional implications when liver disease occurs.

This chapter includes a brief review of the roles played by the liver in major metabolic processes and tests for hepatic function. Alcohol metabolism and its relationship to hepatic disease is discussed, along with the nutritional implications of viral hepatitis and cirrhosis.

18.1   Roles of the Liver

The liver is a vascular organ, its blood supply coming from two major sources, the portal vein and the hepatic arteries. Blood vessels run through the liver in portal canals from which they give off small branches that divide and subdivide between the functional units of the liver, called lobules (Fig. 18.1). The nutrient-rich portal blood and the oxygen-rich arterial blood mix, filter through the sinusoid channels (capillaries) of the lobules, and drain from the centrolobular veins into the inferior vena cava.

The sinusoids pass between columns of parenchyma cells, which are the working, secreting cells of the liver. Some cells, called Kupffer cells, have taken on a phagocytic function that includes destruction of leukocytes and erythrocytes and storage of iron. The Kupffer cells are also important filters for bacteria coming from the colon.

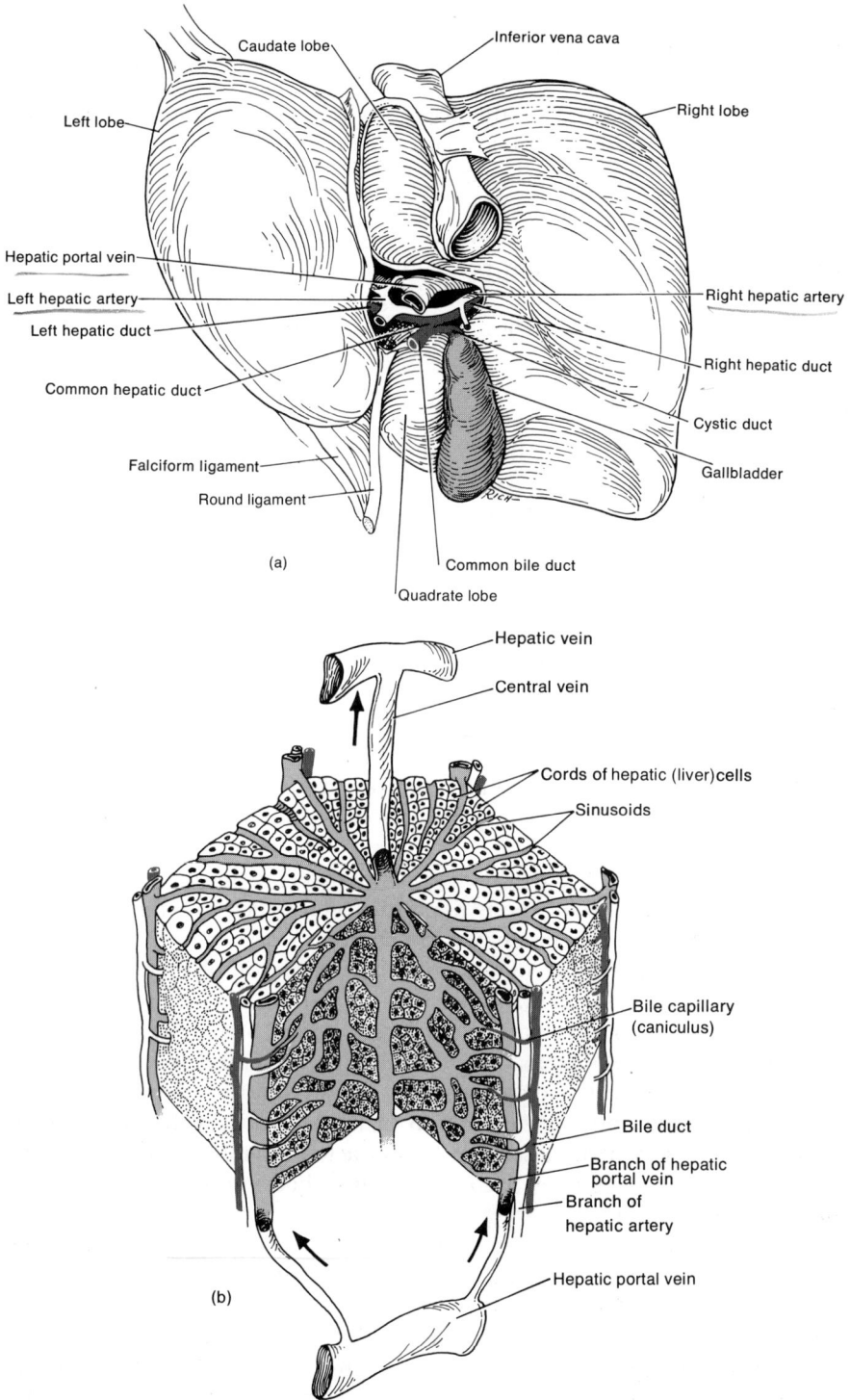

Fig. 18.1 The liver. (a) External anatomy in posteroinferior view. (b) Diagrammatic representation of the microscopic appearance of a lobule. (From Gerard J. Tortora and Nicholas P. Anagnostakos, *Principles of Anatomy and Physiology*, 2d ed., New York: Harper & Row, 1978; by permission of the publisher.)

395

Bile ducts divide and subdivide in tiny canaliculi in the same manner as the portal vein and hepatic arteries. Bile capillaries begin between the hepatic cells, from which bile is secreted. Vacuoles in the cells communicate by tiny intracellular channels with adjoining bile canaliculi.

The lobules of the liver are highly organized, vascularized systems of active cells functioning in many roles. Functions include metabolism, secretion, excretion, detoxification, and storage (glycogen; some amino acids; vitamins A, D, and B_{12}; iron, copper, zinc, molybdenum, and other minerals).

Metabolism

The liver maintains carbohydrate homeostasis by four major pathways: (1) storage of glycogen; (2) synthesis of glucose by gluconeogenesis; (3) release of glucose from glycogen; and (4) conversion of carbohydrate to fat. Glucose is taken up from the portal venous blood and glycogen is synthesized through the action of glycogen synthetase. Glucose is released from glycogen by the phosphorylase enzymes. In the adult, glycogen stores are available for the maintenance of normal blood sugar levels for approximately 24 hours, in the absence of other supplies of glucose. Gluconeogenesis, chiefly from amino acids, is of functional significance when the amount of available carbohydrate is reduced and is increased by glucagon release. The importance of the liver in regulation of carbohydrate homeostasis is shown by the occurrence of fasting hypoglycemia in the presence of mild hepatic injury. More severe hypoglycemia may occur with extensive hepatic damage (Grand and Ulshen, 1975).

Several proteins are synthesized in the liver, including a majority of the plasma proteins, endogenous hepatic proteins such as ferritin, most of the clotting factors (fibrinogen, prothrombin, and so on), transferrin, ceruloplasmin, and several of the components of complement. Albumin, the major circulating protein, is secreted into the plasma within 20 minutes of its synthesis in the liver and its half-life in the blood is 20 days. The synthesis of albumin is probably controlled by the supply of amino acids and its degradation by the absolute serum level (Grand and Ulshen, 1975).

Deamination and transamination of amino acids, with formation of urea and synthesis of nonessential amino acids, occurs in the liver. Ammonia formed in the gut by bacteria and absorbed into the blood is made into urea in the liver.

The liver is the central site for synthesis of cholesterol, although this sterol is produced in small quantities in every cell and in greater amounts in intestinal mucosa. The liver, using cholesterol as a precursor, forms the primary bile acids, cholic acid and chenodeoxycholic acid, conjugates them with taurine or glycine, and secretes them into the bile. The liver controls formation and utilization of fatty acids. Hepatic fatty acids come by transport from adipose tissue, from hydrolysis of triglycerides in the liver, or by synthesis from carbohydrate via pyruvate and acetyl-CoA. These fatty acids can then be utilized for (1) oxidation to CO_2 with the release of energy; (2) synthesis of phospholipid; or (3) resynthesis of triglyceride that is released into the circulation as very low-density (pre-beta) lipoprotein. Some low-density (beta) and high-density (alpha) lipoproteins are also made in the liver. Normally the liver contains approximately 5 percent fat by weight. Accumulation of fat in amounts of 10 to 50 percent, mostly as triglyceride, may result from protein-calorie malnutrition, excessive consumption of alcohol, certain drugs and toxins, and some familial disorders such as cystic fibrosis, galactosemia, and Wilson's disease (Grand and Ulshen, 1975).

Secretion and Excretion

The hepatic cells form and secrete bile, which is collected through the canaliculi and duct system and stored in the gallbladder. The conjugated bile acids combine with Na^+ or K^+ in bile to form bile salts. Bile salts are reabsorbed in the ileum and recycled to the liver.

The liver is the chief organ capable of metabolizing bilirubin. At least 75 percent of the bilirubin produced daily is derived from red blood cells (RBCs), with the remainder from cytochromes and other hepatic heme. Aging RBCs are taken up by the reticuloendothelial system, the heme being first converted to biliverdin and then to bilirubin. Fat-soluble unconjugated bilirubin is bound to albumin in the plasma and delivered to the liver cell membrane, where it is detached from albumin, transported within the cell, conjugated with glucuronide, and excreted into the bile. Normally, conjugated bilirubin is broken down by bacteria in the intestine to urobilinogen, about 10 to 20 percent of which is reabsorbed and taken up by liver cells. Most of this is then reexcreted into the bile, but a small portion escapes into the systemic circulation and is excreted in the urine (Grand and Ulshen, 1975).

Jaundice describes a yellowish tint to the skin and body tissues. The usual cause is the accumulation of large quantities of bilirubin in extracellular fluids.

Detoxification

The liver detoxifies both exogenous substances, such as drugs, and endogenous substances, such as hormones, by two basic processes: (1) toxic substances may be inactivated by reduction, oxidation, or hydroxylation and/or (2) water-insoluble toxic substances may be conjugated with glucuronic acid, sulfate, or other agents to produce water-soluble derivatives that can be excreted into the bile or urine and eliminated from the body. The corticosteroid hormones are first inactivated by a reduction process and then conjugated with glucuronic acid or sulfate before being excreted in the urine. Estrogens are similarly treated in the liver. In liver damage, some drugs will show increased effectiveness or toxicity (Wintrobe et al., 1974, p. 1516).

Several substances found in natural products are liver toxins. Senecio, which grows in the wheat fields of South Africa and may be harvested with the grain, contains a liver toxin. Jamaican bush tea may also produce liver toxicity. Aflatoxin is elaborated by certain molds as they grow on products such as peanuts and cereal grains. It is a powerful liver toxin, as is carbon tetrachloride and other organic solvents. The ability of the liver to detoxify may be easily overwhelmed as these compounds continue to be consumed and liver damage eventually results.

The liver has a limited ability to regenerate itself. It is very susceptible to damage from malnutrition (Kirsch and Saunders, 1972) or lack of certain essential nutrients because of the high activity of its cells.

18.2   Tests for Hepatic Function

Many tests used for measuring hepatic function actually indicate liver cell injury (serum enzyme levels) or the immunologic response to that injury (gamma globulins and tissue antibodies). However, some tests do measure true hepatic function. The sulfobromophthalein (Bromsulphalein or BSP) test and serum bilirubin levels evaluate the liver's handling of organic anions. Serum albumin and prothrombin time determinations measure the liver's ability to synthesize proteins (Burke, 1974). A combination of tests that measure different aspects of hepatic function may be used. No single test is universally satisfactory.

Cell Necrosis
Measurements of serum enzymes have been used to quantify liver damage but most of the tests are nonspecific. Serum glutamicoxaloacetic (SGOT or GOT) and glutamic-pyruvic (SGPT or GPT) transaminases have proved useful as indicators of liver cell necrosis or altered cell permeability, since they are released to the circulation in elevated amounts with damage to hepatic cells. GOT occurs in all body tissues. GPT is present primarily in the liver and to a lesser extent in kidney and skeletal muscle. Although many studies have shown that the height and duration of serum enzyme elevations parallel the extent of liver cell damage, precise quantitative correlations cannot be made in most clinical conditions (Wintrobe et al., 1974, p. 1518). Aspartate aminotransferase, alanine aminotransferase, and ornithyl carbamyl transferase (present primarily in liver) have also been measured as indicators of liver damage (Burke, 1974).

Cholestasis
Alkaline phosphatase is produced by many tissues, particularly bone, intestine, liver, and placenta, and is excreted in bile. Most of the enzyme in normal serum is derived from bone. Synthesis apparently increases and more enzyme is released into the blood with an impaired hepatic excretory function. Therefore, elevated serum alkaline phosphatase activity, in the absence of bone disease and pregnancy, is characteristic of cholestasis. The

enzyme, 5'-nucleotidase, is virtually absent from bone and is also elevated in obstructive biliary disease (Wintrobe et al., 1974, p. 1518).

Organic Anion Transport

Two bilirubin fractions measured in the laboratory are (1) the water-soluble conjugated fraction that gives a *direct reaction* with a diazo reagent and consists largely of bilirubin diglucuronide, and (2) the lipid-soluble fraction that reacts with a diazo reagent after the addition of alcohol (*indirect reaction*) and represents primarily unconjugated bilirubin. The serum of normal adults contains less than 0.25 mg direct-reacting bilirubin per 100 ml and 1 mg or less of total bilirubin per 100 ml serum (Wintrobe et al., 1974, p. 1517).

The BSP test involves infusing 5 mg per kg body weight of sulfobromophthalein dye over 2 to 5 minutes into an arm vein and drawing a blood sample for BSP determination from the opposite arm 45 minutes later. BSP is taken up rapidly by liver cells, concentrated within the cytoplasm, and conjugated enzymatically with glutathione. Both free BSP and BSP-glutathione are secreted into the bile. Normally less than 5 percent of the injected dye remains in the serum after 45 minutes. The test is simple, quantitative, and sensitive but notably nonspecific and often difficult to interpret. It is of no value in the presence of jaundice since retention of the dye will occur regardless of the nature of the underlying disease (Wintrobe et al., 1974, pp. 1517–1518; Burke, 1974).

Protein Synthesis

Albumin, prothrombin, fibrinogen, and several other serum proteins are synthesized exclusively by liver cells, and extensive liver damage leads to decreased blood levels of these proteins. The serum immunoglobulins are produced by lymphocytes and plasma cells and their concentration varies widely in hepatobiliary disease. Serum albumin concentration is normally 3.5 to 5 g and globulin is 2 to 3.5 g/100 ml. Hypoalbuminemia may occur in disorders with significant destruction or replacement of liver cells. Serum albumin level serves as a useful guide to prognosis and therapy (Wintrobe et al., 1974, p. 1519).

Prolongation of the one-stage prothrombin time may occur in severe hepatitis or cirrhosis and in patients with chronic bile duct obstruction. Inadequate vitamin K nutrition may be responsible for an abnormal prothrombin time (Wintrobe et al., 1974, p. 1519).

18.3 Classification of Liver Disorders

There is an abundance of labels for hepatic disorders since etiology and pathogenesis of liver disease is often obscure. A classification in terms of the morphologic character of hepatic lesions may be of more value than one based on etiology and Wintrobe et al. (1974, p. 1512) have classified liver disease in these terms as:

1. Parenchymal
   (a) Hepatitis (viral, drug-induced, toxic)
   (b) Cirrhosis
   (c) Infiltrations (glycogen, fat, amyloid, etc.)
   (d) Space-occupying lesions (hepatoma, abscess, etc.)
   (e) Functional disorders associated with jaundice
2. Hepatobiliary
   (a) Extrahepatic biliary obstruction (by stone, stricture, etc.)
   (b) Cholangitis
3. Vascular

The pathology of destructive processes in various liver disorders involving the parenchyma is similar. It usually includes fatty change, necrosis, and atrophy. These initial changes may lead to fibrous tissue development and scarring.

18.4 Interactions of Nutrition and Liver Disease

Liver cell necrosis has been produced in experimental animals by feeding diets deficient in cystine, vitamin E, and selenium. Choline deficiency alone or in combination with lack of protein leads eventually to diffuse granular cirrhosis in experimental animals (Leevy and Baker, 1970). Alcoholics often develop liver lesions. It has been assumed that this effect in alcoholics is the result of an inadequate diet, but the metabolism of alcohol itself apparently contributes to accumulation of fat and other changes in hepatic cells (Davidson, 1973).

Accumulation of fat in hepatocytes (fatty liver) occurs in rats on diets deficient in choline or its precursors, although this has not been demonstrated in humans. Several conditions in humans can, however, result in fatty liver. This may come from increased lipid mobilization of peripheral fat or several disturbances of lipid transport and metabolism. Protein-calorie malnutrition, particularly kwashiorkor, produces a large, very fatty liver, presumably because of defective synthesis of lipoproteins and consequent decrease in secretion of triglycerides from the liver (Walker and Mathis, 1975). With prompt treatment the condition is reversible. Fatty liver has been observed in patients fed only carbohydrate for long periods (Leevy and Baker, 1970). Some patients who have undergone intestinal bypass surgery for treatment of obesity have developed fatty liver. Untreated massive obesity itself may be reflected in excessive liver fat. During starvation, free fatty acids are mobilized in relatively large quantities from adipose tissue and, in part, esterified in the liver to triglycerides. Problems in peripheral mobilization, along with protein deficiency, may result in fatty liver in starved individuals.

Not only do nutritional deficiencies have the potential for producing liver injury, but established liver disease may affect nutritional state. This may result from (1) failure to store or convert absorbed nutrients into their metabolically active forms; (2) decreased intestinal absorption of ingested nutrients; and (3) failure to ingest increased quantities of nutrients needed to supply normal requirements and repair tissue damage. Patients with active liver disease require extra nutrients to repair damaged tissue, and failure to supply these eventually leads to deficiency states with additional complications (Leevy and Baker, 1970; Leevy et al., 1970; Prasad et al., 1970). Nutritional care of patients with liver disease thus assumes an important place in treatment.

18.5 Alcohol Metabolism and Liver Disease

People in the United States are significant producers and consumers of alcoholic beverages. Approximately 200 million gallons of pure alcohol were contained in the alcoholic products produced in this country in 1972 alone.

Alcohol is absorbed into the bloodstream without digestion, some from the stomach, but the major portion from the small intestine. Pronounced central nervous system effects of alcohol have for many years directed attention to the problems created by alcoholism and its accompanying social influences. However, the problems caused by alcohol consumption also include metabolic processes in the body that eventually result in injury to the liver and other organs (Smuckler, 1975).

Since alcohol is a common component of the U.S. dietary, its intake must be considered in nutritional counseling. In some cases, it must be specifically limited for optimal nutritional effects. Alcoholism is receiving increasing attention as a general health concern, and marked malnutrition often occurs among alcoholics. Therefore, dietitians/nutritionists, as well as other members of the health care team, should be familiar with problems created by the metabolism of alcohol in the body, interrelationships with nutrients, and special problems of the alcoholic.

Metabolism of Alcohol

Ethanol (CH_3CH_2OH) is an energy-yielding substance for the body (approximately 7 kcal per g as measured in the bomb calorimeter), but it has little in common with other energy-rich compounds. Carbohydrates and fats can be synthesized in the cells and stored to varying degrees. Alcohol is essentially foreign to the body, is not effectively stored, and cannot be eliminated to any appreciable degree through the lungs or kidneys. The body can dispose of alcohol only by oxidizing it, and the liver is basically the only tissue with an adequate supply of enzymes to complete this process (Lieber, 1976).

The first reaction in the primary pathway for ethanol metabolism is:

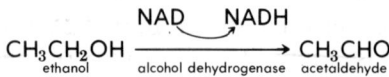

$$CH_3CH_2OH \xrightarrow[\text{alcohol dehydrogenase}]{\text{NAD} \quad \text{NADH}} CH_3CHO$$

ethanol · alcohol dehydrogenase · acetaldehyde

The acetaldehyde is further oxidized to acetyl-CoA. Several metabolic effects of alcohol are directly linked to the products of this first reaction, hydrogen and acetaldehyde. The liver cell must dispose of the excess hydrogen from alcohol metabolism and does so by shunting it into one or more of several pathways dependent on it, sometimes with deleterious effects. One of these pathways involves the reduction of pyruvate to lactate instead of converting pyruvate into glucose through the normal process of gluconeogenesis. Thus gluconeogenesis essentially stops. If an individual has been drinking alcohol and not eating, there will be no dietary carbohydrate and no glycogen stores. The body then becomes dependent on gluconeogenesis to maintain normal blood sugar. Alcohol metabolism takes precedence in the liver cells, however, and gluconeogenesis remains blocked by this diversion of pyruvate to lactate. Hypoglycemia results and may be severe. Hypoglycemia has been induced in humans who were on low-carbohydrate diets for weight reduction after they consumed three 1.5 oz portions of rye whiskey at hourly intervals (McLaughlan et al., 1973 and 1976). Lactic acidosis may occur from lactate buildup in the blood and interfere with excretion of uric acid in kidney tubules, resulting in hyperuricemia (Lieber, 1976; Kreisberg et al., 1971).

Liver cells may dispose of excess hydrogen by formation of fatty acids and alpha-glycerophosphate, which are then combined for triglyceride synthesis. Triglyceride accumulates with resulting fatty liver. If alcohol is ingested along with a diet containing fat, the fat of dietary origin accumulates in the liver, but even on a low-fat diet containing alcohol, fat is deposited in liver cells. Hyperlipidemia is another consequence of alcohol consumption.

A second metabolic pathway found in the microsomal fraction of the cell supplements the basic alcohol dehydrogenase system.

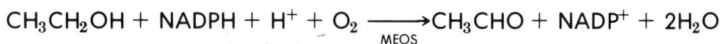

$$CH_3CH_2OH + NADPH + H^+ + O_2 \xrightarrow{\text{MEOS}} CH_3CHO + NADP^+ + 2H_2O$$

The microsomal ethanol-oxidizing system (MEOS) begins to operate after blood alcohol reaches a certain level and adapts to heavy drinking in an attempt to increase alcohol tolerance. Since other drugs share elements of the microsomal system, the metabolism of those drugs is decreased when alcohol is being consumed and their effect on the body is thus enhanced (Lieber, 1976). Heat is produced by the MEOS without efficient conservation of chemical energy in an energy-wasteful process because this system has no known link with energy-conserving mechanisms such as the synthesis of ATP. It requires the uncoupled oxidation of NADPH. When ethanol is consumed in large quantities, the kilocalories from it may be used inefficiently (Pirola and Lieber, 1976).

Metabolism of alcohol by the liver, therefore, stops gluconeogenesis and leads to hypoglycemia when food is not consumed; contributes to lactic acidosis in the blood and retention of uric acid with resulting hyperuricemia; produces fatty liver and hyperlipidemia; and interferes with drug metabolism. In addition, alcohol apparently has a direct toxic effect on liver tissue.

For many years, a controversy existed as to whether or not the injurious effects of alcohol on the liver were indirect nutritional effects resulting from the inadequate diets that often accompanied heavy consumption of alcohol. Experimental proof for a direct toxic effect came through improved methods of feeding alcohol to rats and baboons (Lieber and Decarli, 1976). By feeding ethanol as part of a nutritionally adequate, totally liquid diet, ethanol intake will be sufficient in the animals to produce fatty liver and ethanol dependence. Research on human volunteers showed that ethanol administration caused fatty liver while the subjects were consuming a variety of normal or high-protein diets.

Liver cell mitochondrial swelling and disfiguration have been observed in alcoholics, which may have additional detrimental effects on metabolism, contributing to ketonemia, fatty infiltration, and elevated levels of aldehyde in the blood. Aldehyde is an extremely reactive compound and affects most tissues in the body. It may be responsible for a number of the toxic effects attributed to ethanol (Lieber, 1975). Alcohol depresses myocardial function by decreasing myocardial contractility (Myerson, 1973; Song and Rubin, 1972).

Liver Disease in the Alcoholic

Alcoholics may display complications of liver disease to varying degrees, ranging from reversible fatty liver to alcoholic hepatitis and finally to irreversible cirrhosis. Relationships among these disorders in alcoholics have been the subject of much debate. Cirrhosis appears to be, at least in part, a consequence of the necrosis and inflammation associated with alcoholic hepatitis. That fatty liver may be a precursor of alcoholic hepatitis has been less generally accepted.

Fatty liver is the most common abnormality associated with alcohol ingestion and produces hepatomegaly. It is reversible when alcohol is withdrawn and is not accompanied by signs of liver disease such as ascites, jaundice, and splenomegaly. Alcoholic hepatitis, on the other hand, is a serious and not infrequently fatal illness. It is apparently a unique, toxic, inflammatory response of the liver which occurs in 10 to 20 percent of alcoholics, usually in the setting of an abrupt increase in alcohol intake. The histologic features in the acute phase include hepatocellular necrosis, infiltration of the involved areas with polymorphonuclear leukocytes, and presence of alcoholic hyalin or Mallory's bodies. The Mallory body is a fibrillar intracytoplasmic inclusion distinct from the cellular organelles and usually produces massive necrosis of liver cells. Clinical symptoms and signs of alcoholic hepatitis include anorexia, nausea, vomiting, weakness, weight loss, abdominal pain, diarrhea, fever, jaundice, hepatomegaly, ascites, spider angiomas, and splenomegaly. The death rate in severe alcoholic hepatitis is substantial, and cirrhosis develops in approximately half of the patients who survive. Therapy should include abstinence from alcohol, bed rest, a high-kilocalorie diet with as much protein as the patient can tolerate, vitamin supplementation (including particularly folic acid and thiamin), correction of fluid and electrolyte abnormalities, and caution in the use of sedative drugs or opiates (Lesesne and Fallon, 1973; Jewell et al., 1971).

Cirrhosis was the earliest recognized form of alcoholic liver disease. Only 10 to 25 percent of chronic alcoholics develop cirrhosis, however. Patek et al. (1975) evaluated the alcohol intakes and dietary habits of 304 alcoholic, hospitalized patients. There were 195 with hepatic cirrhosis, 40 precirrhotics, and 69 noncirrhotics. Dietary intakes were assessed for a period of at least 2 years before the presenting illness, and alcohol contributed 50 to 58 percent of total kilocalories during this time. Two-thirds of the patients drank excessively for more than 20 years. There were no statistically significant differences among the patient groups in the duration or degree of alcohol excess. The diets of both cirrhotic and noncirrhotic patients were poor when judged by traditional standards, with a marked imbalance of nutrients. However, noncirrhotics had somewhat higher protein and caloric intakes from food than did the cirrhotics, suggesting that dietary factors played a role, along with the direct toxic effects of alcohol, in the development of severe liver disease. The poor dietary intake of these alcoholics appeared to be due primarily to lack of appetite and not to poverty.

Nutritional Care of Alcoholics

It is probable that a high alcohol intake reduces the availability of many nutrients that are consumed. It interferes with intestinal transport and absorption and impairs the metabolism of lipids, carbohydrates, proteins, and vitamins (Patek et al., 1975). Baker et al. (1975) reported that alcoholics exhibited a significantly lowered absorption of thiamin and vitamin B_6 from yeast than did healthy, nonalcoholic subjects. The alcoholics were also unable to use the polyglutamate form of folic acid found in yeast, although the synthetic monoglutamate form was satisfactorily absorbed. Synthetic thiamin HCl was not well absorbed, but no problems were noted with the absorption of riboflavin and pantothenic acid. These researchers suggested that the folate, vitamin B_6, and thiamin deficiencies so commonly reported in alcoholic liver disease ensue from inability to absorb these specific vitamins from food. Special consideration needs to be given to the chemical forms as well as the amounts of supplemental vitamins for alcoholics. Subnormal levels of magnesium and zinc in body tissues have been associated with alcohol consumption (Wang and Pierson, 1975; Lim and Jacob, 1972; Prasad et al., 1970).

Effective therapy for alcoholics must include abstinence from alcohol in any form. In addition, apparent nutritional deficiencies should be corrected with a well-balanced, vitamin-enriched diet that is sufficiently high in kilocalories to spare protein and restore normal body weight. No specific alterations in diet appear to be routinely necessary for rehabilitation of the alcoholic with the exception of the complications of chronic cirrhosis which are discussed in Sec. 17.7. The present nutritional status and the stage of progression of the alcoholism are of vital importance, however, in outlining a nutritional rehabilitation program on an individual basis.

Since alcoholism is a complex problem, many treatment centers use a team approach. For example, the Zeller Zone Center in Peoria, Illinois, as described by Williamson and Turi (1975), uses a team consisting of a psychologist, social worker, nurse, registered dietitian, hearing and speech specialist, physician, and activity therapist. This program stresses continuity of care and concentrates primarily on medical detoxification of both inpatients and outpatients. Detoxification programs average 30 to 40 days. A new patient is interviewed by each team member during the first few days of treatment, as soon as the patient's physical and psychological condition permits. The dietitian's role is to provide a sound nutritional program for each patient that will arrest or correct injury and digestive tract malfunction sustained thus far. A nutritional history includes information about ethanol intake and is used with the medical history to ascertain whether or not a therapeutic diet is warranted. The condition of the new patient helps determine whether he receives intravenous infusion of vitamin- and mineral-fortified glucose. If he does not require this, he first receives fruit juices and high-calorie fluids, and his diet is progressed to solid foods as soon as possible. Vitamin and mineral supplements are given. Appetites of alcoholic patients usually return to normal soon after detoxification. Later, a nutrition education program for both the patient and family is used to help establish good dietary habits.

Southmayd (1974) reported that close attention to the acceptability of foods served in a hospital for the treatment of chronic alcoholism resulted in excellent food consumption and contributed to the social aspects of a 21-day physical and social rehabilitation program. Patients were served in a cafeteria-type arrangement and lunch was the same hearty type of meal as was dinner.

Guidelines for nutritional care of alcoholics during rehabilitation have been prepared by a Committee of the American Dietetic Association (1971). Nutrition counseling is an important part of this process and may involve (1) group teaching that allows for interaction among members as well as with instructors; (2) nutrition content that will provide for i͘ ͘dual motivation and adequate background knowledge of a nutritiou͘ (3) handling of economic and ethnic considerations that affect t͘ of individual nutritional needs. Nutrition counseling should be the follow-up care of the alcoholic.

18.6   Viral Hepatitis

Viral hepatitis is a generic term that includes at least two etiologically distinct disease forms, each with similar clinical signs but different epidemiological characteristics. Hepatitis Type A, previously known as infectious hepatitis, is the epidemic, community-spread disease ordinarily acquired by ingestion of minute amounts of hepatitis A virus. Hepatitis Type B, previously known as serum hepatitis, is commonly associated with drug abuse and transfusion of blood, but this virus may enter the body either parenterally or orally (Bryan and Pattison, 1976).

Hepatitis A is spread directly by fecal-oral routes or indirectly when contaminated water or food is consumed by susceptible persons. An outbreak in a general hospital that involved 44 clinical and 22 subclinical cases of hepatitis implicated two cafeteria workers (Meyers et al., 1975). In Minneapolis, 107 cases of hepatitis A were traced primarily to consumption of cold sandwiches served in a department store restaurant and prepared by a person with the disease (Levy et al., 1975). Sanitary public health measures are essential in prevention and control. Gamma globulin is used prophylactically and vaccines are being developed against hepatitis viruses.

Typical acute viral hepatitis can be divided into three phases: prodromal, icteric, and recovery. The prodromal phase usually includes malaise, anorexia, nausea, vomiting, and fatigue. Levels of serum GOT and GPT are often abnormal. The icteric phase usually follows in 2 to 4 days and is characterized by jaundice, dark urine, and light stools. Anorexia may be severe during the early part of this phase. Full recovery generally takes 3 to 4 months. Hepatitis may be an acute process from which the patient is expected to recover without sequelae, a fulminant process that may easily lead to early death, or a chronic condition that may persist and ultimately lead to cirrhosis (Milan and Appelman, 1975).

Management of Viral Hepatitis

There is no specific treatment for acute viral hepatitis but general supportive therapy is given. If the patient has persistent vomiting and cannot maintain oral intake in the early stage of the disease, parenteral feeding may be necessary. If anorexia and nausea are severe, tube feeding may be used. Generally, however, normal eating is resumed in a few days to a week. A nutritionally balanced diet should be given and the patient's nutritional state evaluated and maintained on an individual basis.

Modai and Theodor (1970) reported that the bile acid concentration of intestinal contents was significantly lower after a test meal for patients with hepatitis than for those without liver disease. The concentration of lipids in the micellar phase was also lower in hepatitis patients. This study was not sufficient to determine relationships between bile acid concentration and fat malabsorption in hepatitis, but fat digestion may be impaired if bile acid concentration is very low.

Strict bed rest and forced feeding of a high-protein diet have previously been recommended for patients with viral hepatitis, but do not seem necessary. In a 10-year follow-up of American servicemen with viral hepatitis, Nefzger and Chalmers (1963) found no significant differences in mortality rates, cause of death, hospital admission rates, hospital diagnoses, and veteran's disability ratings for those who had been treated with rest and a forced high-kilocalorie, high-protein diet as compared to ad lib rest and diet. Silverberg et al. (1969) evaluated the effect of a low-fat diet in the management of acute infectious hepatitis in children. One group of 49 patients was placed on a low-fat diet (1 g per kg body weight), while another group of 44 subjects consumed fat ad lib. Estimated average daily caloric intake was 1280 kcal on the low-fat diet and 1800 kcal on the liberalized regimen. No evidence was found that the low-fat diet was particularly beneficial to the children with hepatitis, and the more liberal diet was more easily managed. A nutritious diet is recommended for patients with hepatitis but strict limitation of fat is probably unnecessary.

18.7   Cirrhosis and Hepatic Coma

Cirrhosis is a generic term that includes all forms of chronic diffuse liver disease characterized by significant loss of liver cells, collapse and fibrosis of the supporting reticulin network with distortion of the vascular bed, and nodular regeneration of the remaining liver cell masses. The major cause of the lesion is liver cell death with the scarring and regeneration developing secondarily. Clinical signs and symptoms that accompany the changes in cirrhosis of the liver include jaundice, ascites and edema, central nervous system dysfunction or encephalopathy, and cachexia. Excessive fibrosis leads to distortion of the intrahepatic vascular system which then contributes to the development of portal venous hypertension with resultant esophageal and gastric varices and splenomegaly (Wintrobe et al., 1974, p. 1540).

The patient with cirrhosis commonly exhibits malnutrition. Nutritional care should be aimed at correcting existing deficiencies and insuring nutritionally adequate food intake. Electrolyte and fluid disturbances are often present, along with chronic muscle wasting, hypoproteinemia, and ascites. Patients with cirrhosis may have abnormal serum amino acid patterns and impending hepatic coma limits the nourishment that can be given. The major complications of cirrhosis that involve dietary modifications are (1) ascites, with or without edema, (2) hepatic coma, and (3) upper gastrointestinal bleeding.

Ascites
Ascites is the accumulation of massive quantities of fluid in the peritoneal cavity. Although the pathophysiology of ascites is uncertain, patients with

cirrhosis and ascites may be considered as having two principal disorders that may or may not be related. First, they have conditions that can cause transudation of fluid into the peritoneal cavity, namely portal hypertension, hypoalbuminemia, and an increased hepatic lymph production. Second, they have a renal dysfunction characterized by an increased renal tubular sodium resorption. Some patients also have a decreased glomerular filtration rate and an impaired ability to excrete free water (Arroyo and Rodés, 1975). Invariably, total body sodium and water content are increased in cirrhotic patients who have significant ascites or edema, or both. This disturbance of sodium homeostasis must be corrected in treatment (Shear, 1973).

A diet rigidly restricted in sodium to about 11 meq per day (250 mg) will nearly always halt the further accumulation of ascites and may lead to diuresis. Hyponatremia, unless very severe and causing symptoms, should not be a deterrent to dietary salt restriction. In fact, severe sodium restriction enhances water excretion and may thus, paradoxically, lead to a rise in serum sodium concentration. Occasionally, but not routinely, fluid intake may need to be restricted to prevent progressive hyponatremia in patients who cannot excrete water normally (Shear, 1973; Davidson, 1973).

Many potent diuretics are available for use by the physician in combination with sodium restriction. However, they must be used with great care. Shear (1973) suggested that they should be withheld for the first few days after a patient with ascites is hospitalized to permit better evaluation and correction of metabolic complications. A potassium deficiency may be present due to poor diet, abnormal gastrointestinal loss, and abnormal renal loss and may cause complications. Rapid diuresis may produce decreases in plasma volume without absorption of ascitic fluid. Functional renal failure may also occur.

In long-term management, dietary sodium should be kept at or below the level of urinary sodium excretion. Variable degrees of restriction are necessary in individual cases. In some patients, after ascites and edema are gone, dietary sodium restriction may be modest and the intake gradually increased to tolerance. Other patients may require more rigid sodium restriction indefinitely. Diuretic agents may be used intermittently (Shear, 1973).

Hepatic Coma

High protein diets containing at least $1\frac{1}{2}$ to 2 g protein per kg body weight per day were commonly recommended for patients with cirrhosis during the 1940s. This trend began to change during the 1950s, however, when a syndrome clinically indistinguishable from impending hepatic coma was reported to occur with the feeding of dietary protein and to reverse when protein intake was decreased. Abnormalities in ammonium metabolism were later related to the development of hepatic coma, with symptoms including confusion, spasticity, muscle spasms, flapping tremor, and personality change. Clinicians then began to emphasize protein restriction rather than protein feeding. A major problem for the cirrhotic patient continues to be how to provide sufficient protein to insure healing and regeneration of liver tissue while also restricting protein intake to control or prevent the occurrence of hepatic coma (Gabuzda and Shear, 1970).

A high blood ammonium concentration during hepatic coma or pre-coma supported the suggestion that at least one cause was the production of ammonia in the gastrointestinal tract (probably by bacterial action) which then reached the central nervous system because of a failing liver. However, other toxic materials arising in the gastrointestinal tract, such as amines and indole compounds coming from the action of bacteria on the amino acids tyrosine and tryptophan, may also be important in the pathogenesis of hepatic coma (Davidson, 1973).

It has also been suggested that because of a damaged liver and the shunting of blood around the hepatic portal circulation, amines or their precursor amino acids might flood the central nervous system and replace the usual central neurotransmitters by weak or false neurotransmitters that are comparatively inactive. For example, octopamine, a known false adrenergic neurotransmitter that may replace norepinephrine and dopamine, accumulates in the brains of animals with hepatic encephalopathy. In humans a correlation between urinary excretion of octopamine and grade of encephalopathy was noted. The pattern of plasma amino acids appears to be related to the metabolism of central neurotransmitters. In patients with hepatic coma, plasma concentrations of phenylalanine, tyrosine, and tryptophan seem to increase while concentrations of the branched-chain amino acids, valine, leucine, and isoleucine, decrease. Parenteral infusion of an amino acid mixture low in aromatic amino acids and methionine and relatively high in threonine, arginine, and the branched-chain amino acids has been reported to be beneficial in decreasing symptoms of encephalopathy in both experimental animals and humans (Fischer, 1976).

When hepatic coma seems imminent, poorly absorbed antibiotics, such as neomycin, are commonly given to prevent the intestinal production of toxic materials. When these drugs are not sufficiently effective, dietary protein may be reduced. However, since protein is essential for building healthy liver tissue, protein restriction should be continued for as short a time as possible (Davidson, 1973). The minimal protein intake required by patients of average body build to achieve nitrogen equilibrium is 35 to 50 g per day. Positive nitrogen balance is ensured by 65 to 75 g intakes. The beneficial effects of dietary protein in excess of 75 g daily have not been established, although the nitrogen requirements for maximal healing and regeneration of liver and nutritional rehabilitation also remain unknown. At least 1600 kcal daily should be provided to spare protein for building and repair purposes (Gabuzda and Shear, 1970). Rudman et al. (1970) described a formula diet with 35 kcal per kg body weight per day and 2 g protein, containing canned fruits, sucrose, butter, cornstarch, and water, that effectively corrected the plasma amino acid pattern simultaneously with improvement in clinical status for six cirrhotic patients who had a history of hepatic coma.

Upper Gastrointestinal Bleeding

Massive upper gastrointestinal bleeding is a major threat to a cirrhotic patient's life. The bleeding may occur from ruptured esophageal varices, gastritis, or ulcers. The development of esophageal varices is encouraged by the elevated portal hypertension characteristic of cirrhosis. Frequent, small feedings, possibly alternating with an antacid, may be of some benefit to a patient with severe chronic liver disease, even though he or she has not had a massive gastrointestinal bleeding episode. At least, severe gastrointestinal irritants, as well as large meals taken intermittently, should be avoided. The same therapy presumably holds true as soon as a bleeding episode has been stopped, but care must be taken that hepatic coma is not precipitated by overzealous use of protein-containing foods. There is no clear evidence that diet modification will prevent bleeding from superficial gastric erosions or from ruptured esophageal or gastric varices; however, such diet modification may be tried (Davidson, 1973).

18.8　Low Sodium Diets

The average daily adult intake of sodium in the United States is 100 to 300 meq (2000 to 7000 mg), equivalent to 6 to 18 g salt (NaCl). Salt is not the only source of dietary sodium since sodium is present in a number of

Table 18.1　SODIUM IN EXCHANGE LISTS* AND SUGGESTED MEAL PATTERNS FOR CONTROLLED SODIUM DIETS

					Daily Diet Patterns		
Food List†	**Amount**	**Weight (g)**	**Sodium (meq)**	**(mg)**	**11 meq (250 mg)**	**22 meq (500 mg)**	**44 meq (1,000 mg)**
Milk, regular	1 cup	240	5.2	120	none	2 cups	2 cups
Milk, low sodium	1 cup	240	0.0	0	2 cups		
Meat	1 oz	28	1.0	25	5 oz	5 oz	6 oz
Egg	1	50	3.0	70	1	1	1
Vegetable§	½ cup	100	0.4	9	3 servings	ad lib	ad lib
Fruit	1 serving	varies	0.1	2	5 servings	5 servings	ad lib
Bread, unsalted	1 serving	varies	0.2	5	4 servings	4 servings	4 servings‡
Fat, unsalted	1 tsp	5	0.0	0	ad lib	ad lib	ad lib

* See exchange lists in Sec. 2.2.
† Food produced, processed, and prepared without sodium compounds.
‡ 3 servings should be regular salted bread.
§ The following unsalted vegetables contain 2.2 to 4.4 meq (50 to 100 mg) per ½ cup cooked serving and are limited on a strict low sodium diet: beets, beet greens, carrots, celery, chard, collards, kale, mustard greens, spinach, and turnips.

Table 18.2 FOODS WITH RELATIVELY HIGH SODIUM CONTENT

Food Group	Foods High in Sodium	Food Group	Foods High in Sodium
Milk	Buttermilk	Fruit	Candied fruit
	Malted milk		Dried figs and raisins
	Cheese	Bread	Salted crackers
	Cocoa mixes		Yeast breads prepared with salt
Meat	Canned, salted, or smoked meats and fish		Muffins, biscuits, cornbread, etc., prepared with salt and baking powder
	Ham, bacon, sausage, bologna, and lunch meats		Cakes and cookies prepared with salt, soda, or baking powder
	Corned beef		Ready-to-eat cereal
	Frankfurters		Precooked dehydrated cereal
	Meatloaf, stews, casseroles, etc., as usually prepared		Pretzels and snack chips
Vegetable	Regular canned vegetables		Pastry made with salt
	Brine cured vegetables, sauerkraut, pickles	Fat	Regular salad dressings
	Olives		Salted nuts
	Tomato paste		
	Chili sauce		
	Potato chips		
	Frozen green peas and lima beans		

natural foods. Nevertheless, salt is the major source of sodium in the diet. Table 18.1 gives the approximate sodium content of the exchange lists when foods are produced, processed, or prepared without the addition of any sodium compound.

Table 18.1 gives suggested meal patterns for diets containing 11, 22, and 44 meq (250, 500, and 1000 mg) sodium. When foods containing salt are used, an estimation of sodium content becomes more difficult because of wide variations in the amount of salt added. NaCl is 40 percent sodium and $\frac{1}{4}$ tsp salt thus contains 500 mg sodium. Salted bread may range from 125 to 250 mg sodium per slice. Cooked vegetables and mixed food dishes vary considerably. Salted butter or margarine contains about 50 mg sodium per tsp. Regular salted cereal and salted canned vegetables contain about 250 mg sodium per serving. Foods with comparatively high sodium content that must be restricted on low-sodium diets are listed in Table 18.2.

REFERENCES

1. American Dietetic Association. 1971. Guidelines for nutrition care of alcoholics during rehabilitation.

2. Arroyo, V. and J. Rodés. 1975. Treatment of ascites. *Postgrad. Med. J.*, **51**: 558.

3. Baker, H., O. Frank, R. K. Zetterman, K. S. Rajan, W. Hove, and C. M. Leevy. 1975. Inability of chronic alcoholics with liver disease to use food as a source of folates, thiamin and vitamin B₆. *Am. J. Clin. Nutr.*, **28**: 1377.

4. Bryan, J. A. and C. P. Pattison. 1976. Viral hepatitis—a primer. 1. Epidemiology. *Postgrad. Med.,* **59** (No. 1): 66.

5. Burke, M. D. 1974. Hepatic function tests. *Geriatrics,* **29** (Jan.): 75.

6. Davidson, C. S. 1973. Dietary treatment of hepatic diseases. *J. Am. Dietet. Assoc.,* **62:** 515.

7. Fischer, J. E. 1976. Amino acid infusion in hepatic encephalopathy. *Dietet. Currents* (Ross Laboratories), **3** (No. 2): 5.

8. Gabuzda, G. J. and L. Shear. 1970. Metabolism of dietary protein in hepatic cirrhosis. *Am. J. Clin. Nutr.,* **23:** 479.

9. Grand, R. J. and M. H. Ulshen. 1975. Clinical and physiological abnormalities in hepatic function. *Ped. Clin. No. Am.,* **22:** 897.

10. Jewell, L. D., A. Medline, and N. M. Medline. 1971. Alcoholic hepatitis. *Can. Med. Assoc. J.,* **105:** 711.

11. Kirsch, R. E. and S. J. Saunders. 1972. Nutrition and the liver. *So. Afr. Med. J.,* **46:** 2072.

12. Kreisberg, R. A., A. M. Siegal, and W. C. Owen. 1971. Glucose-lactate interrelationships: Effect of ethanol. *J. Clin. Invest.,* **50:** 175.

13. Leevy, C. M. and H. Baker. 1970. Nutritional deficiencies in liver disease. *Med. Clin. No. Am.,* **54:** 467.

14. Leevy, C. M., A. Thompson, and H. Baker. 1970. Vitamins and liver injury. *Am. J. Clin. Nutr.,* **23:** 493.

15. Lesesne, H. R. and H. J. Fallon. 1973. Alcoholic liver disease. *Postgrad. Med.,* **53** (No. 1): 101.

16. Levy, B. S., R. E. Fontaine, C. A. Smith, J. Brinda, G. Hirman, D. B. Nelson, P. M. Johnson, and O. Larson. 1975. A large food-borne outbreak of hepatitis A. *J. Am. Med. Assoc.,* **234:** 289.

17. Lieber, C. S. 1976. The metabolism of alcohol. *Sci. Am.,* **234** (No. 3): 25.

18. Lieber, C. S. 1975. Alcohol and malnutrition in the pathogenesis of liver disease. *J. Am. Med. Assoc.,* **233:** 1077.

19. Lieber, C. S. and L. M. Decarli. 1976. Animal models of ethanol dependence and liver injury in rats and baboons. *Fed. Proc.,* **35:** 1232.

20. Lim, P. and E. Jacob. 1972. Magnesium status of alcoholic patients. *Metabolism,* **21:** 1045.

21. McLaughlan, J. M., F. J. Noel, and C. A. Moodie. 1973. Hypoglycemia in humans induced by alcohol and a low carbohydrate diet. *Nutr. Rep. Internat.,* **8:** 331.

22. McLaughlan, J. M., D. Usher, F. J. Noel, and C. A. Moodie. 1976. Effect of a low-carbohydrate diet and alcohol on perceptual motor skill. *J. Am. Dietet. Assoc.,* **68:** 138.

23. Meyers, J. D., F. J. Romm, W. S. Tihen, and J. A. Bryan. 1975. Food-borne hepatitis A in a general hospital. *J. Am. Med. Assoc.,* **231:** 1049.

24. Milam, W. F. and H. D. Appelman. 1975. Chronic progressive liver disease: Making order out of nosologic chaos. *Geriatrics,* **30** (Mar.): 109.

25. Modai, M. and E. Theodor. 1970. Intestinal contents in patients with viral hepatitis after a lipid meal. *Gastroent.,* **58:** 379.

26. Myerson, R. M. 1973. Metabolic aspects of alcohol and their biological significance. *Med. Clin. No. Am.,* **57:** 925.

27. Nefzger, M. D. and T. C. Chalmers. 1963. The treatment of acute infectious hepatitis. *Am. J. Med.,* **35:** 299.

28. Patek, A. J., Jr., I. G. Toth, M. G. Saunders, G. A. M. Castro, and J. J. Engel. 1975. Alcohol and dietary factors in cirrhosis. *Arch. Int. Med.,* **135:** 1053.

29. Pirola, R. C. and C. S. Lieber. 1976. Hypothesis: energy wastage in alcoholism and drug abuse: possible role of hepatic microsomal enzymes. *Am. J. Clin. Nutr.,* **29:** 90.

30. Prasad, A. S., D. Oberleas, and G. Rajasekaran. 1970. Essential micronutrient elements. Biochemistry and changes in liver disorders. *Am. J. Clin. Nutr.*, **23:** 581.

31. Rudman, D., S. Akgun, J. T. Galambos, A. S. McKinney, A. B. Cullen, G. G. Gerron, and C. H. Howard. 1970. Observations on the nitrogen metabolism of patients with portal cirrhosis. *Am. J. Clin. Nutr.*, **23:** 1203.

32. Shear, L. 1973. Ascites: Pathogenesis and treatment. *Postgrad. Med.*, **53** (No. 1): 165.

33. Silverberg, M., B. Wherrett, E. Worden, and P. Z. Neumann. 1969. An evaluation of rest and low-fat diets in the management of acute infectious hepatitis. *J. Ped.*, **74:** 260.

34. Smuckler, E. A. 1975. Alcoholic drink, its production and effects. *Fed. Proc.*, **34:** 2038.

35. Song, S. K. and E. Rubin. 1972. Ethanol produces muscle damage in human volunteers. *Science*, **175:** 327.

36. Southmayd, E. B. 1974. The role of the dietitian in team therapy for chronic alcoholism. *J. Am. Dietet. Assoc.*, **64:** 184.

37. Walker, W. A. and R. K. Mathis. 1975. Hepatomegaly. *Ped. Clin. No. Am.*, **22:** 929.

38. Wang, J. and R. N. Pierson, Jr. 1975. Distribution of zinc in skeletal muscle and liver tissue in normal and dietary controlled alcoholic rats. *J. Lab. Clin. Med.*, **85:** 50.

39. Williamson, D. and M. E. Turi. 1975. Nutrition in treatment of the alcoholic. *Dietet. Currents* (Ross Laboratories), **2** (No. 1): 1.

40. Wintrobe, M. M., G. W. Thorn, R. D. Adams, E. Braunwald, K. J. Isselbacher, R. G. Petersdorf (Eds.). 1974. *Harrison's Principles of Internal Medicine*, 7th ed. New York: McGraw-Hill.

STUDY GUIDE

The liver plays a central role in the control of metabolic homeostasis.

1. Describe the major functions of the liver as an organ of metabolism; secretion and excretion; detoxification; and storage.

2. List several substances that are toxic to the liver.

Clinical tests may measure true hepatic function but often measure only liver cell injury or immunologic response to that injury.

3. Explain the general principles upon which each of the following hepatic tests is based and discuss the significance of the test in diagnosing liver disorders: serum GOT or GPT; serum alkaline phosphatase; serum bilirubin, direct and total; BSP test; serum albumin; prothrombin time.

Pathological features of several destructive processes are essentially the same when they involve the parenchyma of the liver and may include fatty metamorphosis, necrosis, and simple atrophy.

4. Describe the general type of change occurring in fatty infiltration, necrosis, and atrophy of liver cells.

5. Give possible explanations for the development of fatty liver in kwashiorkor, starvation, massive obesity, and toxic injury from alcohol.

Alcohol is metabolized almost exclusively in the liver, where it profoundly affects the metabolism of other substances.

6. Outline two different pathways for ethanol metabolism and explain why the liver is so important to the body's handling of alcohol.

7. Explain why alcohol taken in a fasting state may produce hypoglycemia.

8. Explain, in terms of hydrogen-containing coenzymes, how metabolism of alcohol adversely influences metabolism of glucose, lactic acid, and fat synthesis in the liver.

9. Explain why hyperuricemia often accompanies excessive alcohol consumption.

Cirrhosis and certain types of hepatitis are more common among alcoholics than among the general population.

10. Distinguish between fatty liver and alcoholic hepatitis in terms of reversibility and usual severity.

11. Make and explain appropriate nutritional suggestions for an alcoholic during detoxification and rehabilitation programs.

Viral hepatitis includes at least two disease forms with similar clinical signs but different epidemiological characteristics.

12. Describe the usual route of infection for viral hepatitis A and B.

13. Describe three phases of the disease for typical acute viral hepatitis.

14. Describe and explain the rationale for appropriate nutritional care in typical acute cases of viral hepatitis.

Cirrhosis of the liver involves complications with nutritional implications for treatment.

15. Explain possible mechanisms whereby each of the following may be produced in cirrhosis: ascites, hepatic coma, and upper gastrointestinal bleeding.

16. Explain the rationale for a strict low-sodium diet in treatment of ascites and/or edema for cirrhotics and describe necessary dietary modifications.

17. Describe and explain common symptoms associated with development of hepatic coma and explain possible relationships between dietary protein and this complication of liver disease.

18. Discuss the dilemma created by the possible need to restrict dietary protein when hepatic coma is imminent.

19. Describe dietary modifications that may be useful for a patient with severe liver disease and esophageal varices or similar upper gastrointestinal problems.

19

Other Metabolic Problems: Hypoglycemia; Gout

19.1 Hypoglycemia

The first recognized case of hypoglycemia due to a pancreatic insulin-producing tumor was reported in 1927, with symptoms similar to those seen in overinsulinized diabetic patients. As blood sugar values were measured more frequently during episodes suggesting hypoglycemia, it became apparent that the more common type of hypoglycemia was a functional, benign disorder and not the result of pancreatic tumor. Various names, i.e., reactive, functional, anxiety hypoglycemia, have been applied to this type (Conn and Pek, 1974). In 1936 Conn demonstrated a stabilizing effect of high-protein meals on the blood sugar of patients with functional hypoglycemia and introduced the high-protein, low-carbohydrate diet. A similar diet is often prescribed today.

Classification

The classification for various types of hypoglycemia has changed over the years as new information and techniques of analysis have become available. Hypoglycemias have been classified into organic and functional; fasting and fed; and according to physiologic mechanisms, clinical circumstances, anatomic lesions, and combinations of these characteristics. One classification according to fasting or fed states is given in Table 19.1. In addition, hypoglycemia may result from exogenous causes, including overinsulinization in treatment of diabetes

Table 19.1 CLASSIFICATION OF SPONTANEOUS HYPOGLYCEMIA
(ENDOGENOUS METABOLIC PROCESSES)*

I. Fasting state hypoglycemia
A. Pancreatic disorders
    1. Islet beta cell hyperfunction (adenoma, carcinoma, hyperplasia); leucine hypersensitivity
    2. Islet alpha cell hypofunction or deficiency
B. Hepatic disorders
    1. Severe liver disease
    2. Enzyme defects (glycogen storage disease, galactosemia, hereditary fructose intolerance, familial galactose and fructose intolerance, maple syrup disease, fructose diphosphatase deficiency)
C. Pituitary-adrenal disorders
D. Central nervous system disease (hypothalamus or brain stem)
E. Nonpancreatic neoplasms
F. Unclassified
    1. Excessive loss or utilization of glucose and/or deficient substrate (prolonged or strenuous exercise, fever, lactation, pregnancy, renal glycosuria, diarrheal states, chronic starvation)
    2. Ketotic hypoglycemia of childhood (idiopathic hypoglycemia of childhood)
II. Postprandial hypoglycemia (reactive to fed state)
A. Early alimentary hypoglycemia (includes GI surgery, peptic disease, and vagotonic personality)
    1. Hyperglycemia-hyperinsulinism
    2. Normoglycemia-hyperinsulinism
B. Late hypoglycemia of early maturity-onset diabetes mellitus
C. Hormonal hypoglycemia (hypopituitarism and deficient reserve of cortisone, epinephrine, glucagon, thyroid, or growth hormone)
D. Idiopathic

* Adapted from Hofeldt et al., 1972.

(iatrogenic) and the deliberate giving of insulin to produce symptoms (factitious hypoglycemia).

Symptoms

Hypoglycemia has been defined as a blood glucose level of less than 40 mg/100 ml or plasma glucose less than 50 mg/100 ml (Hofeldt et al., 1972). When the rate of fall in blood glucose is rapid, the major early symptoms are associated with the compensatory secretion of epinephrine, which attempts to restore normal blood glucose levels by accelerating hepatic glycogenolysis. Symptoms include sweating, weakness, hunger, tachycardia, apprehension, nervousness, and anxiety. If the blood glucose level falls slowly, the symptoms arise primarily from neuroglycopenia and include poor concentration, drowsiness, confusion, lethargy, memory loss, blurred vision, headache, diplopia, incoherent speech, stupor, and coma. The onset and magnitude of all symptoms depend on the severity and duration of hypoglycemia (Hofeldt et al., 1972; Conn and Pek, 1974).

Fasting State Hypoglycemia

Many factors contribute to the maintenance of normoglycemia during fasting. A number of different pathologic states may interfere with normal mechanisms and result in fasting hypoglycemia (Table 19.1). Since normal physiologic mechanisms, particularly in fasting women, often produce blood glucose levels less than 45 mg/100 ml, Merimee and Tyson (1977) suggested the use of elevated insulin/glucose (I/G) ratios rather than blood glucose levels alone for diagnosing pathologic fasting hypoglycemia. Serum insulin levels remain high in cases of beta cell tumors and similar causes of fasting hypoglycemia.

The treatment for fasting hypoglycemia must be aimed at the cause. It cannot be satisfactorily treated by dietary means alone. Insulin-secreting tumors require surgical intervention.

Postprandial or Reactive Hypoglycemia

Hypoglycemia has commonly been employed in recent years to explain the varied symptoms that often occur in daily life. The magnitude of such complaints may lead a physician to be overzealous in searching for a cause to account for the patient's symptoms. Clinical studies of reactive hypoglycemia have been hampered by its vagueness in definition and by the different criteria used in selection of patients. Some investigators use clinical symptoms alone in choosing patients for study, whereas others include patients who have had blood glucose values below a certain arbitrary limit, whether or not concomitant symptoms of hypoglycemia exist. Objective evidence to verify the hypoglycemic symptoms is often not used (Hofeldt et al., 1975).

Because of publicity in the popular press, a special report on hypoglycemia was issued in 1973 by the American Diabetes Association, the Endocrine Society, and the American Medical Association, emphasizing that many persons with the symptoms commonly associated with hypoglycemia do not have hypoglycemia. A great many patients with anxiety reactions present with similar symptoms. Furthermore, it was stated, there is no good evidence that hypoglycemia causes depression, chronic fatigue, allergies, alcoholism, juvenile delinquency, childhood behavior problems, drug addiction, or inadequate sexual performance. Before any patient receives treatment for hypoglycemia, all the following should be present: (1) the documented occurrence of low blood sugar; (2) a demonstrated relationship between the particular symptoms of which the patient complains and hypoglycemia; (3) demonstrated relief of symptoms by ingestion of food or sugar; and (4) establishment of the kind of hypoglycemia producing the symptoms. Treatment depends on the particular kind of reactive hypoglycemia.

According to Hofeldt et al. (1975 and 1972), hypoglycemia exists as a bona fide state only when the patient's symptoms occur simultaneously with the nadir (lowest point) in the blood glucose level. Following this glucose nadir, evidence of hypothalamic-pituitary-adrenal responsiveness must be shown by a substantial rise in plasma cortisol to stress levels. If all these criteria are not met, hypoglycemia should not be diagnosed.

Postprandial blood sugar levels were measured in a normal population by Cahill and Soeldner (1974). They found that 23 percent of these subjects had blood glucose levels of less than 50 mg/100 ml, and an occasional patient had a glucose value as low as 35 mg/100 ml with no apparent symptoms. Burns et al. (1974) measured postprandial blood glucose levels on a continuous basis and showed that approximately 42 percent of normal asymptomatic subjects had glucose values below 50 mg/100 ml. Jung et al. (1971) reported that blood glucose levels of 59 to 42 mg/100 ml in the later hours of a glucose tolerance test were so common among young women, both obese and nonobese, that this must be considered in evaluating for hypoglycemia. The prevalence of low blood glucose levels among normal individuals may encourage the misdiagnosis of hypoglycemia without the use of reasonably strict criteria.

Early Alimentary Hypoglycemia. Alimentary hypoglycemia commonly occurs in patients who have undergone total or partial gastrectomy, gastrojejunostomy, or pyloroplasty with or without vagotomy. It may also occur in patients with overt peptic ulcer disease (Hofeldt et al., 1972), and has been reported by Permutt et al. (1973) in three patients without gastrointestinal disease or surgery.

Alimentary hypoglycemia is characterized by the absorption from jejunal mucosa of ingested carbohydrate within a short period of time. The result is an excessive postprandial rise in blood glucose and this exaggerated stimulus causes substantial increases in plasma insulin. With decreasing absorption of glucose, the hyperinsulinism then produces low blood sugar levels (Conn and Pek, 1974). A few individuals may show alimentary hypoglycemia without a hyperglycemic peak (Hofeldt et al., 1972).

Late Reactive Hypoglycemia of Early Maturity-Onset Diabetes. Some patients in the early stages of mild, maturity-onset diabetes may have symptomatic hypoglycemia 3 to 5 hours after meals supplying substantial amounts of carbohydrate. This is commonly due to a delayed release of insulin in the early stage of response to oral glucose. With normal insulin release in the later stage, hyperinsulinism develops while blood glucose is decreasing, resulting in hypoglycemia (Hofeldt et al., 1972; Conn and Pek, 1974).

Idiopathic Hypoglycemia. Idiopathic hypoglycemia is diagnosed when, during a 5-hour glucose tolerance, there is a symptomatic lowering of blood glucose and the individual shows a significant elevation of cortisol and growth hormone secretion in response to this stress. In addition, no alimentary or hormonal abnormalities are observed that would allow the cause to be categorized with other types of reactive hypoglycemia. The precise cause of idiopathic hypoglycemia cannot be determined by usual procedures.

Hofeldt et al. (1974) studied insulin secretion during an oral glucose tolerance test for 70 patients with reactive hypoglycemia, along with patient controls, disease-matched controls, and normal control subjects. They reported that 32 of 44 patients with idiopathic hypoglycemia showed delayed insulin secretion, regardless of the control group used for comparison. Nine of 44 patients with idiopathic reactive hypoglycemia, however, showed no abnormalities in insulin secretion under conditions of this study. All hypoglycemic patients had been diagnosed according to strict criteria. These results suggest that reactive hypoglycemia, including the idiopathic type, is indeed a syndrome with multiple etiologies.

Dietary Treatment of Reactive Hypoglycemia

A diet high in protein and low in carbohydrate has been used in treatment of reactive hypoglycemia for many years. The recommended protein level for a hypoglycemic adult is usually 110 to 140 g daily or approximately 2 g per kg body weight. Carbohydrate content may be as low as 90 to 100 g and should not exceed 40 percent of total kilocalories. Large carbohydrate loads and free sugar should be avoided. Frequent small feedings, with similar divisions of both protein and carbohydrate throughout the day, should be helpful in avoiding extremes of blood sugar levels. Total kilocalories should be prescribed to achieve or maintain ideal body weight (Conn and Pek, 1974). The exchange lists (see Sec. 2.2) may be used in calculating the carbohydrate content of the diet.

Anderson and Herman (1975) reported that seven patients with reactive hypoglycemia showed deterioration in glucose tolerance after a low-carbohydrate diet, whereas this was not observed in normal subjects. The reasons for these effects were not apparent, but did not seem to be due to decreased insulin secretion. These researchers questioned the wisdom of using a strict low-carbohydrate diet for patients with reactive hypoglycemia. For most of their patients they use a diabetic-type diet that contains approximately 45 percent of kilocalories as carbohydrate and avoids rapidly absorbed sugars such as sucrose. Sekso et al. (1975) found the traditional diet therapy unsatisfactory for their patients with reactive hypoglycemia. They reported satisfactory treatment with buformin (a biguanide) for some obese patients.

19.2 Gout

Gout is an ancient disease that has been discussed in medical literature since the time of Hippocrates. It is an inborn metabolic disorder characterized by hyperuricemia, recurrent attacks of acute arthritis, and deposits of sodium urate crystals (called tophi) in body tissues, particularly around joints. The presence of renal calculi (nephrolithiasis) commonly occurs during the course of the illness. Gout is not a single disease, but rather a syndrome resulting from any one of several different biochemical abnormalities which lead to hyperuricemia (Wintrobe et al., 1974, p. 607). It may develop secondarily as a result of other factors, including the use of thiazides as diuretic agents, lead intoxication, blood dyscrasias, and a type of glycogen storage disease (Talbott, 1970).

Etiology and Pathogenesis

Through the centuries, gout has been considered a hereditary disease primarily because it occurs in family groups. The incidence of hyperuricemia among asymptomatic blood relatives of gouty subjects is about 25 percent. Genetic determinants of hyperuricemia are apparently multifactorial, with some autosomal dominant and some sex-linked dominant factors. Environmental influences, such as diet, alcohol, and drugs, may operate in conjunction with genetic factors in determining hyperuricemia (Wintrobe et al., 1974, p. 609).

Uric acid is formed by oxidation of the purine bases, adenine and guanine, which serve as structural elements of DNA and RNA in body cells. These bases are of both dietary and biosynthetic origin. After several days of reduced purine intake, the body contains about 1200 mg uric acid and turns over about 700 mg per day. Two-thirds of this amount is excreted in the urine and one-third in bile, gastric juice, and intestinal secretions and is destroyed by colonic bacteria. About 20 to 25 percent of gouty subjects synthesize abnormally large amounts of purine and excrete excessive amounts of uric acid. About two-thirds of subjects with gout produce excessive quantities of purine but excrete normal amounts of uric acid in the urine. Several enzymatic abnormalities that are responsible for excessive production of uric acid have been described in gouty families. They include (1) a decreased activity of hypoxanthine-guanine phosphoribosyltransferase and (2) an increased activity of phosphoribosylpyrophosphate synthetase. Each of these enzymes plays a key role in the formation of purine nucleotides (Wintrobe et al., 1974, pp. 609–610).

The kidney filters urate through the glomeruli. About 98 percent of filtered urate is reabsorbed, with excreted urate then being secreted again from the tubules into the urine. In some patients with primary gout without demonstrable overproduction of uric acid, Rieselbach et al. (1970) suggested that there may be insufficient secretory response by renal tubules.

With either increased production or abnormal retention of uric acid, serum levels are elevated. The level in most gouty patients is usually higher than 6.5 to 7.0 mg/100 ml. As the disease develops, sodium urate crystals form, are deposited as tophi in various body tissues, and contribute to joint degeneration (Talbott, 1970). Urate crystals are ingested by phagocytic cells in a foreign-body reaction and inflammation occurs, accompanied by pain. In many cases of gout there is a history of acute onset in a single metatarsophalangeal joint of the big toe (Riccitelli, 1968).

A relationship between elevated serum uric acid level and certain motivations, personality styles, and accomplishments has been suggested. Psychosocial correlates of hyperuricemia have been reported to include high achievement interest and drive, strong competitive and leadership qualities, and impressive professional, academic, or socioeconomic achievement (Katz and Weiner, 1972; Katz et al., 1973). In a study of seven pairs of adult brothers and a pair of first cousins raised together, all with family histories of gout and therefore likely to have hyperuricemia, manifest achievement, achievement orientation, and achievement drive did not reliably predict which brother in each pair possessed the higher uric acid level. However, significant success in prediction occurred when the variable of obesity-dietary content was employed. Obesity and overeating tended to contribute toward hyperuricemia and gout (Katz et al., 1973).

Treatment

The therapeutic aims in treatment of gout are (1) to terminate the acute gouty attack promptly; (2) to prevent recurrences; (3) to prevent or reverse complications resulting from deposition of sodium urate in joints and kidneys; and (4) to prevent formation of uric acid kidney stones. Drugs used in the acute attack may include colchicine, which relieves pain within 24 to 48 hours; phenylbutazone, which has analgesic and antipyretic properties; indomethacin, for the inflammatory process; and hydrocortisone injected into the joint to control inflammation (Wintrobe et al., 1974, p. 615; Riccitelli, 1968).

In the interval between attacks, a gouty patient should avoid high-purine foods in order to lessen the burden of uric acid excretion. However, a severe limitation of purine-containing foods is rarely indicated unless renal function and the ability to excrete uric acid are reduced significantly (Wintrobe et al., 1974, p. 616). Foods are grouped according to purine content in Table 19.2.

Many patients with gout are obese and weight loss should usually be prescribed. However, the weight loss must be gradual since rapid loss may precipitate a gouty attack. In general, moderate levels of dietary protein are desirable in order to avoid an excessive amount of nitrogen that may be used in purine synthesis. Fat may retard excretion of uric acid and should also be moderately low. The diet should be generally well balanced nutritionally. Alcohol consumption, particularly in combination with limited food intake, may increase serum uric acid levels and is associated with gouty attacks.

Table 19.2 PURINE CONTENT OF FOODS PER 100 G*

Group I (0 to 15 mg)	Group II (50 to 150 mg)	Group III (over 150 mg)
Cereals and breads	Beans, dry	Anchovies
Butter and other fats	Peas, dry	Asparagus
Cheese	Lentils	Brains
Milk	Fish and seafood	Sweetbreads
Eggs	Meats	Liver
Fruits	Poultry	Kidney
Vegetables	Spinach	Sardines
Nuts	Oatmeal	Meat extracts and gravies
		Mushrooms

* Adapted from Turner, 1970; Robinson and Lawler, 1977.

A high fluid intake is advisable to maintain a urinary output of 2000 ml per day. This promotes uric acid excretion and lessens the dangers of crystal formation in the kidney or ureter (Wintrobe et al., 1974, p. 616). Urate stones tend to be precipitated in an acid urine.

For patients with chronic gout, the drug allopurinol may be given. This drug is a xanthine oxidase inhibitor and blocks the formation of uric acid from xanthine and hypoxanthine without disrupting the biosynthesis of purines. Uricosuric agents, which increase the excretion of uric acid by blocking tubular reabsorption, may also be given. These include probenecid, sulfinpyrazone, and salicylates (Wintrobe et al., 1974, p. 616; Riccitelli, 1968).

REFERENCES

1. Anderson, J. W. and R. H. Herman. 1975. Effects of carbohydrate restriction on glucose tolerance of normal men and reactive hypoglycemic patients. *Am. J. Clin. Nutr.*, **28:** 748.

2. Burns, T. W., R. Bregant, H. J. Van Teenen, and T. E. Hood. 1965. Observations on blood glucose concentrations of human subjects during continuous sampling. *Diabetes,* **14:** 186.

3. Cahill, G. F. and J. S. Soeldner. 1974. A noneditorial on non-hypoglycemia. *N. Eng. J. Med.,* **291:** 905.

4. Conn, J. W. 1936. The advantage of a high protein diet in the treatment of spontaneous hypoglycemia. *J. Clin. Invest.,* **15:** 673.

5. Conn, J. W. and S. Pek. 1974. Current concepts on spontaneous hypoglycemia. *Scope Monograph* (Upjohn Company).

6. Hofeldt, F. D., R. A. Adler, and R. H. Herman. 1975. Postprandial hypoglycemia. *J. Am. Med. Assoc.,* **233:** 1309.

7. Hofeldt, F. D., S. Dippe, and P. H. Forsham. 1972. Diagnosis and classification of reactive hypoglycemia based on hormonal changes in response to oral and intravenous glucose administration. *Am. J. Clin. Nutr.,* **25:** 1193.

8. Hofeldt, F. D., E. G. Lufkin, L. Hagler, M. B. Block, S. E. Dippe, J. W. Davis, S. R. Levin, P. H. Forsham, and R. H. Herman. 1974. Are abnormalities in insulin secretion responsible for reactive hypoglycemia? *Diabetes,* **23:** 589.

9. Jung, Y., R. C. Khurana, D. G. Corredor, A. Hastillo, R. F. Lain, D. Patrick, P. Turkeltaub, and T. S. Danowski. 1971. Reactive hypoglycemia in women. *Diabetes,* **20:** 428.

10. Katz, J. L. and H. Weiner. 1972. Psychosomatic considerations in hyperuricemia and gout. *Psychosom. Med.,* **34:** 165.

11. Katz, J. L., H. Weiner, A. Gutman, and T. Yu. 1973. Hyperuricemia, gout, and the executive suite. *J. Am. Med. Assoc.,* **224:** 1251.

12. Merimee, T. J. and J. E. Tyson. 1977. Hypoglycemia in man. *Diabetes,* **26:** 161.

13. Permutt, M. A., J. Kelly, R. Bernstein, D. H. Alpers, B. A. Siegel, and D. M. Kipnis. 1973. Alimentary hypoglycemia in the absence of gastrointestinal surgery. *N. Eng. J. Med.,* **288:** 1206.

14. Riccitelli, M. L. 1968. Etiology and treatment of gout—modern concepts. *J. Am. Ger. Soc.,* **16:** 719.

15. Rieselbach, R. E., L. B. Sorensen, W. D. Shelp, and T. H. Steele. 1970. Diminished renal urate secretion per nephron as a basis for primary gout. *Ann. Int. Med.,* **73:** 359.

16. Robinson, C. H. and M. R. Lawler, 1977. *Normal and Therapeutic Nutrition,* 15th ed. New York: Macmillan.

17. Sekso, M., M. Solter, V. Zjačić, and T. Čabrijan. 1975. Treatment of reactive hypoglycemia with buformin. *Am. J. Clin. Nutr.,* **28:** 1271.

18. Special Report. 1973. Statement on hypoglycemia. *Diabetes,* **22:** 137.

19. Talbott, J. H. 1970. Gout. *Med. Clin. No. Am.* **54:** 431.

20. Turner, D. 1970. *Handbook of Diet Therapy,* 5th ed. Chicago: University of Chicago Press.

21. Wintrobe, M. M., G. W. Thorn, R. D. Adams, E. Braunwald, K. J. Isselbacher, and R. G. Petersdorf (Eds.) 1974. *Harrison's Principles of Internal Medicine,* 7th ed. New York: McGraw-Hill.

STUDY GUIDE

Hypoglycemia
Hypoglycemia may result from several different causes and has been classified in various ways.

1. Describe several different types of hypoglycemia and explain the possible cause in each case.

2. Describe the usual symptoms of hypoglycemia that result from neuroglycopenia and those that result from epinephrine discharge.

Reactive hypoglycemia has been widely diagnosed and is commonly treated by diet.

3. Suggest a procedure whereby reactive hypoglycemia might be effectively diagnosed and explain the importance of setting reasonably strict criteria for diagnosis.

4. Distinguish among early alimentary hypoglycemia, late reactive hypoglycemia of early maturity-onset diabetes, and idiopathic hypoglycemia in terms of probable causes and general management.

5. Make and explain appropriate dietary recommendations for a newly diagnosed patient with reactive hypoglycemia, including suggested levels of dietary protein and carbohydrate.

Gout
Gout is an ancient familial disease involving abnormal purine metabolism.

1. Describe characteristic biochemical and clinical manifestations of gout and explain their relationship to the disease process.

Treatment of gout may include both drugs and dietary modification.

2. Describe the major effect of each of the following drugs in the treatment of gout:
    (*a*) Cholchicine
    (*b*) Adrenal steroids
    (*c*) Allopurinol
    (*d*) Probenecid

3. List seven to eight foods that are comparatively high in purines and should probably be avoided by patients with gout.

4. Make and explain appropriate nutritional suggestions for a patient with acute or chronic gout concerning caloric level, fluid intake, protein and fat levels, and alcohol consumption.

UNIT 6

Cardiovascular and Renal Disorders

20

Hyperlipo-proteinemias

Fats play important roles in the diet and in body metabolism. However, excessive consumption of total dietary fat or of certain types of fat and/or abnormal metabolic handling of fat in the body may result in disease conditions that affect the circulatory system and heart. An elevation of lipid levels in the blood, called *hyperlipidemia*, is characteristic of these disease states. Elevated serum cholesterol is called *hypercholesterolemia* and *hypertriglyceridemia* designates an increased level of triglycerides. Lipid substances, being insoluble in water, are solubilized in the blood by combination in various proportions with proteins and phospholipids and the resulting particles are called lipoproteins. An elevation of lipoproteins in the blood is referred to as hyperlipoproteinemia.

Interest in the hyperlipidemias or hyperlipoproteinemias in recent years has developed, to a large extent, because of their association with coronary heart disease (CHD). Hypercholesterolemia, and possibly hypertriglyceridemia, create an increased risk of developing premature CHD. Hyperlipidemia is frequently genetically determined and early screening of populations is indicated to identify and treat individuals with hyperlipidemias before CHD can occur. As an aid in the diagnosis and treatment of hyperlipoproteinemias, a system of classification of these disorders was developed by Fredrickson et al. (1967). This chapter discusses the classification and treatment of hyperlipoproteinemias. A discussion of atherosclerosis and CHD and various factors that appear to influence the development and course of this disease state is in Chap. 21. As background for the discussion of hyperlipoproteinemias, a review of normal lipid metabolism is presented.

20.1   Blood Lipids

Chylomicrons enter the small lymph vessels (lacteals) from the intestinal mucosal cells and are released into the blood via the thoracic duct. Suchy and Sullivan (1975) followed the fatty acid composition of chylomicrons for 10 normal male subjects from fasting to 8 hours after consumption of 50 ml corn oil. Data collected during this experiment suggest that dietary triglyceride fatty acids incorporated into chylomicrons during absorption are rapidly released in the serum as free fatty acids and subsequently utilized in hepatic lipoprotein production and secretion. The data also indicate that a small but constant amount of triglyceride fatty acids in chylomicrons comes from an endogenous source rather than a dietary source. In other words, the intestinal cell is capable of synthesizing small amounts of lipoproteins even when dietary fat is not being consumed.

Hyperlipidemia, as hyperchylomicronemia, occurs normally after every fat-containing meal, reaching a peak in about 4 hours, and clearing from the blood within 8 to 12 hours. Chylomicrons do not normally appear in significant amounts in the blood of an individual who has not eaten for 12 to 16 hours.

Since blood, an aqueous system, contains appreciable amounts of water-insoluble lipids, it is interesting to consider how the lipids are dispersed. There is some lipid in the red blood cells, but almost all of this is in the stroma or framework of the cells as an essential part of the structure of the cell membrane. These lipids are quite constant in amount and are not influenced to any important degree by diet. A tiny fraction of plasma lipid consists of fatty acids attached to plasma albumin molecules, commonly called free fatty acid (FFA) or nonesterified fatty acid (NEFA), which changes rapidly in response to such influences as levels of blood glucose, insulin, exercise, and exposure to cold. It is evidently not critical in relation to the development of atherosclerosis and CHD. Most of the remainder of the lipids in the blood are combined with varying amounts of protein and dispersed as lipoproteins. This solubilizes them and allows their transport in aqueous blood.

Lipoproteins contain protein, triglycerides, cholesterol, cholesteryl esters, and phospholipids in variable proportions. Four particle systems of serum lipoproteins have been characterized by use of laboratory methods involving both ultracentrifugation and electrophoresis. Different terms have been used to describe the lipoprotein particles separated by each of these methods (see Fig. 20.1). Separation by ultracentrifugation depends on differences in density among the various particles, with those highest in protein being most dense. Separation by electrophoresis is affected by differences in electrical charge. The protein portion of the lipoprotein usually contributes the greatest charge, and highly charged particles tend to move rapidly in an electric field, although the charge and movement are influenced by conditions under which the separation is made.

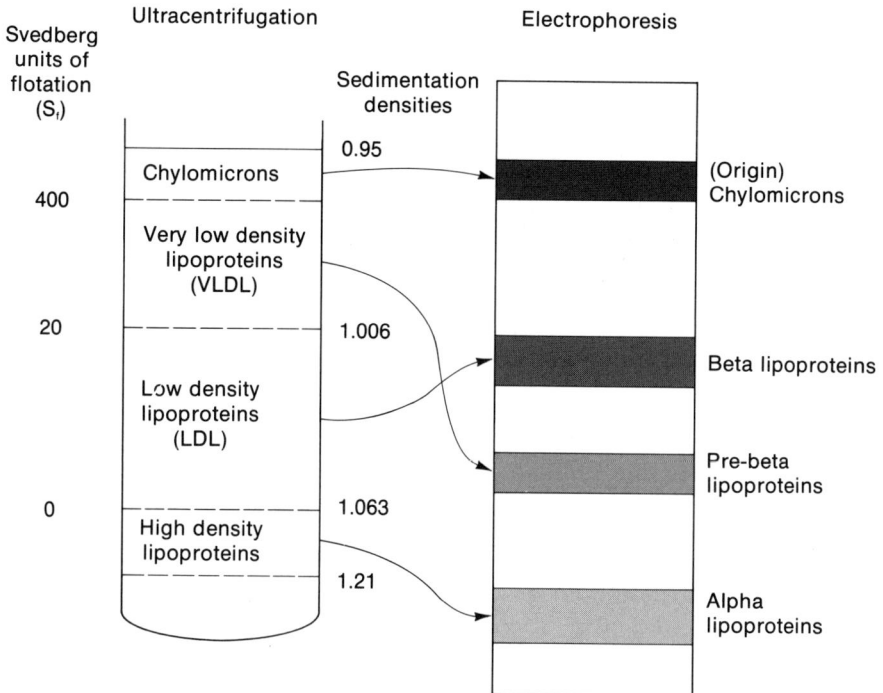

Fig. 20.1 Classification of blood lipoproteins by ultracentrifugation and lipoprotein electrophoresis. (Adapted from W. P. Castelli and R. F. Moran, "Lipid Studies for Assessing the Risk of Cardiovascular Disease and Hyperlipidemia," *Human Pathology*, **2**: 153, 1971.)

Some of the chylomicrons in the blood stream may be taken up immediately by adipose tissue cells. However, most of the chylomicrons apparently reach the liver where they are taken up by the cells, modified, and released back into the circulation as very-low-density lipoproteins (VLDL) and low-density lipoproteins (LDL). The liver cells also synthesize triglycerides from 2-carbon fragments, dietary carbohydrate, and fatty acids circulating in the blood, incorporating them into VLDL. The VLDL and LDL produced by the liver and released into the circulation are called *endogenous lipoproteins,* whereas chylomicrons, coming more directly from dietary fat, are labeled *exogenous lipoproteins,* although, as previously noted, the intestinal cell may synthesize a small amount of endogenous chylomicron-like particles. VLDL are probably the major source of plasma LDL, apparently through the formation of a transient intermediate low density lipoprotein form (ILDL). Conversion of VLDL to LDL involves the loss of core triglyceride and surface apoproteins (Levy et al., 1974).

Both endogenous and exogenous lipoproteins must be "cleared" from the blood. It is thought that a group of enzymes called *postheparin lipolytic activity* or *lipoprotein lipase* are involved in the breakup of large glyceride-containing particles into smaller more soluble lipoproteins and fatty acids which are rapidly assimilated by adipose and muscle cells (Levy, 1971).

Lipoproteins rich in triglycerides, as VLDL and chylomicrons, function primarily in the body as part of a transport system for energy metabolism. It has been suggested that lipoproteins rich in cholesterol and cholesteryl esters, particularly LDL, might have some transport function in sterol metabolism. Phospholipids and proteins in lipoproteins probably function primarily to stabilize the insoluble triglycerides and cholesterol in plasma (Nichols, 1970). Although the size and composition of lipoprotein particles vary, the usual range is presented in Table 20.1.

It is a less complicated laboratory procedure to measure total serum cholesterol and/or triglycerides than it is to measure the various types of blood lipoproteins. Serum cholesterol measurements are often made routinely. Since cholesterol and triglycerides do not circulate free in plasma, but rather are bound together with the other components of the lipoprotein particles, a measurement of these lipids does not give precise information as to the various lipoprotein levels in the blood. However, since LDL or beta lipoproteins contain 47 to 50 percent cholesterol, if this lipoprotein fraction is elevated it will be reflected in abnormally high serum cholesterol levels. Likewise, high serum triglyceride levels in fasting blood will be associated with elevated VLDL since this lipoprotein fraction contains 50 to 60 percent triglyceride. Therefore, the less expensive and less complicated measurements of serum cholesterol and triglycerides are more widely used in clinical practice than is the measurement of a lipoprotein profile directly.

There is some disagreement among both researchers and practitioners as to what constitutes a normal or desirable serum cholesterol level in humans. An uppermost acceptable level of 240 mg/100 ml has been sug-

Table 20.1 USUAL SIZE AND LIPID COMPOSITION OF VARIOUS LIPOPROTEIN PARTICLES*

		Lipid Composition (%)			Protein
Lipoprotein	**Size (nm)**	**Triglyceride**	**Cholesterol**	**Phospholipid**	**Composition (%)**
Chylomicrons	70–100	85–90	5–8	3–5	2
Very-low-density lipoproteins (VLDL)	30–100	50–60	12–15	18	8–10
Intermediate density (ILDL)	25–40	40	30	20	10
Low-density lipoproteins (LDL)	20	9–10	47–50	15–20	22–25
High-density lipoproteins (HDL)	7.5–10	5–8	18–20	25–27	46–50

* Castelli and Moran, 1971; Keys, 1967; Levy et al., 1974.

gested by some. However, a more desirable or optimal level for retardation of atherosclerosis is probably under 200 mg/100 ml. Even lower levels (170 to 200 mg/100 ml) for longer periods of time may be necessary to bring about regression of atherosclerotic lesions (Wright, 1976). Values for serum cholesterol vary somewhat in any one individual from time to time and are influenced by diet and change in weight. A seasonal variation in serum cholesterol has been reported, especially for women (Bleiler et al., 1963). Concentration of serum lipids increases with age. An upper limit for fasting serum triglycerides may be 150 mg/100 ml.

20.2 Cholesterol Metabolism

Cholesterol is a structural component of cell membranes and, therefore, vital to cell growth and survival. However, excessive amounts of cholesterol in the body can be detrimental. Mammalian cells must cope with the need to provide sufficient cholesterol for essential processes while, at the same time, avoiding excessive accumulation. Control of cholesterol metabolism by some type of feedback mechanism has been suggested, although the precise mechanism has not been clarified. From data collected in a study of cultured human fibroblasts, Brown and Goldstein (1976) postulated that a specific LDL receptor at the cell surface may participate in a feedback mechanism for cholesterol control, the surface receptor binding LDL of plasma and regulating the rate at which this lipoprotein transfers its cholesterol into the cell. The LDL receptor itself is under feedback regulation so that the cell increases the number of receptor sites in order to obtain cholesterol and suppresses the synthesis of LDL receptors to protect itself against an overaccumulation. Additional research is needed to confirm these mechanisms in humans.

Adipose tissue is a major site of cholesterol storage (Angel and Farkas, 1974). The total body pool of cholesterol is regulated by the interaction of absorption, synthesis, and excretion. Cholesterol taken in food is esterified with long-chain fatty acids, absorbed into the mucosal cell, and incorporated into chylomicrons. It eventually reaches the liver where it is incorporated into lipoproteins and released again into the plasma. The liver is apparently the main source of cholesterol that is synthesized in the body, although the intestines synthesize some. The main route for excretion of cholesterol from the body is bile, both as cholesterol and as bile acids. There is also a constant loss and replacement of cells lining the small intestine, leading to removal of some cholesterol in this way. Some of the cholesterol excreted in bile is reabsorbed, after mixing with cholesterol present in food that has been consumed.

Conflicting results have been reported concerning relationships among absorption, excretion, and synthesis of cholesterol in humans. Kaplan et al. (1963) and Wilson and Lindsey (1965) concluded that regardless of the amount of dietary cholesterol, the maximal absorption was generally at or below 300 mg per day. However, Quintão et al. (1971) reported that absorption of dietary cholesterol from liquid-formula diets given to patients in a metabolic ward increased with intake. Up to 1 g of cholesterol was absorbed in patients fed as much as 3 g per day. In most subjects, accumulation of cholesterol in body pools was small because of compensating decreases in synthesis and reexcretion of excess cholesterol. However, large dietary cholesterol intakes did not inhibit body synthesis of cholesterol in all subjects and large amounts of cholesterol could accumulate in the body in some cases. In this study, cholesterol accumulation in the body was not necessarily reflected in elevated plasma cholesterol levels. Kudchodkar et al. (1973), in a study of cholesterol absorption in 10 hyperlipemic subjects consuming normal foods, found that the amount of dietary cholesterol absorbed correlated well with dietary intake (401 to 1214 mg per day). The mean percentage absorption was 37 ± 5 percent. These later studies indicate that within the normal range of dietary cholesterol intake in North America, the amounts absorbed are proportional to intake. Compensatory regulation of cholesterol synthesis with increased dietary intake may not occur in all individuals.

20.3   Classification of Hyperlipoproteinemias

The terms hypercholesterolemia, hypertriglyceridemia, and hyperlipidemia do not indicate precisely which of the lipoprotein families is elevated. For example, hypertriglyceridemia can result from increased concentrations of chylomicrons, VLDL, or ILDL alone, or in various combinations. In 1967 Fredrickson, Levy, and Lees offered a classification of hyperlipoproteinemias that was based on a quantitative assessment of the lipoprotein systems using a preparative ultracentrifuge and standard lipoprotein separations with paper electrophoresis. Five patterns or types were described originally and more recently one of these types has been subdivided into two. Each type represents a shorthand term to describe which lipoproteins are increased in the plasma. The classifications are (Levy et al., 1974):

> Type I. Increased chylomicrons
> Type IIa. Increased LDL
> Type IIb. Increased LDL and VLDL
> Type III. Increased ILDL
> Type IV. Increased VLDL
> Type V. Increased chylomicrons and VLDL

The lipoprotein families each have distinct biochemical features that are summarized in Table 20.2. Some lipoproteins, upon elevation, produce a milky, turbid plasma that can be seen with the naked eye after the plasma has stood overnight in the refrigerator. It has been found with experience

Table 20.2 BIOCHEMICAL FEATURES OF THE LIPOPROTEIN FAMILIES*

Family	Origin	Function	Catabolism	Plasma Appearance
Chylomicrons	Intestine, from dietary fat	Transport of dietary fat	Lipoprotein lipase at tissue sites; chylomicron remnant cleared by liver	Creamy supernate—clear infranate
VLDL	Liver and small bowel, from carbohydrate, FFA, medium chain triglycerides	Transport of endogenous triglycerides	Complex—probably requires lipoprotein lipase for degradation	Turbid
ILDL	VLDL	Unknown	Unclear—degradation to LDL	Turbid
LDL	VLDL-ILDL (Possible alternate source)	Unknown	Unclear—primary site of removal appears to be liver	Clear
HDL	Liver (Possibly in intestine also)	Unknown	Possibly facilitates cholesterol-ester metabolism	Clear

* Adapted from Levy et al., 1974.

in clinical practice that the appearance of the plasma, along with accurate determinations of cholesterol and triglyceride levels, will usually be sufficient to "type" the hyperlipoproteinemia. The patient's history and clinical features will also help to distinguish the type of pattern. Sometimes additional procedures, such as ultracentrifugation or the determination of HDL concentrations, or both, may be necessary to establish the lipoprotein type.

Once the lipoprotein pattern has been typed, it is necessary to determine whether the hyperlipoproteinemia is primary or secondary to other disorders, such as myxedema, alcoholism, liver disease, renal disease, or diabetes mellitus. If it is secondary, treatment of the primary disorder will usually correct the hyperlipoproteinemia. If it is primary it may be familial, in which case family screening should be done.

A summary of the types of hyperlipoproteinemia is given in Table 20.3. None of the patterns indicates a specific mechanism of disease. The abnormalities could result from overproduction of various lipoproteins or from decreased clearance or catabolism.

Type I

The Type I disorder is indicative of the body's inability to clear chylomicrons from the blood. It is nearly always familial, recessively transmitted, diagnosed in young patients, and extremely rare. The basic defect appears

Table 20.3 TYPES OF HYPERLIPOPROTEINEMIA*

Features	Type I	Type IIa	Type IIb	Type III	Type IV	Type V
Incidence	Very rare	Common	Common	Relatively uncommon	Common	Uncommon
Lipoprotein abnormality	↑ fasting chylomicrons	↑ LDL	↑ LDL ↑ VLDL	↑ ILDL	↑ VLDL	↑ fasting chylomicrons ↑ VLDL
Plasma cholesterol	Normal or elevated	Elevated	Elevated	Elevated	Normal or elevated	Elevated or normal
Plasma triglycerides	Greatly elevated	Normal	Elevated	Usually elevated	Elevated	Elevated to greatly elevated
Clinical signs	Lipemia retinalis, eruptive xanthomas, hepatosplenomegaly, abdominal pain; childhood expression	Tendon and tuberous xanthomas, xanthelasma, juvenilis corneal arcus accelerated coronary atherosclerosis, detected in early childhood in severe cases		Planar, tuberoeruptive and tendon xanthomas; accelerated atherosclerosis of coronary and peripheral vessels, detected in adults	Accelerated coronary vessel disease, abnormal glucose tolerance, hyperuricemia, detected in adults	Lipemia retinalis, eruptive xanthomas, hepatosplenomegaly, abdominal pain, hyperglycemia, hyperuricemia, detected in early adulthood
Inheritance, if primary	Recessive, deficiency in lipoprotein lipase	Dominant, sporadic		Recessive	Dominant, sporadic	Dominant, sporadic
Secondary causes	Dysgammaglobulinemia, insulinopenic diabetes, myxedema	Myxedema, myeloma, porphyria, nephrosis, obstructive liver disease, excess dietary cholesterol		Myxedema, dysgammaglobulinemia	Diabetes, nephrosis, pancreatitis, glycogen storage disease	Nephrosis, myeloma, diabetic acidosis, alcoholism, pancreatitis

* Adapted from Levy, 1971; LaRosa, 1972a.

to be a deficiency of one or more of the lipoprotein lipase enzymes. A discrete creamy top layer forms on plasma from Type I patients after the plasma stands in the cold. Eruptive xanthomas are common in Type I but are not usually painful and may be overlooked by the patient. They disappear when high plasma triglyceride levels are decreased. Bouts of abdominal pain usually occur. Since patients with this disorder cannot handle dietary fat, it must be decreased to a very low level. Medium chain triglycerides may be used since these are not incorporated into chylomicrons.

Type II

Type II is fairly common and may be found in all ages. It is often familial, transmitted as a dominant trait with almost complete penetrance, and is associated with the development of premature coronary artery disease. Therefore, family members of the patient with Type II should be screened and treated for hyperlipoproteinemia when this is present. Elevated LDL will be reflected in high levels of serum cholesterol. Type IIa shows elevated serum cholesterol but normal triglyceride levels. Type IIb is characterized by elevation of VLDL, as well as LDL, and usually shows abnormally high levels of both serum triglycerides and cholesterol. Mild forms of Type IIa may be due to excessive dietary intake of cholesterol. The Type IIa and IIb patterns alternate in relatives affected with "monogenic" familial Type II. Patients with Type IIb resemble Type IV patients in blood lipid patterns and response to diet, particularly in mild cases.

Clinical symptoms include xanthomas over tendons in familial Type II. The Achilles tendon is most commonly affected although the extensor tendons of the hands, feet, knees, and elbows are often involved. Tuberous xanthomas occur in the skin and are prominent in areas where minor trauma is greatest, as over elbows and buttocks. Xanthelasma are cutaneous cholesterol deposits around the eyelids. Corneal arcus, which is a whitish band just inside the outer rim of the cornea, represents cholesterol deposition in the area where the cornea becomes avascular, and may occur in Type II hyperlipoproteinemia. Xanthelasma and corneal arcus may also occur without lipoprotein abnormality (LaRosa, 1972a).

Type III

The Type III pattern is relatively uncommon. It was first described as an abnormal beta lipoprotein form ("floating" or "broad beta") and has more recently been associated with an increase in ILDL (Levy et al., 1974). Both plasma cholesterol and triglycerides are elevated and the plasma may appear clear, cloudy, or milky. Type III is usually familial and is transmitted as a recessive trait. The defect seems to be in the mechanism for conversion or breakdown of large glyceride-containing lipoprotein complexes into the smaller more soluble lipoproteins (Levy, 1971). Planar xanthomas (orange-yellow lipid deposits in the palms of the hands) and tuberoeruptive xanthomas are common in Type III and contribute to diagnosis. There is accelerated atherosclerosis of coronary and peripheral vessels.

Type IV

The Type IV pattern is relatively common, frequently diagnosed in adults, and associated with abnormal glucose tolerance and premature atherosclerosis. It is characterized by increased VLDL and, therefore, plasma triglyceride levels are elevated. The plasma is clear, cloudy, or milky depending on the level of triglyceride. Plasma cholesterol levels are often normal and there are no external signs of the disorder. This pattern sometimes reflects a familial disorder transmitted apparently as a dominant trait with delayed expression. Several different mutations may be responsible for the Type IV pattern (Levy, 1971). Whether primary or secondary to other disorders, it is usually exacerbated by obesity. Reduction to normal weight is, therefore, of vital importance in treatment. The triglyceridemia seems to be particularly responsive to dietary carbohydrate, which should be limited in the diet.

Type V

The Type V abnormality is characterized by excessive amounts of both chylomicrons and VLDL. This pattern may be familial, but is most commonly secondary to acute metabolic disturbances such as diabetic acidosis, pancreatitis, alcoholism, and nephrosis. It has similar features to Type I, with creamy plasma, hepatosplenomegaly, and bouts of abdominal pain. Plasma triglyceride levels may be extremely high because of the presence of chylomicrons and elevated VLDL levels. Serum cholesterol may also be elevated. Abnormal glucose tolerance and hyperuricemia are frequently associated with this pattern. Restriction of fat is necessary to control the chylomicron level and the VLDL fraction is sensitive to dietary carbohydrate. Both of these nutrients must be limited in the diet.

20.4   Treatment of Hyperlipoproteinemias

Since there is no single cause for hyperlipidemia, there is no single all-embracing treatment. However, on an individual basis, each type of hyperlipoproteinemia may be treated substantially or totally. A number of benefits accrue from treatment. Correction of chylomicronemia will prevent attacks of abdominal pain and pancreatitis that are commonly associated with Types I and V hyperlipoproteinemia. Xanthomas and similar clinical signs should regress with treatment. It has been hypothesized that treating Types II, III, and IV will decrease the risk of developing CHD. This hypothesis is strongly supported by epidemiological evidence although direct experimental proof is lacking for humans (Levy et al., 1974).

Dietary treatment constitutes the basis of serum lipoprotein-lowering therapy and lifelong dietary modifications are desirable. In general, the following dietary modifications will be appropriate for the various lipoprotein abnormalities:

Lipoprotein abnormality	Dietary modification
Increased chylomicrons (Types I and V)	Low fat (25 to 35 g per day) Medium-chain triglycerides may be used
Increased VLDL (Types IIb, IV, and V)	Weight reduction to ideal Controlled amounts of carbohydrate and alcohol
Increased ILDL (Type III)	Weight reduction to ideal Controlled amounts of carbohydrate Low cholesterol and saturated fat (empirical)
Increased LDL (Types IIa and IIb)	Low cholesterol High ratio polyunsaturated to saturated fat

Two categories of drugs that may be used in combination with diet therapy for the treatment of hyperlipoproteinemia are (1) those that decrease lipoprotein synthesis and (2) those that increase lipoprotein catabolism. Nicotinic acid and possibly clofibrate (Atromid-S) belong to the first group. Clofibrate has also been shown to enhance the catabolism of VLDL. Cholestyramine (Questran), d-thyroxine (Choloxin), and probably sitosterol (Cytellin) belong to the second group. All of these drugs have been approved by the Food and Drug Administration for use as hypolipidemic agents (Levy et al., 1974).

Nicotinic acid is primarily indicated in cases of elevated VLDL. However, it is also useful in patients with increased levels of ILDL and LDL. Side effects include cutaneous flushing and pruritus. Development of fatty liver occurs on long-term administration but choline may prevent this. Clofibrate is indicated when increased levels of VLDL and ILDL are present. It probably has little value with LDL. Serious side effects do not usually accompany the administration of clofibrate. Cholestyramine remains completely unabsorbed in the gastrointestinal tract. In the small intestine it exchanges its chloride ions for bile acids and thus increases bile acid excretion by interrupting the enterohepatic circulation. Cholestyramine is indicated only when increased levels of LDL are present. Gastrointestinal symptoms, including constipation, nausea, vomiting, abdominal distention, and cramps, may occur as side effects. With increased levels of LDL, and possibly increased ILDL, d-thyroxine is useful. Its use in therapy is limited, however, because of its cardiotoxic effects, particularly in subjects with existing coronary artery disease. Sitosterol is an emulsion of plant sterols that have structures similar to cholesterol but are not absorbed in humans. They have been shown to inhibit cholesterol absorption on a competitive basis. Sitosterol is only indicated for states characterized by increased LDL. It may have a mild laxative effect and sometimes causes nausea and diarrhea. Combinations of drugs may sometimes be used (Levy et al., 1974).

The mechanisms by which dietary measures accomplish their lipid-lowering effects are not fully understood, some being used on an empirical basis. Decreased dietary cholesterol has been shown to decrease intestinal absorption and increased synthesis may not always compensate for the lesser amount absorbed. A low-cholesterol diet may also increase catabolism of LDL (Vessby et al., 1975).

Using sterol balance techniques, some researchers have reported an increase in sterol excretion in humans with diets high in polyunsaturated fatty acids (PUFA) (Connor et al., 1969; Nestel et al., 1973). This effect is greater on high- than low-cholesterol diets and more pronounced during the early than later stages of the experimental period (Nestel et al., 1975). However, Grundy and Ahrens (1970) concluded from studies in humans that the total amount of body cholesterol can increase when PUFA are consumed in comparatively large amounts and the plasma cholesterol concentration is falling. It has also been suggested that PUFA may reduce the cholesterol carrying capacity of apoprotein B in the LDL because of steric hindrance (Spritz and Mishkel, 1969).

Restriction of simple carbohydrate and weight reduction will result in decreased hepatic triglyceride synthesis. It is not clear if this is due to the decreased amount of triglyceride precursors, reduced insulin levels, decreased insulin resistance, or some other effect (Vessby et al., 1975).

Table 20.4 presents a summary of the diets suggested by Fredrickson et al. (1973). Detailed information on these diets and lists of foods to be included and excluded has been compiled in a Handbook for Physicians and Dietitians and also in a series of pamphlets for use in counseling patients with hyperlipoproteinemia.

Long-term effects of diet therapy in lowering serum lipids have been significant but often the effect is not extremely large. A review by Berkowitz (1973) of nine dietary trials in outpatients showed that a reduction in serum cholesterol of 14 percent was the maximum effect obtained. A 25 percent mean decrease in plasma cholesterol was reported in 12 normal volunteers on a low cholesterol high P/S ratio diet (Levy et al., 1972). Mean serum LDL level fell by 11 percent in a group of hypertriglyceridemic men on the American Heart Association's fat-modified diet for 6 months. It decreased another 7 percent when these subjects were then placed on a 30 percent carbohydrate diet for another 6 months. The mean VLDL level of these subjects decreased 14 percent during the first 6 months on the American Heart Association diet and decreased an additional 21 percent on the low-carbohydrate regimen (Hulley et al., 1972). Glueck et al. (1977) reported an overall reduction by diet of total and LDL cholesterol levels between 6 percent and 15 percent in 2- to 7-year-old children with familial hypercholesterolemia. Effective diet counseling is important in helping patients to understand and follow diets for hyperlipoproteinemias. Gotto et al. (1977) reported that over a 2-year period, 103 patients with Type IV hyper-

Table 20.4 SUMMARY OF DIETS FOR TYPES I–V HYPERLIPOPROTEINEMIA*

	Type I	Type IIa	Type IIb and Type III	Type IV	Type V
Diet Prescription	Low fat 25– 35 g	Low cholesterol Polyunsaturated fat increased	Low cholesterol Approximately: 20% kcal Protein 40% kcal Fat 40% kcal CHO	Controlled CHO Approximately 45% of kcal Moderately restricted cholesterol	Restricted fat 30% of kcal Controlled CHO 50% of kcal Moderately restricted cholesterol
Calories	Not restricted	Not restricted	Achieve and maintain "ideal" weight, i.e., reduction diet if necessary	Achieve and maintain "ideal" weight, i.e., reduction diet if necessary	Achieve and maintain "ideal" weight, i.e., reduction diet if necessary
Protein	Total protein intake is not limited	Total protein intake is not limited	High protein	Not limited other than control of patient's weight	High protein
Fat	Restricted to 25– 35 g	Saturated fat intake limited Polyunsaturated fat intake increased	Controlled to 40% kcal. (PUF recommended in preference to saturated fats)	Not limited other than control of patient's weight (PUF recommended in preference to saturated fats)	Restricted to 30% of kcal (PUF recommended in preference to saturated fats)
Cholesterol	Not restricted	As low as possible; the only source of cholesterol is the meat in the diet	Less than 300 mg—the only source of cholesterol is the meat in the diet	Moderately restricted to 300– 500 mg	Moderately restricted to 300– 500 mg
Carbohydrate	Not limited	Not limited	Controlled—concentrated sweets are restricted	Controlled—concentrated sweets are restricted	Controlled—concentrated sweets are restricted
Alcohol	Not recommended	May be used with discretion	Limited to 2 servings (substituted for carbohydrate)	Limited to 2 servings (substituted for carbohydrate)	Not recommended

* Fredrickson et al., 1973.

lipoproteinemia who received regular dietary counseling by a dietitian and physician showed significantly decreased levels of serum triglycerides in comparison to 175 patients with the same diagnosis who received similar written diets but little counseling. Diet therapy is the first line of defense in the treatment of hyperlipoproteinemia because it is generally more effective than drug therapy and has fewer side effects. Lowering of plasma lipid levels to normal may result from dietary therapy alone but rarely does this happen with drugs alone (LaRosa, 1972b). A reduction of 15 percent or greater in serum cholesterol or triglyceride concentration means that the dietary treatment is successful.

Type I
Metabolism of chylomicrons is better understood than is that for any of the other lipoproteins. Diet therapy for Type I hyperlipoproteinemia is aimed at reducing the load of exogenous fat to accommodate the defective chylomicron clearing mechanism of the body. To keep the serum triglyceride level near the normal range, it is necessary to drastically restrict dietary fat to 25 to 35 g per day. All sources of fat in the food must be considered in calculating the diet. Since low-fat diets tend to be somewhat dry and not very acceptable, it may be desirable to include medium-chain triglyceride (MCT) oil in the regimen. MCTs are discussed in Secs. 12.1 and 13.5.

The diet for Type I, as outlined by the National Heart and Lung Institute, does not restrict cholesterol and does not calculate P/S ratio. Carbohydrate and protein intakes are not limited. Reduction of fat is accomplished by:

> Eliminating all separated fats, such as butter, margarine, oils, and so on
> Eliminating nuts
> Using lean meats
> Avoiding many baked goods
> Restricting dairy products containing fat

A sample menu pattern for an adult with Type I hyperlipoproteinemia is shown in Table 20.5.

Type IIa
The major characteristics of the diet for Type IIa hyperlipoproteinemia are decreased dietary cholesterol and modification in type of fat to produce an increased P/S ratio. In calculating the P/S ratio, the total grams of linoleic acid in the diet are divided by total grams of saturated fatty acids.

$$\text{P/S ratio} = \frac{\text{linoleic acid}}{\text{saturated fatty acids}}$$

The P/S ratio should be at least 2 or higher. This requires that lean meats are used and that 1 tsp PUF is consumed for each ounce of meat in the diet. The cholesterol is restricted to no more than 300 mg per day. No egg yolk

Table 20.5 SAMPLE MENU PATTERNS FOR TYPES I TO V
HYPERLIPOPROTEINEMIA*

Sample menu for adult with Type I; 1700 to 2000 kcal

Daily Food Plan	Sample Menu Pattern
1 qt skim milk	Breakfast:
5 oz cooked poultry, fish, or lean trimmed meat	Citrus fruit or juice
5 servings vegetable and fruit	Cereal
6 or more servings bread or cereal	Toast
1 or more servings potato, rice, etc.	Jelly and sugar
Allowed desserts	Skim milk
Sugar, sweets	Coffee or tea if desired
	Lunch:
	2 oz cooked poultry, fish, or lean meat
	Potato, rice, spaghetti, or noodles
	Vegetable
	Bread
	Jelly and sugar
	Fruit
	Allowed dessert
	Skim milk
	Dinner:
	3 oz cooked poultry, fish, or lean meat
	Potato, rice, or noodles
	Vegetable
	Bread
	Jelly and sugar
	Allowed dessert
	Skim milk
	Between-Meal Snack:
	Skim milk
	Fruit or allowed dessert
	Bread with jam or jelly

Sample menu for adult with Type IIa; 1700 to 2000 kcal

Daily Food Plan	Sample Menu Pattern
1 pt or more skim milk	Breakfast:
Cooked poultry, fish, or lean trimmed meat	Citrus fruit or juice
5 servings vegetable and fruit; include:	Cereal
1 serving citrus	Toast
1 serving dark green or deep yellow vegetable	Allowed fat
7 or more servings whole grain or enriched bread	Jelly and sugar
or cereal	Skim milk
1 or more servings potato, rice, etc.	Coffee or tea if desired
Allowed fat	Lunch:
Allowed desserts and sweets	Poultry, fish, or lean meat
	Potato or substitute
	Vegetables
	Bread
	Allowed fat
	Fruit or allowed dessert
	Skim milk

Table 20.5 SAMPLE MENU PATTERNS FOR TYPES I TO V HYPERLIPOPROTEINEMIA* (cont'd.)

Sample menu for adult with Type IIa; 1700 to 2000 kcal

	Sample Menu Pattern
	Dinner:
	Poultry, fish, or lean meat
	Potato or substitute
	Vegetable
	Bread
	Allowed fat
	Fruit or allowed dessert
	Skim milk
	Between-Meal Snack:
	Fruit
	Skim milk

Sample menu for adult with Type IIb or Type III; 2000 kcal maintenance diet plan

Daily Food Plan	Sample Menu Pattern
2 servings poultry, fish, or lean trimmed meat	Breakfast:
3 servings skim milk	1 serving citrus fruit or juice
8 servings bread, cereal, etc.	2 servings cereal or toast
15 servings allowed fat	3 servings allowed fat
3 servings fruit	1 serving skim milk
Vegetables as desired	
	Lunch:
	1 serving poultry, fish, or lean trimmed meat
	1 serving potato or substitute
	Vegetables
	2 servings bread
	6 servings allowed fat
	1 serving fruit
	1 serving skim milk
	Dinner:
	1 serving poultry, fish, or lean trimmed meat
	1 serving potato or substitute
	Vegetables
	2 servings bread
	6 servings allowed fat
	1 serving fruit
	1 serving skim milk

Sample menu for adult with Type IV; 1800 kcal maintenance diet plan†

Daily Food Plan	Sample Menu Pattern
Servings poultry, fish, or lean trimmed meat	Breakfast:
2 servings skim milk	2 servings citrus fruit or juice
8 servings bread, cereal, etc.	2 servings cereal or toast
Allowed fat	Allowed fat
6 servings fruit	1 serving skim milk
Vegetables as desired	

Table 20.5 SAMPLE MENU PATTERNS FOR TYPES I TO V
HYPERLIPOPROTEINEMIA* (*cont'd.*)

Sample menu for adult with Type IV; 1800 kcal maintenance diet plan†

Sample Menu Pattern

Lunch:

    Serving poultry, fish, or lean trimmed meat
    1 serving potato or substitute
    Vegetables
    2 servings bread
    Allowed fat
    2 servings fruit

Dinner:

    Serving poultry, fish, or lean trimmed meat
    1 serving potato or substitute
    Vegetables
    2 servings bread
    Allowed fat
    2 servings fruit
    1 serving skim milk

Sample menu for adult with Type V; 1800 kcal maintenance diet plan

---

Daily Food Plan	Sample Menu Pattern
2 servings poultry, fish, or lean trimmed meat	Breakfast:
4 servings skim milk	1 serving citrus fruit or juice
10 servings bread, cereal, etc.	3 servings cereal or toast
6 servings allowed fat	2 servings allowed fat
3 servings fruit	1 serving skim milk
Vegetables as desired	Lunch:
	1 serving poultry, fish, or lean trimmed meat
	1 serving potato or substitute
	Vegetables
	2 servings bread
	2 servings allowed fat
	1 serving fruit
	1 serving skim milk
	Dinner:
	1 serving poultry, fish, or lean trimmed meat
	1 serving potato or substitute
	Vegetables
	2 servings bread
	2 servings allowed fat
	1 serving fruit
	1 serving skim milk
	P.M. Snack:
	1 serving skim milk
	1 serving bread or cereal

---

* Fredrickson et al., 1973.

† Limit skim milk, breads, cereals, etc., and fruit as designated. This diet controls only carbohydrate foods. If patient not able to follow this relatively free diet (an indication might be weight gain), the more strictly controlled Type III diet may be prescribed.

or organ meats are allowed. Up to 9 oz of fish, shellfish (except shrimp), poultry, and veal may be consumed per day, but beef, lamb, ham, and pork are limited to a 3-oz portion three times each week. Oils can be used in the preparation of meats, in salad dressings, sauces, vegetables, and baked products. A sample menu pattern for an adult with Type IIa hyper-lipoproteinemia is shown in Table 20.5.

Types IIb and III

Dietary treatment for Types IIb and III is similar and usually successful in normalizing blood lipoproteins. In individuals who are obese, the first step is to reduce the daily caloric intake so that weight reduction occurs and ideal body weight is achieved. Serum triglycerides are usually decreased by decreasing obesity. Once the individual has reached ideal weight, the main-tenance diet is balanced in fat and carbohydrate (40 percent of kilocalories coming from each) and is also low in cholesterol (less than 300 mg per day). The most important characteristic of the reduction diet is its limitation of kilocalories; any nutritionally balanced low-kilocalorie diet may be used. The maintenance diet must control the level of carbohydrate, particularly, to maintain normal plasma triglyceride concentration since excessive dietary car-bohydrate tends to increase production of VLDL. Carbohydrate intake should not exceed 4 g per kg body weight. Fat intake should not exceed $1\frac{1}{2}$ to 2 g per kg body weight and PUF should be substituted for saturated fat as much as possible. Cholesterol intake is restricted to control the level of serum LDL. All high-cholesterol foods such as egg yolk and organ meats are eliminated from the diet. Most concentrated sweets are also eliminated. Protein makes up 18 to 21 percent of total kilocalories in this high-protein diet ($1\frac{1}{2}$ to 2 g per kg body weight). Alcohol may be substituted for car-bohydrate food in limited amounts at the discretion of the nutrition coun-selor and physician. A sample menu pattern for an adult with Type IIb or III is shown in Table 20.5.

Type IV

Diet therapy in Type IV hyperlipoproteinemia emphasizes reduction to ideal body weight. At ideal weight the patient almost always has serum triglyceride levels reduced from those present when he is heavier. Any nutritionally balanced low-kilocalorie diet may be used for weight reduc-tion. After ideal weight is achieved, the diet is designed to avoid an excess of carbohydrate and alcohol since either tends to increase levels of VLDL in the blood and, therefore, serum triglycerides. The carbohydrate intake is controlled at about 45 percent of kilocalories. Concentrated sweets are restricted, and the total carbohydrate intake should not exceed 4 to 5 g per kg body weight. Protein and fat intakes are not limited except to control the caloric level for ideal weight maintenance. PUF is substituted for saturated fat at reasonable levels, and cholesterol intake is moderately restricted (less than 500 mg/day). Alcohol in limited amounts may be substituted for carbohydrate, at the discretion of the nutrition counselor and physician. Type IV hyperlipoproteinemia is often associated with diabetes mellitus, and dietary treatment as outlined helps control diabetes, when present. A sample menu pattern for an adult with Type IV is shown in Table 20.5.

Type V

A mixed hyperlipidemia, with elevated exogenous (chylomicrons) and endogenous (VLDL) lipids in fasting plasma, is characteristic of Type V. Patients with familial Type V may have all the features of Type I. On an unrestricted diet, plasma triglycerides may range from 1000 to 6000 mg/100 ml. Diet therapy emphasizes caloric restriction and reduction to ideal body weight. After attainment of ideal weight, the maintenance diet is limited in both fat and carbohydrate, allowing plasma triglyceride concentrations to be maintained below 300 to 600 mg/100 ml. The diet is high in protein. Fat content is approximately 30 percent of kilocalories, carbohydrate approximately 50 percent, and protein about 20 percent. Cholesterol intake is moderately restricted to less than 500 mg per day. Dietary fat is limited in order to help control the chylomicronemia. The carbohydrate is limited to control the production of VLDL, and thus plasma triglycerides. PUF should be used where possible but the total amount that can be consumed is limited by total fat restriction. This is a difficult diet for most patients to follow and they require a great deal of encouragement and counsel. Table 20.5 shows a sample menu pattern for an adult.

Prescription of a diet is the beginning and not the end of treatment for a patient with hyperlipoproteinemia. Such patients should be followed at regular intervals, with particular attention to adherence, changes in weight, associated symptoms, and levels of plasma lipids. Patients may need considerable counsel and help in the early stages of diet therapy (LaRosa, 1972b).

Surgical Treatment

When diet and drugs fail to control hyperlipoproteinemia in patients with a high risk of CHD, surgery for an ileal bypass may be performed to increase excretion of bile acids and sterols. This produces a direct loss of normally absorbed (exogenous) cholesterol and reabsorbed (endogenous) cholesterol. It may also produce an indirect metabolic drain on the cholesterol pools of the body (Scott, 1972). Buchwald et al. (1974) reported data on the management of 101 consecutive patients with hyperlipidemias followed for at least 3 months before ileal bypass. The surgical procedure was effective in patients having poor or no response to diet and/or drug therapy. The average reduction in serum cholesterol from the preoperative but postdietary baseline was 40 percent; reduction in serum triglycerides ranged from 2 percent to 41 percent.

20.5 Screening for Hyperlipoproteinemia

The prevalence of various forms of serum lipid abnormalities has been reported by several researchers. Wood et al. (1972) studied 1118 free-living volunteers, 25 to 79 years of age, from eight counties of the Central Valley in California. Type IV lipoproteinemia was the most common abnormality found within the entire normal population (8.6 percent) and was 2.7 times as common in men as in women. Type II was less common (3.7 percent) and more frequent in women than men. Types III and V were very uncommon and Type I was not found.

Gibson and Whorton (1973) screened a population sample of 142 men and 148 women, aged 40 to 69 years, in Chittenden County, Vermont for blood lipid abnormalities. Type II hyperlipoproteinemia was present in 3.5 percent of the men and 6 percent of the women, whereas Type IV was found in 21 percent of the men and 10 percent of the women. Brown and Daudiss (1973) found no patients with Type I or V hyperlipoproteinemia among 1301 male and female blood donors, aged 18 to 64 years, in Albany, New York and only three patients with Type III. Type IV was the most prevalent hyperlipoproteinemia in this study and was significantly more prevalent in males than females (261 per 1000 versus 81 per 1000). The prevalence rate for Type II in male and female subjects was 87 per 1000 and 104 per 1000, respectively. Subjects with Type IV hyperlipoproteinemia, but not those with Type II, were significantly more obese than normal. In all three studies, Type IV was found to be most prevalent and Type II second. More males than females were found with Type IV, whereas the opposite was true for Type II. Gibson and Whorton (1973) speculated that it may be inappropriate without further study to recommend nationwide dietary modifications that aim primarily at hypercholesterolemia when Type IV, with elevated serum triglycerides, is possibly the most common type of abnormality.

Wilson et al. (1970) studied 98 adult-onset diabetic patients selected at random from an ambulatory clinic in Boston. They found that 37.8 percent of this sample had hyperlipidemia. In follow-up examination of the hyperlipidemia patients, 23 percent had Type II, 58 percent Type IV, 13 percent a combined Type with elevated LDL and VLDL, and 6 percent had reverted to normal values. The Type IV patients were distinguished by greater relative body weight and hyperglycemia.

Tamir et al. (1972) followed 64 men in Israel who were under the age of 41 years and had survived for more than 6 months after a myocardial infarction. They also studied their children. Of this group, 26 fathers and all of their 55 children had normal serum lipids and lipoprotein patterns. Normal serum lipid concentration and abnormal lipoprotein patterns were found in 38 fathers. Of these, 23 had Type IIa, 11 had Type IIb, and four had Type IV hyperlipoproteinemia. Thirty of the 85 children whose fathers had abnormal lipoproteins were found to have Type II hyperlipoproteinemia.

Glueck et al. (1974) studied 223 children from 70 families where one parent had a myocardial infarction before age 50. Familial hyperlipoproteinemia was documented in 60 of 70 (85 percent) of the families with predominant phenotypes for IIa, IIb, and IV hyperlipoproteinemia in 14, 18, and 28 families, respectively. Familial hyperlipoproteinemia was documented in 69 of 223 (31 percent) of children from the myocardial infarction families, with phenotypes IIa, IIb, and IV hyperlipoproteinemia in 34, 10, and 25 children, respectively. The common occurrence of familial hyperlipoproteinemia in progeny of parents with myocardial infarction before age 50 makes screening of their families a logical process in order to identify and treat those individuals with hyperlipoproteinemia. Glueck et al. (1977) reported that dietary treatment seemed to be most effective when instituted in children at ages 1 or 2. Measurement of umbilical cord blood cholesterol offers promise in early diagnosis of familial Type II hyperlipoproteinemia in the neonate (Glueck et al., 1971). CHD in adulthood has its origin in infancy and childhood and early detection and treatment are indicated.

REFERENCES

1. Angel, A. and J. Farkas. 1974. Regulation of cholesterol storage in adipose tissue. *Lipid Res.*, **15:** 491.

2. Berkowitz, D. 1973. Management of the hyperlipidemic patient. *Med. Clinics N. Am.*, **57:** 881.

3. Bleiler, R. E., E. S. Yearick, S. S. Schnur, I. L. Singson, and M. A. Ohlson. 1963. Seasonal variation of cholesterol in serum of men and women. *Am. J. Clin. Nutr.*, **12:** 12.

4. Brown, D. F. and K. Daudiss. 1973. Hyperlipoproteinemia. Prevalence in a free-living population in Albany, New York. *Circulation*, **47:** 558.

5. Brown, M. S. and J. L. Goldstein. 1976. Receptor-mediated control of cholesterol metabolism. *Science*, **191:** 150.

6. Buchwald, H., R. B. Morre, and R. L. Varco. 1974. Surgical treatment of hyperlipidemia. *Circulation*, 49 (Supplement No. I).

7. Castelli, W. P. and R. F. Moran. 1971. Lipid studies for assessing the risk of cardiovascular disease and hyperlipidemia. *Human Pathology*, **2:** 153.

8. Connor, W. E., D. T. Witiak, D. B. Stone, and M. L. Armstrong. 1969. Cholesterol balance and bile acid excretion in normal men fed dietary fats of different fatty acid composition. *J. Clin. Invest.*, **48:** 1363.

9. Fredrickson, D. S., R. I. Levy, M. Bonnel, and N. Ernst. 1973. *Dietary Management of Hyperlipoproteinemia*. Bethesda, Md.: U.S. Department of Health, Education and Welfare, National Heart and Lung Institute.

10. Fredrickson, D. S., R. I. Levy, and R. S. Lees. 1967. Fat transport in lipoproteins—an integrated approach to mechanisms and disorders. *N. Eng. J. Med.*, **276:** 34.

11. Gibson, T. C. and E. B. Whorton. 1973. The prevalence of hyperlipidemia in a natural community. *J. Chron. Dis.*, **26:** 227.

12. Glueck, C. J., R. C. Tsang, R. W. Fallat, and M. J. Mellies. 1977. Diet in children heterozygous for familial hypercholesterolemia. *Am. J. Dis. Child.*, **131:** 162.

13. Glueck, C. J., R. W. Fallat, R. Tsang, and C. R. Buncher. 1974. Hyperlipemia in progeny of parents with myocardial infarction before age 50. *Am. J. Dis. Child.*, **127:** 70.

14. Glueck, C. J., F. Heckman, M. Schoenfeld, P. Steiner, and W. Pearce. 1971. Neonatal familial type II hyperlipoproteinemia: Cord blood cholesterol in 1800 births. *Metabolism,* **20:** 597.

15. Gotto, A. M., Jr., M. E. DeBakey, J. P. Foreyt, L. W. Scott, and J. I. Thornby. 1977. Dietary treatment of type IV hyperlipoproteinemia. *J. Am. Med. Assoc.,* **237:** 1212.

16. Grundy, S. M. and E. H. Ahrens, Jr. 1970. The effects of unsaturated dietary fats on absorption, excretion, synthesis, and distribution of cholesterol in man. *J. Clin. Invest.,* **49:** 1135.

17. Hulley, S. B., W. S. Wilson, M. I. Burrows, and M. Z. Nichaman. 1972. Lipid and lipoprotein responses of hypertriglyceridaemic outpatients to a low-carbohydrate modification of the A.H.A. fat-controlled diet. *Lancet,* **2** (Sep. 16): 551.

18. Kaplan, J. A., G. E. Cox, and C. B. Taylor. 1963. Cholesterol metabolism in man: Studies on absorption. *Arch. Pathol.,* **76:** 359.

19. Keys, A. 1967. Blood lipids in man—A brief review. *J. Am. Dietet. Assoc.,* **51:** 508.

20. Kudchodkar, B. J., H. S. Sodhi, and L. Horlick. 1973. Absorption of dietary cholesterol in man. *Metabolism,* **22:** 155.

21. LaRosa, J. C. 1972a. Hyperlipoproteinemia. 1. Diagnosis and clinical significance. *Postgrad. Med.,* **51:** 62.

22. LaRosa, J. C. 1972b. Hyperlipoproteinemia. 2. Dietary management. *Postgrad. Med.,* **52:** 75.

23. Levy, R. I. 1971. Classification and etiology of hyperlipoproteinemias. *Fed. Proc.,* **30:** 829.

24. Levy, R. I., D. S. Fredrickson, R. Shulman, D. W. Bilheimer, J. L. Breslow, N. J. Stone, S. E. Lux, H. R. Sloan, R. M. Krauss, and P. N. Herbert. 1972. Dietary and drug treatment of primary hyperlipoproteinemia. *Ann. Int. Med.,* **77:** 267.

25. Levy, R. I., J. Morganroth, and B. M. Rifkind. 1974. Treatment of hyperlipidemia. *N. Eng. J. Med.,* **290:** 1295.

26. Nestel, P. J., N. Havenstein, Y. Homma, T. W. Scott, and L. J. Cook. 1975. Increased sterol excretion with polyunsaturated-fat high-cholesterol diets. *Metabolism,* **24:** 189.

27. Nestel, P. J., N. Havenstein, H. M. Whyte, T. J. Scott, and L. J. Cook. 1973. Lowering of plasma cholesterol and enhanced sterol excretion with the consumption of polyunsaturated ruminant fats. *N. Eng. J. Med.,* **288:** 379.

28. Nichols, A. V. 1970. Functions and interrelationships of different classes of plasma lipoproteins. *Proc. Nat. Acad. Sci.,* **64:** 1128.

29. Quintão, E., S. M. Grundy, and E. H. Ahrens, Jr. 1971. Effects of dietary cholesterol on the regulation of total body cholesterol in man. *J. Lipid Res.,* **12:** 233.

30. Scott, H. W., Jr. 1972. Metabolic surgery for hyperlipidemia and atherosclerosis. *Am. J. Surgery,* **123:** 3.

31. Spritz, N. and M. A. Mishkel. 1969. Effects of dietary fats on plasma lipids and lipoproteins: An hypothesis for the lipid-lowering effect of unsaturated fatty acids. *J. Clin. Invest.,* **48:** 78.

32. Suchy, N. and J. F. Sullivan. 1975. Endogenous fatty acids in alimentary triglyceridemia in normolipemic young males. *Am. J. Clin. Nutr.,* **28:** 36.

33. Tamir, I., Y. Bojanower, O. Levtow, D. Heldenberg, Z. Dickerman, and B. Werbin. 1972. Serum lipids and lipoproteins in children from families with early coronary heart disease. *Arch. Dis. Childhood,* **47:** 808.

34. Vessby, B., H. Lithell, and I. Gustafsson. 1975. Effects of dietary treatment on lipoprotein levels in hyperlipoproteinaemia. *Postgrad. Med. J.,* **51** (Supplement 8): 52.

35. Wilson, D. E., P. H. Schreibman, V. C. Day, and R. A. Arky. 1970. Hyperlipidemia in an adult diabetic population. *J. Chron. Dis.*, **23:** 501.

36. Wilson, J. D. and C. A. Lindsey, Jr. 1965. Studies on the influence of dietary cholesterol on cholesterol metabolism in the isotopic steady state in man. *J. Clin. Invest.*, **44:** 1805.

37. Wood, P. D. S., M. P. Stern, A. Silvers, G. M. Reaven, and J. von der Groeben. 1972. Prevalence of plasma lipoprotein abnormalities in a free-living population of the Central Valley, California. *Circulation*, **45:** 114.

38. Wright, I. S. 1976. Correct levels of serum cholesterol: Average vs. normal vs. optimal. *J. Am. Med. Assoc.*, **236:** 261.

STUDY GUIDE

Lipids circulate in the blood as part of lipoprotein complexes.

1. Describe five fractions of blood lipoproteins, indicating for each the probable origin, composition, and whether exogenous or endogenous.

2. Describe relationships between the measurement of serum cholesterol and triglyceride levels and that of serum lipoproteins. Evaluate the use of each measurement in clinical practice.

3. List normal values for serum cholesterol and triglycerides.

4. Discuss general relationships among cholesterol intake, absorption, excretion, and synthesis in the body of normal man and indicate how cholesterol is generally distributed throughout the body.

Hyperlipoproteinemias have been classified into types on the basis of specific serum lipoprotein abnormalities.

5. For each type or subtype of hyperlipoproteinemia, describe and discuss:
   (*a*) Comparative frequency or incidence (rare or common)
   (*b*) Typical blood lipid abnormalities, including appearance of plasma
   (*c*) Major clinical symptoms or abnormalities that may occur
   (*d*) Whether or not there is an increased tendency toward the development of premature CHD
   (*e*) Probable mode of inheritance, if familial

6. Explain what is meant by primary and secondary causes and give examples of secondary causes for various types of hyperlipoproteinemia.

Dietary treatment constitutes the basis of lipid-lowering therapy in hyperlipoproteinemias.

7. For each type or subtype of hyperlipoproteinemia describe and discuss rationale for treatment, with emphasis on dietary treatment.

8. Describe and discuss some possible mechanisms by which diets high in PUFA may act to lower serum cholesterol levels.

9. What is the usual magnitude of the effect diet therapy may be expected to have on lowering serum lipids?

10. Write appropriate diet patterns and menus for each of the types of hyperlipoproteinemias, adapting them to individual needs and cultural patterns.

11. List drugs sometimes effectively used in combination with diet therapy and describe their probable effect in lowering serum lipids.

A few studies have estimated the prevalence of hyperlipoproteinemias in free-living populations.

12. Discuss the probable relative prevalence of the various types of hyperlipoproteinemias in the United States and the possible significance of this for public health programs.

Many cases of hyperlipoproteinemia are apparently familial in nature.

13. Describe the general results of studies on the incidence of hyperlipoproteinemia among families of patients with early myocardial infarction and discuss the significance of these findings for possible prevention of CHD.

21

Atherosclerosis and Coronary Heart Disease

Atherosclerosis is characterized by accumulation of cholesterol and other fatty substances in the walls of large blood vessels, and persons with extensive lesioning of the cornary arteries become prime candidates for heart attacks (myocardial infarctions) and angina pectoris (pain from deficient blood supply to heart muscle). A similar type of atherosclerotic process may affect the cerebral arteries and result in stroke. The high frequency and poor clinical course of atherosclerotic artery disease and its complications has turned attention to prevention as the best means of lessening the impact on populations.

Diet is one of several factors that is apparently involved in the pathogenesis of atherosclerotic vascular disease (AVD). However, considerable controversy has arisen over the precise role played. Elevated levels of dietary saturated fat and cholesterol have been most widely accepted as critical factors influencing the atherosclerotic process, although there are still "unbelievers" in the scientific community (Reiser, 1973; Keys et al., 1974; Kaunitz, 1975). Dietary sugars, fiber, minerals, and vitamins have all been suggested as important factors contributing to the cause. Nondietary factors, including cigarette smoking, heredity, personality type, and lack of physical exercise, also play critical roles in the "risk" associated with susceptibility to coronary heart disease (CHD). With so many factors involved, yet unclarified, it is understandable that the state of knowledge in prevention of CHD is often viewed as a "tangled web of evidence."

This chapter discusses some theories concerning the development of atherosclerotic lesions and their relationship to myocardial infarction (MI). It also considers several factors that are thought to increase the risk of developing AVD, with emphasis on dietary influences. (Lipid substances in the blood and hyperlipoproteinemias were discussed in Chap. 20.)

21.1 Epidemiology of Coronary Heart Disease and Risk Factors

CHD has reached an epidemic stage among males in many industrialized countries of the world. Fig. 21.1 shows death rates from arteriosclerotic and degenerative heart disease and from all causes for men aged 45 to 54 years in selected countries during 1967. The United States ranked second for

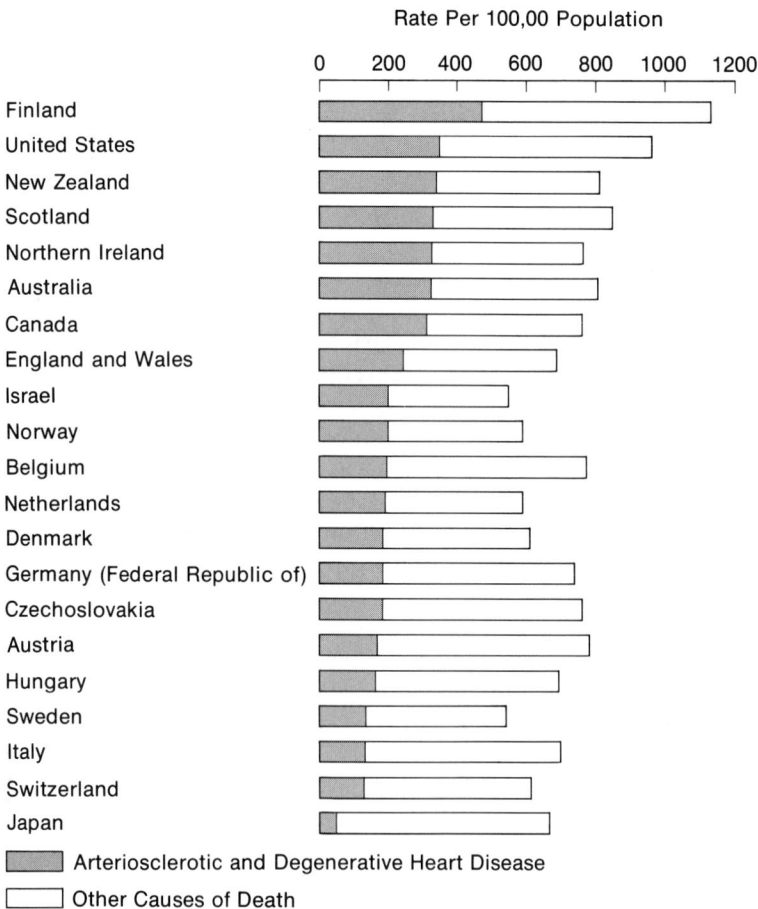

Fig. 21.1 Death rates from arteriosclerotic and degenerative heart disease and from all causes; selected countries, 1967—men aged 45 to 54 years. (From "Arteriosclerosis, Report by National Heart and Lung Institute Task Force on Arteriosclerosis," *World Health Statistics Annual*, 1967.)

deaths from CHD with consequent high rates for mortality from all causes (Task Force on Arteriosclerosis, 1971b). Data indicate that the epidemic is still increasing in several European countries, although CHD has not increased in the United States in recent years (Stamler, 1973).

Epidemiology is the scientific study of factors that influence the frequency and distribution of diseases in humans. It has been applied traditionally to the study of infectious diseases. The first contribution of epidemiology to the study of atherosclerosis and associated CHD was to identify it as an epidemic, i.e., a disease affecting populations, and not a natural and unavoidable adjunct of the aging process in people. The next step was to relate the differences among populations in frequency and extent of disease to other population attributes in order to identify probable causes of the disorder and provide information relevant to its prevention (Strasser, 1972). Many epidemiological studies on atherosclerosis and CHD have been reported, but no single cause has been discovered. Instead, the concept of multifactored cause has gradually become accepted.

Epidemiological data relating to CHD have been collected for populations of white, Bantu, and other racial groups in Africa; various ethnic subdivisions in Israel; groups in India, Japan, China, the Pacific area, South and Central America, the United States, and Europe. In general, the frequency of CHD is greater among groups with higher socioeconomic standards than among those living in less developed and industrialized communities. Factors related to the socioeconomic gradient must be identified to make this general relationship meaningful (Epstein, 1965) and many have been suggested. A concept of "risk factors"—those habits, traits, and abnormalities associated with a 100 percent or more increase in susceptibility to CHD—has developed out of epidemiological studies (Stamler, 1973).

Varying methodologies have undoubtedly contributed to different results in some epidemiological studies. However, many common findings have surfaced, and it has been generalized by the Task Force on Arteriosclerosis (1971a) that CHD occurs with increased frequency in association with the following major risk factors: (1) elevated serum lipids, specifically cholesterol and probably triglycerides; (2) hypertension; (3) cigarette smoking; and (4) elevated blood sugar (diabetes mellitus). Other risk factors for which there is some evidence include increased pulse rate, sedentary living, personality factors, certain patterns of behavior, and a family history of premature clinical atherosclerosis. The concept of risk factors is useful because it is possible to identify those individuals especially susceptible to atherosclerosis and its complications and to develop programs of primary prevention.

It is not possible to review in this chapter a sizeable portion of the epidemiological reports on CHD. A few studies will be described in order to give a general impression of approaches and results in these types of studies.

Lopez-S et al. (1966) reported on the relationship between death rate per 100,000 population and food intake for 15 different European countries, using valid statistical information obtained from publications of the World Health Organization (WHO) and the Food and Agriculture Organization (FAO) of the United Nations. From 1934 to 1959 there was (1) no appreciable change in consumption of protein; (2) an increase in consumption of fats, with proportional increases in the consumption of saturated, mono-, and polyunsaturated fatty acids (PUFA); (3) a slight decrease in the total consumption of carbohydrates; and (4) a marked decrease in the amount of complex carbohydrate consumed with a proportional increase in simple carbohydrate. The mortality rate from arteriosclerotic heart disease (AHD) increased in the European countries from 1948 to 1959, although this increase was not uniformly consistent from one country to another. Caloric intake was closely related to AHD death rate, although calories did not significantly correlate with the increase in death rate in each of the 3-year periods for which correlations were calculated. No correlation was found between protein consumption and death rate. A high correlation was found between the percent of kilocalories from saturated fat and the death rate, but a low correlation between the percent of kilocalories derived from PUFA and death rate. The highest correlation coefficient in the study was found between the percent of kilocalories derived from simple carbohydrate and the death rate from AHD. Both saturated fat and simple carbohydrate intake were correlated with death rate in this study.

Prior and his coworkers (1971) observed the gradual emergence of civilization's pattern of organic diseases among the Maori people in both New Zealand and the islands of the Pacific from which they came. In Pukapuka and the Tokelau Islands life is barely changed from what it was 200 years ago. Rarotonga, in the Cook Islands, is representative of a halfway station between the simple life and the complicated Europeanized life of the Maori in New Zealand. In general, mean caloric intake increased for adults from 1800 to 2100 to 2560 kcal in these three groups, respectively, as the society became more and more westernized. Fat intake also tended to increase, along with incidence of obesity, especially in women. Mean daily sucrose consumption increased from 9 to 35 to 71 g per person as the level of industrialization increased. Sodium increased from 50 to 70 meq, to 120 to 140 meq, to 188 meq. The incidence of ischaemic heart disease (IHD) in males increased from 2 percent to 4.3 percent to 4.9 percent, whereas in women it increased from 1.4 percent to 5.5 percent to 8.9 percent in the three groups studied. The results of these investigations supported the hypothesis that a low-salt intake, not only in infancy and childhood but in adult life, is probably an important factor in lessening the increase in blood pressure that usually occurs with age.

The mortality rate from CHD for the Japanese in Hawaii has been reported to be lower than that for Hawaiians but is not as low as the rate for Japanese in Japan (Bassett et al., 1969; Keys et al., 1958). The chief differences in diet that might contribute to the higher incidence of risk factors observed in the Hawaiians than Japanese and might account for the higher CHD mortality were (1) a history of sporadic heavy caloric intake, (2) a greater day-to-day variation in caloric intake (modified feast-or-famine type of eating pattern), and (3) higher intakes of saturated and total fat in the Hawaiian group. Robertson et al. (1977) reported a higher incidence of MI and death from CHD for Japanese men in California than those in Hawaii. The incidence rate was lowest among Japanese men in Japan.

There has been an increase in CHD mortality rates in Japan since 1949 and also a substantial increase in fat and cholesterol consumption by Japanese citizens. Wen and Gershoff (1973), using data from the 1949 to 1968 national nutrition household survey in Japan, calculated the amounts of cholesterol and fatty acids consumed per person and estimated the changes in serum cholesterol that would be expected from the dietary changes. Two different formulas were used for this estimation. The expected increase in serum cholesterol was 21 mg/100 ml with one formula and 14 mg/100 ml with the other. The equation derived from the multivariate analysis of data for the Framingham epidemiological study was used to estimate the effect of serum cholesterol changes on the risk of developing CHD. For this estimation it was assumed that all other risk factors remained the same during the 18-year period. An increased risk of CHD of 18.4 percent was calculated while the actual CHD mortality rate in a comparable age group rose from 39.3 to 69.1 per 100,000 during this period, an increase of 75.9 percent. Thus the calculated dietary lipid increases in Japan could, at best, account for only 24.3 percent of the increase in CHD. Kahn (1970) performed similar calculations using USDA estimates of food "disappearing" into civilian channels from 1909 to 1965 in the United States. An 8 percent increase in risk of CHD was calculated, much below the actual increase in mortality from CHD in the United States during this same time period. It was concluded from these studies that the long-term change in dietary fat intake was not consistent with the reported increased risk of CHD.

Using data on per capita food supplies at the retail level, Antar et al. (1964) reported that the main changes in the American diet over the past 70 to 80 years have been (1) a considerable decrease in the consumption of total carbohydrates with a greater progressive decline in the intake of complex carbohydrate from flours, cereals, and potatoes and a concurrent dramatic increase of simple sugars, and (2) a slight increase in total fat consumption contributed mainly by the increase of unsaturated fatty acids. The P/S ratio has increased about 37 percent since 1909. The change in type of carbohydrate was suggested by the researchers as a possible factor in the increased incidence of CHD in the United States.

A long-term international cooperative study on cardiovascular epidemiology was organized primarily to answer questions about the portent for future CHD of characteristics and mode of life of middle-aged men in contrasting population samples and began with preliminary trials in 1956 to 1957 (Keys et al., 1970). International teams examined 12,770 men, including 11 cohorts of 500 to 1000 each in rural Yugoslavia, Japan, Finland, Italy, and Greece, using standard methods and criteria. A group in the Netherlands and a group of railroad employees in Minnesota were also included. A report of entry and 5-year follow-up covered 64,000 man-years of experience.

The examination procedure included standard questionnaires on family status, work, personal habits, and medical history. Anthropometric measurements included subcutaneous fat. Physical examination by internists used a standardized protocol and record forms, blood sample, and qualitative urinalysis. Diagnoses and classification in regard to disease incidence among the populations were based on medical history, physical examinations, and electrocardiographic data obtained by the examining teams in the field situation. Men with CHD in the entry examination were removed from the major study project so that a CHD-free sample could be the focus of the long-term study. An important part of the study was the diet and its possible relationship to the etiology of CHD. Average diets of all cohorts except the U.S. railroad men were estimated from surveys on random samples of the cohorts. The dietary surveys involved weighing all items consumed during seven days of the survey and were repeated in different seasons. Nutrients were estimated from chemical analyses of composites of replicate meals and menus as well as from tables of food composition developed to cover local foodstuffs. The diets of the U.S. railroad men were estimated by calculation from dietary interview and recall records, supplemented by visits to homes of a small subsample.

Men in Finland, Zutphen (Netherlands), and Crete, and the U.S. railroad employees consumed diets classified as high in fat. Men from Slavonia (Yugoslavia) and Corfu (Greece) consumed diets a little lower in fat; the diets of rural Italy and Velika Krsna (Serbia) were low in fat by American standards. The Japanese diet, with only 10 percent or less of the energy supplied from fats, was considered very low fat. In none of the diets did PUFA provide a substantial fraction of the caloric value. The U.S. railroad men and the men of Finland and Zutphen (Netherlands) ate diets that seldom provided less than 15 percent of the kilocalories from saturated fatty acids, usually provided 18 to 20 percent, and not infrequently provided as much as 25 percent. The other European cohorts were in an intermediate class in consumption of saturated fatty acids, and the Japanese diet provided a very small amount of saturates in comparison. A correlation coefficient of 0.89 was found between the average percentage of kilocalories supplied by saturated fatty acids in the subsample for which chemical analyses were done and the median serum cholesterol levels of the total cohorts at the time of the entry examinations. Observed differences in serum cholesterol levels between the cohorts of the study could not all be accounted for by predicting effects of dietary saturated fatty acids and cholesterol, however. Other factors, possibly including dietary differences in complex carbohydrates and in leguminous seeds, undoubtedly contributed to the differences. A correlation between the total fat in the diet and incidence of CHD (from the entry-level, CHD-free group) was low and not significant. However, the correlation between dietary saturated fatty acids and CHD incidence was high (0.84). Such findings do not prove that dietary saturated fatty acids play a major role in the development of CHD, but the data are consistent with that hypothesis. No relationship was found between dietary protein and average serum cholesterol concentration or CHD incidence rate.

The prevalence rates of CHD tended to be directly related to characteristics of the cohorts in regard to blood pressure and serum cholesterol but not in regard to relative body weight, body fatness, or smoking habits. During 5 years there were 588 deaths in the entire study population, 158 from CHD. Among the U.S. railroad men 62 of 125 deaths were due to CHD; in Finland 38 of 111 deaths were due to CHD; in the Netherlands 16 out of 50 deaths were thus accounted for. For all other cohorts combined, only one out of eight deaths was due to CHD. In most cases, low CHD death rates were associated with low death rates from all causes. Examination of the representation in the several cohorts of the so-called risk factors showed that most of these factors, whatever their influence within cohorts, could not explain the observed differences in the incidence of CHD among the various populations. Cigarette smoking habits did not differ much between the various cohorts. Differences between cohorts in the proportion of men who were sedentary or physically inactive did not explain the differences in incidence of CHD and neither did obesity nor relative weight differences. The U.S. railroad men tended to be relatively much heavier and fatter than the men in any of the other groups, but the thin and relatively lightweight Finns matched the Americans in CHD incidence. The Italians were far more obese than the Finns, yet they were much less prone to CHD than were either the Finns or the Americans. There was some tendency for the incidence of CHD to be related to the prevalence of hypertension in the cohorts. The incidence rate of CHD tended to be directly related to the distributions of serum cholesterol values, and the average serum cholesterol levels tended to be directly related to the average proportion of calories provided by saturated fats in the diet.

CHD incidence was significantly related to smoking habits in the U.S. railroad men but not in the European cohorts. In the U.S. cohort, the CHD incidence rate of the men in sedentary occupations was about 16 percent higher than the rate of the physically more active switchmen, but the difference was not statistically significant. In the other cohorts, no statistically significant relationships between habitual physical activity and any measure of CHD incidence rate were found.

A comparative epidemiological study attempting to explain the higher mortality rate from AHD in Massachusetts than in Ireland was done by Brown et al. (1970). More than 500 pairs of brothers, one of whom lived in Ireland and the other in Boston, were included in the 1994 middle-aged men studied. The dietary intake of kilocalories, complex carbohydrates, magnesium, and fluoride (from tea) was higher in Ireland. The proportion of kilocalories derived from fat and saturated fat, serum cholesterol, blood pressure levels, and amount of cigarette smoking did not differ markedly between the two groups. The weight, skin-fold thickness, and number of abnormal electrocardiograms were higher in Boston subjects. A study of the pathology of coronary arteries and aortas from autopsies showed much earlier serious atheromatous involvement in the Boston subjects than in the specimens from Ireland. Increased physical activity appeared to be important in reducing the risk of CHD in Ireland. The implications of this study are that food intake is of less importance when the subjects are active and expending the extra kilocalories consumed in physical activity.

One of the largest and longest epidemiological studies of cardiovascular diseases is the Framingham Study (Gordon and Kannel, 1968–1970). It was begun in 1949 in Framingham, Massachusetts. In this study, 5127 men and women, aged 30 to 62 years and free of clinical evidence of coronary disease when the study began, were examined every other year for the development of CHD and other atherosclerotic conditions. After 14 years of follow-up, Kannel et al. (1971) reported that 323 men and 169 women had developed for the first time some clinical manifestation of CHD. The incidence increased with age in both sexes with a striking male predominance in younger victims but with less difference between sexes as age advanced. The mean level of each of the major serum lipids and lipoproteins was higher at the initial examination in those who went on to develop CHD than it was for other subjects in the study who remained free of CHD. In men, the risk of developing CHD could be estimated by using serum cholesterol, pre-beta lipoproteins, or beta lipoproteins. None were superior to the more convenient serum cholesterol determination, however. Knowledge of the associated lipoprotein pattern in hypercholesterolemic men may be important for determining the type of hyperlipidemia and selecting the most appropriate therapy, but its contribution to assessing risk of CHD remains to be determined, according to these investigators.

Gordon and Kannel (1972) reported from a 16-year follow-up examination of Framingham subjects that high blood pressure, elevated serum cholesterol, cigarette smoking, electrocardiographic evidence of left ventricular hypertrophy, and glucose intolerance were precursors common to atherosclerotic brain infarction, CHD, and intermittent claudication. None of these factors, however, was clearly dominant for CHD. Glucose intolerance was only weakly related to CHD. The investigators claimed as the most striking conclusion that all three atherosclerotic diseases appeared to share a common set of precursors and that this was true in either sex.

In 1957 to 1960 a diet assessment was undertaken for a sample of the Framingham Study population on their fifth biennial examination (Gordon and Kannel, 1968–1970, Section 24). A dietary interview directed toward evaluating the "usual" long-term food intake of each person was used. A sample of 1049 persons was drawn according to an elaborate sampling scheme. Only 912 yielded successful interviews. The object of this study was to collect information to test the hypotheses that "the regulation of the level of serum cholesterol and the development of CHD are related to: (1)

caloric balance, (2) level of animal fat intake, (3) level of vegetable fat intake, (4) level of protein intake, (5) level of cholesterol intake, and (6) level of the ratio of complex to simple carbohydrate. No relationship could be discerned within the study between food intake and serum cholesterol level, except for a weak negative association between caloric intake and serum cholesterol level in men. Neither could any relationship be found between diet and the subsequent development of CHD, despite a distinct elevation of serum cholesterol in men from this sample who developed CHD. These findings mean that in the Framingham Study Group, diet (as measured here) was not associated with concurrent differentials in serum cholesterol level. These findings do not mean that the difference between Framingham and another population (such as the Japanese) in serum cholesterol level is unrelated to differences between these populations in diet. Neither do they mean that serum cholesterol levels cannot be changed by changes in dietary intake. On the other hand, these findings suggest caution with respect to hypotheses relating diet to serum cholesterol levels in the United States. Other techniques for measuring dietary intake or measuring some other dietary parameters than this study measured might yield different conclusions.

Although varying results have been reported for epidemiological studies throughout the world, when these findings were considered, along with those from laboratory and clinical studies, by the Task Force on Arteriosclerosis (1971a) appointed by the U.S. Department of Health, Education and Welfare, they concluded that there are certain associations that indicate risk of developing CHD. An association has been demonstrated between the amount and type of fat and the amount of cholesterol in the diet, on the one hand, and the level of serum lipoproteins and the development of atherosclerosis, on the other hand. With few exceptions, populations consuming large quantities of saturated fat and cholesterol have a relatively high concentration of serum cholesterol and a high mortality from CHD. Conversely, the serum cholesterol levels and the mortality from CHD are low in populations with a low consumption of saturated fat and cholesterol. There appears to be a continuous relationship between CHD, coronary mortality, and the concentration of serum cholesterol. There is also a progressive increase in CHD with increasing blood pressure, even in the range generally regarded as normal. In the United States there is a significant positive association between cigarette smoking and susceptibility to CHD. CHD occurs with greater frequency among diabetics than among nondiabetics, especially in young age groups. There are also some families in which premature and often fatal heart attacks occur with greater frequency than in others. It is uncertain to what extent this tendency is caused by genetic factors and how much is due to a similar mode of life and the same type of diet. A relationship between increased risk of dying from clinical complications of atherosclerosis and extreme obesity appears to be present. Other risk factors also appear to be of some importance.

Two or more risk factors are commonly present in one individual. Persons with three, four, or more definite risk factors form an especially high-risk group. The incidence of acute heart attacks in this high-risk group is far greater than in persons with no risk factors or only one (Task Force on Arteriosclerosis, 1971a).

21.2 Atherogenesis, Atherosclerotic Lesions, and Myocardial Infarction

Atherosclerosis is apparently a very old disease, the aortas of Egyptian mummies entombed for centuries showing typical atherosclerotic lesions. The name atherosclerosis is derived from two Greek words: *athere,* meaning "porridge" or "mush," and *skleros,* meaning "hard." The atherosclerotic lesion begins as a soft area and hardens as it develops. At one stage in its development a fatty gruel-like material is present in the lesion. *Arteriosclerosis* is a general term indicating hardening of the arteries from any cause. Atherosclerosis is a particular type of hardening that involves the infiltration of fatty materials. Lesions in atherosclerosis may occur in many of the large and medium-sized arteries of the body, but the principal locations are the aorta, its major branches, the coronary arteries, and the larger arteries of the brain. The coronary circulation is shown in Fig. 21.2.

The normal artery wall is described as having three layers: (1) tunica interna or intima, (2) tunica media, and (3) tunica externa or adventitia. Fig. 21.3 shows these layers. The intima, or innermost layer, consists of a narrow region bounded on the luminal side by a single continuous layer of

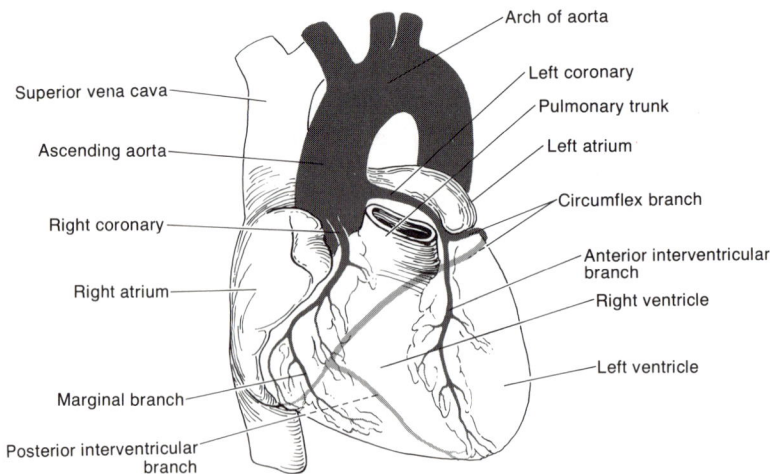

Fig. 21.2 Coronary circulation. Anterior view of arterial distribution. (From Gerard J. Tortora and Nicholas P. Anagnostakos, *Principles of Anatomy and Physiology,* 2d ed., New York: Harper & Row; by permission of the publisher.)

endothelial cells and on the other side by a fenestrated sheet of elastic fibers called the internal elastic membrane. Between these boundaries are various components of extracellular connective tissue matrix. The intact endothelial layer acts as a barrier for the passage of blood constituents into the artery wall. In children there are only occasional smooth muscle cells in the intimal area but, with increasing age, more smooth muscle cells and extracellular material, including collagen and mucopolysaccharide-containing ground substance, slowly accumulate. The media, or middle layer, consists of diagonally oriented smooth muscle cells, surrounded by variable amounts of collagen, small elastic fibers, and mucopolysaccharides. The morphology of the media does not usually change with age. The adventitia, the outermost layer, consists mainly of longitudinally directed bundles of collagen fibers. In addition, there are fibroblasts, some elastic fibers, nerve bundles, and small blood vessels (vasa vasorum). In most arteries the vasa vasorum does not penetrate more than halfway into the media and the layers of arterial wall from there to the endothelium are nourished from the lumen (Ross and Glomset, 1976a).

The lesions of atherosclerosis involve chiefly the intima of the artery, although the media may be involved in secondary changes. Three types of lesions have been described as the fatty streak, the fibrous plaque, and the complicated lesion. Fatty streaks occur in childhood and are produced by lipid deposits, mostly cholesterol and cholesteryl esters, in and around small numbers of smooth muscle cells in the intima. They are yellowish in color and are flat or only slightly elevated. Thus they do not significantly narrow the lumen of blood vessels (Ross and Glomset, 1976a).

Strong et al. (1973) found aortic fatty streaks in many New Orleans children under age 3 and in all of the group of children over that age. Coronary fatty streaks were rare before age 10 but became much more frequent in the second decade of life and were nearly always present after age 20.

The fibrous plaque is a firm, elevated intimal lesion that protrudes into the lumen of the artery. Lipid accumulates in and around intimal smooth muscle cells. The cells are also surrounded by collagen, elastic fibers, and mucopolysaccharides, and a fibrous cap is formed that covers a large, deeper deposit of free extracellular lipid intermixed with cell debris (Ross and Glomset, 1976a). Fig. 21.4 shows the possible distribution of lipid and connective tissue matrix in a raised atherosclerotic lesion.

Although direct proof is not available, the panel of pathologists appearing before the Task Force on Arteriosclerosis (1971b) felt strongly that fatty streaks are an early stage of fibrous plaque formation. They expressed the opinion that fatty streaks vary in their potential, i.e., some regress, some are static, and some progress to plaques.

The complicated lesion is a fibrous plaque with various degrees of degenerative change such as hemorrhage into the lesion, mural thrombosis, cell necrosis, ulceration, and calcification. This type of lesion is often associated with occlusion of the arterial lumen.

In a healthy human coronary artery the lumen is wide and allows normal flow of blood through the artery. In early stages of atherosclerosis, the intima becomes thickened and the lumen decreases somewhat in size. As a fibrous plaque continues to enlarge and becomes a complicated lesion, the lumen becomes very small and passage of blood through the artery is restricted. This narrowed channel may be easily blocked by a thrombus (blood clot). When this occurs in a coronary artery that nourishes the heart muscle, it is called a *coronary occlusion*. It cuts off the supply of oxygen and nutrients to those cells beyond the occluded artery and they die. The area of necrosis in the heart muscle is called a *myocardial infarct*. A myocardial

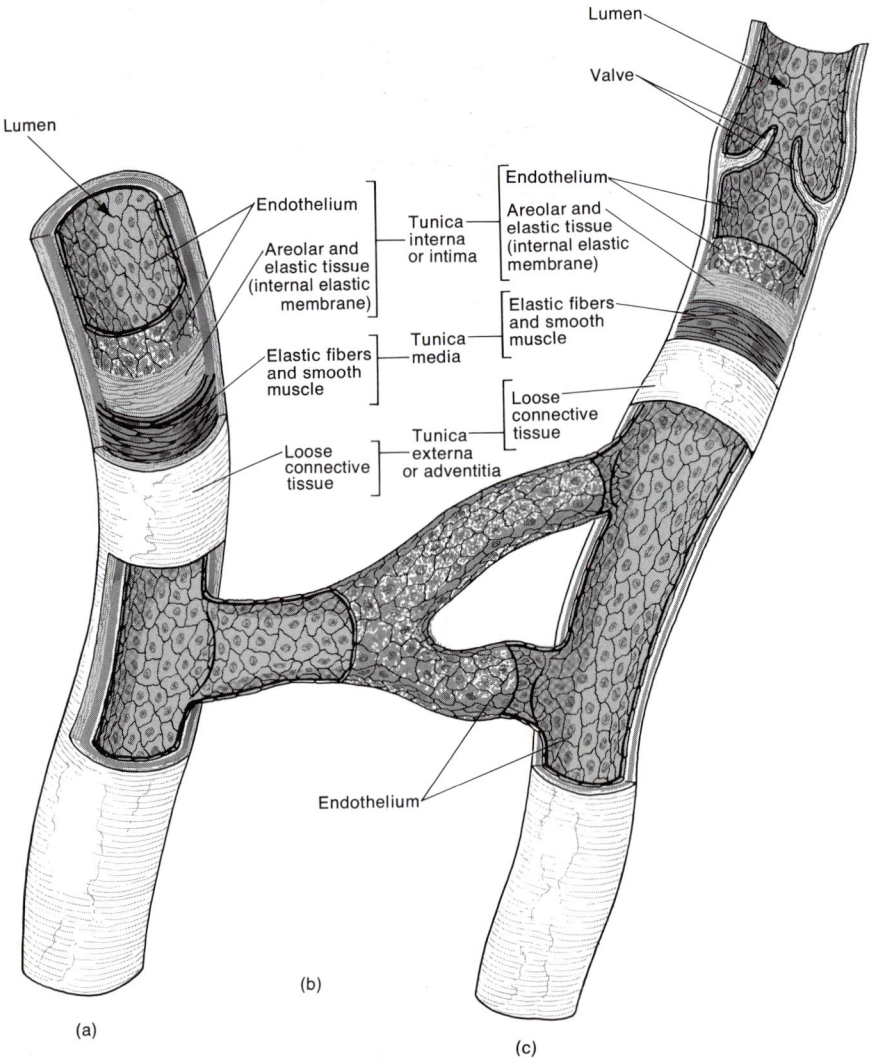

infarction (MI) is commonly called a *heart attack*. The various stages of artery occlusion by atherosclerotic lesions are illustrated in Fig. 21.5.

If this same atherosclerotic process occurs in arteries of the brain and one of these arteries is occluded, certain areas of the brain are without oxygen and nutrients. The result is a stroke and often paralysis of parts of the body occurs. Particularly when hypertension is present along with the atherosclerotic lesion, hemorrhaging may occur into brain tissue. Part of the brain may be destroyed by compression.

If severe atherosclerosis occurs in the aorta, it may weaken the walls of this large artery to produce an aneurysm. The artery balloons out in the area of the aneurysm as blood is forcefully pumped through the artery. An aortic aneurysm can often be repaired surgically.

Several theories have been proposed to explain atherogenesis. An early suggestion was the sterol hypothesis, which proposed that plasma-derived cholesterol was deposited in the arterial wall (Frantz and Moore, 1969). Very early, cholesterol and its esters were found to be the major constituent of the atherosclerotic plaque. Later, plasma beta lipoprotein was shown to accumulate in intimal lesions (Watts, 1971). In 1913

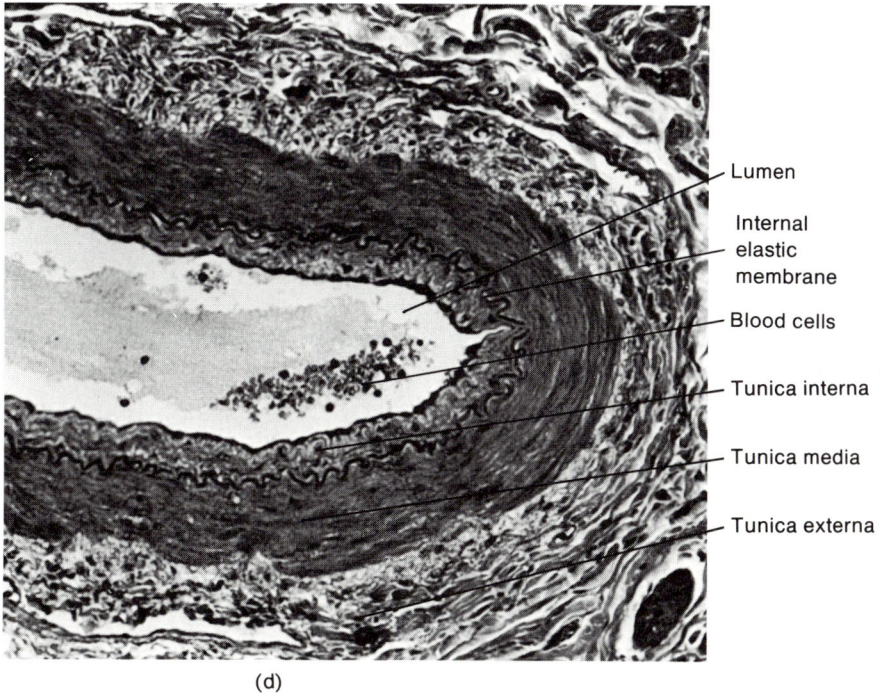

(d)

Fig. 21.3 (a) to (c): Structure of blood vessels. (a) Artery. (b) Capillary. (c) Vein. The relative size of the capillary is enlarged for emphasis. (d) Cross section of an artery at a magnification of × 50. (From Gerard J. Tortora and Nicholas P. Anagnostakos, *Principles of Anatomy and Physiology*, 2d ed., New York: Harper & Row, 1978; by permission of the publisher.)

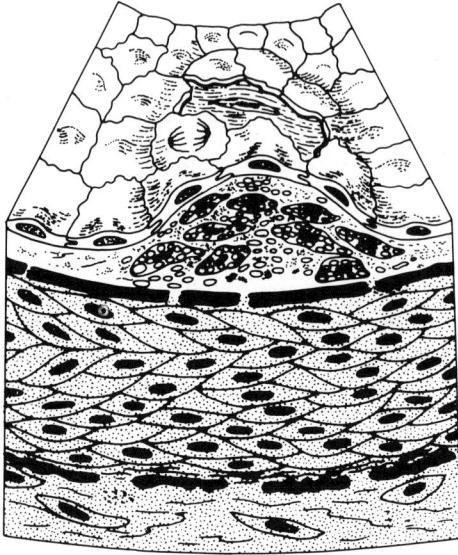

Fig. 21.4 Characteristic lipid deposition within the cells and their surrounding connective matrix if lesion progression continues. This process results in a proliferative lesion of cells and connective tissue surrounding a pool of lipid derived from deposition of lipids in connective tissue and debris resulting from smooth-muscle necrosis. (From Ross Russell, and John A. Glomset, "The Pathogenesis of Atherosclerosis." Reprinted, by permission, from the *New England Journal of Medicine,* **295:** 422, 1976.)

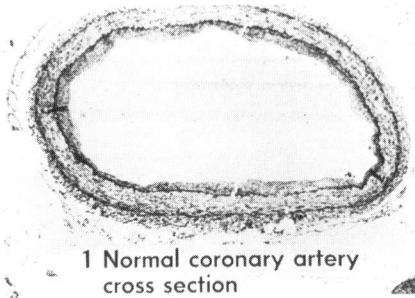

1 Normal coronary artery cross section

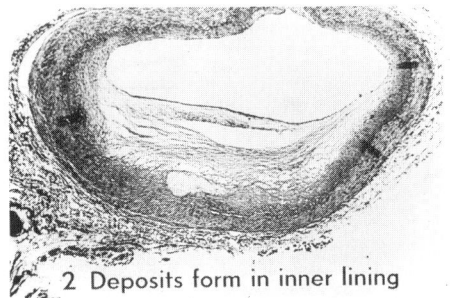

2 Deposits form in inner lining

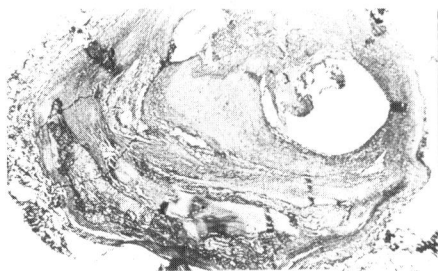

3 Deposits harden

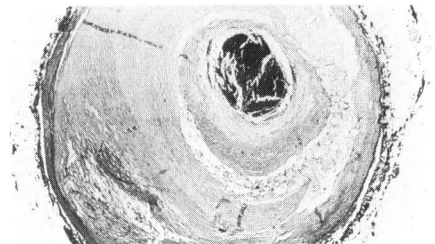

4 Narrowed channel blocked by blood clot

Fig. 21.5 Stages of artery clogging with atherosclerosis. (Courtesy American Heart Association.)

Anitschkow described the induction of atherosclerosis in rabbits by feeding pure cholesterol dissolved in oil. The disease has since been induced in many other species by similar methods. Epidemiologic evidence for an association between elevated plasma cholesterol levels and consumption of saturated fat and cholesterol has supported the sterol hypothesis. Although cholesterol synthesis occurs in the wall of the artery, it is generally believed to be too slow to contribute appreciably to the buildup of sterols in the plaque and the blood is thought to be the major source of plaque cholesterol. The sterol theory of atherogenesis still leaves many unresolved questions concerning mechanisms.

The response-to-injury hypothesis of atherogenesis has been modified and extended by a number of investigators over the years (Ross and Glomset, 1976b). This theory proposes that various factors, such as hyperlipidemia, hormone dysfunction, and increased shear stress from hypertension, may injure the endothelial lining of the artery. Focal desquamation of the endothelium in this way exposes the underlying subendothelial connective tissue to platelets and other elements in the circulation. Platelets adhere to subendothelial collagen, aggregate, and release the contents of their granules. Massive infiltration of platelet factors, plasma lipoproteins, and other plasma constituents such as hormones at sites of injury apparently causes focal proliferation of arterial smooth muscle cells, which then leads to formation of large amounts of connective tissue matrix by these cells and to deposition of lipids. Restoration of the endothelial barrier will ultimately occur and the lesions regress if both the injury and the tissue response to it are limited. However, if injury to the endothelium is continuous or is repeated, the lesion may enlarge.

Other theories of atherogenesis include the thrombogenic theory that plaques result from transformation of small blood clots on the arterial wall (mural thrombi); the theory that an immune-complex induces atherosclerosis (Poston and Davies, 1974); and the monoclonal or monotypic hypothesis that each lesion of atherosclerosis is derived from a single smooth muscle cell that serves as a progenitor for the remaining proliferative cells (Ross and Glomset, 1976b).

Thrombosis is intimately related to atherogenesis. It contributes to the progression of atherosclerotic lesions and is also responsible for many of the clinical complications of atherosclerosis, as a thrombus may occlude a coronary artery causing acute MI. The basic mechanism of thrombosis includes (1) fibrin coagulation, (2) platelet adhesion and aggregation, and (3) decreased fibrinolysis. Injury to the endothelial lining of an artery wall may trigger thrombosis. Platelet aggregates and fibrin may then be incorporated into the atherosclerotic lesion. Coagulation and fibrinolytic factors are altered in patients with atherosclerosis and IHD. Reduction in inhibitors of coagulation and increased platelet stickiness have been reported (Task Force on Arteriosclerosis, 1971b). Anticoagulant therapy is often used in the treatment of MI although advantages of this treatment have not always been evident (Vigran, 1969; Seaman et al., 1964).

21.3 Diet and Serum Lipids

A statement on Diet and Coronary Heart Disease, prepared jointly by the Food and Nutrition Board, National Academy of Sciences-National Research Council, and the Council on Foods and Nutrition of the American Medical Association (1972), emphasized that the risk of developing CHD is positively correlated with the level of plasma cholesterol and that the level of plasma cholesterol can be lowered in most people by appropriate dietary modification. The statement further indicated that such lowering can generally be achieved by partial replacement of dietary sources of saturated fat with sources of unsaturated fat, especially those rich in PUFA, and by a reduction in the consumption of foods rich in cholesterol. However, appropriate dietary advice should be given on an individual basis in line with the nature of the blood lipid profile.

Several dietary components have been shown to affect plasma lipid levels, although the emphasis has most often been on fat and cholesterol since these have appeared to affect plasma lipids most markedly. Although much evidence exists to relate dietary factors to serum lipid levels, it must be remembered that the relationships between diet and CHD are less clear. CHD is a condition of multifactored origin, and serum cholesterol, with its relationship to diet, is only one of the several factors that may influence the development of the disease.

Dietary Fat and Cholesterol

The amount of fat in the diet is not as important quantitatively in affecting serum cholesterol levels as is the type of fat—saturated or polyunsaturated (Brown, 1971). Many investigators have confirmed that substitution of unsaturated vegetable oils for animal fats in the diet produces a substantial lowering of the plasma cholesterol level. All the saturated fatty acids are not equally active in elevating plasma cholesterol. The C14 myristic acid and C12 lauric acid components of saturated fat are apparently responsible to a large extent for the serum cholesterol-raising effect (Grande et al., 1961; Hegsted et al., 1965a). Palmitic acid (C16) probably also raises serum cholesterol, although cocoa butter at a level of 80 percent of total fat in the diet had no effect on serum cholesterol in humans, and cocoa butter contains about 25 percent palmitic acid (Grande et al., 1970). Fatty acids with less than 12 carbon atoms do not influence serum lipid levels. Stearic acid (C18) seems to have little or no influence on serum cholesterol, and this is also the case for the monounsaturated C18 oleic acid (Brown, 1971).

Formulas have been developed, from experimental data, to calculate the expected effect on serum cholesterol in humans of varying amounts of dietary saturated fatty acids, PUFA, and cholesterol (Keys et al., 1965; Hegsted et al., 1965b; Keys and Parlin, 1966). Saturates are about twice as effective in increasing serum cholesterol levels as polyunsaturates are in reducing them. Dietary saturated fatty acids come chiefly from products containing animal fat, such as meat, fish, poultry, whole milk, cheese, butter, and so on. Coconut fat also contains relatively large amounts of saturated fatty acids. This is a notable exception for plant sources of fat, which usually contain large proportions of unsaturated fatty acids.

The usual process of hydrogenation of oils changes the configuration of some of the unsaturated fatty acids from *cis* to *trans*. With partial hydrogenation of a vegetable oil, *trans* double bonds may occur in either monounsaturated or diunsaturated acids, with the monounsaturated acids usually predominating. Mattson et al. (1975) studied the effect on blood lipids in males, aged 24 to 41 years, of the *trans* monounsaturated acids as the only dietary variable. With over 60 percent of the monounsaturated fatty acids in the diet having the *trans* configuration, the levels of plasma cholesterol and triglyceride were found to be the same as with all *cis* monounsaturated fatty acids.

Linoleic acid occurs most frequently of the PUFA in foods. However, all straight-chain fatty acids with two or more double bonds are equally effective in reducing serum cholesterol. Serum cholesterol decreases as PUFA increases in the diet (Brown, 1971). The mechanism by which this occurs is not clarified.

A linear relationship exists between dietary and serum cholesterol (Hegsted et al., 1965b; Keys et al., 1965). Unless cholesterol is dissolved in fat or eaten with fat, however, it is not readily absorbed and thus has less effect on serum cholesterol. A maximum effect of dietary cholesterol on the serum level is probably obtained with about 750 mg per day. The effect on serum cholesterol of dietary cholesterol is apparently independent of the fatty acid composition of the diet. Each exerts its own separate influence. However, relationships between dietary quantities of cholesterol and of saturated and PUFA do affect serum cholesterol. To obtain an appreciable reduction in serum cholesterol, the PUFA requirement increases as the dietary cholesterol rises. For a reduction of 18 to 22 percent in serum cholesterol, a diet with 200 mg cholesterol requires 15 percent of kilocalories as PUFA and one with 550 mg requires 23 percent (Brown, 1971).

The fatty acid composition of the diet at which a change from partial to full effectiveness in serum cholesterol reduction occurs (compared with a standard diet) has been called the critical limit. Critical limits for a diet having 38 percent kilocalories as fat and 200 mg cholesterol were 13 percent of kilocalories for saturated fatty acids and 14 percent for PUFA (Brown and Page, 1966; Brown et al., 1966). Diets that are effective in lowering serum cholesterol have contained 5 to 12 percent of kilocalories as saturates and 14 to 22 percent as polyunsaturates. In considering these figures in terms of proportions of the total fatty acids in the diet, they were 33 percent or less of saturates, 42 percent or more of polyunsaturates, and approximately 25 percent of monounsaturates. With reduction in total dietary fat, the critical limits, expressed in percent kilocalories, drop to 5 percent saturates and 6 percent polyunsaturates with 15 percent total fat, yet the critical fatty acid composition in percent total fat remains the same

(Brown, 1971). It is difficult to express in simple terms the composition of dietary fat necessary for serum cholesterol reduction, particularly when working with fat-modified diets for research studies.

A number of investigators have followed the change in serum lipid concentrations of free-living subjects consuming practical fat-modified diets. Wilson et al. (1971) reported on 59 nonobese normal and hyperlipidemic men, with a mean age of 43 years, who were instructed in an isocaloric American Heart Association fat-controlled diet and followed monthly for 6 months. Mean responses were similar in both normal and hyperlipidemic subjects. A comparison of the diets (based on a 7-day recall dietary history) before and after the 6-month period showed that the percentage of total kilocalories supplied by saturated fat was reduced from 14.8 to 9.8 percent and the percentage from PUF increased from 5.1 to 15.2 percent. The dietary cholesterol was reduced from 464 to 227 mg per day. At the end of 6 months, the mean serum cholesterol level had decreased 9.6 percent, beta lipoprotein 15.6 percent, triglyceride 11.7 percent, and pre-beta lipoprotein 5.7 percent. These changes were statistically significant.

Shorey et al. (1974) followed 58 married hyperlipidemic males, mean age of 28.8 years, in a 3-month program stressing diet modification based on the diagnosis of Type IIa, IIb, or IV hyperlipoproteinemia. A 19 percent mean reduction in serum cholesterol was achieved by all groups, and a 57 percent mean decrease in serum triglyceride levels was achieved by the group with Type IV hyperlipoproteinemia. The major modifications in intake of specific nutrients for the Type IIa and IIb groups involved cholesterol, type and amount of fat, and kilocalories, whereas the major modification for the group with Type IV was in caloric intake, largely achieved by reduction in the consumption of simple carbohydrates.

Hill and Wynder (1976) reported a significant reduction in serum cholesterol of approximately 25 mg/100 ml in 45 nonobese healthy medical students and their wives, aged 20 to 30 years, on diets with P/S ratios of 0.3, 0.7, or 1.2. Dietary cholesterol intake was 250 mg per day and 33 percent of the total kilocalories were from fat. A significant change in serum triglycerides was not observed.

Hodges et al. (1975) reported that 25 healthy young couples varied in their responses to diets containing either regular beef, lamb, and dairy products or polyunsaturated beef, lamb, and dairy products produced by feeding ruminant animals "protected lipid" feeds. High responders showed a mean decrease of 10.7 mg/100 ml in serum cholesterol on the PUF diet and an increase of 7.8 mg/100 ml on the saturated fat diet.

These and other studies have shown that serum cholesterol may be decreased with dietary modification by 10 to 20 percent, but the significance of these reductions is still controversial. Many of the healthy young subjects studied had prestudy serum cholesterol levels below 200 to 220 mg/100 ml. Reiser (1976) questioned the need to recommend dietary changes that will reduce this level by 10 to 20 percent, particularly when the modified diet may be expensive or difficult to follow. On the other hand, any reduction of serum cholesterol in a hypercholesterolemic subject is usually desirable. The hyperlipidemic individuals should be identified so that they may be counseled. Practical fat- and kilocalorie-controlled diets can be planned for serum lipid reduction.

Plant Sterols

Three plant sterols of importance quantitatively are sitosterol, stigmasterol, and campesterol. Chemical structures of these compounds, along with that of cholesterol, are shown in Fig. 21.6. Cholesterol is the major source of sterol in animal foods but small amounts of other sterols may be present (Connor, 1968).

Interest in plant sterols stemmed from observations on both animals and humans that the increase in plasma cholesterol produced by feeding cholesterol can be prevented or modified by including plant sterols in the diet, and plant sterols (Cytellin) are available for therapeutic use. Plant sterols are absorbed to a considerably lesser extent than is cholesterol, but there are differences in the amounts absorbed among the plant sterols. Inhibition of cholesterol absorption by plant sterols may not be the only mechanism of plant sterol action that influences serum cholesterol levels (Subbiah, 1973).

Pollak (1953) reported a 20 to 40 percent decrease in serum cholesterol in humans fed up to 10 g sitosterol per day. A 10 to 25 percent

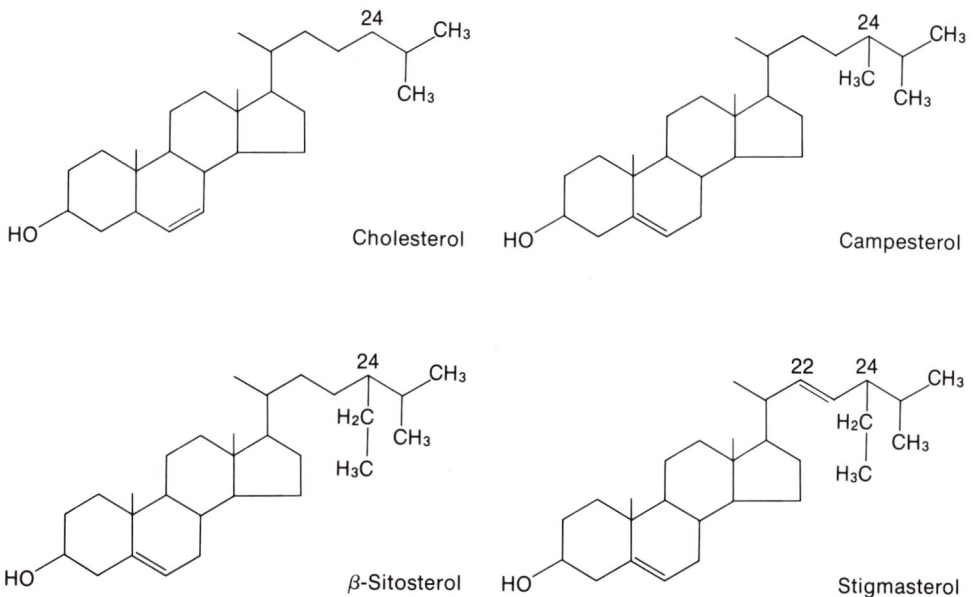

Fig. 21.6 Chemical structures for cholesterol and plant sterols.

decrease in hypercholesterolemic subjects has been noted by feeding 5 to 9 g per day (Subbiah, 1968). Kudchodkar et al. (1976) found a mean decrease of 9 ± 4 percent in the plasma cholesterol of 3 normal and 3 hyperlipemic subjects fed Cytellin (3 g t.i.d.) for periods of 12 or 15 days. Treatment with plant sterols markedly increased the fecal excretion of steroids. Using ^{14}C-cholesterol to label endogenous cholesterol, it was found that the increase in fecal excretion of endogenous cholesterol and its metabolites was much greater than the decrease in plasma cholesterol pools. The extra cholesterol could have been derived from decreased absorption of endogenous cholesterol, increased endogenous cholesterol synthesis, and/or mobilization of cholesterol from tissues. More information concerning plant sterol absorption and metabolism is desirable if plant sterols continue to be used as therapeutic agents in hypercholesterolemia.

Dietary Carbohydrate

Some epidemiological data have related the increasing death rates from CHD in industrialized nations to an increased dietary intake of carbohydrate, particularly sucrose. Controversy has continued for several years over dietary fat or sucrose as possible causative agents in development of AHD. Yudkin (1964) reviewed patterns and trends in carbohydrate consumption throughout the world and concluded that wealthier nations with the highest death rate from CHD consumed the most sugar. Yudkin and Morland (1967) used a questionnaire to assess sugar intake of men who had recently had a first known MI and compared the results with the sugar intake of two groups of control subjects. This study confirmed their earlier findings that MI occurred in men whose habitual consumption of sugar was about twice that of men with no history of MI. Other researchers have found that coronary patients ate more sucrose than control subjects prior to their first attack, but the differences were not as great as those reported by Yudkin (R. A. Ahrens, 1974). Finegan et al. (1968) did not find any difference in sugar intake of coronary patients and controls, but they measured only "added" sugar.

In 1961 E. H. Ahrens et al. identified a hyperlipemia that was "induced" by dietary carbohydrate. A number of other researchers since that time have reported similar results, particularly with high-sucrose diets (Herman et al., 1970). Palumbo et al. (1977) reported that 2 g of simple carbohydrate per kg body weight had no effect on serum triglycerides but diets containing 4 g simple carbohydrate (predominantly sucrose) produced a significant rise in serum triglycerides that was greater in CHD patients than normal controls. Fructose appeared to contribute to the sucrose sensitivity. On the other hand, R. A. Ahrens (1974) pointed out that the basic theory of carbohydrate induction is invalid because: (1) the elevated serum triglyceride levels produced by switching to a high-carbohydrate, low-fat diet have been shown to be temporary; (2) populations that routinely consume such diets have low serum triglyceride levels;

and (3) most studies have measured fasting serum triglyceride levels and these are daily maximal levels for subjects on high-carbohydrate diets, whereas subjects on high-fat, Western-type diets characteristically have higher serum triglyceride levels over the day. In spite of these findings suggesting little or no dietary carbohydrate induction of elevated serum triglycerides, high-sucrose diets apparently do produce some basic metabolic changes that are not transitory. Serum triglyceride levels were elevated in adult male subjects eating a high-sucrose diet for 25 days in comparison to the ingestion of a high-starch diet under similar circumstances (Macdonald and Braithwaite, 1964). Also, a sucrose-free diet consumed by men who had relatively high triglyceride levels while on a "normal" diet, caused a significant decrease in these serum lipids, whereas no significant change in triglyceride levels occurred in men whose initial levels were low (Roberts, 1973). The mechanism for the elevation of serum triglycerides by dietary sucrose is apparently complex and needs further clarification.

Dietary carbohydrates have been shown to have lesser effects on serum cholesterol than on triglycerides (Grande, 1967). McGandy et al. (1966) concluded that manipulation of the source of dietary carbohydrate would appear to add little to the dietary regulation of blood cholesterol. Others have argued that serum triglyceride elevation, which may occur with high-carbohydrate diets, is not an independent risk factor in the development of CHD (Heyden, 1975). On the other hand, there are proponents of the concept that hypertriglyceridemia is a significant and independent risk factor in AHD (Albrink, 1973). There are also those who feel that consumption of high levels of sucrose can be shown, through both epidemiological and experimental evidence, to be a major factor in the development of CHD (Yudkin, 1972; R. A. Ahrens, 1974). It is difficult at the present time to relate research findings on dietary carbohydrate to nutritional counseling on a practical basis.

Dietary Fiber

It has been suggested that the amount of fiber in the diet is related to the incidence of IHD in a population (Trowell, 1972; Klevay, 1974; Moore et al., 1976; Burkitt, 1976). Dietary fiber has been defined as the skeletal remains of plant cells that are resistant to hydrolysis by human enzymes and is synonymous with "unavailable carbohydrate." It includes cellulose, pentosans or hemicelluloses, pectic substances, and the noncarbohydrate lignin. Crude fiber, given in most food tables, is a measurement of what remains after boiling plant foods in acid and alkali and is not the same as dietary fiber. Crude fiber contains lignin and part of the cellulose (Trowell, 1972).

Moore et al. (1976), in a retrospective study of 253 deceased New Orleans men, reported a positive association between dietary intakes during the terminal year of life of crude fiber (as well as protein of vegetable origin, total carbohydrate, and starch) and the extent of raised lesion involvement in coronary arteries. Trowell (1972) pointed out that modern Western society consumes more refined and less starchy carbohydrate fiber-carrying foods than do various African groups, who often consume large quantities of lightly milled grains. Serum cholesterol levels are generally low in the African tribal groups and IHD very uncommon. Substitution of 140 g rolled oats for 300 g bread was made for 21 male Dutch subjects for a 3-week period, and a mean decrease in serum cholesterol levels from 258 mg/100 ml to 226 mg/100 ml was noted (deGroot et al., 1963). However, the addition of 13 g cellulose per day to a controlled diet of natural foods for five healthy young women during 4-week periods had no significant effect on serum cholesterol levels (Prather, 1964). No change was seen in serum cholesterol and triglyceride levels of six young male subjects on metabolically controlled diets fed 36 g wheat fiber per day for 3 weeks (Jenkins et al., 1975). Plasma cholesterol concentration was reduced by 13 percent when 15 g per day of citrus pectin were added to metabolically controlled diets in 9 young subjects (Kay and Truswell, 1977).

A possible mechanism by which dietary fiber protects against CHD is to decrease reabsorption of bile salts from the intestine. Apparently, however, all fiber components do not have the same effect in binding bile salts. Story and Kritchevsky (1976) reported that cellulose bound only negligible amounts (1.4 percent) of a mixture of bile salts *in vitro,* while lignin bound 29.2 percent. Alfalfa bound 15.9 percent and bran 9.0 percent bile salts. Pectin was shown by Tsai et al. (1976) to have the greatest hypocholesterolemic effect on rats of any fibers tested, which also included cellulose, wheat bran, carragheenan, agar, and gum arabic. The authors concluded that the effect of dietary fiber is dependent on the composition of the diet as well as on the fiber itself. Additional research is necessary to further define dietary fiber and clarify its relationship to serum lipids and CHD.

Feeding Patterns

The effects of frequency of eating on metabolic processes in the body are discussed in Sec. 4.4. Increased body-fat synthesis appears to be encouraged by large, infrequent meals, at least in experimental animals. Prevalence of hypercholesterolemia tended to decrease in Czechoslovakian men as meal frequency increased (Hejda and Fábry, 1964). Consumption of six meals a day by five medical students and the wife of one student produced a fall in serum cholesterol concentration in comparison with the levels on a three-meals-per-day pattern (Cohn, 1964). Gwinup et al. (1963) reported there was an increase in serum lipids of hyperlipidemic and normal subjects during a one-meal-per-day experimental period (gorging) and a decrease during a 10-meal-per-day period (nibbling).

Animal studies on a number of species have shown similar responses of increased serum cholesterol levels to decreased feeding frequency. Not many data are available on humans, and few long-term studies have been done. Possibly feeding frequency could be one factor influencing serum lipid levels and consequent CHD but, based on available data, it is not likely to be a major influence.

Dietary Protein

Significant interactions between type of dietary fat, presence of cholesterol, and type and feeding level of protein were noted by Lofland et al. (1966) in a study of serum lipid levels and aortic atherosclerosis in pigeons. Carrol and Hamilton (1975) also reported that the hypercholesterolemia that develops in rabbits on cholesterol-free, semisynthetic diets appears to be primarily dependent on the protein component of these diets. The thrombotic syndrome induced in the rat by a hyperlipemic diet containing laboratory chow, sodium cholate, butter, and cholesterol was found by Renaud and Allard (1964) to be prevented by increasing the protein content of the diet.

Studies on the effect of dietary protein on serum lipid levels in humans have yielded controversial results. Keys and Anderson (1957) reported that varying the protein level from 11 to 20 percent of the caloric intake had no significant effect on serum cholesterol concentration. However, Olson et al. (1958) found that diets containing 25 g protein per day produced a 20 percent decrease in serum cholesterol concentration in human subjects after they had been subsisting on diets containing 100 g protein per day. Olson et al. (1970) reported that formula diets given to eight healthy normocholesteremic male subjects caused a marked fall in serum cholesterol when they contained the eight essential amino acids plus glutamate as a source of nonessential nitrogen to provide a total nitrogen intake of 16 g. When glycine was used instead of glutamate, the hypocholesteremic effect was not present (Garlich et al., 1970).

Hodges et al. (1967) fed a low-fat, cholesterol-free diet, containing vegetable oils and either sugar or complex carbohydrate, to six hypercholesterolemic male volunteers. When vegetable protein, primarily from isolated soybean protein products, replaced animal protein in the diet, serum cholesterol levels were reported to decrease markedly and remain low regardless of the source of carbohydrate (sugar versus starch) or the level of fat (15 percent versus 45 percent of kilocalories), although Keys (1967) has criticized some aspects of this study. Elson et al. (1971) fed two dietary protein levels, 48 and 141 g, to six healthy college students maintaining a constant ratio of the essential amino acids, cystine, and tyrosine in the diets. The ratios of fat to carbohydrate and simple to complex carbohydrates were also constant. Serum cholesterol levels were significantly lower and phospholipid levels higher when the subjects were fed the 48 g protein diet than when they consumed the 141-g diet. Campbell et al. (1965) found that substitution of wheat gluten for a casein-lactalbumin mixture in diets containing 6.5 g nitrogen per day produced somewhat less nitrogen retention in human subjects. However, ingestion of the two diets differing in kind and quality of protein did not have any effect on levels of various serum lipid fractions. This was true whether the diet contained 12 percent or 40 percent linoleic acid.

Vitamins

Low serum cholesterol levels have been reported to occur in patients with macrocytic anemia due to folic acid or vitamin B_{12} deficiency or both. A statistical correlation between serum cholesterol levels and serum folate levels up to 6.2 pcg per ml was established by Bazzano (1969) for folate-deficient patients. Williams et al. (1966) concluded from a study on pyridoxine-deficient rats that the deficiency significantly altered metabolism of dietary and endogenous cholesterol. Bring et al. (1965) showed that increasing the dietary vitamin A in cholesterol-fed rats decreased serum and liver total cholesterol concentrations in these animals.

Ginter et al. (1969) reported that chronic hypovitaminosis C increased liver cholesterol levels in guinea pigs. Ginter (1973) also showed that the catabolism of cholesterol to bile acids was significantly decreased in guinea pigs with a low level ascorbic acid deficiency. Human studies on the effect of oral ascorbic acid on plasma cholesterol have yielded variable results. In subjects with normal serum cholesterol levels, several researchers have been unable to demonstrate any effect of ascorbic acid therapy on serum cholesterol levels (Anderson et al., 1972; Sokoloff et al., 1966). However, Spittle (1971), in a study of 58 volunteers, reported a tendency for serum cholesterol levels to fall after administration of 1 g vitamin C daily to individuals under 25 years of age. There was little change in the 25 to 45 year age group, whereas some subjects over age 45 showed a rise in serum cholesterol on this regimen.

In hypercholesterolemic subjects treated with oral ascorbic acid (1 to 6 g per day) for 5 to 16 weeks, no effect was found by Samuel and Shalchi (1964) on seven males and six females with an age range of 9 to 56 years. One additional male patient in this study showed a substantial decrease in serum cholesterol. Peterson et al. (1975) treated nine hypercholesterolemic subjects with 4 g per day ascorbic acid for 2 months and found no significant change in plasma cholesterol or triglyceride levels. On the other hand, Myasnikov (1958) reported that administration of high doses of vitamin C reduced serum cholesterol levels in patients with hypercholesterolemia. Sokoloff et al. (1966) also found decreased cholesterol levels with oral ascorbic acid supplements to hypercholesterolemic individuals. Ginter et al. (1970) found decreased plasma cholesterol levels after oral ascorbic acid supplementation in hypercholesterolemic subjects with initial low blood ascorbic acid levels. A potential role of ascorbic acid deficiency in atherogenesis has been suggested by Shaffer (1970). The conflicting data presently available do not support a clear statement on the effect of ascorbic acid on serum lipid levels or CHD.

Much enthusiasm has been generated in the public sector of the United States for vitamin E supplementation in CHD. Hodges (1973) reviewed some of the studies in this area with the conclusion that the weight of evidence fails to support the hypothesis that large doses of alpha-tocopherol may benefit patients with CHD. Olson (1973) arrived at a similar conclusion. Anderson et al. (1974) conducted a double-blind study on 50 patients with angina pectoris using a daily dosage of 3200 IU of vitamin E or a placebo with no statistically convincing evidence that the vitamin-treated group fared better than the placebo group. Serum levels of tocopherol apparently increase in hypercholesterolemic animals and humans and may be a reflection of the increased lipid-carrying property of the plasma proteins rather than an indication of vitamin E status (Marshall et al., 1973; Horwitt et al., 1972).

21.4   Minerals and Cardiovascular Disease

An association has been suggested between hardness of drinking water and cardiovascular death rates, but mechanisms to explain this association have not been clarified. Schroeder (1960) used data from the 1950 U.S. census to show that death rates from hypertensive and arteriosclerotic heart diseases were inversely related to hardness of drinking water. This association persisted in 1960 (Schroeder, 1966). Morris et al. (1961) have shown a similar association in Great Britain and reports from other countries have confirmed these findings (Perry, 1973). Three matched Los Angeles communities supplied by water of different hardnesses did not show consistent differences in death rates from heart disease (Allwright et al., 1974). Neither were significant correlations between total water hardness and cardiovascular disease death rates found in a study of Oklahoma by counties (Lindeman and Assenzo, 1964).

To explain the effects of water, it has been suggested that (1) the roles of calcium and/or magnesium may be primary in maintaining heart rhythm during ischemia, or (2) soft water is corrosive and may dissolve toxic substances, such as cadmium, which may be an active factor in some human hypertension (Perry, 1973; Schroeder, 1966; Seelig and Heggtveit, 1974). Stitt et al. (1973) found that mean values for blood pressure, plasma cholesterol, and heart rate were higher in a group of 245 middle-aged males living in soft-water areas than were those for 244 similar men living in hard-water areas. They suggested that these observed differences could be important in explaining a substantial part of the difference in cardiovascular mortality between these areas. However, Bierenbaum et al. (1973) found serum cholesterol levels to be diet-related and higher in the hard-water communities of Omaha, Nebraska and London, England than in the soft-water communities of Winston-Salem, North Carolina and Glasgow, Scotland even though lower cardiovascular mortality rates were found in the hard-water areas than in the soft-water areas. Cardiovascular death rates were inversely related to serum levels of magnesium and calcium.

This study probably raised more questions than it answered and further studies are indicated.

Klevay (1975) suggested a zinc/copper hypothesis, postulating that a metabolic imbalance of zinc and copper is a major factor in the etiology of CHD. The imbalance is either a relative or an absolute deficiency of copper characterized by a high ratio of zinc to copper and produces hypercholesterolemia. Klevay and Forbush (1976) reported that there was probably less copper in human foods in the United States in 1966 than in 1942, this decrease being consonant with the zinc/copper hypothesis. However, Kime and Sifri (1976) pointed out that this hypothesis has not been proven experimentally and is based upon a great deal of speculation.

21.5 Behavior Patterns, Stress, and Coronary Heart Disease

Several observations that suggest a relationship between long-term stress and CHD have been summarized by Syme (1970). Studies made in North Dakota showed that the incidence of CHD among men who were first reared on a farm and then moved to the city to take a white-collar job was three times higher than among men who remained on the farm. However, in men from the farm who moved to the city to take a blue-collar job, the increase in risk of CHD was not significant. Differences in CHD incidence were not due to differences in diet, smoking habits, physical activity, obesity, blood pressure, age, or familial longevity. Findings in two studies made in California were similar and suggested that the risk of CHD increases as men move up in the world of work. The risk of CHD has been found to be higher in men whose life situation during adulthood changed frequently, as moving to a new residence or taking a new job, than in those who made fewer changes. The risk of CHD is higher in men who live in urban industrialized areas. In a study in North Carolina, the mortality rate from CHD increased among the original residents of many rural communities as the communities became urbanized.

Russek and Russek (1972) reported that young coronary patients accustomed to a "typical" American diet could be differentiated from healthy controls far more readily by dimensions of occupational emotional stress than by differences in heredity, diet, obesity, tobacco consumption, or physical exercise. At the time of their attacks, 91 of 100 coronary patients (as compared with 20 percent of healthy controls) had been holding two or more jobs, working more than 60 hours per week, or experiencing unusual insecurity, discontent, or frustration in relation to employment. These authors suggested that the lethality of a high-fat diet in Western society may actually be dependent on the "catalytic" influence of stressful living. Bruhn et al. (1966) reported that educational and occupational mobility in male subjects were variables in a study of social characteristics of patients with

CHD that distinguished most meaningfully the patients from control subjects.

In the Western Collaborative Group study initiated by Rosenman et al. (1964), comprehensive studies of overt behavior pattern, blood lipids and coagulation, body measurements, socioeconomic factors, individual habits, and cardiovascular status were obtained annually beginning in 1960 for 3524 men, aged 30 to 59 years. As part of the study, an overt behavior pattern was assessed with the use of a tape-recorded personal interview requiring 30 minutes and a psychophysiological test. The researchers described a Behavior Pattern Type A that was characterized by personality traits such as aggressiveness, ambition, drive, competitiveness, and a profound sense of time urgency. Locomotion and mannerisms were rapid. Speech usually was forceful, fast, often explosively uneven and emphatic, and accompanied by sudden gestures such as fist-clenching and taut facial grimaces. Men with behavior pattern Type A appeared excessively and willingly driven to achievement; to getting things done. They were simultaneously unable to overcome the inflexibility of time or the competing and obstructing effects of other persons and things. A Type B behavior pattern was also identified in which the Type A characteristics were present to a much lesser degree. Subjects with this pattern were more CHD-resistant (Rosenman and Friedman, 1971).

During the first 2 years of follow-up, 70 subjects developed manifest CHD. Findings of the study published at this time indicated that the presence of (1) abnormalities in lipoprotein pattern, (2) hypertension, or (3) exhibition of a Type A behavior pattern each possessed significant prognostic value for CHD (Rosenman et al., 1966). Clinical CHD had occurred in 257 subjects at the time of 8 to 9 years of follow-up (Rosenman et al., 1975). Incidence of CHD was reported to be significantly associated with parental CHD, reported diabetes, schooling, smoking habits, overt behavior pattern, blood pressure, and serum cholesterol, triglyceride, and beta lipoproteins. The Type A behavior pattern was strongly related to the CHD incidence and this association could not be explained by association of the behavior pattern with any single predictive risk factor or with any combination of them. The researchers concluded that behavior pattern Type A indicates a pathogenetic force for the development of CHD that is different from and operates in addition to, as well as in conjunction with, the classical risk factors.

Jenkins et al. (1974) developed an easily used computer-scored test questionnaire that attempts to measure the coronary-prone Type A behavior pattern. Kenigsberg et al. (1974) reported that hospitalized CHD patients scored more in the Type A direction on this questionnaire than did those with other health crises. However, Type A behavior pattern as a major risk factor requires further testing to confirm its independent role in CHD development.

Wardwell and Bahnson (1973) studied behavioral variables among 114 survivors of MI and 114 hospitalized controls without cardiovascular disease in the Southeastern Connecticut Heart Study. Their findings did not support hypotheses relating to situational stress, cultural mobility, religious affiliation, commitment to social norms, anxiety, alienation, and psychopathological tendencies. However, the patients with MI scored higher than either the hospitalized control subjects or normal nonhospitalized subjects on a scale designed to measure the Type A behavior pattern. They also scored higher on a scale of somatization, i.e., the tendency to translate conflict and affect into bodily symptoms. The major conclusion of this study was that what counts in the production of MI may not be the amount of situational or intrapsychic stress a person is subjected to but the way he copes with it—his defensive style.

21.6 Treatment of Atherosclerosis and Coronary Heart Disease

Heart attacks are intensively treated once they have occurred. However, they do not usually "just happen," but develop over a period of time. When possible signs of impending heart attack, such as angina pectoris, are observed, they may be treated in some cases by surgery. The use of drugs to lower serum lipids is discussed in Sec. 20.4.

Coronary Bypass Surgery

Since 1967 coronary artery bypass surgery has been performed in selected cases of coronary atherosclerosis to produce direct myocardial revascularization. Vessels from other parts of the body, such as the saphenous vein or the internal mammary artery, are used to bypass the diseased areas of the coronary arteries. The objective is complete revascularization of the myocardium by placement of as many grafts as are necessary. In the past few years, double and triple bypass procedures have made up 65 percent of the operations performed, and quadruple bypass has become almost as common as single bypass (Mills and Ochsner, 1975). The desired effects of coronary artery surgery are to allow the patients to lead more nearly normal lives and to prevent MI.

Excellent symptomatic results in terms of relief or reduction in angina pectoris after bypass surgery have been reported. Clinical manifestations of congestive heart failure have generally improved. Although there are few controlled randomized studies comparing long-term survival in medically versus surgically treated patients with coronary artery disease, there appears to be a higher survival rate in the surgically treated groups (Mundth and Austen, 1975). Further evaluation of the effects of bypass surgery is continuing.

Peterson (1976) reported on one hospital's plan for nutrition counseling of patients admitted for coronary artery bypass surgery. Those admitted for work-up are offered counseling for a low-saturated-fat, low-cholesterol diet of an appropriate caloric level during hospitalization. In the immediate postoperative period, the dietary order is individualized but usually includes a 500 mg sodium and 1500 ml fluid restriction, in addition to fat modification, which progresses to a "no-added-salt" diet without fluid limitation in 2 to 5 days. When lipoprotein typing is done on a patient, more precise dietary modifications may be made.

Myocardial Infarction

The levels of certain enzymes may increase in the blood as a result of acute damage to heart muscle, and enzyme assays to confirm the diagnosis of MI have become part of the routine course of events in the diagnostic work-up. After damage to heart muscle, enzymes escape from the cells into the interstitium. Some enzymes are denatured here and never reach the circulation. However, others are transported by the lymphatic and coronary circulations and appear in the blood. There are varying rates at which this occurs for different enzymes and there are also differences in their clearance from the general circulation. Therefore, various enzymes reach peak levels of serum activity at different times following MI. The major cardiac enzymes of diagnostic value are (Galen, 1975):

1. Creatine phosphokinase (ATP : Creatine phosphotransferase). Serum creatine phosphokinase (CPK) activity begins to rise 4 to 8 hours following MI, reaching levels five to 10 times the upper limit of normal. Peak activity is usually reached 24 hours following the onset of chest pain and activity returns to normal by the fifth day. Measurements of CPK are more specific in detecting heart muscle damage than are most of the other enzymes except in the presence of skeletal muscle injury.

2. Glutamic oxalacetic transaminase (L-Aspartate: 2-Oxoglutarate aminotransferase).
   Glutamic oxalacetic transaminase (GOT) is more properly referred to as aspartate aminotransferase. Its activity begins to rise 8 to 12 hours following MI, reaching levels two to three times the upper limit of normal. Peak activity is usually reached 24 hours following chest pain and returns to normal by the fifth day.

3. Lactate dehydrogenase (L-Lactate : NAD oxidoreductase).
   Lactate dehydrogenase (LDH) activity can be found in virtually all human tissues. The liver and skeletal muscle have the greatest concentration, followed by the heart. The level of LDH begins to rise 12 to 24 hours following MI, frequently reaching levels two to three times the upper limit of normal. Peak activity is usually reached on the third day following onset of chest pain and activity may remain elevated for as long as 10 days after infarction.

Isoenzymes (multiple molecular forms) may also be separated and their activity measured. The specificity of an isoenzyme is greater than that of the total activity of the enzyme and a particular isoenzyme may be organ specific. Hydroxybutyrate dehydrogenase (Hydroxybutyrate : NAD oxidoreductase), an isoenzyme expression of LDH, has been used for diagnosis of MI. Its activity parallels that of LDH.

Acute MI produces some lowering of glucose tolerance through an increased release of catecholamines, steroids, and glucagon, and a decreased release of insulin. Overt hyperglycemia or abnormal glucose tolerance curves have been found in 50 to 100 percent of patients with MI during the first ten days following the acute attack. Ravid et al. (1975) followed 169 patients with acute MI and found elevated fasting blood glucose levels in 47.5 percent with reduced oral glucose tolerance in 72.5 percent. Of 32 patients who died in the hospital, fasting blood glucose was elevated in 72 percent and oral glucose tolerance was abnormal in 89 percent.

A number of other metabolic changes accompany MI. Metabolic acidosis is often present and may influence cardiac arrhythmias. Metabolic changes in the handling of fat and carbohydrate may occur in ischemic heart muscle. Administration of glucagon has been reported to have a positive effect on the force of cardiac contractions in patients with acute MI and was thought to be of value in the shock syndromes associated with MI (Christakis and Winston, 1973). The nutritional plan for a patient with acute MI should be regarded as part of total patient care, according to Christakis and Winston (1973), and should be integrated with the patient's unique pattern of metabolic response to the stress of MI. They have suggested appropriate nutritional care for the acute, subacute, and rehabilitative phases of the MI patient's illness.

Acute Phase. Some form of liquid diet, with a daily volume of 1000 to 1500 ml, is often used for the first few days. A 500 to 800-kcal diet for the remainder of the acute phase may be appropriate. The liquid diet may reduce the risk of cardiac arrest by avoidance of gagging on food boluses and may help to avoid food aspiration. Fluids may include fruit juice, skim milk, clear soups, gingerale, and water. Extremes in temperature of liquids should be avoided in order to avert possible precipitation of arrhythmias via neural mechanisms. Coffee and tea are commonly eliminated since they contain stimulants that may increase the heart rate. Every precaution should be taken to avoid abdominal distension in patients who cannot tolerate milk, excessive amounts of fruit juices, and carbonated beverages. Low-sodium milk may be tolerated in some cases. The sodium and potassium content of the diet may need adjustment for some patients. Sodium is restricted if there is evidence of congestive heart failure. If patients cannot consume liquids by mouth, appropriate parenteral feeding may be desirable; however, the use of unrestricted intravenous infusions is contraindicated because of the reduced efficiency of a damaged myocardium and the hazard of pulmonary edema due to fluid overload.

Subacute Phase. Once the acute phase is past, more solid food may be given. A 1000- to 1200-kcal diet is usually reasonable, composed of approximately 20 percent protein, 45 percent carbohydrate, and 30 to 35 percent fat, with no more than 300 mg cholesterol. The goal is to provide sufficient kilocalories for basal metabolism and optimal levels of essential nutrients for maintenance of good nutritional status without inducing an increase in oxygen uptake. Foods that are easily digested, free of gastric irritants, soft, and low in roughage are preferred. Flatus and constipation should be avoided if at all possible. Appropriate foods may include skim milk; tender lean cuts of meat, fish, and poultry; tender cooked or canned vegetables and fruits; plain breads and cooked cereals; and simple puddings and gelatin desserts. Coffee and tea may be permitted in moderation if they do not increase restlessness or sleeplessness. Frequent small feedings may be desirable. Moderate sodium restriction may be suggested on an individual basis.

Rehabilitative Phase. As a patient resumes moderate activity, a wider variety of food may be used. However, the principles of the fat-controlled diet should usually continue to be applied, with sodium restriction when necessary. Optimal weight should be maintained or achieved. Weight reduction, if necessary, should be done slowly. The patient may be relatively inactive for 2 to 3 months and this will influence caloric needs. Diet patterns may be individualized after serum lipid levels have stabilized and a lipid profile is determined. A firm diagnostic determination of type of hyperlipoproteinemia may sometimes not be made for 6 months to 1 year after a MI. The hospitalization provides an excellent opportunity for nutrition counseling and instruction of both the patient and family.

21.7 Prevention of Atherosclerosis and Coronary Heart Disease

The Task Force on Arteriosclerosis stated that

> *prevention, rather than treatment, of arteriosclerosis offers the greatest promise of reducing mortality. Once the clinical manifestations of arteriosclerosis are apparent, the consequences may be difficult, if not impossible, to correct. Since at least half of the patients who develop heart attacks die before receiving medical care, only primary prevention can affect a significant reduction in the number of sudden deaths.*

The Joint Statement of the Food and Nutrition Board and the Council on Foods and Nutrition (1972) also points out:

> *Preliminary evidence suggests that faithful and continued consumption of a cholesterol-lowering diet over a period of years can reduce the coronary attack rate in middle-aged men. As would be expected in dealing with a chronic disease of this kind, early intervention appears to be more effective than intervention after the disease is evident.*

Primary prevention refers to prevention of overt CHD in people free of apparent manifestations of CHD at the start of a program. Secondary prevention, on the other hand, refers to prevention of additional clinical signs in persons who have already shown clinical complications of coronary atherosclerosis, such as a single nonfatal MI (Dayton and Pearce, 1969). Long-term prevention trials are expensive and difficult to implement. It is most important that experimental and control groups be established that are basically equivalent at the beginning of the study. It is also important that the treatment under study is the only variable present during the trial. A double-blind study design is desirable. One of the earliest primary prevention trials in the United States was the anticoronary club program conducted by the Bureau of Nutrition of the New York City Department of Health, beginning in 1957 (Christakis et al., 1966; Jolliffe et al., 1959). Free-living healthy male volunteers, 40 to 59 years of age, were requested from all segments of the population. There were 941 active participants and 532 who started the program but did not return for regular check-ups nor adhere well to the fat-controlled diet. A control group of 457 men was recruited about 2 years after the formation of the original anticoronary club. These control subjects were comparable demographically and with respect to hypercholesterolemia but the experimental group had a somewhat larger amount of initial obesity and hypertension. The experimental diet used was low in animal fat and cholesterol with an increased use of PUFA. For normal weight persons, the recommended diet contained, on a daily basis, 130 to 150 g protein, 66 to 97 g fat, 225 to 280 g carbohydrate, and 2,000 to 2,700 kcal. Fat made up 30 to 38 percent of total kilocalories, contained 20 to 33 g PUFA, and 19 to 21 g saturated fatty acids for a P/S ratio of 1.3 to 1.5. When appropriate, a low-fat reducing diet was recommended. This provided 140 g protein, 34 g fat, 180 g carbohydrate on a daily basis, with fat making up 19 percent of kilocalories and with 8.3 g PUFA, 13.8 g saturated fatty acids, and a P/S value of 0.6. Diet was the only intervention in this study and adherence was judged to be good to excellent on the basis of change in weight, serum cholesterol, and adipose tissue analysis of active participants. Endpoint criteria for the study included MI, coronary thrombosis, coronary sclerosis, electrocardiographic abnormalities, and angina pectoris. A summary of morbidity and mortality data reported by Christakis and Rinzler (1969) and Rinzler (1968) is:

	Fat-controlled Diet	Inactive Subjects	Unmodified Diet
Total persons at risk	941	532	457
Confirmed new events	17	24	32
Incidence per 1000 man-years	4.3	7.5	10.3

The risk factors considered in the study were hypercholesterolemia, obesity, and hypertension. At the time of entry into the study, 32 percent of the experimental subjects showed at least two of these risk factors, whereas only 17 percent had none. Two and 4 years later, these percentages had changed to 6 and 60, respectively. Incidence of obesity and hypertension was reduced in later years over the first 4 years of the study in experimental subjects, whereas it remained stable for the control group. It was suggested that the unusual degree of success in reducing the weight of obese subjects might be attributable to the intense nutritional guidance given the subjects by the study's public health nutritionists. Normal weight subjects as well as those in the weight-reduction program were seen every 6 weeks at a minimum. During the phase of weight reduction they were seen weekly.

A coronary prevention evaluation program was also conducted by Stamler et al. (1966) for the Chicago Board of Health. The main nutritional emphasis in this program was the control of dietary saturated fat and cholesterol intake in order to reduce serum cholesterol levels. Subjects with higher initial levels of serum cholesterol experienced the greatest decrease on the modified diet, with sometimes over a 30 percent decline in serum cholesterol. Obesity and hypertension were reduced in subjects on the program. The trend in morbidity and mortality favored the experimental participants over dropouts of the program.

Dayton and Pearce (1969) conducted a double-blind, 8-year prevention trial involving a mixed group of men, some with but most without overt evidence of occlusive atherosclerosis. The participants were middle-aged and elderly men living in a veterans' home in Los Angeles, California and were allocated at random either to a control (422 men) or an experimental group (424 men). The experimental diet was similar in total fat content to the control diet, but the type of fat was adjusted so that a P/S ratio of about 1.7 was achieved. The P/S ratio of the control diet was 0.2. The fat-controlled diet averaged 97 g protein, 108 g fat, 365 mg cholesterol, and 2500 kcal daily. Fat made up 39 percent of total kilocalories. The control diet averaged 96 g protein, 111 g fat, 653 mg cholesterol, and 2500 kcal, with 40 percent of total kilocalories as fat. Adherence was estimated to be 56 percent among controls and 49 percent in the experimental group. The mean serum cholesterol level decreased significantly in the experimental group. Among the 424 subjects on fat-controlled diets, there were 48 deaths ascribable to vascular disease, whereas there were 70 deaths among the 422 persons on unmodified diets. The number with clinical events that could be evaluated in a relatively objective fashion was:

	Control	Experimental
Definite MI, by electrocardiogram only	4	9
Definite MI, overt	47	33
Sudden death due to CHD	27	18
Definite cerebral infarct	25	13
Ruptured aneurysm	5	2
Amputation for gangrene	5	7
Miscellaneous	6	3
Total	119	85

There was a difference in the endpoint of the study favorable to the experimental diet group, but it was not statistically significant. However, when these data were pooled with those for definite cerebral infarction, a significant difference was shown (Dayton and Pearce, 1969).

Turpeinen, Miettinen, and their coworkers have reported on a 12-year primary prevention trial for CHD among Finnish subjects in two mental hospitals, each serving as a control for 6 years (Miettinen et al., 1972; Miettinen, 1975; Turpeinen et al., 1968). The mortality from CHD was studied in all patients irrespective of previous CHD. In men, the use of a cholesterol-lowering diet was accompanied by significantly reduced mortality from CHD. In women, the mortality from CHD also appeared to be lower during the diet period but the differences were small and not statistically significant. A detailed analysis was made of middle-aged patients whose initial electrocardiogram was free from the coronary pattern. The endpoint was the intermediate or major coronary electrocardiogram pattern or coronary death. In this more pure primary prevention study, the incidence of CHD was lower in both men and women during the diet periods.

Several studies have involved dietary treatment in the secondary prevention of CHD. Many of the early reports in this area have been criticized because of faulty statistical design and incomplete reporting although many of them showed a favorable effect of diet (Anderson et al., 1973). A study by Leren (1970) in Oslo, Norway involved 412 men below 68 years of age who had survived a MI for an average of 20 months before being admitted to the study. The men were randomly assigned to control and dietary treatment groups, with the experimental diet being designed to decrease the intake of saturated fat and cholesterol and to increase consumption of PUFA. Patients were instructed to consume $\frac{1}{2}$ liter of soybean oil per week mixed with skim milk powder as a substitute for butter, in baking and cooking, in salad dressings, and in daily amounts of 15 to 30 g as "medicine." Adherence to the experimental diet was apparently good except for the failure of many patients to consume the soybean oil "medicine." During 5 years, there were significantly fewer recurrences of MI and deaths from infarctions among the experimental group as compared with controls.

A National Diet-Heart Study Feasibility Trial was begun in the United States in 1960 with the support of the National Heart Institute of the U.S. Public Health Service. An overall purpose for a Diet-Heart Study had been outlined to design and conduct large-scale field trials in order to test the hypothesis that premature primary heart disease may be prevented by diet. However, such a study would require approximately 100,000 men followed for at least 5 years. The Feasibility Trial was a pilot study to ascertain: how to obtain sufficient numbers of participants for a definitive study; how to measure the extent of their cooperation; how to plan and conduct an effective experiment; what the most suitable diets would be and the place special foods had in implementing them; whether a uniform program could be used in a study comprising centers widely separated geographically; what personnel and physical facilities would be required and the cost of such a project; whether a decrease in blood cholesterol could not only be obtained but maintained for a year or longer; and whether data from all study centers could be pooled. The Feasibility Trials were conducted in five urban centers with free-living participants and in one institutional center, a mental hospital. A total of 2400 men took part in the study, 1400 the first year and 1000 the second. Several different diets were developed, using food specially prepared by the food industry, and the design was double-blind. The study was successfully managed, adherence was reasonable, and the overall reduction in blood cholesterol was 11 percent (Brown, 1968). A large-scale study has not yet been completed. Under federal funding, the National Heart and Lung Institute has established a number of Lipid Research Clinics in various parts of the United States. These centers will participate in intervention studies in which diet may be appropriately modified or observed and drugs prescribed.

Several booklets have been prepared as aids to nutritional counseling for the prevention of CHD. In addition to those published by the National Heart and Lung Institute for the dietary management of hyperlipoproteinemia, the American Heart Association has published booklets outlining fat-controlled meal patterns (American Heart Association, 1966 and 1967). These diets limit beef, lamb, pork, or ham to 3 servings per week with one serving being designated to contain 3 oz cooked weight. Chicken, turkey, fish, and veal may be used for the other 11 lunch and dinner meals consumed during a week. The diets also limit eggs to no more than 3 egg yolks per week, although some researchers have reported no effect on serum cholesterol levels from adding 1 to 2 eggs daily to a usual diet (Kummerow et al., 1977; Porter et al., 1977). Four or more tablespoons of vegetable oil per day are required in the diet pattern, with some substitution of special margarine or shortening allowed. Skim milk is used and no cheeses other than low-fat cottage cheese are eaten. Saturated fat in baked products and other foods is to be avoided. Kilocalories may also be restricted on an individual basis. Recipe booklets for fat-controlled, low-cholesterol meals are published by the American Heart Association (American Heart Association, 1975).

A Subcommittee on Diet and Hyperlipidemia, Council on Arteriosclerosis, American Heart Association, has prepared a series of booklets entitled "A Maximal Approach to the Dietary Treatment of the Hyperlipidemias." These booklets describe the following diets:

Diet A: The low-cholesterol (100 mg), moderately low-fat diet
Diet B: The low-cholesterol (200 mg), moderately low-fat diet
Diet C: The low-cholesterol, high-polyunsaturated-fat diet
Diet D: The extremely low-fat diet

The booklets are available to patients through their physicians. The diet patterns are very restrictive in order to achieve maximal effect.

The dietitian/nutritionist and the physician may design many different diet patterns for the control of hyperlipidemia and the possible prevention of atherosclerosis and CHD. Most commonly, the type of fat is modified to restrict animal products containing saturated fats and to encourage the use of foods containing vegetable oils. The liberal use of vegetables and fruits is usually encouraged, both because they are low in fat and because of their content of vitamins, minerals, and fiber. Whole grain breads and cereals may also contribute dietary fiber and certain vitamins and minerals without adding substantial amounts of fat to the diet. The total amount of fat is often preferably decreased from the average intake in the United States, although extremely low-fat diets are not usually recommended. Skim milk and low-fat dairy products are used. Kilocalories and simple sugars are restricted on an individual basis. The diet must be adequate in all essential nutrients. A number of food products specially designed for use in fat-modified diets are available commercially. These include various egg substitutes, trimmed meats that are relatively low in fat, imitation cheese and ice cream containing vegetable oils, margarines containing comparatively large amounts of nonhydrogenated vegetable oil, and fabricated meat analogs made with soy protein products. Meats and milk containing more than the usual amounts of PUFA have been produced by feeding ruminants polyunsaturated oil that is encapsulated with protein and denatured with formalin in order to make the oil unavailable to the hydrogenating action of bacteria in the rumen of the animal (Food and Nutrition Board, 1976; Brown et al., 1976; Mattos and Palmquist, 1974).

Dietary measures and appropriate physical exercise to control hyperlipidemia and obesity, drugs and diet to control hypertension, desisting from smoking, and learning to adapt effectively to the stress of living all offer promise to control the epidemic of CHD among the populations of industrialized countries. Since the cause of atherosclerosis and CHD appears to be multifactored, prevention will also require a multifactored approach.

REFERENCES

1. Ahrens, E. H., Jr., J. Hirsch, K. Oette, J. W. Farquhar, and Y. Stein. 1961. Carbohydrate-induced and fat-induced lipemia. *Trans. Assoc. Am. Phys.,* **74:** 134.

2. Ahrens, R. A. 1974. Sucrose, hypertension, and heart disease: An historical perspective. *Am. J. Clin. Nutr.,* **27:** 403.

3. Albrink, M. J. 1973. Triglyceridemia. *J. Am. Dietet. Assoc.,* **62:** 626.

4. Allwright, S. P. A., A. Coulson, R. Detels, and C. E. Porter. 1974. Mortality and water-hardness in three matched communities in Los Angeles. *Lancet,* **2:** 860.

5. American Heart Association. 1975. Recipes for fat-controlled, low cholesterol meals.

6. American Heart Association. 1967. Planning fat-controlled meals for approximately 2000–2600 calories.

7. American Heart Association. 1966. Planning fat-controlled meals for 1200 and 1800 calories.

8. Anderson, J. T., F. Grande, and A. Keys. 1973. Cholesterol-lowering diets. *J. Am. Dietet. Assoc.*, **62:** 133.

9. Anderson, T. W. and D. B. W. Reid. 1974. A double-blind trial of vitamin E in angina pectoris. *Am. J. Clin. Nutr.*, **27:** 1174.

10. Anderson, T. W., D. B. W. Reid, and G. H. Beaton. 1972. Vitamin C and serum cholesterol. *Lancet*, **2:** 876.

11. Antar, M. A., M. A. Ohlson, and R. E. Hodges. 1964. Changes in retail market food supplies in the United States in the last seventy years in relation to the incidence of coronary heart disease, with special reference to dietary carbohydrates and essential fatty acids. *Am. J. Clin. Nutr.*, **14:** 169.

12. Bassett, D. R., M. Abel, R. C. Moellering, Jr., G. Rosenblatt, and J. Stokes III. 1969. Coronary heart disease in Hawaii: Dietary intake, depot fat, "stress", smoking, and energy balance in Hawaiian and Japanese men. *Am. J. Clin. Nutr.*, **22:** 1483.

13. Bazzano, G. 1969. Effects of folic acid metabolism on serum cholesterol levels. *Arch. Int. Med.*, **124:** 710.

14. Bierenbaum, M. L., A. I. Fleischman, J. P. Dunn, T. Hayton, D. C. Pattison, and P. B. Watson. 1973. Serum parameters in hard and soft water communities. *Am. J. Pub. Health*, **63:** 169.

15. Bring, S. V., C. A. Ricard, and M. V. Zaehringer. 1965. Relationship between cholesterol and vitamin A metabolism in rats fed at different levels of vitamin A. *J. Nutr.*, **85:** 400.

16. Brown, H. B. 1971. Food patterns that lower blood lipids in man. *J. Am. Dietet. Assoc.*, **58:** 303.

17. Brown, H. B. 1968. The National Diet-Heart Study—Implications for dietitians and nutritionists. *J. Am. Dietet. Assoc.*, **52:** 279.

18. Brown, H. B., V. G. deWolfe, H. K. Naito, W. J. Harper, and D. L. Palmquist. 1976. Polyunsaturated meat and dairy products in fat-modified food patterns for hyperlipidemia. *J. Am. Dietet. Assoc.*, **69:** 235.

19. Brown, H. B., M. E. Farrand, and I. H. Page. 1966. Design of practical fat-controlled diets. Foods, fat composition, and serum cholesterol content. *J. Am. Med. Assoc.*, **196:** 205.

20. Brown, H. B. and I. H. Page. 1966. Practical diets for serum cholesterol reduction. *Proc. 2nd Intl. Cong. Nutr., Hamburg*, **5:** 429.

21. Brown, J., G. J. Bourke, G. F. Gearty, A. Finnegan, M. Hill, F. C. Heffernan-Fox, D. E. Fitzgerald, J. Kennedy, R. W. Childers, W. J. E. Jessop, M. F. Trulson, M. C. Latham, S. Cronin, M. B. McCann, R. E. Clancy, I. Gore, H. W. Stoudt, D. M. Hegsted, and F. J. Stare. 1970. Nutritional and epidemiologic factors related to heart disease. *World Rev. Nutr. Dietet.*, **12:** 1.

22. Bruhn, J. G., B. Chandler, T. N. Lynn, and S. Wolf. 1966. Social characteristics of patients with coronary heart disease. *Am. J. Med. Sci.*, **251:** 629.

23. Burkitt, D. P. 1976. Economic development—not all bonus. *Nutr. Today*, **11** (No. 1): 6.

24. Campbell, A. M., M. E. Swendseid, W. H. Griffith, and S. G. Tuttle. 1965. Serum lipids of men fed diets differing in protein quality and linoleic acid content. *Am. J. Clin. Nutr.*, **17:** 83.

25. Carroll, K. K. and R. M. G. Hamilton. 1975. Effects of dietary protein and carbohydrate on plasma cholesterol levels in relation to atherosclerosis. *J. Food Sci.*, **40:** 18.

26. Christakis, G. and S. H. Rinzler. 1969. Diet. In *Atherosclerosis*, F. G. Schettler and G. S. Boyd (Eds.). New York: Elsevier.

27. Christakis, G., S. H. Rinzler, M. Archer, and A. Kraus. 1966. Effect of the anti-coronary club program on coronary heart disease risk-factor status. *J. Am. Med. Assoc.,* **198:** 597.

28. Christakis, G. and M. Winston. 1973. Nutritional therapy in acute myocardial infarction. *J. Am. Dietet. Assoc.,* **63:** 233.

29. Cohn, C. 1964. Feeding patterns and some aspects of cholesterol metabolism. *Fed. Proc.,* **23:** 76.

30. Connor, W. E. 1968. Dietary sterols: Their relationship to atherosclerosis. *J. Am. Dietet. Assoc.,* **52:** 202.

31. Council on Foods and Nutrition. 1972. Diet and coronary heart disease. *J. Am. Med. Assoc.,* **222:** 1645.

32. Dayton, S. and M. L. Pearce. 1969. Prevention of coronary heart disease and other complications of atherosclerosis by modified diet. *Am. J. Med.,* **46:** 751.

33. de Groot, A. P., R. Luyken, and N. A. Pikaar. 1963. Cholesterol-lowering effect of rolled oats. *Lancet,* **2:** 303.

34. Elson, C. E., E. Humleker, and L. Pascal. 1971. Dietary protein level and serum and erythrocyte lipids in young adult males. *Am. J. Clin. Nutr.,* **24:** 194.

35. Epstein, F. H. 1965. The epidemiology of coronary heart disease. *J. Chron. Dis.,* **18:** 735.

36. Finegan, A., N. Hickey, B. Maurer, and R. Mulcahy. 1968. Diet and coronary heart disease: Dietary analysis on 100 male patients. *Am. J. Clin. Nutr.,* **21:** 143.

37. Food and Nutrition Board and Board on Agriculture and Renewable Resources. 1976. *Fat Content and Composition of Animal Products.* Washington, D.C.: National Research Council, National Academy of Sciences.

38. Frantz, I. D., Jr. and R. B. Moore. 1969. The sterol hypothesis in atherogenesis. *Am. J. Med.,* **46:** 684.

39. Galen, R. S. 1975. The enzyme diagnosis of myocardial infarction. *Human Path.,* **6:** 141.

40. Garlich, J. D., G. Bazzano, and R. E. Olson. 1970. Changes in plasma free amino acid concentrations in human subjects on hypocholesteremic diets. *Am. J. Clin. Nutr.,* **23:** 1626.

41. Ginter, E. 1973. Cholesterol: Vitamin C controls its transformation to bile acids. *Science,* **179:** 702.

42. Ginter, E., I. Kajaba, and O. Nizner. 1970. The effect of ascorbic acid on cholesterolemia in healthy subjects with seasonal deficit of vitamin C. *Nutr. Metabol.,* **12:** 76.

43. Ginter, E., R. Ondreicka, P. Bobek, and V. Šimko. 1969. The influence of chronic vitamin C deficiency on fatty acid composition of blood serum, liver triglycerides and cholesterol esters in guinea pigs. *J. Nutr.,* **99:** 261.

44. Gordon, T. and W. B. Kannel. 1972. Predisposition to atherosclerosis in the head, heart, and legs. *J. Am. Med. Assoc.,* **221:** 661.

45. Gordon, T. and W. B. Kannel (Eds.). 1968–1970. The Framingham Study. An epidemiological investigation of cardiovascular disease. Bethesda, Maryland, National Heart and Lung Institute, Monograph Sections 1–26.

46. Grande, F. 1967. Dietary carbohydrates and serum cholesterol. *Am. J. Clin. Nutr.,* **20:** 176.

47. Grande, F., J. T. Anderson, and A. Keys. 1970. Comparison of effects of palmitic and stearic acids in the diet on serum cholesterol in man. *Am. J. Clin. Nutr.,* **23:** 1184.

48. Grande, F., J. T. Anderson, and A. Keys. 1961. The influence of chain length of the saturated fatty acids on their effect on serum cholesterol concentration in man. *J. Nutr.,* **74:** 420.

49. Gwinup, G., R. C. Byron, W. H. Roush, F. A. Kruger, and G. J. Hamwi. 1963. Effect of nibbling versus gorging on serum lipids in man. *Am. J. Clin. Nutr.,* **13:** 209.

50. Hegsted, D. M., R. B. McGandy, M. L. Myers, and F. J. Stare. 1965a. Dietary fatty acids and changes in serum cholesterol. (Abstract). *Fed. Proc.,* **24:** 262.

51. Hegsted, D. M., R. B. McGandy, M. L. Myers, and F. J. Stare. 1965b. Quantitative effects of dietary fat on serum cholesterol in man. *Am. J. Clin. Nutr.,* **17:** 281.

52. Hejda, S. and P. Fábry. 1964. Frequency of food intake in relation to some parameters of the nutritional status. *Nutr. Dieta,* **6:** 216.

53. Herman, R. H., D. Zakim, and F. B. Stifel. 1970. Effect of diet on lipid metabolism in experimental animals and man. *Fed. Proc.,* **29:** 1302.

54. Heyden, S. 1975. The problem with triglycerides. *Nutr. Metabol.,* **18:** 1.

55. Hill, P. and E. L. Wynder. 1976. Dietary regulation of serum lipids in healthy young adults. *J. Am. Dietet. Assoc.,* **68:** 25.

56. Hodges, R. E. 1973. Vitamin E and coronary heart disease. *J. Am. Dietet. Assoc.,* **62:** 638.

57. Hodges, R. E., W. A. Krehl, D. B. Stone, and A. Lopez. 1967. Dietary carbohydrates and low cholesterol diets: Effects on serum lipids of man. *Am. J. Clin. Nutr.,* **20:** 198.

58. Hodges, R. E., A. F. Salel, W. L. Dunkley, R. Zelis, P. F. McDonagh, C. Clifford, R. K. Hobbs, L. M. Smith, A. Fan, D. T. Mason, and C. Lykke. 1975. Plasma lipid changes in young adult couples consuming polyunsaturated meats and dairy products. *Am. J. Clin. Nutr.,* **28:** 1126.

59. Horwitt, M. K., C. C. Harvey, C. H. Dahn, Jr., and M. T. Searcy. 1972. Relationship between tocopherol and serum lipid levels for determination of nutritional adequacy. *Ann. N.Y. Acad. Sci.,* **203:** 223.

60. Jenkins, C. D., R. H. Rosenman, and S. J. Zyzanski. 1974. Prediction of clinical coronary heart disease by a test for the coronary-prone behavior pattern. *N. Eng. J. Med.,* **290:** 1271.

61. Jenkins, D. J. A., M. S. Hill, and J. H. Cummings. 1975. Effect of wheat fiber on blood lipids, fecal steroid excretion and serum iron. *Am. J. Clin. Nutr.,* **28:** 1408.

62. Jolliffe, N., S. H. Rinzler, and M. Archer. 1959. The anti-coronary club; including a discussion of the effects of a prudent diet on the serum cholesterol level of middle-aged men. *Am. J. Clin. Nutr.,* **7:** 451.

63. Kahn, H. A. 1970. Change in serum cholesterol associated with changes in the United States civilian diet, 1909–1965. *Am. J. Clin. Nutr.,* **23:** 879.

64. Kannel, W. B., W. P. Castelli, T. Gordon, and P. M. McNamara. 1971. Serum cholesterol, lipoproteins, and the risk of coronary heart disease. *Ann. Int. Med.,* **74:** 1.

65. Kaunitz, H. 1975. Dietary lipids and arteriosclerosis. *J. Am. Oil Chem. Soc.,* **52:** 293.

66. Kay, R. M. and A. S. Truswell. 1977. Effect of citrus pectin on blood lipids and fecal steroid excretion in man. *Am. J. Clin. Nutr.,* **30:** 171.

67. Kenigsberg, D., S. J. Zyzanski, C. D. Jenkins, W. I. Wardwell, and A. T. Licciardello. 1974. The coronary-prone behavior pattern in hospitalized patients with and without coronary heart disease. *Psychosom. Med.,* **36:** 344.

68. Keys, A. (Ed.). 1970. Coronary heart disease in 7 countries. *Circulation* **41** (Supplement No. I.): I-1.

69. Keys, A. 1967. Effects on serum lipids of different dietary proteins and carbohydrates. (Letter). *Am. J. Clin. Nutr.,* **20:** 1249.

70. Keys, A. and J. T. Anderson. 1957. Dietary protein and the serum cholesterol level in man. *Am. J. Clin. Nutr.,* **5:** 29.

71. Keys, A., J. T. Anderson, and F. Grande. 1965. Serum cholesterol response to changes in the diet. *Metabolism,* **14:** 747.

72. Keys, A., F. Grande, and J. T. Anderson. 1974. Bias and misrepresentation revisited: Perspective on saturated fat. *Am. J. Clin. Nutr.,* **27:** 188.

73. Keys, A., N. Kimura, A. Kusakawa, B. Bronte-Stewart, N. Larsen, and M. H. Keys. 1958. Lessons from serum cholesterol studies in Japan, Hawaii, and Los Angeles. *Ann. Internat. Med.,* **48:** 83.

74. Keys, A. and R. W. Parlin. 1966. Serum cholesterol response to changes in dietary lipids. *Am. J. Clin. Nutr.,* **19:** 175.

75. Kime, Z. R. and M. Sifri. 1976. Objections to the Klevay hypothesis. (Letter). *Am. J. Clin. Nutr.,* **29:** 1065.

76. Klevay, L. M. 1975. Coronary heart disease: The zinc/copper hypothesis. *Am. J. Clin. Nutr.,* **28:** 764.

77. Klevay, L. M. and J. Forbush. 1976. Copper metabolism and the epidemiology of coronary heart disease. *Nutr. Rep. Internat.,* **14:** 221.

78. Kudchodkar, B. J., L. Horlick, and H. S. Sodhi. 1976. Effects of plant sterols on cholesterol metabolism in man. *Atherosclerosis,* **23:** 239.

79. Kummerow, F. A., Y. Kim, A. Hull, J. Pollard, P. Ilinov, D. L. Dorossiev, and J. Valek. 1977. The influence of egg consumption on the serum cholesterol level in human subjects. *Am. J. Clin. Nutr.,* **30:** 664.

80. Leren, P. 1970. The Oslo diet heart study, eleven-year report. *Circulation,* **42:** 935.

81. Lindeman, R. D. and J. R. Assenzo. 1964. Correlations between water hardness and cardiovascular deaths in Oklahoma counties. *Am. J. Pub. Health,* **54:** 1071.

82. Lofland, H. B., T. B. Clarkson, L. Rhyne, and H. O. Goodman. 1966. Interrelated effects of dietary fats and proteins on atherosclerosis in the pigeon. *J. Atheroscl. Res.,* **6:** 395.

83. Lopez-S, A., W. A. Krehl, R. E. Hodges, and E. I. Good. 1966. Relationship between food consumption and mortality from atherosclerotic heart disease in Europe. *Am. J. Clin. Nutr.,* **19:** 361.

84. Macdonald, I. and D. M. Braithwaite. 1964. The influence of dietary carbohydrates on the lipid pattern in serum and in adipose tissue. *Clin. Sci.,* **27:** 23.

85. Marshall, M. W., J. Lehmann, M. Haubrich, and V. A. Washington. 1973. Elevated plasma tochopherols associated with elevated lipids and low biotin status in adult hypercholesterolemic rats. *Nutr. Rep. Internat.,* **8:** 371.

86. Mattos, W. and D. L. Palmquist. 1974. Increased polyunsaturated fatty acid yields in milk of cows fed protected fat. *J. Dairy Sci.,* **57:** 1050.

87. Mattson, F. H., D. J. Hollenbach, and A. M. Kligman. 1975. Effect of hydrogenated fat on the plasma cholesterol and triglyceride levels of man. *Am. J. Clin. Nutr.,* **28:** 726.

88. Miettinen, M. 1975. Prevention of coronary heart disease by cholesterol lowering diet. *Postgrad. Med. J.,* **51** (Supplement 8): 47.

89. Miettinen, M., O. Turpeinen, M. J. Karvonen, R. Elosuo, and E. Paavilainen. 1972. Effect of cholesterol-lowering diet on mortality from coronary heart disease and other causes. A twelve-year clinical trial in men and women. *Lancet,* **2:** 835.

90. Mills, N. L. and J. L. Ochsner. 1975. Concepts of coronary bypass surgery. *Postgrad. Med.,* **57:** 97.

91. Moore, M. C., M. A. Guzman, P. E. Schilling, and J. P. Strong. 1976. Dietary-atherosclerosis study on deceased persons. *J. Am. Dietet. Assoc.,* **68:** 216.

92. Morris, J., M. D. Crawford, and J. A. Heady. 1961. Hardness of local water supplies and mortality from cardiovascular disease. *Lancet,* **1:** 860.

93. Mundth, E. D. and W. G. Austen. 1975. Surgical measures for coronary heart disease. *N. Eng. J. Med.,* **293:** 13.

94. Myasnikov, A. L. 1958. Influence of some factors on development of experimental cholesterol atherosclerosis. *Circulation,* **17:** 99.

95. McGandy, R. B., D. M. Hegsted, M. L. Myers, and F. J. Stare. 1966. Dietary carbohydrate and serum cholesterol levels in man. *Am. J. Clin. Nutr.*, **18**: 237.

96. Olson, R. E. 1973. Vitamin E and its relation to heart disease. *Circulation*, **48**: 179.

97. Olson, R. E., M. Z. Nichaman, J. Nittka, and J. A. Eagles. 1970. Effect of amino acid diets upon serum lipids in man. *Am. J. Clin. Nutr.*, **23**: 1614.

98. Olson, R. E., J. W. Vester, D. Gursey, N. Davis, and D. Longman. 1958. The effect of low-protein diets upon serum cholesterol in man. *Am. J. Clin. Nutr.*, **6**: 310.

99. Palumbo, P. J., E. R. Briones, R. A. Nelson, and B. A. Kottke. 1977. Sucrose sensitivity of patients with coronary-artery disease. *Am. J. Clin. Nutr.*, **30**: 394.

100. Perry, H. M., Jr. 1973. Minerals in cardiovascular disease. *J. Am. Dietet. Assoc.*, **62**: 631.

101. Peterson, C. R. 1976. Dietary counseling for patients admitted for coronary artery bypass graft. *J. Am. Dietet. Assoc.*, **68**: 158.

102. Peterson, V. E., P. A. Crapo, J. Weininger, H. Ginsberg, and J. Olefsky. 1975. Quantification of plasma cholesterol and triglyceride levels in hypercholesterolemic subjects receiving ascorbic acid supplements. *Am. J. Clin. Nutr.*, **28**: 584.

103. Pollak, O. J. 1953. Reduction of blood cholesterol in man. *Circulation*, **7**: 702.

104. Porter, M. W., W. Yamanaka, S. D. Carlson, and M. A. Flynn. 1977. Effect of dietary egg on serum cholesterol and triglyceride of human males. *Am. J. Clin. Nutr.*, **30**: 490.

105. Poston, R. N. and D. F. Davies. 1974. Immunity and inflammation in the pathogenesis of atherosclerosis. *Atherosclerosis*, **19**: 353.

106. Prather, E. S. 1964. Effect of cellulose on serum lipids in young women. *J. Am. Dietet. Assoc.*, **45**: 230.

107. Prior, I. A. M. 1971. The price of civilization. *Nutr. Today*, **6** (No. 4): 2.

108. Ravid, M., M. Berkowicz, and E. Sohar. 1975. Hyperglycemia during acute myocardial infarction. *J. Am. Med. Assoc.*, **233**: 807.

109. Reiser, R. 1976. Plasma lipid changes in young adult couples consuming polyunsaturated meat and dairy products. (Letter). *Am. J. Clin. Nutr.*, **29**: 237.

110. Reiser, R. 1973. Saturated fat in the diet and serum cholesterol concentration: A critical examination of the literature. *Am. J. Clin. Nutr.*, **26**: 524.

111. Renaud, S. and C. Allard. 1964. Effect of dietary protein level on cholesterolemia, thrombosis, atherosclerosis and hypertension in the rat. *J. Nutr.*, **83**: 149.

112. Rinzler, S. H. 1968. Primary prevention of coronary heart disease by diet. *Bull. N.Y. Acad. Med.*, **4**: 936.

113. Roberts, A. M. 1973. Effects of a sucrose-free diet on the serum-lipid levels of men in Antarctica. *Lancet*, **1**: 1201.

114. Robertson, T. L., H. Kato, G. G. Rhoads, A. Kagan, M. Marmot, S. Leonard, T. Gordon, R. M. Worth, J. L. Belsky, D. S. Dock, M. Miyanishi, and S. Kawamoto. 1977. Epidemiologic studies of coronary heart disease and stroke in Japanese men living in Japan, Hawaii and California. *Am. J. Card.*, **39**: 239.

115. Rosenman, R. H., R. J. Brand, C. D. Jenkins, M. Friedman, R. Straus, and M. Wurm. 1975. Coronary heart disease in the Western Collaborative Group Study. *J. Am. Med. Assoc.*, **233**: 872.

116. Rosenman, R. H. and M. Friedman. 1971. Observations on the pathogenesis of coronary heart disease. *Nutr. News* (Nat. Dairy Council), **34** (No. 3): 9.

117. Rosenman, R. H., M. Friedman, R. Straus, M. Wurm, C. D. Jenkins, H. B. Messinger, R. Kositchek, W. Hahn, and N. T. Werthessen. 1966. Coronary heart disease in the Western Collaborative Group Study. *J. Am. Med. Assoc.*, **195**: 86.

118. Rosenman, R. H., M. Friedman, R. Straus, M. Wurm, R. Kositchek, W. Hahn, and N. T.

Werthessen. 1964. A predictive study of coronary heart disease. *J. Am. Med. Assoc.*, **189:** 15.

119. Ross, R. and J. A. Glomset. 1976a. The pathogenesis of atherosclerosis. *N. Eng. J. Med.*, **295:** 369.

120. Ross, R. and J. A. Glomset. 1976b. The pathogenesis of atherosclerosis. *N. Eng. J. Med.*, **295:** 420.

121. Russek, H. I. and L. G. Russek. 1972. Etiologic factors in ischemic heart disease. *Geriatrics*, **27:** 81.

122. Samuel, P. and O. B. Shalchi. 1964. Effect of vitamin C on serum cholesterol in patients with hypercholesterolemia and arteriosclerosis. *Circulation*, **29:** 24.

123. Schroeder, H. A. 1966. Municipal drinking water and cardiovascular death rates. *J. Am. Med. Assoc.*, **195:** 81.

124. Schroeder, H. A. 1960. Relations between hardness of water and death rates from certain chronic and degenerative diseases in the United States. *J. Chron. Dis.*, **12:** 586.

125. Seaman, A. J., H. E. Griswold, R. B. Reaume, and L. W. Ritzman. 1964. Prophylactic anticoagulant therapy for coronary artery disease. *J. Am. Med. Assoc.*, **189:** 183.

126. Seelig, M. S. and H. A. Heggtveit. 1974. Magnesium interrelationships in ischemic heart disease: A review. *Am. J. Clin. Nutr.*, **27:** 59.

127. Shaffer, C. F. 1970. Ascorbic acid and atherosclerosis. *Am. J. Clin. Nutr.*, **23:** 27.

128. Shorey, R. L., K. Brewton, B. Sewell, and M. O'Brien. 1974. Alteration of serum lipids in a group of free-living adult males. *Am. J. Clin. Nutr.*, **27:** 268.

129. Sokoloff, B., M. Hori, C. C. Saelhof, T. Wroolek, and T. Imai. 1966. Aging, atherosclerosis, and ascorbic acid metabolism. *J. Am. Geriat. Soc.*, **14:** 1239.

130. Spittle, C. R. 1971. Atherosclerosis and vitamin C. *Lancet*, **2:** 1280.

131. Stamler, J. 1973. Epidemiology of coronary heart disease. *Med. Clinics No. Am.*, **57:** 5.

132. Stamler, J., D. M. Berkson, M. Levinson, H. A. Lindberg, L. Mojonnier, W. A. Miller, Y. Hall, and S. L. Andelman. 1966. Coronary artery disease—status of preventive efforts. *Arch. Envir. Health*, **13:** 322.

133. Stitt, F. W., D. G. Clayton, M. D. Crawford, and J. N. Morris. 1973. Clinical and biochemical indicators of cardiovascular disease among men living in hard and soft water areas. *Lancet*, **1:** 122.

134. Story, J. A. and D. Kritchevsky. 1976. Comparison of the binding of various bile acids and bile salts *in vitro* by several types of fiber. *J. Nutr.*, **106:** 1292.

135. Strasser, T. 1972. Atherosclerosis and coronary heart disease: The contribution of epidemiology. *WHO Chronicle*, **26:** 7.

136. Strong, J. P., D. A. Eggen, M. C. Oalmann, M. L. Richards, and R. E. Tracy. 1973. Pathology and epidemiology of atherosclerosis. *J. Am. Dietet. Assoc.*, **62:** 262.

137. Subbiah, M. T. R. 1973. Dietary plant sterols: Current status in human and animal sterol metabolism. *Am. J. Clin. Nutr.*, **26:** 219.

138. Syme, S. L. 1970. Stress and coronary heart disease. *Postgrad. Med.*, **48:** 123.

139. Task Force on Arteriosclerosis. 1971a. Arteriosclerosis. National Heart and Lung Institute. DHEW Publication No. (NIH) 72–137, vol. I.

140. Task Force on Arteriosclerosis. 1971b. Arteriosclerosis. National Heart and Lung Institute. DHEW Publication No. (NIH) 72–219, vol. II.

141. Trowell, H. 1972. Ischemic heart disease and dietary fiber. *Am. J. Clin. Nutr.*, **25:** 926.

142. Tsai, A. C., J. Elias, J. J. Kelley, R. C. Lin, and J. R. K. Robson. 1976. Influence of certain dietary fibers on serum and tissue cholesterol levels in rats. *J. Nutr.*, **106:** 118.

143. Turpeinen, O., M. Miettinen, M. J. Karvonen, P. Roine, M. Pekkarinen, E. J. Lehtosuo, and P. Alivirta. 1968. Dietary prevention of coronary heart disease: Long-term experiment. *Am. J. Clin. Nutr.*, **21:** 255.

144. Vigran, I. M. 1969. Basis for using anticoagulants in coronary artery disease. *Postgrad. Med.*, **45:** 75.

145. Wardwell, W. I. and C. B. Bahnson. 1973. Behavioral variables and myocardial infarction in the southeastern Connecticut heart study. *J. Chron. Dis.*, **26:** 447.

146. Watts, H. F. 1971. Basic aspects of the pathogenesis of human atherosclerosis. *Human Pathology*, **2:** 31.

147. Wen, C. and S. N. Gershoff. 1973. Changes in serum cholesterol and coronary heart disease mortality associated with changes in the postwar Japanese diet. *Am. J. Clin. Nutr.*, **26:** 616.

148. Williams, M. A., D. J. McIntosh, and I. Hincenbergs. 1966. Changes in fatty acid composition in liver lipid fractions of pyridoxine-deficient rats fed cholesterol. *J. Nutr.*, **88:** 193.

149. Wilson, W. S., S. B. Hulley, M. I. Burrows, and M. Z. Nichaman. 1971. Serial lipid and lipoprotein responses to the American Heart Association fat-controlled diet. *Am. J. Med.*, **51:** 491.

150. Yudkin, J. 1972. Sucrose and cardiovascular disease. *Proc. Nutr. Soc.*, **31:** 331.

151. Yudkin, J. 1964. Patterns and trends in carbohydrate consumption and their relation to disease. *Proc. Nutr. Soc.*, **23:** 149.

152. Yudkin, J. and J. Morland. 1967. Sugar intake and myocardial infarction. *Am. J. Clin. Nutr.*, **20:** 503.

CLIENT REFERENCES

1. American Heart Association. 1975. Recipes for fat-controlled, low-cholesterol meals.

2. American Heart Association. 1973. *The American Heart Association Cookbook.* New York: David McKay.

3. American Heart Association. 1969. Programed instruction for fat-controlled diet, 1800 calories. Also, guidelines for professional personnel on use of programed instruction for fat-controlled diet, 1800 calories.

4. American Heart Association. 1967. Planning fat-controlled meals for approximately 2000–2600 calories.

5. American Heart Association. 1966. Planning fat-controlled meals for 1200 and 1800 calories.

6. Buller, A. L. 1973. The what, why, how of hyperlipidemia. Developed under sponsorship of Northern New England Regional Medical Program and Vermont Heart Association.

   Type II
   Type IIB
   Type IV

7. Fredrickson, D. S., R. I. Levy, M. Bonnell, and N. Ernst. 1973. Dietary management of hyperlipoproteinemia. National Heart and Lung Institute, Bethesda, Maryland. DHEW Publication No. (NIH) 73–110.

   Diet 1. For dietary management of hyperchylomicronemia. DHEW Publication No. (NIH) 73–111

   Diet 2. For dietary management of hypercholesterolemia. DHEW Publication No. (NIH) 73–112

Diet 3. For dietary management of hypercholesterolemia with endogenous hyperglyceridemia. DHEW Publication No. (NIH) 73–113

Diet 4. For dietary management of endogenous hyperglyceridemia. DHEW Publication No. (NIH) 73–114

Diet 5. For dietary management of mixed hyperglyceridemia. DHEW Publication No. (NIH) 73–115

8. Kraus, B. 1975. *The Barbara Kraus Guide to Fiber in Foods.* New York: New American Library.

9. Revell, D. 1961. *Cholesterol Control Cookery.* New York: Berkley Publishing.

10. Stone, D. B., W. E. Connor, J. A. Lichty, et al. 1968. A low cholesterol diet manual. Iowa City, Iowa: The University of Iowa, Department of Internal Medicine, College of Medicine.

11. Subcommittee on Diet and Hyperlipidemia. 1973. A Maximal approach to the dietary treatment of the hyperlipidemias.

Diet A: The low cholesterol (100 mg) moderately low fat diet
Diet B: The low cholesterol (200 mg) moderately low fat diet
Diet C: The low cholesterol, high polyunsaturated fat diet
Diet D: The extremely low fat diet

STUDY GUIDE

Epidemiological studies have probed for clues to the cause(s) of atherosclerosis and CHD.

1. Describe examples of epidemiological studies concerned with CHD and discuss the contributions of this type of research in probing cause(s) of atherosclerosis and CHD.

2. Explain the concept of "risk factors" in the development of CHD and discuss possible relationships for several of these factors in the development of atherosclerosis and CHD.

3. Discuss possible reasons why investigators in the Framingham Study did not find significant associations among serum lipids, development of CHD, and dietary intake in subjects studied, whereas associations of this type have been found in international studies.

Atherosclerotic lesions in human arteries have been observed in various stages of development.

4. Describe major characteristics of fatty streaks, fibrous plaques, and complicated lesions.

5. Discuss possible relationships between fatty streaks and fibrous plaques.

6. Describe several theories that have been suggested to explain atherogenesis.

Advanced atherosclerotic lesions in coronary and brain arteries, particularly in connection with thrombosis, may lead to heart attacks or strokes.

7. Explain probable relationships among the development of large or ruptured lesions in coronary arteries or arteries of the brain, thrombosis, and MI or stroke.

Dietary fat and sterols and other dietary components have been shown, in experimental studies with both animals and humans, to affect serum lipids.

8. Give examples and discuss reported research findings and implications for nutrition counseling in relation to atherosclerosis and CHD for each of the following dietary components: quantity of fat; type of fat (saturated, monounsaturated, polyunsaturated); cholesterol; plant sterols; simple and complex carbohydrate, particularly sucrose; dietary fiber; minerals; and vitamins.

9. What is meant by carbohydrate-induced hyperlipidemia? Discuss pros and cons for the theory of carbohydrate induction as a factor in the development of CHD.

10. Discuss possible explanations for associations that have been reported between hardness of drinking water and CHD.

Behavior patterns and stress have been suggested as important factors in the development of CHD.

11. Describe the Type A behavior pattern and discuss its possible relationship to coronary proneness.

Diet has been used to maintain normal levels of serum lipids in an attempt to prevent the development of atherosclerosis and CHD.

12. Distinguish between primary and secondary coronary prevention trials.

13. Describe examples of both primary and secondary coronary disease prevention studies and discuss the implications of the results of these studies for public health programs.

14. Make and justify general recommendations for diet in a program aimed at the prevention of CHD and discuss the practicality of adherence to dietary modifications in free-living populations.

15. Discuss some of the unanswered questions and need for further research, particularly concerning diet, in the prevention of CHD.

Coronary artery bypass surgery may be successful in selected cases.

16. Describe the usual purpose and procedure used in coronary artery bypass surgery.

17. What type of nutritional care may be desirable for a patient having coronary bypass surgery, both during hospitalization and after discharge? Explain.

Nutritional therapy for the patient with an acute myocardial infarction should be part of the total treatment program.

18. Describe how and why the measurement of serum enzyme activity may be used in the diagnosis of MI. What enzymes are most useful?

19. Outline and explain a general nutritional plan that might be effective for the acute, subacute, and rehabilitative phases in the treatment of patients with MI.

22

Congestive Heart Failure

The term congestive heart failure describes a clinical syndrome that results from the inability of heart muscle to contract adequately when presented with a work load. The basic underlying cause of heart failure may be either a congenital or an acquired lesion and may exist for many years with little disability. An acute disturbance that places an additional load on the heart can initiate further deterioration of cardiac function, however, and precipitate congestive heart failure.

Congestive heart failure may influence the nutritional state of the body in various ways. In turn, nutritional factors may influence heart failure. This chapter discusses some of these nutritional implications for congestive heart failure, following a discussion of the clinical syndrome itself and some information on diuretics, which are commonly used in treatment.

22.1   The Process of Heart Failure

The primary functions of the heart are to propel unoxygenated blood to the lungs and deliver the resulting oxygenated product to peripheral tissues in accordance with their metabolic requirements, which vary from moment to moment. For example, heavy exercise produces a greatly increased requirement for oxygen within a short period of several seconds. There must be an integrated response of the heart and peripheral vascular system to provide and distribute this additional oxygen to appropriate tissues (Braunwald, 1974). The activity of the heart is regulated in an important way by the needs of peripheral tissues.

The heart consists of two pumps, the right and the left heart (Fig. 22.1). When the left side does not function properly, congestion develops in the pulmonary veins and blood backs up into the lungs, causing dyspnea (labored breathing). Right-sided failure (cor pulmonale) causes congestion in the superior and inferior vena cava, liver, spleen, and other organs. The inadequacy of circulation from either type of failure triggers a complex sequence of adjustments that eventually results in accumulation of fluid in the body. Although many of the clinical manifestations of heart failure are secondary to this excessive retention of fluid, the abnormal fluid accumulation represents an important compensatory mechanism that tends to maintain cardiac output by increasing blood volume. The adjustments to heart pump failure are both hemodynamic and hormonal ones which promote reduced renal sodium and water excretion by lowering renal cortical blood flow and glomerular filtration rate. The renin-angiotensin system is activated and stimulates aldosterone secretion by the adrenal cortex, increasing the reabsorption of sodium ion (Na^+) in the distal renal tubule. Another factor contributing to aldosterone excess may be a congested liver in which the metabolism of aldosterone is impaired. Increased aldosterone activity is reflected in low concentrations of sodium in the urine, sweat, and saliva (Wintrobe et al., 1974, pp. 1119–1120).

Dyspnea, or respiratory distress, at first is present only on exertion, but as congestive heart failure increases, dyspnea may occur even when the patient is at rest. Orthopnea results in blood from the lower extremities and the splanchnic bed is redistributed to the lungs when the patient is lying down. When orthopnea is present, the patient may sleep with several pillows to elevate the head. Lack of oxygenated hemoglobin in the blood produces a bluish discoloration of the skin and mucous membranes called *cyanosis*. Fatigue and weakness are common nonspecific symptoms of heart failure. Anorexia and nausea associated with abdominal pain and fullness are frequent complaints during severe attacks and may be related to an enlarged, congested liver. Vascular congestion of the gastric mucosa may contribute to anorexia and postprandial gastric distress. Edema usually occurs symmetrically in the legs of ambulatory patients and in the sacral region of individuals at bed rest (Wintrobe et al., 1974, pp. 1120–1121).

22.2 Diuretics

Several drugs may be used to promote diuresis in conditions characterized by sodium and water retention. The first effective oral diuretics were thiazide compounds, discovered in 1957. Diuretics reduce edema by increasing the excretion of sodium, with a parallel excretion of water, so that output exceeds intake. They act at various points on the renal tubule (see Fig. 24.2).

Types of Diuretics

Diuretics include (1) organic mercurials, (2) carbonic anhydrase inhibitors, (3) thiazides, (4) furosemide and ethacrynic acid, and (5) aldosterone antagonists.

Organic mercurials apparently release inorganic mercury within the tubule cell, which then combines with sulfhydryl enzymes essential for Na$^+$ reabsorption, thus decreasing it. An increased amount of Na$^+$ becomes available for exchange with potassium in the distal tubule (Wintrobe et al., 1974, p. 1125). Mercurial diuretics are about twice as effective as the thiazides but must be given by injection (Remmers et al., 1973).

Carbonic anhydrase in the renal tubule cell is responsible for generating hydrogen ion (H$^+$), which is exchanged for Na$^+$ from the tubular lumen. This takes place primarily in the proximal tubule and to a lesser extent in the distal tubule. Acetazolamide inhibits carbonic anhydrase and results in a mild increase in sodium, potassium, and bicarbonate excretion

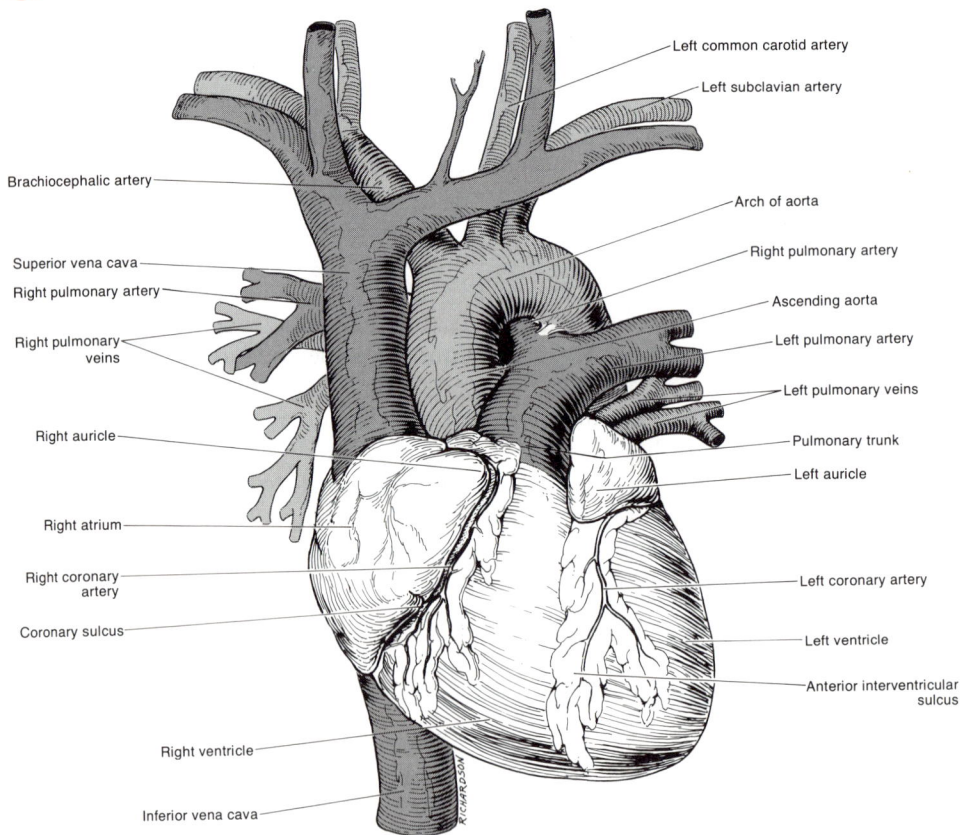

Fig. 22.1   The structure of the heart. (*a*) Anterior external view. (*b*) Anterior internal view. (*c*) Path of blood through the heart. (From Gerard J. Tortora and Nicholas P. Anagnostakos, *Principles of Anatomy and Physiology*, 2d ed., New York: Harper & Row, 1978; by permission of the publisher.)

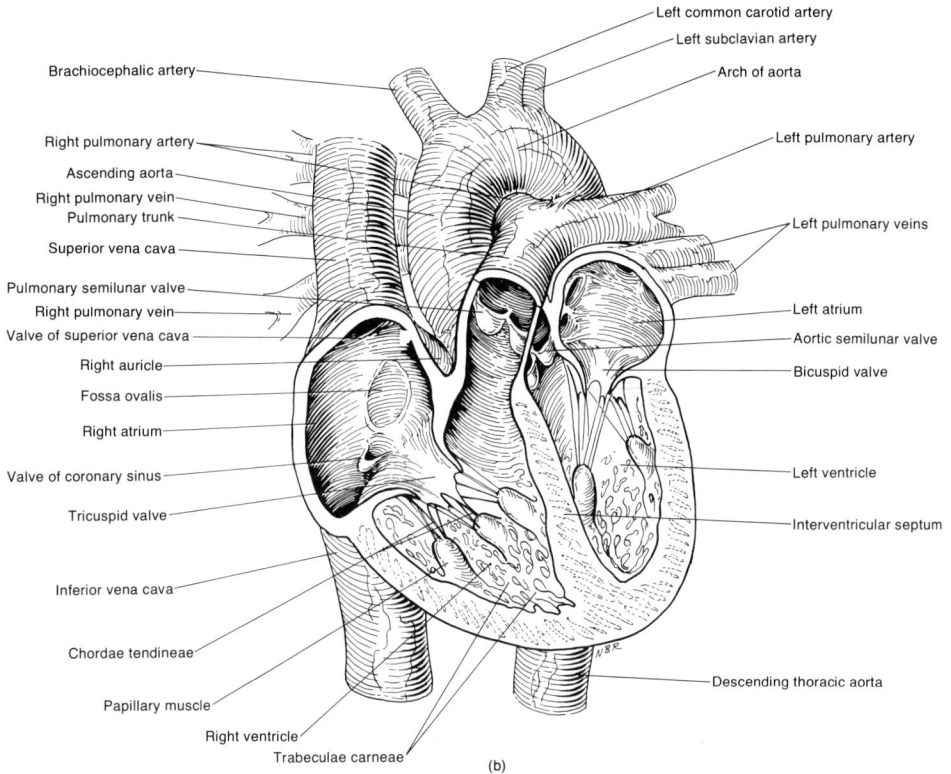

Brachiocephalic artery—

Left common carotid artery
Left subclavian artery
Arch of aorta

Right pulmonary artery—
Ascending aorta—
Right pulmonary vein—
Pulmonary trunk—
Superior vena cava—

Left pulmonary artery

Pulmonary semilunar valve—
Right pulmonary vein—
Valve of superior vena cava—
Right auricle—
Fossa ovalis—
Right atrium—

Left pulmonary veins

Left atrium
Aortic semilunar valve
Bicuspid valve

Valve of coronary sinus—
Tricuspid valve—

Left ventricle
Interventricular septum

Inferior vena cava—

Chordae tendineae—
Papillary muscle—
Right ventricle—
Trabeculae carneae—

Descending thoracic aorta

(b)

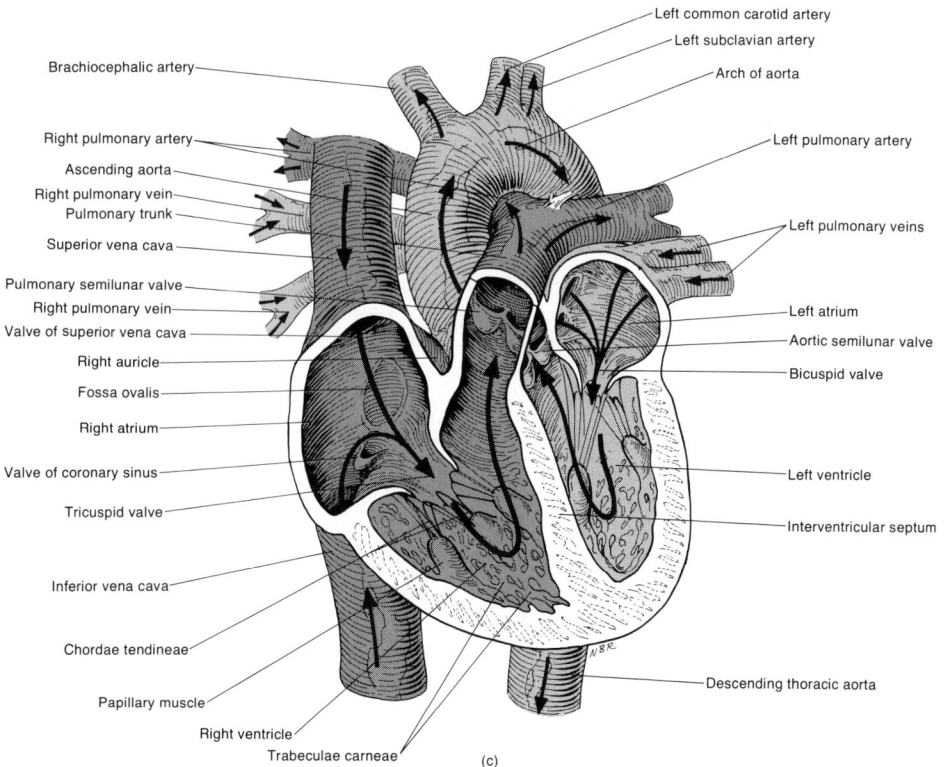

Brachiocephalic artery—

Left common carotid artery
Left subclavian artery
Arch of aorta

Right pulmonary artery—
Ascending aorta—
Right pulmonary vein—
Pulmonary trunk—
Superior vena cava—

Left pulmonary artery

Pulmonary semilunar valve—
Right pulmonary vein—
Valve of superior vena cava—
Right auricle—
Fossa ovalis—
Right atrium—

Left pulmonary veins

Left atrium
Aortic semilunar valve
Bicuspid valve

Valve of coronary sinus—
Tricuspid valve—

Left ventricle
Interventricular septum

Inferior vena cava—

Chordae tendineae—
Papillary muscle—
Right ventricle—
Trabeculae carneae—

Descending thoracic aorta

(c)

and a reduction in H^+ excretion. The urine becomes alkaline and mild systemic metabolic acidosis is induced. Its diuretic action is mild (Remmers et al., 1973).

The thiazides, including chlorothiazide and its derivatives, are widely used oral agents. They reduce the reabsorption of Na^+ in the proximal tubule. Chloride and water follow the unreabsorbed Na^+ into the more distal tubule. Here, potassium-sodium exchange is enhanced because of the large amount of Na^+ present, resulting in increased excretion of potassium.

Potassium depletion is the major adverse effect of the use of thiazides for prolonged periods and may enhance the dangers of digitalis intoxication and affect heart function. Clinical signs of potassium depletion include anorexia, nausea, vomiting, muscle weakness, ileus, respiratory depression, and cardiac dysrhythmia (MacLeod, 1975). Oral supplements of potassium chloride solution have been given since the use of enteric-coated tablets was reported to cause gastrointestinal ulceration and stenosis (Baker et al., 1964). However, these solutions are unpalatable and may be hazardous for patients with renal failure because of resulting hyperkalemia (Hultgren et al., 1975; Shapiro et al., 1971). Patients may take liquid potassium supplements, prescribed in moderation, by adding them to fruit juices to mask their salty taste. A tablet containing potassium chloride crystals suspended in a waxy matrix apparently overcomes the drawbacks of the enteric-coated tablets and may be useful in some cases (Rider et al., 1975). An intermittent dosage schedule that substitutes a potassium-retaining diuretic (such as aldosterone antagonists) for the thiazide every third day may be followed (Wintrobe et al., 1974, p. 1125). Although it is difficult to consume large amounts of potassium through food alone, some useful increase in potassium intake may be accomplished by counseling patients concerning high-potassium foods. The incidence of iatrogenic hyperkalemia from unwise use of supplements may be decreased by emphasis on dietary potassium along with judicious use of supplements. The usual dietary intake of potassium is 50 to 100 meq per day (1950 to 3900 mg). About 40 meq (1560 mg) is required (MacLeod, 1975). Table 22.1 contains a list of foods that are good sources of potassium.

Furosemide and ethacrynic acid are powerful diuretics that inhibit Na^+ reabsorption throughout the nephron, but especially in the ascending limb of the loop of Henle, thereby reducing urinary concentration. Because of their potency, complications with their use may be high. Alkalosis is produced by a large increase in the urinary excretion of chloride, hydrogen, and potassium ions. Hyperuricemia may occur, as well as hypokalemia and hyponatremia. Hyperuricemia may also occur with the use of thiazide diuretics (Wintrobe et al., 1974, pp. 1125–1126).

Aldosterone antagonists resemble aldosterone in chemical structure and act on the distal renal tubule by competitive inhibition of aldosterone. They tend to produce potassium retention. Spironolactones and spironolactone-like drugs are included in this group (Wintrobe et al., 1974, p. 1125).

Table 22.1 POTASSIUM IN SELECTED FOODS*

Food	Weight (g)	Measure	Potassium (meq)	Potassium (mg)
Apricots, canned, sweetened	192	4 apricots; 4 tbsp liquid	11	422
Bananas, sliced	150	1 cup	14	555
Beans, red kidney, cooked	185	1 cup	16	629
Beet greens, cooked†	145	1 cup	12	481
Cantaloupe, diced	160	1 cup	10	402
Dates, pitted	80	10 dates	13	518
Figs, raw	200	4 medium	10	388
Grapefruit juice	246	1 cup	10	399
Orange juice	248	1 cup	13	496
Peaches, canned, sweetened	256	1 cup	9	333
Pineapple juice	250	1 cup	10	373
Potatoes, baked in skin	250	1 potato; $4\frac{3}{4}''$ long	20	782
Potatoes, boiled in skin, diced	155	1 cup	16	631
Prunes, dried, uncooked, pitted	75	10 prunes	18	708
Prune juice	256	1 cup	15	602
Raisins, uncooked, not packed	145	1 cup	28	1106
Spinach, boiled, leaves†	180	1 cup	15	583
Squash, winter, baked, mashed	205	1 cup	24	945
Sweet potatoes, cooked, mashed	255	1 cup	16	620
Tomatoes, cooked	241	1 cup	18	692
Tomato juice	243	1 cup	14	552

* Adams, 1975.
† Also contains 4 to 5 meq (90 to 110 mg) sodium.

22.3 Effect of Obesity on Heart Failure

Extreme obesity is capable of causing congestive heart failure in the absence of definite intrinsic disease of the heart or lungs. This syndrome is called the "Pickwickian syndrome," in honor of a Dickens character with similar tendencies, and includes alveolar hypoventilation with hypoxemia, hypercapnia, secondary polycythemia, cyanosis, right ventricular hypertrophy, and right heart failure (Jones, 1966).

Alexander and Pettigrove (1967) surveyed autopsy records at the Veterans Administration Hospital, Houston, Texas from 1959 to 1965 for obesity and congestive heart failure. Nine individuals with body weights of 300 lb or more (range 300 to 467 lb) were found in 3514 consecutive autopsies. All but one had severe congestion and edema of the lungs and other viscera, including the heart, at postmortem examination. High cardiac output at rest, together with increased plasma and blood volume, are well documented in very obese subjects. A high output state occurs in rough proportion to degree of overweight and brings about a significant increase in the work of the heart at rest, as well as for a given level of activity. Alexander and Pettigrove (1967) suggested that this work load leads to the development of myocardial hypertrophy and myocardial failure.

22.4 Treatment of Congestive Heart Failure

It is important to remove the precipitating cause and correct the basic underlying cause of congestive heart failure whenever possible. In any case, however, treatment is aimed at control of the heart failure. This control may center on (1) reducing the cardiac work load, (2) enhancing myocardial contractility, and (3) controlling excessive fluid retention. Following satisfactory treatment, recurrence of heart failure may be prevented by continuing the measures that were originally effective (Wintrobe et al., 1974, p. 1123).

Reduction of Cardiac Work Load

Physical activity is curtailed for patients with congestive heart failure in order to decrease the work load of the heart, the degree depending upon the severity of failure. Patients are often anxious and need to be reassured since emotional rest also tends to lower arterial pressure, slow heart rate, and reduce the cardiac stress. Meals should be small in quantity to avoid the strain on the heart that may result from an overloaded stomach. Large meals may increase vascular congestion in the gastrointestinal tract during digestion and produce distress. Soft, easily chewed foods help to limit stress associated with eating.

Gradual weight reduction in the obese patient will decrease the work load of the heart and is a desirable goal. It is well to maintain weight in patients with congestive heart failure slightly below what is usually considered to be ideal weight. However, care must be exercised to assure a nutritionally adequate diet with reduced caloric intake. Obesity can cause elevation of the diaphragm, decreased volume of the lungs, and change in position of the heart. Fat on the heart itself impairs myocardial function.

Enhancement of Cardiac Contractility

Cardiac glycosides, from the genus digitalis, are commonly employed to improve myocardial contractility. Some of these drugs are involved in an enterohepatic recirculation. For example, the portion of digitoxin not metabolized in the liver is excreted by way of the bile into the intestine and then reabsorbed. Malabsorption and other gastrointestinal disorders can modify the degree of reabsorption and thus affect the action of the drug (DeGraff, 1974). Potassium depletion, which may occur with diuretic therapy, causes increased sensitization of the heart to the action of digitalis.

Control of Excessive Fluid Retention

Fluid retention is commonly controlled in patients with heart failure by a combination of sodium-restricted diet and diuretic therapy. When the failure is mild, considerable improvement may result from the simple reduction of sodium intake, particularly if this is accompanied by bed rest. Sodium restriction must be more rigid, even when accompanied by drug therapy, if the failure is severe. Following recovery from a bout with congestive heart failure, at least moderate sodium restriction should be maintained (Wintrobe et al., 1974, p. 1124).

The average sodium intake in the United States of 100 to 300 meq (2300 to 7000 mg) may be reduced to 100 to 150 meq (2300 to 3500 mg) simply by excluding salt-rich foods and avoiding the addition of salt at the table. If all salt is omitted in cooking, the sodium content of the diet may be decreased to approximately 50 meq (1150 mg). Low-sodium diets are outlined in Sec. 18.8. Sodium in drinking water and in various drug preparations should be considered in planning, especially when dietary restriction is severe (Visconti, 1977).

In severe congestive heart failure, dietary sodium may be restricted to as low as 11 to 22 meq (250 to 500 mg). This is not usual, however, since diuretic therapy is also commonly employed. Milk must be eliminated, or a low-sodium product substituted, on a sodium level of 11 meq. Dietary sodium levels of 22 to 35 meq (500 to 800 mg) may be appropriate when therapy is being initiated or when diuretics are not being used extensively. With diuretic therapy, and also between attacks, 44 to 174 meq (1000 to 4000 mg) sodium may be prescribed daily on an individual basis. Constant monitoring for potassium adequacy must be maintained. With potassium-losing diuretics, high-potassium foods should be useful, as discussed in Sec. 22.2.

The natural history of congestive heart failure was studied over a 16-year period in connection with the Framingham Heart Study by McKee et al. (1971). Over this period, overt evidence of congestive heart failure developed in 142 of 5192 subjects. Hypertension was the most frequently encountered precursor of congestive heart failure in this study. Aging was associated with a strikingly increased risk for development.

The prognosis for a patient with congestive heart failure is often poor. Especially in the older population, there is failure to maintain the necessary medical and dietary regimen for control. Farag and Mozar (1967) reported on a project for prevention of congestive heart failure recurrences through a comprehensive health education and follow-up program. A nutritionist, a nurse, and a health educator separately visited selected patients in their homes over a 12-month period, each health worker averaging six to seven visits. The patients responded well to the visitors. As they learned how their symptoms were related to the heart and to therapy, adherence to the prescribed regimen improved. During the year of observation, eight of 69 study patients and 28 of 66 control patients required hospitalization for treatment of congestive heart failure. The number of hospital days for congestive heart failure during the 12 months of the study was 23 days for the study patients and 212 days for the controls. There was less edema, less difficulty with breathing, and fewer other symptoms in the study patients than in the unvisited control subjects at the end of the year. Although the number of visits was high in this study, the program was designed not only to control heart failure but also to discover the problems encountered in follow-up care. The researchers concluded that the education effort was effective in improving the control of congestive heart failure and also that subprofessional workers, trained by paramedical personnel, may be effectively used in this type of program.

REFERENCES

1. Adams, C. F. 1975. *Nutritive Value of American Foods.* U.S. Department of Agriculture.

2. Alexander, J. K. and J. R. Pettigrove. 1967. Obesity and congestive heart failure. *Geriatrics,* **22** (July): 101.

3. Baker, D. R., W. H. Schrader, and D. R. Hitchcock. 1964. Small-bowel ulceration apparently associated with thiazide and potassium therapy. *J. Am. Med. Assoc.,* **190:** 586.

4. Braunwald, E. 1974. Regulation of the circulation. *N. Eng. J. Med.,* **290:** 1124.

5. DeGraff, A. C. 1974. Drug therapy of cardiovascular disease. *Geriatrics,* **29** (June): 51.

6. Farag, S. A. and H. N. Mozar. 1967. Preventing recurrences of congestive heart failure. *J. Am. Dietet. Assoc.,* **51:** 26.

7. Hultgren, H. N., R. Swenson, and G. Wettach. 1975. Cardiac arrest due to oral potassium administration. *Am. J. Med.,* **58:** 139.

8. Jones, R. J. 1966. Nutrition in congestive heart failure. *Med. Clin. No. Am.,* **50:** 301.

9. MacLeod, S. M. 1975. The rational use of potassium supplements. *Postgrad. Med.,* **57** (No. 2): 123.

10. McKee, P. A., W. P. Castelli, P. M. McNamara, and W. B. Kannel. 1971. The natural history of congestive heart failure: The Framingham study. *N. Eng. J. Med.,* **285:** 1441.

11. Remmers, A. R., Jr., G. A. Beathard, J. D. Lindley, and H. E. Sarles. 1973. Diuretics. *Am. Fam. Physician,* **8** (No. 4): 209.

12. Rider, J. A., R. J. Manner, and J. I. Swader. 1975. Potassium chloride preparations and fecal blood loss. *J. Am. Med. Assoc.,* **231:** 836.

13. Shapiro, S., D. Slone, G. P. Lewis, and H. Jick. 1971. Fatal drug reactions among medical inpatients. *J. Am. Med. Assoc.,* **216:** 467.

14. Visconti, J. A. May 1977. Drug-food interaction. *Nutrition in Disease* (Ross Laboratories).

15. Wintrobe, M. M., G. W. Thorn, R. D. Adams, E. Braunwald, K. J. Isselbacher, R. G. Petersdorf (Eds.). 1974. Harrison's Principles of Internal Medicine, 7th ed. New York: McGraw-Hill.

STUDY GUIDE

Congestive heart failure is a clinical syndrome resulting from the inability of the myocardium to adequately propell blood through the circulatory system.

1. Explain, on the basis of underlying physiological abnormalities, major characteristic symptoms or signs of congestive heart failure.

2. Describe the probable role of the kidney in the fluid retention that is characteristic of congestive heart failure.

Diuretics may be prescribed for a variety of conditions and an understanding of their effects on the kidney is essential for most effective use.

3. For each of the following, describe site and mode of action in the nephron and discuss advantages or disadvantages of their use: organic mercurials; carbonic anhydrase inhibitors; thiazides; furosemide and ethacrynic acid; and aldosterone antagonists.

Treatment of congestive heart failure is aimed at decreasing the work load of the heart, enhancing myocardial contractility, and controlling fluid retention.

4. Explain the roles of each of the following in meeting the goals of treatment: controlled physical activity; diuretics; size of meals and consistency of food; dietary sodium intake; body weight; and digitalis.

5. Describe and explain nutritional objectives that would usually be appropriate for a patient with moderately severe congestive heart disease.

6. Explain why potassium supplementation may be desirable for a patient during prolonged or intensive therapy with thiazides and suggest satisfactory ways to achieve this supplementation.

23

Hypertension

High blood pressure, or hypertension, is in many cases an undiscovered asymptomatic disorder until the complications of cardiovascular-renal damage have occurred. An estimated 24 million persons in the United States have undetected, untreated, or inadequately treated high blood pressure (Stamler et al., 1976). Strasser (1972) suggested that about 10 percent of adults in various societies at all levels of affluence may have hypertension. Although there is no sharp dividing line between normal and elevated blood pressure, an arterial pressure in a resting adult of 160/95 mmHg or higher may be considered to be elevated (Wintrobe et al., 1974, p. 1236).

Hypertension may be primary or secondary. Secondary hypertension is due to a clearly definable cause, such as kidney disease with inflammatory, fibrotic, or obstructive changes. Aldosteronism, the excessive secretion of aldosterone by the adrenal cortex, may also cause secondary hypertension. A tumor of the adrenal glands, called pheochromocytoma, produces and releases into the blood large quantities of epinephrine and norepinephrine. These hormones may cause secondary hypertension by cardiac stimulation and peripheral blood vessel constriction. The particular cause of secondary hypertension is treated.

If a specific organic cause cannot be found for hypertension, the condition is said to be primary. It is often called essential hypertension. Approximately 85 to 90 percent of all hypertension is in this category. Although a precise cause of primary hypertension has not been identified, a number of psychosocial and neuroendocrine mechanisms have been implicated in the early pathophysiology of this disorder.

Primary hypertension can be treated. Drug therapy is very effective, although there may be side effects. Aagaard (1973) suggested that general measures for management of mild hypertension should include education, weight control, sodium restriction, exercise, relaxation, and control of life style. This chapter focuses on the nutritional aspects of the prevention and treatment of essential hypertension.

23.1   Control of Blood Pressure

The level of blood pressure is determined to a large extent by the rate of blood flow or cardiac output, the volume of circulating blood, and the capacity of the blood vessels. The resistance to blood flow offered by vessels in the peripheral vascular bed, particularly the arterioles, plays an important role in the control of blood pressure as it affects the capacity of the vascular system. The walls of the arterioles contain muscle fibers that may excessively contract and constrict these vessels, thus increasing resistance to blood flow and raising blood pressure. A slight constriction of blood vessels is normally maintained largely by the activity of the sympathetic nervous system but humoral systems, including secretion of norepinephrine, epinephrine, antidiuretic hormone (ADH), adrenocorticotropic hormone (ACTH), renin-angiotensin, and aldosterone, are also involved. The kidneys play a pivotal role in long-term arterial pressure regulation (Guyton et al., 1972). A number of baroreceptors are present in the walls of arteries, with the most important ones being found in the carotid sinuses and aortic arch. They continuously monitor blood pressure and initiate appropriate compensatory reflexes. Thus, a number of mechanisms normally operate to regulate heart performance and systemic blood pressure. In essential hypertension, some phase of this regulatory system fails to function satisfactorily.

Blood pressure, as normally measured, refers to the pressure exerted against the walls of the arteries. It is expressed in two numbers. The first number is the *systolic pressure* recorded during the heart's pumping stroke, or systole. The second number represents the pressure while the heart relaxes and refills and is called the *diastolic pressure*. The normal aging process often causes an increase in the systolic pressure because of a general decrease in elasticity of artery walls. However, in essential hypertension the diastolic pressure is raised, as well as and often somewhat more than the systolic pressure. The small arterioles are very much involved in this case.

23.2   The Renin-Angiotensin System and Hypertension

The kidney plays an important role in the hypertensive process through (1) regulation of extracellular fluid volume and (2) elaboration of both prohypertensive (renin) and antihypertensive (prostaglandins) humoral agents (Tobian, 1974). Since the beginning of the twentieth century, much research in physiology, biochemistry, and clinical medicine has contributed to an understanding of the role of the renin-angiotensin system in the control of blood pressure and in regulation of salt and water metabolism. Laragh et al. (1977) recently described the present state of knowledge on this system. Renin is an enzyme that is secreted by the juxtaglomerular cells of the kidneys. Fig. 23.1 shows a nephron with the juxtaglomerular apparatus which includes juxtaglomerular cells of the afferent arteriole and adjacent

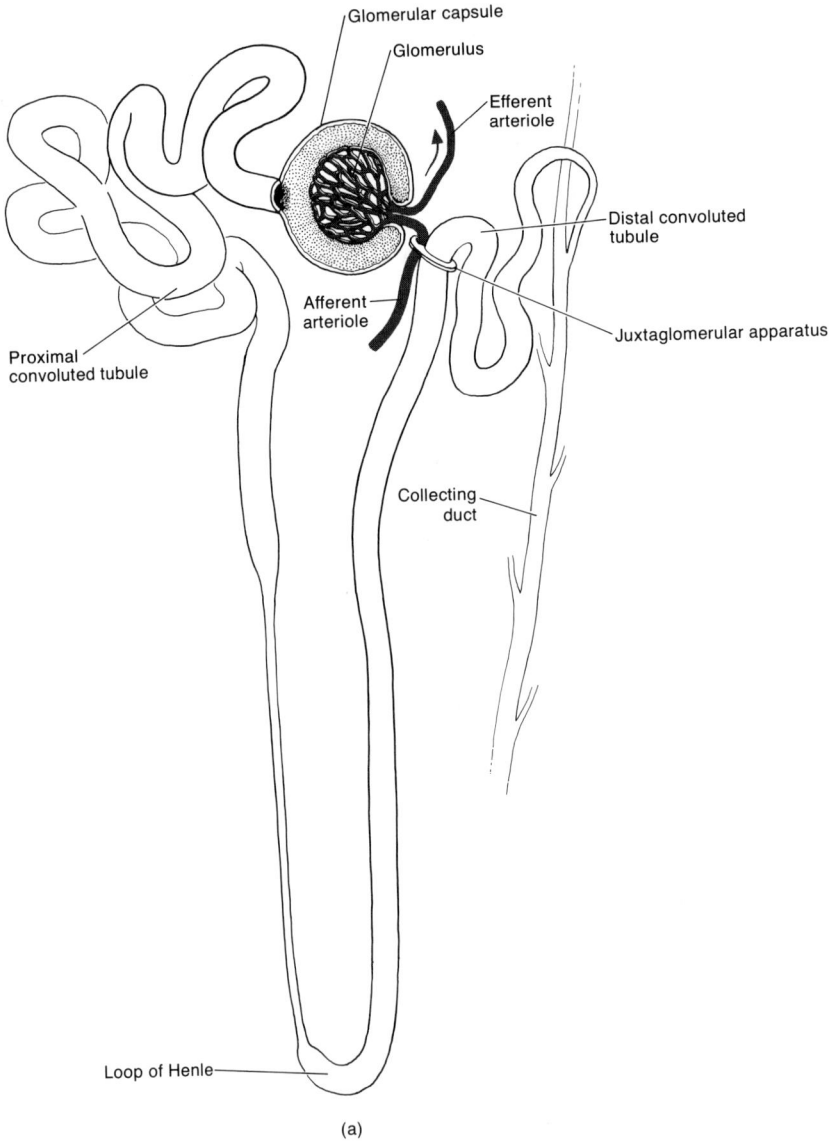

(a)

Fig. 23.1 The juxtaglomerular apparatus. (*a*) The juxtaglomerular apparatus as it appears externally. (*b*) The cells of the juxtaglomerular apparatus. (From Gerard J. Tortora and Nicholas P. Anagnostakos, *Principles of Anatomy and Physiology,* 2d ed., New York: Harper & Row, 1978; by permission of the publisher.)

cells in the distal convoluted tubule that are known as the macula densa. Renin acts on an alpha$_2$-globulin substrate, that was produced in the liver and released to the general circulation, to yield a decapeptide called angiotensin I. Angiotensin I is biologically inactive, but in passage through the lungs it encounters pulmonary converting enzymes that hydrolyze it into the octapeptide angiotensin II. This substance has potent pressor effects that act immediately to produce vasoconstriction and increase blood pressure. At the same time, but in a slower and more prolonged manner, angiotensin II stimulates adrenocortical release of aldosterone, a hormone that acts on the distal renal tubule to increase sodium resorption and fluid retention. Both the vasoconstriction and the increased blood volume tend to raise blood pressure.

Several factors are known to regulate the release of renin (Ganong, 1977). Two local factors include a baroreceptor mechanism in the juxtaglomerular cells and a macula densa mechanism that makes renin secretion inversely proportional to the rate of sodium or chloride transport across its cells. Two humoral factors include inhibition of renin secretion by angiotensin II and by vasopressin (ADH). An additional factor is stimulation of the juxtaglomerular cells through the sympathetic nervous system. Renin secretion is controlled by several feedback mechanisms (Oparil and Haber, 1974). Another hormonal system involving a prostaglandin E compound apparently has an opposite effect on renal blood flow to that of the renin-angiotensin system, the prostaglandin system producing a high level of flow and angiotensin depressing flow (Itskovitz and McGiff, 1974; McGiff et al., 1974). With several systems involved in renal function and blood pressure regulation, many complex interactions result.

The role of the renin-angiotensin system has not been clearly defined in the pathogenesis and maintenance of essential hypertension. Plasma renin activity, along with sodium balance or 24-hour urinary sodium excretion to help interpret renin values, has been measured in hypertensive, as

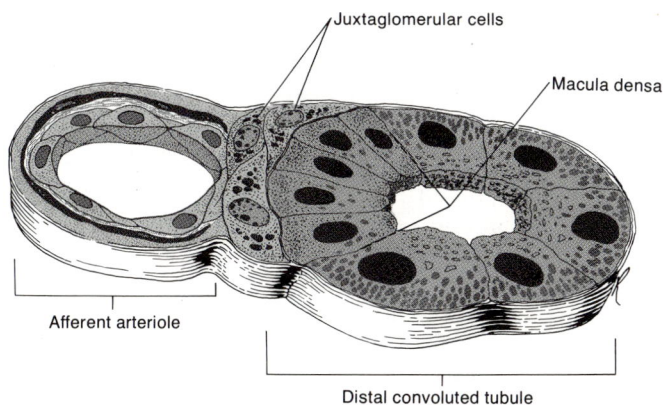

(b)

well as normal, subjects and found to vary considerably among the hypertensives (Laragh et al., 1977; Oparil and Haber, 1974). Some patients exhibit a low, some normal, and some a high renin/sodium index. Laragh et al. (1977), using drugs to block the renin-angiotensin system at different points, concluded that an absolute or relative excess of renin-angiotensin is actively involved in maintenance of the elevated blood pressure of about 70 percent of all patients with essential hypertension. This includes nearly all those with high or "normal" renin/sodium profiles. In the remaining 30 percent, the renin system apparently acts appropriately and a low renin/ sodium profile is found. These studies did not indicate, however, if the excessive renin secretion was the primary cause of the hypertension. Freis (1976) hypothesized that an expanded extracellular fluid (ECF) volume is closely related to an elevation in arterial blood pressure and that the renin-angiotensin system plays a secondary role in the pathogenesis of hypertension. In any case, the measurement of the renin/sodium profile should be a useful tool in screening and applying therapies for hypertensive patients.

23.3 Pathogenesis

A mosaic or multifactored theory for the pathophysiology of primary hypertension was suggested by Page as early as 1949 (Page, 1974). One of the factors is heredity since hypertension is observed to run in families. Miall (1971) concluded that polygenic inheritance is the most likely possibility, but that familial factors account for only a third of the variance of systolic pressure and a fifth of that for diastolic. Nonfamilial environmental factors presumably account for the remainder. There are some racial differences in incidence of hypertension. Blacks are particularly prone to develop the disorder.

Psychosocial stimulation as an initial factor in the pathogenesis of essential hypertension has been reviewed by Henry (1976). He has suggested that interactions and confrontations occur as an individual moves within the social milieu in search of the necessities and luxuries of life. The effects of genetically determined sensitivity and early life experiences, taken in conjunction with social assets, determine the effectiveness of the individual's coping defenses in response to the problems encountered. A dominant coping pattern of aggression or a subordinate pattern of depression may be adopted. The dominant pattern is expressed through the sympathetic adrenal medullary system and results in increases in sympathetic stimulus, initial cardiac output, peripheral resistance, blood pressure, plasma fatty acids, glycogenolysis, and catecholamine synthetic enzymes. The subordinate pattern is expressed through the pituitary adrenal cortical systems and is associated with increases in ACTH, vagal activity, gluconeogenesis, blood pressure, and pepsin. Animal studies have shown that the consequences of sustained and frequent arousal of the dominant or defense response include secondary structural adaptation of blood vessels with thickening of the walls, increased adrenal medullary catecholamine-synthesizing enzymes, loss of sensitivity of baroreceptors in artery walls, and increased release of renin as a result of the increase in catecholamines. The subordinate or depression response may be even more physiologically damaging than the defense response with its involvement of the ACTH-adrenal cortical mechanisms producing adrenal cortical hyperplasia. In any case, a state of positive feedback eventually develops to maintain hypertension. In genetically and socially susceptible individuals, therefore, this sequence of events may lead to changes that are initially reversible but gradually become irreversible and ultimately result in complications such as cerebrovascular accidents and myocardial or renal failure.

An association has been noted between blood pressure and body weight in United States populations (Chiang et al., 1969). Hypertension is more common among the obese than among the nonobese and, conversely, a significant proportion of hypertensive persons in the population are overweight. Weight reduction has been shown to lower blood pressure and it may bring about a more favorable prognosis in obese hypertensive persons. However, Dahl (1975) postulated that the real effect on decreasing blood pressure of a weight-reduction program is from restriction of salt rather than from restriction of kilocalories. Although the underlying mechanisms responsible for the association between obesity and blood pressure have not been clarified, the metabolic and hemodynamic effects of the obesity itself impose an extra burden and strain on the circulatory system of the hypertensive patient. A relationship between body weight and blood pressure does not seem to hold among primitive societies (Freis, 1976).

Ingestion of 50 to 100 g licorice per day has been observed to produce a reversible form of hypertension that is associated with hypokalemia and low plasma renin activity. The hypertensive effects are apparently related to the presence in licorice of glycyrrhizinic acid which has a mineralocorticoid effect.

The renin-angiotensin system in hypertension has been discussed in Sec. 23.2. Sodium balance is intimately involved in the adjustments of this system and may also exert direct effects on vascular reactivity and hypertension (Gavras et al., 1976; Abboud, 1974).

Sodium and Hypertension

Historically, salt was a relatively rare and valued commodity. Today, however, salt is plentiful and widely used in the developed countries of the world. Most processed foods contain relatively large quantities of salt and the mean intake of American adults has been estimated to be 10 to 14 g per day (Dahl, 1975).

Actually, very little sodium is needed by the human adult who is not subjected to unusual salt depletion by sweating or loss of other body fluids. Metabolic equilibrium can be maintained with sodium intake ranging from 40 to 200 mg (1.7 to 8.7 meq) per day. Some highland New Guinea natives have lived for generations on sodium intake levels of approximately 40 mg per day (Dahl, 1975). However, an appetite for salt can be acquired and the body is able to adapt to comparatively large quantities of sodium. This is accomplished by adjustments in the renal-endocrine system, although considerable genetically determined variation in the ability to adjust is apparently present among individuals (Holliday, 1974).

Epidemiological studies in various societies have shown a correlation between chronically high salt intake and prevalence of hypertension. Primitive societies where salt is not used in the diet are free of hypertension and blood pressure does not rise with age in these populations (Freis, 1976). Dahl (1975) reported average salt intakes to range from about 4 g per day by Eskimo of Anaktuvik Pass in Alaska to about 26 g by inhabitants of the Akita region in northern Japan, with Marshall Islanders, northern U.S. Americans, and southern Japanese ranging in between. As group mean salt intake increased, group incidence of hypertension also increased. Individual susceptibility was not assessed within each of the groups.

Schechter et al. (1974 and 1973) reported that hypertensive patients on a constant dry diet containing 9 meq sodium per day drank a significantly greater proportion of their total fluid as saline and drank a greater total volume of fluid than did normotensive volunteers. The total amount of sodium consumed by hypertensive patients in these studies was 4.8 to 7.3 times greater than that of the control subjects, although all subjects exhibited normal detection and recognition thresholds for the taste of sodium chloride. In pilot explorations, Dahl (1972) made crude assessments of sodium chloride intake by questioning individuals concerning their use of saltshakers at the table. Those who never added salt were classified as low-salt intake, those who tasted food before adding salt were classified as average intake, and those who always added salt without tasting food were classified as high intake. In spite of the obvious shortcomings of this type of study for accurate assessment of sodium intake, a significant difference in the prevalence of hypertension was found between the groups classified as low- and high-salt intake. Others have not confirmed these findings and further clarification is needed.

Evidence relating salt intake to hypertension in humans is circumstantial, and a direct cause and effect relationship has been debated. However, animal studies have provided evidence for a direct relationship in several species. Dahl (1972) and his coworkers have studied more than 40,000 rats over more than 20 years. Thousands of rats have developed hypertension from chronic salt feeding. It was noted during the course of these studies that a genetic influence was important in determining whether or not blood pressure became chronically elevated from salt ingestion since it did not occur in all cases. Through selective breeding, salt-sensitive and salt-resistant strains of rats were developed.

The value of salt restriction in the treatment of hypertension was reported by Allen in 1925. It was not commonly applied in medical practice, however, until renewed interest was kindled by Kempner's (1948) use

1948

of the rice diet. The rice diet contained approximately 2000 kcal, not more than 5 g fat, about 20 g protein, and 150 mg (6.5 meq) sodium derived from rice and fruit only. The low-sodium level appeared to be the primary factor in producing a decrease in blood pressure when the diet was consumed. Since that time, it has been demonstrated that sodium restriction leads to a marked drop in blood pressure in approximately one-third of patients so treated, a modest decrease in another one-third, but no significant fall in pressure for the remaining third (Dahl, 1975). Sodium chloride restriction to about 1 g per day is necessary for significant lowering of blood pressure to occur. Freis (1976) suggested that the antihypertensive effect of sodium restriction depends upon the maintenance of a reduced volume of ECF. The decreased volume load permits the hypertensive kidney to operate at a lower level of arterial blood pressure and still maintain homeostasis of the ECF. The use of diuretics in the treatment of hypertension has a similar effect to sodium restriction on ECF.

A Committee on Nutrition of the American Academy of Pediatrics reviewed data on salt intake of infants and children in relation to blood pressure (Holliday, 1974). As a result of this review, they recommended the development of guidelines for restraining the use of salt by food processors and suggested that consumers need more information on the salt content of their diets. They did not recommend that salt should be restricted for all members of the U.S. population. For the normotensive 80 percent of this group, present salt intake has apparently not been harmful. For persons at risk from developing hypertension, however, they concluded that there is a reasonable possibility that a low-sodium intake begun early in life may give protection.

23.4   Treatment

For many years, asymptomatic elevated blood pressure was considered to be a benign condition. Specific therapy was not available and the disease was largely ignored (Moser and Wood, 1976). Gradually over two or three decades, however, the realization developed that hypertension was one of the greatest killers in industrialized countries because of its damage to the cardiovascular-renal system. The pharmaceutical industry began to produce a large variety of antihypertensive drugs that made treatment possible and programs were initiated in the areas of both professionals and public education. Enthusiasm for detection and treatment of hypertension has grown (Page, 1976).

Conclusive evidence that treatment markedly reduces the major complications of hypertension was reported from the Veterans Administration Cooperative Study Group (1967, 1970, and 1972). This study followed 523 male hypertensive patients for periods up to $5\frac{1}{2}$ years in a double-blind design that randomly assigned subjects to an active treatment (hydrochlorothiazide plus reserpine plus hydralazine) or a placebo group.

Significantly fewer complications occurred in the treated than in the control groups. Data from this study, further analyzed by Taguchi and Freis (1974), also suggested that considerable therapeutic benefit may be obtained from treatment even if the blood pressure is reduced only partially and does not return completely to normal.

Treatment should be individualized. However, drug treatment for individuals over 60 years of age is probably less important than for those under 60, according to Fry (1974). He studied 704 hypertensives over a period of 20 years and found that most of the excessive mortality affected the younger hypertensives.

A number of antihypertensive drugs are available to the physician and have been reviewed by Hayes and Schneck (1976). The mainstay of all antihypertensive regimens is a diuretic. As many as one-third of patients with mild and moderate hypertension respond adequately to a diuretic alone or a diuretic plus dietary sodium restriction. Depletion of sodium appears to be responsible in large part for the antihypertensive effect of diuretic treatment. If hypokalemia becomes a problem from use of potassium-losing diuretics such as the thiazides, a potassium-sparing diuretic, e.g., spironolactone, may be tried. Diuretics are discussed in Sec. 22.2.

Additional drugs that may be used with diuretics in the treatment of hypertension include (1) substances that inhibit the sympathetic nervous system at various points, and (2) vasodilating compounds. Drugs in the first category include the rauwolfia alkaloids, methyldopa, and pargyline. The vasodilators lower blood pressure by directly dilating arterioles, causing a fall in peripheral vascular resistance. Hydralazine is the only direct vasodilator available for oral administration (Hayes and Schneck, 1976).

Essential hypertensive patients who respond to diuretic drugs also respond well to low-sodium diets (Dustan et al., 1974). This suggests that control of hypertension with both of these measures results from some aspect of the negative salt and water balance that is produced during treatment. Control is maintained to some degree as long as treatment is continued. When low-sodium diets are used alone in the treatment of hypertension, the sodium level probably needs to be less than 400 to 500 mg (17 to 22 meq) to have a significant effect in reducing blood pressure. This is a very restrictive diet to be followed over long periods of time in free-living populations, and many patients have not been willing or able to maintain this level of sodium intake. Moderate dietary sodium restriction, however, may be used in combination with diuretic therapy for hypertension to produce an additional blood pressure lowering effect over that due to the drug action alone. Parijs et al. (1973), in a cross-over type study with 22 mild hypertensive patients, found that moderate sodium restriction (avoiding foods with sodium added during preparation) and diuretics produced a statistically significantly greater blood pressure reduction than did the same diuretic treatment in combination with a regular diet. Instruction on the sodium content of the diet should routinely be part of the management process for hypertensive patients. The low-sodium diet is discussed in Sec. 18.8.

For hypertensive patients, the ideal body weight should be a lean weight (Aagaard, 1973). A weight-control program should be part of the nutritional care for these patients. Individualized exercise programs should also be followed.

REFERENCES

1. Aagaard, G. N. 1973. The management of hypertension. *J. Am. Med. Assoc.*, **224:** 329.

2. Abboud, F. M. 1974. Effects of sodium, angiotensin, and steroids on vascular reactivity in man. *Fed. Proc.*, **33:** 143.

3. Allen, F. M. 1925. Treatment of kidney diseases and high blood pressure. Morristown, N.J.: The Psychiatric Institute.

4. Chiang, B. N., L. V. Perlman, and F. H. Epstein. 1969. Overweight and hypertension. *Circulation*, **39:** 403.

5. Dahl, L. K. 1975. Salt intake and hypertension. *Dietetic Currents* (Ross Laboratories), **2** (No. 4): 1.

6. Dahl, L. K. 1972. Salt and hypertension. *Am. J. Clin. Nutr.*, **25:** 231.

7. Dustan, H. R., R. C. Tarazi, and E. L. Bravo. 1974. Diuretic and diet treatment of hypertension. *Arch. Int. Med.*, **133:** 1007.

8. Freis, E. D. 1976. Salt, volume and the prevention of hypertension. *Circulation*, **53:** 589.

9. Fry, J. 1974. Natural history of hypertension. A case for selective non-treatment. *Lancet*, **2:** 431.

10. Ganong, W. F. 1977. The renin-angiotensin system and the central nervous system. *Fed. Proc.*, **36:** 1771.

11. Gavras, H., A. B. Ribeiro, I. Gavras, and H. R. Brunner. 1976. Reciprocal relation between renin dependency and sodium dependency in essential hypertension. *N. Eng. J. Med.*, **295:** 1278.

12. Guyton, A. C., T. G. Coleman, A. W. Cowley, Jr., K. W. Scheel, R. D. Manning, Jr., and R. A. Norman, Jr. 1972. Arterial pressure regulation. *Am. J. Med.*, **52:** 584.

13. Hayes, A. H., Jr. and D. W. Schneck. 1976. Antihypertensive pharmacotherapy. *Postgrad. Med.*, **59** (No. 5): 155.

14. Henry, J. P. 1976. Understanding the early pathophysiology of essential hypertension. *Geriatrics*, **31** (No. 1): 59.

15. Holliday, M. A. 1974. Salt intake and eating patterns of infants and children in relation to blood pressure. *Pediatrics*, **53:** 115.

16. Itskovitz, H. D. and J. C. McGiff. 1974. Hormonal regulation of the renal circulation. *Circ. Res.*, **34** and **35** (Supplement 1): I-65.

17. Kempner, W. 1948. Treatment of hypertensive vascular disease with rice diet. *Am. J. Med.*, **4:** 545.

18. Laragh, J. H., D. B. Case, J. M. Wallace, and H. Keim. 1977. Blockade of renin or angiotensin for understanding human hypertension: a comparison of propranolol, saralasin and converting enzyme blockade. *Fed. Proc.*, **36:** 1781.

19. McGiff, J. C., K. Crowshaw, and H. D. Itskovitz. 1974. Prostaglandins and renal function. *Fed. Proc.*, **33:** 39.

20. Miall, W. E. 1971. Heredity and hypertension. *The Practitioner,* **207:** 20.

21. Moser, M. and D. Wood. 1976. Management of hypertension. *J. Am. Med. Assoc.,* **235:** 2297.

22. Oparil, S. and E. Haber. 1974. The renin-angiotensin system. *N. Eng. J. Med.,* **291:** 389.

23. Page, I. H. 1976. Hypertension. A strange case of neglect. *J. Am. Med. Assoc.,* **235:** 809.

24. Page, I. H. 1974. Arterial hypertension in retrospect. *Circ. Res.,* **34:** 133.

25. Parijs, J., J. V. Joossens, L. Van der Linden, G. Verstreken, and A. K. P. C. Amery. 1973. Moderate sodium restriction and diuretics in the treatment of hypertension. *Am. Heart J.,* **85:** 22.

26. Schechter, P. J., D. Horwitz, and R. I. Henkin. 1974. Salt preference in patients with untreated and treated essential hypertension. *Am. J. Med. Sci.,* **267:** 320.

27. Schechter, P. J., D. Horwitz, and R. I. Henkin. 1973. Sodium chloride preference in essential hypertension. *J. Am. Med. Assoc.,* **225:** 1311.

28. Stamler, J., R. Stamler, W. F. Riedlinger, G. Algera, and R. H. Roberts. 1976. Hypertension screening of 1 million Americans. *J. Am. Med. Assoc.,* **235:** 2299.

29. Strasser, T. 1972. Pilot programmes for the control of hypertension. *WHO Chronicle,* **26:** 451.

30. Taguchi, J. and E. D. Freis. 1974. Partial reduction of blood pressure and prevention of complications in hypertension. *N. Eng. J. Med.,* **291:** 329.

31. Tobian, L., Jr. 1974. Hypertension and the kidney. *Arch. Intern. Med.,* **133:** 959.

32. Veterans Administration Cooperative Study Group on Antihypertensive Agents. 1967. Effects of treatment on morbidity in hypertension: results in patients with diastolic blood pressures averaging 115 through 129 mm Hg. *J. Am. Med. Assoc.,* **202:** 1028.

33. Veterans Administration Cooperative Study Group on Antihypertensive Agents. 1970. Effects of treatment on morbidity in hypertension. II. Results in patients with diastolic blood pressure averaging 90 through 114 mm Hg. *J. Am. Med. Assoc.,* **213:** 1143.

34. Veterans Administration Cooperative Study Group on Antihypertensive Agents. 1972. Effects of treatment on morbidity in hypertension. III. Influence of age, diastolic pressure, and prior cardiovascular disease: further analysis of side effects. *Circulation,* **45:** 991.

35. Wintrobe, M. M., G. W. Thorn, R. D. Adams, E. Braunwald, K. J. Isselbacher, and R. G. Petersdorf (Eds.). 1974. *Harrison's Principles of Internal Medicine,* 7th ed. New York: McGraw-Hill.

STUDY GUIDE

Hypertension may be a symptom of several disorders or it may occur persistently with no known cause and be labeled primary or essential hypertension.

1. Describe conditions that may produce hypertension as a secondary symptom.

2. Describe characteristic physiological and structural changes that occur eventually in patients with progressive primary hypertension.

The cause of essential hypertension is not known but several contributing factors have been suggested in a "mosaic" or multifactored hypothesis.

3. Discuss possible roles of heredity, psychosocial stimulation, and obesity in the pathogenesis and maintenance of hypertension.

4. Outline the sequence of events that is involved in the operation of the renin-angiotensin system and discuss possible relationships of this system to the pathogenesis and maintenance of hypertension.

5. Describe and evaluate evidence that relates dietary salt intake to essential hypertension.

6. Make and justify dietary recommendations for children and adults who are at high risk of developing hypertension.

Dietary treatment is of value, in combination with drugs, for patients with hypertension.

7. Describe major changes in trends since the 1920s for the use of low-salt or low-sodium diets with hypertensive patients.

8. Explain the rationale behind dietary sodium restriction for treatment of essential hypertension and suggest appropriate sodium levels.

9. Cite evidence that treatment markedly reduces major complications of hypertension.

10. Describe the general action of several types of drugs found to be effective in the treatment of essential hypertension.

11. Explain why reduction of obesity is desirable in a hypertensive patient.

24

Renal Disorders

The kidneys have the major responsibility for regulating volume and composition of body fluids. They do this by filtering and reabsorption processes that operate at the rate of about 125 ml of fluid per minute or 180 liters per day. The two kidneys in humans, although accounting for less than 0.5 percent of the body weight, receive about 20 percent of the total blood volume pumped by the heart. Because of the great importance of these organs to homeostasis and the body's well-being, diseases of the kidneys may produce serious consequences.

Maintenance of an adequate nutritional state in patients with renal disease has received much attention in recent years. Renal dialysis and transplant procedures have been developed, and the lives of many with chronic renal disease have been prolonged. This chapter focuses on the role of dietary modification in medical therapy for the control of renal disease. A review of kidney anatomy, function, and tests for measuring functional adequacy is also included.

24.1   Renal Anatomy and Function

The kidneys are extremely complex organs from the standpoint of both structure and function. They operate to maintain an appropriate interior milieu for the functioning of all body cells. The chief operation involved in performing this function is excretion of water and nonmetabolized solute in appropriate proportions through highly selective filters.

Figure 24.1 diagrams a section through the center of a kidney and shows gross structure. The outer portion of the kidney is called the

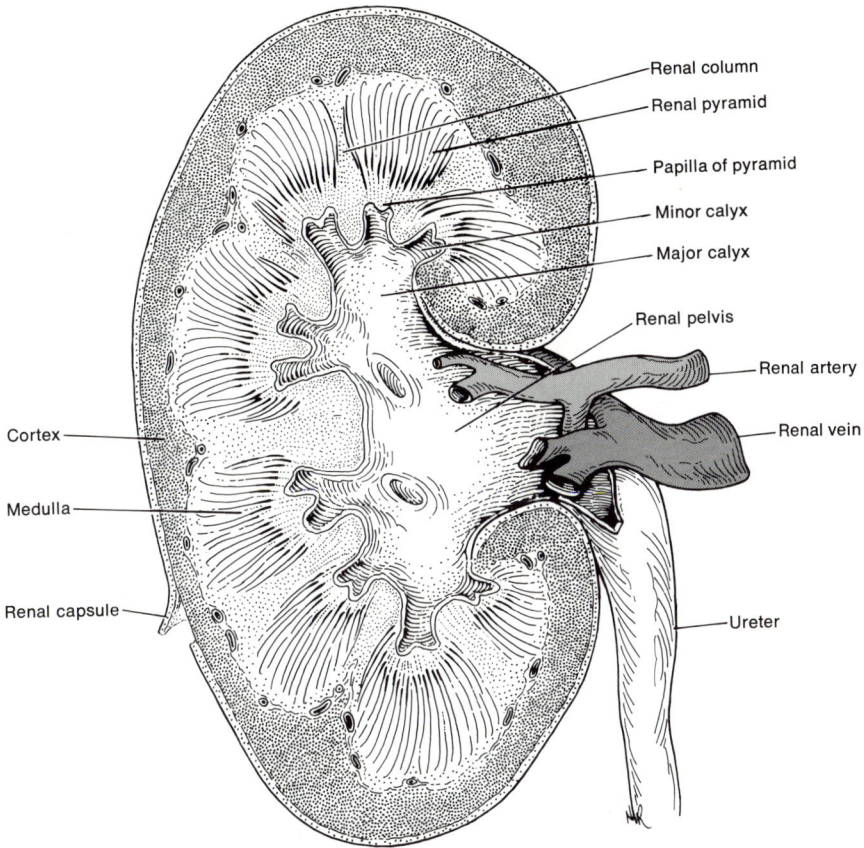

Fig. 24.1 Coronal section through the right kidney illustrating gross internal anatomy. (From Gerard J. Tortora and Nicholas P. Anagnostakos, *Principles of Anatomy and Physiology*, 2d ed., New York: Harper & Row, 1978; by permission of the publisher.)

cortex and the region next to it is the medulla. The physiological units of the kidney, the nephrons, are found primarily in the cortex, with part of their tubular system extending into the medulla. Collecting tubules from the nephrons traverse the medulla to the minor calyces which collect urine as it forms. The urine then drains from the major calyces into the pelvis of the kidney and out through the ureter to the bladder.

A diagram of nephrons is shown in Fig. 24.2. They are the filters of the kidney and approximately one million of these tiny units are found in each of the two organs. In the filtering process, the afferent arteriole takes blood into a capillary network called the *glomerulus*. Water and solutes of the blood filter through these capillary walls into the glomerular or Bowman's capsule which surrounds the glomerulus. From here the filtrate drains into a tubule, which is subdivided for classification purposes into several sections. The specific gravity of the filtrate is approximately the same as plasma (normally 1.022 to 1.031) as it is first filtered but it is almost

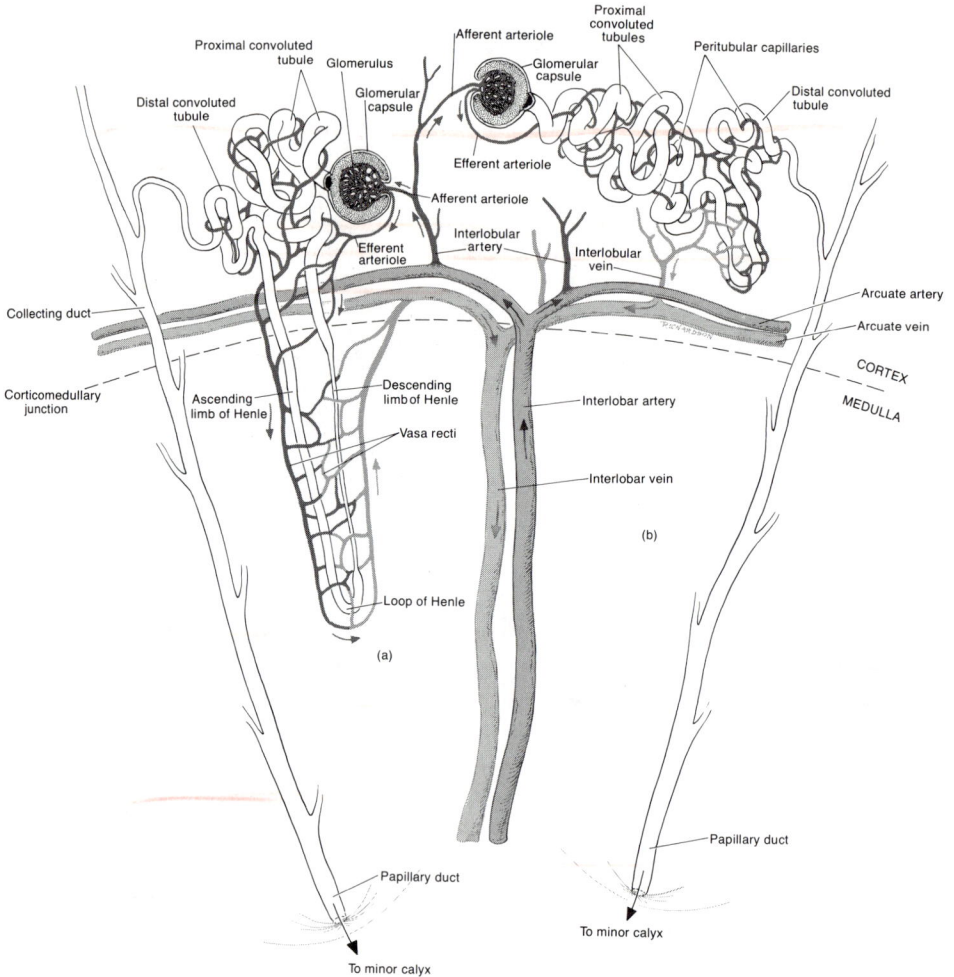

Fig. 24.2 Nephrons. (a) Juxtamedullary nephron. (b) Cortical nephron. (From Gerard J. Tortora and Nicholas P. Anagnostakos, *Principles of Anatomy and Physiology*, 2d ed., New York: Harper & Row, 1978; by permission of the publisher.

protein-free. As the filtrate goes through the proximal convoluted tubule, a large portion of the water is passively reabsorbed into the blood vessels that surround the tubule. In addition, glucose, amino acids, potassium, phosphate, sulfate, sodium, chloride, bicarbonate, urea, and other solutes are reabsorbed in varying degrees. Some of these solutes are actively absorbed, requiring energy, while others are passively absorbed. The filtrate is isotonic with the extracellular fluid by the time it reaches the end of the proximal tubule.

The kidneys have a remarkable ability to concentrate and thus regulate the amount of fluid excreted as urine. Although approximately 180 liters of fluid are filtered each day, only 1 to 2 liters are normally excreted.

[handwritten margin notes: descend, [ ] cug NaClin', H₂O out / ascend, dilute cug NaCl out, H₂O in]

The urinary concentrating mechanism responsible for this process has been studied for many years. Jamison and Maffly (1976) reviewed the current status of knowledge concerning this mechanism. As the glomerular filtrate goes from the proximal convoluted tubule into the thin descending limb of the loop of Henle, which is located in the outer medulla, it becomes more concentrated. This is the result of water being extracted across its permeable wall by the high osmolality of the interstitial fluid. The high osmolality is produced by active reabsorption of sodium chloride (NaCl) from the thick ascending limb which has an extremely low-water permeability. The chloride rather than sodium ion is actively reabsorbed and sodium is then passively removed. The active chloride ion pump supplies necessary energy for the concentrating system which has been hypothesized to work on a countercurrent principle. Urea also accumulates in the interstitium of the medulla and plays an important role in the extraction of water from the descending limb because of its contribution, along with NaCl, to the high osmolality of this interstitial fluid.

As the filtrate enters the distal tubule from the ascending limb of the loop of Henle, it is hypo-osmotic to the surrounding interstitium of the cortex. With the action of antidiuretic hormone (ADH) on the distal tubule, water is reabsorbed until the filtrate is isotonic to the interstitial fluid. The collecting tubules then take the filtrate a second and final time through the medulla and more water is reabsorbed because of the hyperosmotic interstitial fluid in this area of the kidney. Urea is also reabsorbed from the collecting tubule and some of it reenters the loop of Henle as part of its recycling process. Thus, through a complex process involving countercurrent flow in the two limbs of the loop of Henle, active transport of NaCl from the ascending limb, recycling of urea, differences in water permeability for various parts of the renal tubule, and the action of ADH, the glomerular filtrate is normally concentrated to a urine volume of 1 to 2 liters with a specific gravity that normally ranges from 1.003 to 1.030.

In the renal tubule, some important mechanisms for regulating acid-base balance also operate. These are discussed in Sec. 10.2. The renin-angiotensin system initiated in the kidney is discussed in Sec. 23.2.

Clinical Tests of Renal Function

Several different measurements may be used to estimate the efficiency with which the kidney performs its functions. Serial tests may be of value in following the progress of renal disease.

Measurement of Glomerular Filtration Rate. The glomerular filtration rate (GFR) can be measured by determining the plasma clearance of a substance, such as inulin, which appears in the glomerular filtrate in the same concentration as in the plasma but which is not reabsorbed nor secreted by the renal tubules. The clearance of a substance is given by the following equation (Wintrobe et al., 1974, p. 1371).

$$\text{Clearance} = \frac{\text{excretion rate}}{\text{plasma concentration}} = \frac{\text{mg/ml urine} \times \text{ml urine/min}}{\text{mg/ml plasma}}$$

A normal range for GFR in males is 110 to 150 ml per min; in females it is 105 to 132 ml per min. Clearance values are corrected to a standard body surface area (1.73 sq m) before being compared with standards.

A rough estimate of GFR may be made by measuring the endogenous creatinine clearance. Plasma creatinine concentration is determined by the production rate and the excretion rate. The production rate is closely related to muscle mass and is relatively stable over a 24-hour period. With the collection of a 24-hour urine sample and a single plasma sample for cretinine determination, creatinine clearance may be calculated (Beeson and McDermott, 1975, p. 1091).

Phenolsulfonphthalein Excretion.   The injected dye, phenolsulfonphthalein (PSP), is secreted into the urine primarily by the proximal tubules. Only a small percentage of that reaching the bladder is filtered through the glomeruli. Excretion is rapid in normal kidneys and approximately 70 percent of an injected dose will be detected in the urine after 2 hours with approximately 35 percent being excreted within 15 minutes. The rate of excretion is limited by renal plasma flow and, in severely impaired kidneys, by proximal tubule function (Wintrobe et al., 1974, p. 1372).

Urinary Concentration.   When fluid is withheld for 24 hours or more, the normal kidneys can concentrate urine to 750 to 1400 mOsm/l. In many patients with renal disease, this degree of dehydration may be undesirable or dangerous. Concentrating ability may also be tested by measuring urinary specific gravity or osmolarity after an intramuscular injection of 5 units of vasopressin (ADH) in oil. On a practical basis, if the specific gravity of a casual urine sample, one obtained after a short dehydration period, or one obtained after vasopressin injection reaches 1.022 or more, concentrating ability may be considered to be intact (Wintrobe et al., 1974, p. 1372).

Proteinuria.   Very little protein is filtered by normal glomeruli and essentially none appears in the urine. When glomeruli are damaged by renal disease, protein, primarily albumin, passes into the urine. Damage to proximal tubules may also be responsible for loss of low-molecular-weight proteins that are normally filtered and reabsorbed (Wintrobe et al., 1974, p. 1371). Small amounts of protein may appear in the urine of normal individuals after exercise, chilling, or trauma such as surgery and hemorrhage.

24.2   Renal Disease

Classification of renal disease is difficult and variable. The etiology of a renal disorder is often unclear and classification on the basis of autopsy findings alone is not satisfactory. Disease may initially attack a specific area of the kidney, such as the glomerulus or the tubules. However, as the disease progresses, general impairment of renal function usually occurs and there is a common end-stage in chronic renal failure.

Maintenance of an adequate nutritional state is important for a patient with any type of renal disorder. However, dietary intake is of particular concern in the control of body fluid composition for patients with renal failure and for those undergoing dialysis. Special nutritional measures may also be valuable in the management of glomerulonephritis, the nephrotic syndrome, and renal calculi. Nutritional implications for these disorders are discussed later.

24.3   Glomerulonephritis

Glomerulonephritis refers to forms of renal disease characterized by inflammation of the glomeruli or immune glomerular injury (Beeson and McDermott, 1975, p. 1126). A number of different conditions may produce glomerular problems. Therefore, the terms *acute* and *chronic glomerulonephritis* should be regarded as general patterns of reaction of the kidneys rather than as individual diseases with specific causes (Wintrobe et al., 1974, p. 1388).

Acute glomerulonephritis sometimes follows an infection with the group A, beta-hemolytic streptococcus or other infections. An average of 10 to 14 days elapses between the streptococcal infection and the first symptoms of nephritis. Antibodies to the streptococcal antigens are produced and antigen-antibody complexes form in the kidneys. Clinical signs and symptoms include fatigue, anorexia, abdominal pain, edema of face and legs, hypertension, and congestive heart failure. Changes in renal function may include decreased GFR, elevated blood urea nitrogen (BUN), blood in the urine (hematuria), oliguria or anuria, and some proteinuria (Wintrobe et al., 1974, p. 1390).

Most children with acute glomerulonephritis recover completely. A larger number of adults with the disease may develop a chronic disorder, which can be inactive for long periods of time.

Chronic glomerulonephritis represents a variety of different diseases and does not commonly come from acute nephritis following infection. Its clinical pattern varies widely, sometimes progressing slowly over many years and sometimes following a short explosive course.

Nutritional Care in Glomerulonephritis

Nutritional care is particularly important if edema, hypertension, persistent proteinuria, and/or oliguria are present. The appropriate level of dietary protein in glomerulonephritis has been discussed over the years. At one time it was thought that a low-protein diet was desirable in order to decrease the work load of the kidney involved in excretion of urea as a waste product of protein metabolism. It is now known, however, that urea is generally reabsorbed in a passive and nonenergy-requiring process. Severe protein restriction is unnecessary for patients with glomerulonephritis unless oliguria or anuria develops (Goodhart and Shils, 1973, p. 873). Burton (1974b) suggested that in cases of acute glomerulonephritis, because of anorexia and nausea, the diet is best limited for the first few days of illness to 2 to 3 oz of fruit juices every hour. The total volume should not exceed the fluid allowance, which is manipulated according to the volume of urine excreted. Usually 500 to 1000 ml per day more fluid than the total urinary output of the previous day is allowed. After the first few days, Burton (1974b) recommended a daily diet of approximately 40 g protein and 500 mg (22 meq) sodium with gradual individualized liberalization over the next 10 to 15 days. Nutritional care in chronic glomerulonephritis that has progressed to renal failure is discussed in Sec. 24.5.

If hypertension and edema are problems in patients with glomerulonephritis, dietary sodium levels may be adjusted. The level of restriction will depend on the severity of symptoms and other aspects of treatment. The low-sodium diet is discussed in Sec. 18.8.

24.4   The Nephrotic Syndrome

The nephrotic syndrome, as generally defined, refers to a clinical condition that includes the triad of massive proteinuria, hypoalbuminemia, and edema. Hypercholesterolemia and hypertension often are also present but are not necessary in the definition of this syndrome. The nephrotic syndrome results from glomerular injury which may develop from many different causes.

As a result of glomerular injury, permeability is increased and protein molecules are filtered through the glomeruli. Albumin is the smallest plasma protein and is lost in the urine in largest quantity. Hypoalbuminemia is the primary result of this loss since albumin synthesis is usually normal. There is a consequent fall in the oncotic pressure of plasma with resulting transudation of plasma fluid into interstitial spaces and development of edema. An additional sequence of events may contribute to the edema. With plasma fluid loss, blood volume decreases and renal blood flow is reduced. This may activate the renin-angiotensin system (discussed in Sec. 23.2) and produce an increase in aldosterone secretion. Sodium reabsorption is thus increased by aldosterone with an additional retention of water in the body.

The usual serum albumin value in nephrotic syndrome is between 1.0 and 3.0 g/100 ml but may occasionally be as low as 0.5 g/100 ml. Plasma proteins other than albumin may be normal or decreased. Serum levels of transferrin and ceruloplasmin are also reduced since these are relatively small molecules and easily filtered through damaged glomeruli. Protein loss in the urine may range from 4 or 5 g daily to as high as 20 or 30 g.

The mechanism for the hyperlipidemia that commonly accompanies the nephrotic syndrome is obscure but seems to be linked to the low concentration of albumin in the blood (Beeson and McDermott, 1975, p. 1126). The basal metabolic rate is usually low in patients with nephrotic syndrome. This may be a result of malnutrition or failure to correct for edema fluid in estimating body weight (Wintrobe et al., 1974, p. 1398).

Nutritional Care in the Nephrotic Syndrome

The specific cause of the nephrotic syndrome should be identified and treated whenever possible. Otherwise, treatment is directed toward the edema, which is usually the patient's chief complaint. When edema is severe, both diuretics and sodium restriction may be used to control it. Dietary sodium levels may be 22 to 44 meq per day (500 to 1000 mg) with diuretic therapy. Since secondary hyperaldosteronism is often part of the clinical features of nephrotic syndrome, aldosterone antagonists, such as spironolactone, may be most effective as diuretics (Goodhart and Shils, 1973, p. 876).

The efficacy of high-protein diets in the treatment of patients with nephrotic syndrome has been discussed for many years. Urinary protein losses are increased with high dietary protein intake. However, positive nitrogen balances as a result of diets containing 65 to 200 g protein daily have been demonstrated in some patients with long-standing proteinuria (Goodhart and Shils, 1973, p. 876). This indicates that there is a body protein deficit of which the low serum protein level is but one manifestation. Dietary protein levels of approximately 120 g per day, along with a high-kilocalorie intake, should provide for steady replenishment of wasted tissues. Appetites are often poor in edematous patients and constant encouragement is usually necessary to ensure consumption of the prescribed diets.

Since many high-protein foods contain considerable amounts of sodium, high-protein and low-sodium diets are not always compatible and require careful planning. Low-sodium milk may be used to increase the protein level without additional sodium. However, sodium restriction is an emergency measure to control edema and is not indicated during convalescence from the nephrotic syndrome or when edema is minimal (Wintrobe et al., 1974, p. 1399).

24.5 Chronic Renal Failure

There are many different initial causes of chronic renal failure. These include chronic pyelonephritis resulting from recurrent infections of the kidney, chronic glomerulonephritis, vascular kidney diseases, congenital abnormalities, diabetes mellitus, and drug toxicities. However, the syndrome that develops as the end-stage in most cases is the same. It is called the *uremic syndrome* or *uremia* and occurs when the kidneys have lost most of their function. As kidney disease develops and many nephrons cease functioning, it is hypothesized that a small number of surviving nephrons carry on the processes of excretion by increasing the volume of glomerular filtrate and by hypertrophy of the tubules to handle the extra filtrate. Thus, chronically diseased kidneys may adapt to maintain some degree of function and life support until 90 to 99 percent of their normal glomerular filtration has been lost (Beeson and McDermott, 1975, p. 1096).

Pathophysiology of Chronic Renal Failure

Uremia is characterized by (1) retention of urea, creatinine, and other products of protein metabolism in the blood and tissues; (2) progressive acidosis; (3) inability to excrete a water load within a brief period; and (4) various electrolyte disturbances (Burton, 1974a). In the initial stages of renal insufficiency as adaptation occurs by the functioning nephrons, the kidney's ability to concentrate fluid is impaired and polyuria develops. The patient must drink and excrete increased amounts of water in order to handle the usual solute load. Nocturia is common and dehydration may readily occur. Increased loss of urinary sodium accompanies the polyuria. Polyuria reaches a peak, however, as GFR is declining through the range of 25 to 5 ml per minute, and then oliguria develops in the preterminal phase of chronic renal failure (Beeson and McDermott, 1975, p. 1096). When oliguria or anuria is present, retention of sodium and potassium occurs.

As the GFR gradually decreases in renal failure, increased phosphate is retained in the body. Increased serum phosphate causes decreased serum calcium and secondary hyperparathyroidism results. Parathyroid hormone acts on the renal tubule, where approximately 80 percent of the filtered phosphate is normally reabsorbed, and reduces its reabsorption, thus tending to restore serum phosphate and calcium levels to normal. When GFR decreases to about 20 ml per minute, however, serum phosphate cannot be kept within normal limits in spite of increased secretion of parathyroid hormone. Demineralization of bone eventually develops from the action of parathyroid hormone. Giving aluminum hydroxide or aluminum carbonate gels retards the absorption of phosphate in the gastrointestinal tract and helps to control abnormal parathyroid secretion resulting from phosphate retention.

An additional factor contributing to low serum calcium levels and osteodystrophy (which may include osteomalacia, osteitis fibrosa, osteoporosis, and osteosclerosis) in renal failure is reduced intestinal absorption of calcium. Coburn et al. (1976) reviewed the metabolism of vitamin D as it pertains to chronic renal failure. They pointed out many clinical similarities between renal osteodystrophy and nutritional rickets. Massive quantities of vitamin D have been shown to bring about healing of osteomalacia in certain patients with advanced renal disease who do not respond to lesser amounts of this vitamin. The kidney is the site of synthesis of an active metabolite of vitamin D_3 (1,25-dihydroxy-vitamin D_3) from 25-hydroxyvitamin D_3, which is first produced in the liver from vitamin D. The administration of the active vitamin D analogs to uremic patients with symptomatic bone disease is capable of reversing many of the abnormalities of the skeleton. These analogs are becoming available for clinical use.

Anemia may develop early in the course of uremia. It is usually a normocytic, normochromic anemia and the mechanism of its development is complex. It involves toxic suppression of red blood cell production in the bone marrow, toxic shortening of the life span of erythrocytes, and impaired production of the bone marrow-stimulating hormone, erythropoietin, by the nonfunctioning kidney (Burton, 1974a).

Gastrointestinal manifestations complicate advanced uremia. These may include mouth ulcers which are related to bacterial breakdown to ammonia of the urea present in high concentration in saliva. Ulcers may occur throughout the gastrointestinal tract. Common symptoms include anorexia, nausea, vomiting, and abdominal pain. Mental clouding, inability to concentrate, drowsiness, and lethargy usually occur in advanced renal failure. The hypertension and hypertensive heart disease that are often associated with chronic renal failure are responsible for the development of congestive heart failure.

Nutritional Implications of Renal Failure

Dietary intervention for patients with chronic renal failure may become important when residual kidney function has reached 25 percent or less of normal and definite symptoms are discernible. At this point, diet modification can aid in maintaining metabolic balance and lessening many of the unpleasant uremic symptoms. Burton (1977) emphasized that dietary intervention, custom-tailored to the specific circumstances of the patient, may prolong the patient's normal and productive existence for many months. Once the residual renal function approaches roughly 3 percent of normal (GFR of about 3.5 ml per min), however, dietary treatment can no longer help and dialysis or renal transplantation must be instituted. Dietary control is also very important for patients undergoing dialysis, although less restrictive than that for nondialyzed patients.

According to Burton (1977), the basic principles of dietary treatment for chronic renal failure are (1) judicious regulation of protein intake; (2) regulation of fluid intake to balance fluid output and insensible water loss; (3) regulation of sodium intake to balance its output; (4) restriction of potassium and phosphate; (5) insistence on an adequate caloric intake; and (6) supplementation with appropriate vitamins.

Protein Intake.   Urea, creatinine, and uric acid are nitrogenous end-products of protein and nucleic acid metabolism in the body. High levels of dietary protein foods cause accumulation of these nitrogenous wastes in individuals whose kidneys are not functioning properly, with progressively toxic effects. A new era in dietary treatment of patients with chronic renal failure began with Giordano's report in 1963 that feeding uremic patients a total of only 2 g of nitrogen from essential amino acids, along with adequate caloric intake from carbohydrate and fat, vitamins, and minerals, was associated with a decrease in BUN and a reduction in endogenous protein catabolism. Many of the uremic symptoms disappeared. Apparently, endogenous urea could be used by the body in the synthesis of nonessential amino acids as long as the essential amino acids were supplied in adequate amounts.

Giovannetti and Maggiore (1964) reported similar effects with uremic patients using high-calorie, low-protein foods and either an essential amino acid mixture or egg albumin to supply approximately 2 g nitrogen per day. In 1965 Berlyne et al. reported on a British modification of the Giovannetti diet in which egg and milk supplied 12 g of the 18 to 21 g of total protein in the diet. Methionine (500 mg per day) was also given as a supplement. Bread and other special products made from low-protein flour or starch were used in supplying adequate kilocalories.

Since these early dietary trials, the low-protein diet (often called the Giordono-Giovannetti or G-G diet) has been widely applied with varying degrees of success (Franklin et al., 1967; Bailey and Sullivan, 1968; Lonergan and Lange, 1968; Wright et al., 1970; Carmena and Shapiro, 1972). As commonly used, the diet includes one egg, $\frac{3}{4}$ cup milk, an occasional substitution of 1 to 2 oz of meat, fish, or poultry, a multivitamin preparation, and iron-containing tablets (Burton, 1974b). It is very important that the approximately 20 g of protein given daily be of high biological value in order to supply the essential amino acids with a minimum quantity of nonessential ones. Proteins from grains and vegetables are avoided. Adequate caloric intake (2000 to 3000 kcal) must be supplied, primarily as carbohydrate and fat, to avoid breakdown of body tissues. Low-protein bread and other wheat starch products are given to supply kilocalories without protein. The bread may be used as a carrier for fats (butter or margarine) and sugars (jellies, honey, and syrups). Low-protein, low-potassium fruits and vegetables are also included in measured amounts.

The 20-g protein diet is monotonous and restrictive and patient compliance is not always satisfactory. Patients should be selected for motivation and cooperation and receive careful follow-up. As more patients have been placed on dialysis in recent years, the 20-g protein diet has been less widely prescribed. The diet is not curative and is used primarily to maintain life in greater comfort for a prolonged period of time.

Kopple and Swendseid (1974) fed three men with advanced chronic renal failure a diet containing 21 g of the eight free essential amino acids and no more than 2 g of additional protein. Their observations on nitrogen balance suggested that the diet may not be adequate for the maintenance of good nutritional status in renal failure. They suggested that the addition of histidine and possibly a source of nonspecific nitrogen may enhance the nutritional value of this diet. The study supported the findings of others that most nonessential amino acids can be readily synthesized on the low-protein diet.

Regulation of Fluid Intake.   Fluid intake for patients with renal failure must be individualized in line with urinary output. Burton (1974a) suggested that they consume 2 to 3 cups of fluids more than their 24-hour urine output. This will provide for the insensible daily losses of water from the lungs and skin and for water eliminated in the feces.

Regulation of Sodium Intake.   The sodium intake for patients with renal failure should be adjusted on an individual basis to prevent sodium retention in the body and consequent edema. Measurements of the sodium level in serum and urine, if urine is being excreted, should be made regularly as a guide in dietary sodium prescription.

Restriction of Potassium and Phosphate.   Hyperkalemia poses a real danger of cardiac arrhythmias and eventual failure of the heart. Potassium intake should not exceed that lost from the body in order to avoid an excess. As with sodium, repeated measurement of the potassium level in serum and urine should act as a guide in setting the dietary prescription.

Hyperphosphatemia and hypocalcemia are characteristic of uremia, because of phosphate retention and decreased calcium absorption, and produce secondary hyperparathyroidism. This eventually leads to osteodystrophy. On low-protein diets, phosphates are also likely to be limited. When higher protein intakes are appropriate, as in the case of patients undergoing dialysis, dietary phosphorus may need to be decreased somewhat by limiting milk and milk products. From metabolic studies of uremic patients fed low-protein diets, Kopple and Coburn (1973) reported that the point of neutral balance on daily phosphorus intake occurred at a level of 700 mg. Calcium intakes were low in these patients, however.

Schoolwerth and Engle (1975) recommended restriction of dietary phosphorus, possibly in a stepwise fashion proportional to the decrease in GFR. This can be achieved through reduction in dietary protein or by giving aluminum hydroxide or aluminum carbonate gels. Popovtzer et al. (1975) maintained normal serum calcium and phosphorus levels of three patients with advanced renal disease by use of phosphate-binding gels and orally given calcium carbonate.

Adequate Caloric Intake.   With inadequate caloric intake, catabolism of the body's protein tissue occurs, adding to the burden of nitrogenous wastes in the uremic patient. The end products of metabolism for fats and carbohydrates are carbon dioxide and water and thus no additional burden for excretion is imposed when these nutrients are consumed in relatively large amounts. The renal patient must be encouraged to consume an appropriate caloric level.

Hypertriglyceridemia has been reported to occur in patients with moderate or severe uremia as well as in those undergoing chronic hemodialysis. A decrease in lipoprotein lipase activity has also been demonstrated. McCosh et al. (1975) found that both very low density lipoproteins and chylomicrons contributed to the hypertriglyceridemia in patients who had not undergone dialysis. Much of the carbohydrate in the low-protein diets often consumed by these patients is from disaccharides, particularly sucrose. It was suggested that dietary carbohydrate may influence the development of hypertriglyceridemia although other factors may also contribute.

Vitamin Nutrition.   Low-protein diets often do not supply recommended amounts of essential vitamins and supplementation is usual. Since at least some water-soluble vitamins are lost from the blood during hemodialysis, patients undergoing this treatment should receive vitamin supplements.

Some special problems of vitamin nutrition have been noted in renal failure. Vitamin D deficiency results from the inability of the damaged kidney to produce the active analog, 1,25-dihydroxyvitamin D_3. Administration of this compound to patients with renal failure has been reported to increase calcium absorption, decrease plasma parathyroid hormone levels, and improve lesions of osteomalacia (Brickman et al., 1974a and b). From a study of 22 patients with chronic renal failure, Eastwood et al. (1976) concluded that osteomalacia results from a lack of 25-hydroxyvitamin D_3 superimposed on an existing deficiency of 1,25-dihydroxyvitamin D_3, rather than from lack of the latter compound alone. Potter et al. (1974) have reported on the successful treatment of bone disease in 17 dialyzed children by doses of vitamin D ranging from 32,000 to 57,000 IU per day over periods of 5 to 13 months.

Metabolism of vitamin B_6 may be altered in renal failure and the requirement for this vitamin may be increased. Reduced plasma levels of pyridoxal phosphate (PLP) and glutamic oxaloacetic transaminase (which requires PLP as a cofactor), as well as erythrocyte levels of glutamic pyruvic transminase have been reported in uremic patients, both dialyzed and undialyzed (Stone et al., 1975). For dialyzed patients, 5 mg pyridoxine per day, in addition to that found in the food consumed, appears to be an optimal dosage (Swendseid, 1977).

The anemia commonly associated with renal failure is apparently not due to folic acid deficiency (Paine et al., 1976). Lack of erythropoietin production by the kidney is the major factor in its development. Although no replacement for renal erythropoietin is available, and the anemia is refractory to treatment, Higgins et al. (1977) suggested that substantial improvement in hemoglobin concentration can be achieved by use of dialyzers with low residual blood volumes to minimize blood loss during dialysis, avoidance of bilateral nephrectomy wherever possible, and use of deionized water for dialysis. Use of tap water containing chloramine (oxidant compounds containing chlorine and ammonia, used as bactericidal agents in urban water supplies) was reported to contribute to erythrocyte destruction.

Dietary Management of Children with Uremia

Treatment of children with chronic renal failure presents special problems, both physiologically and psychologically. Young children cannot understand the importance of dietary compliance and often their parents find it difficult to enforce strict control (Berger, 1977). Diets should be adapted to the individual needs of the child with consideration for social and cultural differences.

Growth retardation is characteristic of children with chronic renal insufficiency. Spinozzi and Grupe (1977) listed several factors that may contribute to this impaired growth. They include undernutrition; osteodystrophy; acidosis; hyposthenuria (decreased osmolality of the urine); depletion of sodium, phosphate, magnesium, zinc, and potassium; chronic infection; and hypertension. Since growth is an energy-requiring process, it is extremely important that adequate caloric intake be maintained. Adequate protein intake will not provide for normal growth unless caloric levels are also adequate.

Spinozzi and Grupe (1977) suggested that the nutritional rehabilitation of children with renal insufficiency requires a caloric intake of at least 80 percent of the recommended allowances and probably more; protein intake of 1.5 to 2 g per kg per day with emphasis on protein foods of high biological value; and prompt attention to renal osteodystrophy by appropriate control of vitamin D, calcium, phosphorus, and acidosis. The ability of the kidney to handle salt, osmoles, and fluid must also be considered as well as the usual presence of anorexia. This requires the active involvement of sensitive, knowledgeable personnel.

24.6 Dialysis

Dialysis involves the diffusion of dissolved particles across a semipermeable membrane from one fluid compartment to another. Two different types of dialysis processes have been used for patients with renal failure. Hemodialysis is most commonly employed, with a semipermeable membrane separating the blood from a dialysate bath as the blood circulates outside the body. In peritoneal dialysis, the peritoneum may be considered a semipermeable membrane. A dialyzing solution is instilled into the peritoneal cavity and an exchange of solutes and water across the peritoneal membrane occurs. Indwelling peritoneal tubes may be placed. Although peritoneal dialysis is much less widely used than hemodialysis, there are occasions when it is the most appropriate treatment for selected patients with chronic renal failure (Rae and Pendray, 1973).

Hemodialysis

In hemodialysis, the patient's blood is cleansed of accumulated waste products by pumping it through a semipermeable membrane compartment that has dialysate solution circulating around the outside. By-products of cellular metabolism are removed from the blood by processes of diffusion, osmosis, and ultrafiltration. The dialysate solution contains a certain concentration of electrolytes, usually similar to that found in extracellular fluid. When these substances are present in higher concentrations in the patient's blood, they diffuse into the dialysate, which is constantly or periodically changed to maintain a lower concentration. Urea, uric acid, and creatinine diffuse from the blood into the dialysate solution. Applying a negative pressure to the dialysate will pull extra water from the patient's blood by ultrafiltration.

Several types of dialyzers are available (Kolff, 1972; U.S. Department of Health, Education and Welfare, 1971). These include (1) parallel-flow or flat-plate dialyzers with cellophane envelopes arranged in parallel and held between rigid supports; (2) coil dialyzers with one or two long cellophane (or other membrane) tubes held by plastic mesh and rolled into small, compact coils; and (3) capillary dialyzers with specially made fine capillaries attached in parallel in the blood circuit allowing a small volume of blood to be exposed to a very large dialyzing surface area.

There must be adequate access to the circulation for repeated hemodialysis. One method is to surgically insert one end of a silastic teflon cannula into an artery in the arm or leg and the other end in a nearby vein. Blood then flows continuously through the cannula from the artery to the vein. During dialysis the connection is opened and the patient is attached to the dialyzer. A second method employs a surgically created subcutaneous arterial-venous fistula between an artery and a nearby vein in either the arm or the leg. Blood is shunted from the artery to the vein thus producing veins engorged with a high-blood flow which can then be easily punctured with large-bore needles. At the time of dialysis, two needles are inserted into the vein as the patient is attached to the dialyzer.

A number of dialysis centers have been established to handle patients with renal failure. Many patients, however, are dialyzed less expensively at home after an appropriate training program (Blagg, 1972; Rae et al., 1972).

Dietary Management of the Dialyzed Patient.   Approximately 32,000 patients were on maintenance hemodialysis in 1977, with predictions that this number will increase to about 55,000 within a few years (Burton, 1977). Personalized and careful dietary supervision is necessary for successful dialysis treatment, which usually involves three weekly dialyses. Nitrogenous waste products and excess fluid accumulate in the body when renal function is severely impaired and are removed by dialysis. Large amounts of dietary protein will increase the nitrogenous waste load. Sodium and potassium should be maintained at desirable levels by diet. All or most of renal function is usually lost after maintenance dialysis has been instituted.

A protein intake of 1 g per kg ideal body weight will maintain positive nitrogen balance, replace amino acids lost in dialysis, and will not produce excessive amounts of nitrogenous waste products between periods of dialysis (Burton, 1974b; Comty, 1968). At least three-fourths of the protein should come from sources of high biological value, such as eggs, meat, poultry, and fish. Milk is used only in small amounts because of its high potassium, sodium, phosphate, and fluid content. Wineman et al. (1977) pointed out the relationship between the patient's net urea generation rate and his protein catabolic rate which, assuming nitrogen balance, is related to his dietary protein intake. They have successfully used these relationships in dietary control and counseling of patients on maintenance dialysis.

Carbohydrates and fats must be generously supplied to provide energy for daily activities and to spare protein. Tissue building and weight gain can usually be achieved with 45 kcal per kg ideal body weight and 35 to 45 kcal per kg are often prescribed (Burton, 1974b). Carbohydrate foods of low-protein content should be chosen since protein in grains and starchy vegetables is usually of relatively low biological value. Soybeans are an exception.

Dietary potassium is commonly restricted to 52 meq (2028 mg) daily if the dialysate bath contains 2.6 meq potassium (Burton, 1974b). Sodium restriction is individualized to prevent extracellular overhydration leading to hypertension and heart failure (Comty, 1968). Levels of dietary sodium between 65 and 87 meq (1500 to 2000 mg) daily are often prescribed. Potassium restriction is difficult because most foods contain potassium. Fruits and vegetables are fairly high in both potassium and fluid and must be carefully selected and measured. Tsaltas (1969) described a procedure for leaching vegetables in water for 2 hours before cooking in five volumes of water to remove substantial amounts of potassium. The vegetables may then be prepared in any manner desired. Potatoes were very successfully treated in this manner. When they were sliced before leaching, the potassium content decreased from 200 to 300 mg/100 g to 90 mg/100 g.

Fluid restriction is extremely important and often very difficult for the dialysis patient. Usually 300 to 500 ml are permitted daily, plus an amount equal to urine output (if any) (Burton, 1974b). A daily weight gain of 1 lb between dialyses usually results from mild fluid retention.

Since the water-soluble vitamins are relatively small molecules, it has been suspected that many of them are lost through the dialysis membrane. Vitamin supplements are commonly given to dialyzed patients. Sullivan and Eisenstein (1972) reported a decline in plasma and leukocyte ascorbic acid levels in 16 patients receiving long-term hemodialysis therapy. This loss could be prevented by addition of the vitamin to the dialysate concentrate. Rostand (1976) found that serum vitamin B_{12} concentrations of 60 patients undergoing hemodialysis were significantly lower than those of a nondialyzed group with renal failure. However, Niwa et al. (1975) reported that plasma thiamin levels in patients on long-term hemodialysis were not different from those found in normal subjects.

Potential renal osteodystrophy remains an important problem for the dialyzed patient (Goldsmith and Johnson, 1973). Elevated plasma phosphorus can be controlled by giving aluminum hydroxide or aluminum carbonate orally to bind phosphate in the gut and/or by dietary restriction. Serum calcium can be controlled by providing oral supplements of calcium, treatment with vitamin D or its active analogs, and/or by increasing the amount of calcium in the dialysate bath (up to 7 to 8 mg/100 ml).

Cardiovascular disease is the leading cause of death among patients undergoing chronic hemodialysis therapy. Between 40 and 60 percent of all such deaths have been from cardiovascular causes (Lowrie et al., 1974; Lindner et al., 1974). The reasons for these complications are not clear but many cardiovascular risk factors have a high prevalence among the dialyzed population. These include hypertension, hyperlipidemia, hyperuricemia, glucose intolerance, and vascular calcification due to secondary hyperparathyroidism. The phenotypic Type IV pattern of plasma lipids is often found although other types have been noted. Hyperlipidemia is also a frequent finding in pediatric patients treated with maintenance hemodialysis (Pennisi et al., 1976). Further investigation into the metabolic abnormalities that lead to hyperlipidemia would be helpful.

24.7   Basic Diet Patterns

Compliance with dietary and fluid instructions is extremely important for a patient on dialysis since the consequences of noncompliance may be life-threatening. Blackburn (1977) reported that in a population of 53 subjects, approximately 75 percent were compliant as indicated by serum potassium levels; 60 percent were compliant as indicated by serum phosphorus levels; and 49 percent were compliant as indicated by between-dialyses weight gains. She suggested that the problem confronting the medical team caring for patients in dialysis seems to be one of motivation. The problem of how to motivate patients to comply has not been solved. Effective dietary instruction may be of some help but many other factors are undoubtedly involved. Lawson et al. (1976) found that some positive behavioral changes in dietary adherence were apparent among 16 dialyzed patients after completing an audiotutorial program on diet.

In order to improve patient dietary compliance and simplify the nutritional instruction process, various basic diet patterns and groupings of foods in terms of protein, sodium, and potassium content have been developed (Robinson and Paulbitski, 1972; Stein and Winn, 1972; de St. Jeor et al., 1970; de St. Jeor et al., 1969; Jordan et al., 1967). Table 24.1 lists one such grouping of foods which may be used in developing individualized diet patterns for patients with renal insufficiency, with or without dialysis.

Table 24.1 FOOD GROUPINGS FOR APPROXIMATE EQUIVALENCY IN PROTEIN, SODIUM, AND POTASSIUM[a] (Food within each group may be exchanged or substituted for one another.)

Food Groups				
Exchanges	**Amount**	**Protein (g)**	**Sodium (mg)**	**Potassium (mg)**
Milk	$\frac{1}{2}$ cup	4.0	60	170
Vegetables				
Group 1	Varies	1.0	Negligible[b]	120
Group 2	Varies	1.0	Negligible[b]	240
Fruit				
Group 1	Varies	0.5	Negligible	100
Group 2	Varies	0.5	Negligible	200
Bread, starch, and cereal	Varies	2.0	Negligible[b]	70
Meat				
Group 1	Varies	6.0	40	70
Group 2	Varies	8.0	25	120
Fats	As desired			
Miscellaneous	As desired			

Food Exchange Lists for Controlled Protein, Sodium, Potassium Diets

Exchange	**Amount**	**Exchange**	**Amount**
Milk		**Vegetables[d]**	
Cream, light	$\frac{1}{2}$ cup	Group 1	
Cream, heavy	$\frac{3}{4}$ cup	Beans, green or wax, fresh or	
Cream, sour	$\frac{1}{2}$ cup	frozen	$\frac{1}{2}$ cup
Half & half	$\frac{1}{2}$ cup	Beans, green or wax, canned	$\frac{1}{2}$ cup
Ice cream, any flavor, without		Bean sprouts, cooked	$\frac{1}{2}$ cup
nuts	$\frac{2}{3}$ cup	Beets, canned	$\frac{1}{2}$ cup
Milk, evaporated	$\frac{1}{4}$ cup	Carrots, canned	$\frac{1}{2}$ cup
Milk, whole	$\frac{1}{2}$ cup	Corn, canned	$\frac{1}{2}$ cup
Yogurt, plain	$\frac{1}{2}$ cup	Corn, frozen	$\frac{1}{2}$ cup
Bread and Starch		Cucumbers, raw	$\frac{1}{2}$ medium
Beans:		Lettuce, iceberg	$\frac{3}{4}$ cup,
White	2 tbs		1 med.
Red	2 tbs		wedge
Pinto, Calico	2 tbs	Lettuce, loose leaf	$\frac{1}{2}$ cup
Bread, LS[c]	1 slice	Mushrooms, raw	$\frac{1}{2}$ cup
Cooked cereals:		Onion, cooked	$\frac{1}{2}$ cup
Cornmeal, LS	$\frac{3}{4}$ cup	Onion, green, raw	2–5″ long
Farina (Cream of Wheat), LS	$\frac{2}{3}$ cup	Parsley	15 small
Malt-o-Meal, LS	$\frac{1}{2}$ cup		sprigs
Maypo, instant, LS	$\frac{1}{4}$ cup	Peas, canned	$\frac{1}{2}$ cup
Oatmeal, LS	$\frac{1}{2}$ cup	Peas, fresh, cooked	$\frac{1}{3}$ cup
Pettijohns, LS	$\frac{1}{2}$ cup	Peas, frozen	$\frac{1}{2}$ cup

Table 24.1 FOOD GROUPINGS FOR APPROXIMATE EQUIVALENCY IN PROTEIN, SODIUM, AND POTASSIUM (cont'd.)

Food Exchange Lists for Controlled Protein, Sodium, Potassium Diets

Exchange	Amount	Exchange	Amount
Bread and Starch		**Vegetables**	
Cooked Cereals (cont'd.)		Group 1 (cont'd.)	
Ralston, LS	$\frac{1}{2}$ cup	Rutabagas, fresh, cooked	$\frac{1}{2}$ cup
Rice Cereal, LS	1 cup	Watercress	30 sprigs
Wheat, whole, cracked, LS	$\frac{1}{3}$ cup		
Dry cereals:		**Group 2**	
Corn Flakes, LS	1 cup	Asparagus, canned or fresh	$\frac{1}{2}$ cup
Puffed Rice	2 cups	Beets[e], red, fresh, cooked	$\frac{1}{2}$ cup
Puffed Wheat	1 cup	Broccoli	$\frac{1}{4}$ cup
Rice Flakes, LS	$1\frac{1}{3}$ cup	Cabbage, cooked	$\frac{1}{2}$ cup
Rice Krispies, LS	1 cup	Cabbage, raw	$\frac{2}{3}$ cup
Shredded Wheat	1 biscuit	Carrots[e], cooked	$\frac{1}{2}$ cup
Wheat Flakes, LS	$\frac{2}{3}$ cup	Cauliflower, cooked, frozen	$\frac{1}{2}$ cup
Crackers, LS	3 crackers	Corn, fresh	1–4'' cob
Macaroni, LS	$\frac{1}{4}$ cup	Eggplant	$\frac{1}{2}$ cup
Noodles, LS	$\frac{1}{4}$ cup	Greens[e] (chard, kale, mustard,	
Rice, LS	$\frac{2}{3}$ cup	spinach)	$\frac{1}{4}$ cup
Spaghetti, LS	$\frac{1}{3}$ cup	Lima beans	$\frac{1}{2}$ cup
		Pepper, green, raw	1 large shell
Fruit		Potato, boiled, and mashed	$\frac{1}{3}$ cup
Group 1		Squash, summer	$\frac{1}{2}$ cup
Fruits:		Squash, winter, boiled	$\frac{1}{3}$ cup
Apple, raw	1 small	Sweet potato, canned	$\frac{1}{2}$ cup
Applesauce	$\frac{1}{2}$ cup	Tomato, fresh	1 small
Blueberries, canned, fresh,		Tomato, canned	$\frac{1}{2}$ cup
frozen	$\frac{1}{2}$ cup	Turnip, boiled	$\frac{2}{3}$ cup
Boysenberries, frozen	$\frac{1}{2}$ cup	**Meat**	
Cherries, Bing or Royal Ann,		**Group 1**	
canned	$\frac{1}{2}$ cup	Egg	1 medium
	(10 cherries)	Tuna and salmon, canned in	
Cranberries, fresh	1 cup	water	$\frac{1}{4}$ cup
Cranberry sauce	1 cup	Lobster or shrimp, fresh or	
Gooseberries, canned	$\frac{1}{2}$ cup	canned in water	1 oz
Loganberries, canned	$\frac{1}{3}$ cup	Oysters, canned	2 oz
Pears, canned	2 halves	Clams	$1\frac{1}{2}$ oz
Pineapple, canned	1 large ring		
Pineapple, fresh, frozen	$\frac{1}{2}$ cup	**Group 2**	
Peaches, canned or frozen	$\frac{1}{3}$ cup or	Beef, lamb, liver	1 oz
	2 med.	Chicken, turkey	1 oz
	halves	Fish, fresh water	1 oz
Raspberries, red, fresh,		Cod	1 oz
frozen	$\frac{1}{3}$ cup	Salmon	1 oz
Tangerine, fresh	1 medium	Cheese, Cellu low sodium	1 oz
Watermelon	$\frac{1}{2}$ cup	Cottage cheese, low sodium	$\frac{1}{4}$ cup
Fruit Juices:		Fats[f] (use as desired)	
Apple juice	$\frac{1}{3}$ cup	Unsalted butter or margarine	
Cranberry juice	2 cups	Oil	
Grape juice drink	1 cup	Unsalted shortening	
Lemonade	1 cup	Salad dressing: oil and vinegar	

Table 24.1 FOOD GROUPINGS FOR APPROXIMATE EQUIVALENCY IN PROTEIN, SODIUM, AND POTASSIUM (*cont'd.*)

Food Exchange Lists for Controlled Protein, Sodium, Potassium Diets

Exchange	Amount	Exchange	Amount
Fruit		**Fruit**	
Group 1 (cont'd.)		Group 2 (cont'd.)	
Peach nectar	$\frac{1}{2}$ cup	Fruit Juices:	
Pear nectar	1 cup	Apricot nectar	$\frac{1}{2}$ cup
Pineapple-grapefruit drink	$\frac{2}{3}$ cup	Grape juice, canned, frozen	$\frac{2}{3}$ cup
Pineapple-orange drink	$\frac{1}{2}$ cup	Grapefruit juice	$\frac{1}{2}$ cup
		Orange juice	$\frac{1}{2}$ cup
Group 2		Pineapple juice	$\frac{1}{2}$ cup
Fruits:			
Apricots, canned	3 med. halves	**Miscellaneous**[f] (use as desired)	
Blackberries, canned, fresh,		Coffee or tea (limit according to sodium content	
frozen	$\frac{3}{4}$ cup	of water)	
Cherries, Bing or Royal Anne,		Gingerale, Coca Cola, root beer, 7-Up,	
fresh, frozen	$\frac{3}{4}$ cup	lemonade, limeade, Pepsi Cola, Royal Crown	
Figs, canned	3 medium	Cola	
Figs, fresh	2 medium	Tapioca, dry	
Fruit cocktail, canned	$\frac{1}{2}$ cup	Hard candy, gum drops, jelly beans, fondants,	
Grapes, canned, fresh	$\frac{3}{4}$ cup	lollipops	
Grapefruit, canned	$\frac{1}{2}$ cup	Honey, jams, jellies	
Lemon, peeled, fresh	1 medium	Popsicles	
Nectarine, fresh	1 medium	Sugar, corn syrup	
Peach, fresh	1 medium	Vinegar	
Pear, fresh	1 small	Spices not containing sodium	
Plums, canned	3 medium	Herbs	
Plums, fresh	2	Pepper	
Rhubarb, fresh, frozen	$\frac{1}{3}$ cup	Low-protein bread, muffins	
Strawberries, fresh, frozen	$\frac{3}{4}$ cup	Wheatstarch cookies	

[a] Adapted from Utah Dietetic Association. 1977. *Handbook of Clinical Dietetics*, 2d ed. Salt Lake City, Utah: c/o Utah Hospital Association, Suite 10, 455 East 400 South.

[b] Low sodium

[c] LS = low sodium

[d] Vegetables are to be frozen, fresh, or low sodium canned. Potassium is leached from vegetables boiled, without skin, cut in slices, and cooked in large amounts of water.

[e] These vegetables contain an average of 25 mg sodium per serving.

[f] Foods in these groups contain only small amounts of protein, sodium, and potassium but are important sources of calories.

24.8 Renal Calculi (Kidney stones)

Renal calculi represent one of the oldest known medical afflictions. However, much yet remains to be learned about their pathogenesis and treatment. They are found throughout the world. No race or geographic area has been entirely free of them but the incidence is greatest in southern China, parts of India, northern Thailand, Arabia, and Iraq (Boyce, 1960). A large series of studies on bladder stone disease in Thailand have been published in recent years (Valyasevi et al., 1973; Halstead and Valyasevi,

1967). In the United States, nephrolithiasis (presence of renal calculi) accounts for one hospitalization per 1000. In addition there are numerous office and emergency-room visits for renal colic (Williams, 1974).

A large proportion of patients who form renal calculi have no recognized local or systemic disease that would account for them. Diet has been suggested as a possible factor in the etiology of such calculi but specific data are few. A protein-poor, predominantly rice diet among villagers in parts of Thailand has been associated with a high incidence of renal calculi, especially among male children. In experimental animals, urinary calculi have been produced by deficiencies of vitamin A, thiamin, magnesium, or phosphate (Boyce, 1960).

Composition of Calculi

Calculi consist of a matrix and crystalline material. It is not known whether the matrix component can be formed entirely from nonspecific proteinaceous material and cellular debris present in urine or requires specific compounds. Several crystalloids, e.g., calcium, magnesium, phosphate, oxalate, and urate, are present in urine in concentrations exceeding those achievable in water, thus creating a supersaturated state. Other urinary constituents, including urea, sodium, potassium, chloride, and organic acids, contribute to the maintenance of the supersaturation without precipitation and certain inhibitors to crystallization of calcium salts have also been detected in urine. The formation of stones may depend on the presence of metastable concentrations of crystalloids and also on a component to promote the aggregation of crystals (Beeson and McDermott, 1975, p. 1165).

In the United States, two-thirds of all renal stones are composed of either calcium oxalate or calcium oxalate mixed with calcium phosphate in the form of hydroxyapatite. Stones composed of magnesium ammonium phosphate (struvite) account for 15 percent of all renal calculi. They usually occur in patients with recurrent urinary tract infections and persistently alkaline urine. About 10 percent of stones contain uric acid or cystine as the major component (Williams, 1974).

Pathogenesis

Several theories have been proposed to explain the formation and growth of renal calculi and have been reviewed by Williams (1974). The precipitation-crystallization theory suggests that supersaturation of urinary crystalloids eventually leads to their precipitation and growth. The matrix-nucleation theory assumes that some matrix substance forms an initial nucleus for subsequent stone growth by precipitation. The inhibitor-absence theory suggests that stones form because of the absence in the urine of inhibitors of crystal formation such as pyrophosphate, mucopolysaccharides, small polypeptides, certain amino acids, magnesium, and so on. The precipitation-crystallization theory is probably most widely accepted but additional data are needed to support each of the theories.

morbid state of unknown cause

Dietary Implications of Treatment

The crystalline composition of renal calculi should be determined as an indication of pathogenesis and guide to treatment. However, regardless of the type of stone, dilution of the urine by an increased fluid intake, particularly at night, is an important component of treatment.

When idiopathic hypercalciuria is present in a recurrent stone-former, dietary treatment may include a low-calcium, low-vitamin-D regimen. Milk, cheese, and other milk products are limited to the equivalent of a maximum of 2 cups of milk daily and foods fortified with vitamin D are excluded (Mayer, 1969).

When hypercalciuria is not present in patients who form calcium oxalate stones, lowering dietary calcium intake as the only dietary modification is probably undesirable since this type of diet tends to raise urine oxalate levels (Williams, 1974). Dietary oxalate, as well as calcium, should probably be decreased in this case. Marshall et al. (1972), in a short-term study involving both normal and renal-stone-forming subjects, found that a significant fall in the urinary calcium oxalate activity product was produced by a low-calcium, low-oxalate diet. In this study, the daily calcium intake was 250 mg and that of oxalate was 50 mg. The optimum level of dietary calcium has not been determined.

In the genetic syndromes of primary hyperoxaluria there appears to be increased biosynthesis of oxalate (Hagler and Herman, 1973). Treatment has been directed toward inhibiting stone formation by giving pyrophosphate or magnesium oxide. Pyridoxine is a cofactor in transmination reactions that affect oxalate metabolism and deficiency of this vitamin may lead to increased oxalate production in the body. High-dose pyridoxine therapy reduces oxalate excretion in some patients (Williams, 1974).

Small bowell disease causes an increase in oxalate absorption with secondary hyperoxaluria. Reduction in dietary oxalate intake should be useful in this case. Piepmeyer (1974) reviewed the problems of obtaining accurate information on the oxalate content of food. Highest concentrations of oxalic acid are found in tea leaves, spinach, rhubarb, parsley, beetroot, and cocoa.

Altering the urinary pH by medication and also by the use of acid- or alkaline-ash diets has been tried for many years. Uric acid and cystine stones are soluble in alkaline urine and alkalinization of the urine is effective in retarding formation of these stones. Decreased dietary purine intake may also be of some value in the control of urate stones (see Table 19.2 for purine content of food). Acidification of the urine is appropriate for recurrent magnesium ammonium phosphate stone formers, along with treatment of any urinary tract infections. The urinary pH probably has little effect on calcium oxalate stones (Williams, 1974).

Although the use of medication is more effective than diet alone in acidifying or alkalizing the urine, the diet should support the medication. The ash of a diet, after oxidation in the body of organic components, may be predominantly base-forming elements, such as sodium, potassium, calcium, magnesium, and so forth, or it may be chiefly acid-forming end-products such as phosphates and sulfates. Foods with alkaline ash include fruits and vegetables (with the exception of prunes, plums, cranberries, and corn), navy and lima beans, molasses, and almonds. The ash of milk has a slight alkaline preponderance. On an alkaline-ash diet these foods should be emphasized, whereas breads, cereals, meat, fish, and poultry should be limited.

Foods with acid ash include breads, cereals, peanuts, walnuts, lentils, meat, fish, poultry, corn, prunes, plums, and cranberries. Daily intake should include no more than 2 cups of milk, 2 servings of fruits, and 2 servings of vegetables. No products containing soda or baking powder should be consumed.

REFERENCES

1. Bailey, G. L. and N. R. Sullivan. 1968. Selected-protein diet in terminal uremia. *J. Am. Dietet. Assoc.*, **52:** 125.

2. Beeson, P. B. and W. McDermott (Eds.). 1975. Textbook of Medicine, vol. II, 14th ed. Philadelphia: Saunders.

3. Berger, M. 1977. Dietary management of children with uremia. *J. Am. Dietet. Assoc.*, **70:** 498.

4. Berlyne, G. M., A. B. Shaw, and S. Nilwarangkur. 1965. Dietary treatment of chronic renal failure: Experiences with a modified Giovannetti diet. *Nephron*, **2:** 129.

5. Blackburn, S. L. 1977. Dietary compliance of chronic hemodialysis patients. *J. Am. Dietet. Assoc.*, **70:** 31.

6. Blagg, C. R. 1972. Home hemodialysis. *Am. J. Med. Sci.* **264:** 168.

7. Boyce, W. H. 1960. Nutrition and the formation of urinary calculi. *Borden's Review of Nutrition Research*, **21** (No. 3): 27.

8. Brickman, A. S., J. W. Coburn, S. G. Massry, and A. W. Norman. 1974a. 1,25 dihydroxy-vitamin D_3 in normal man and patients with renal failure. *Ann. Int. Med.*, **80:** 161.

9. Brickman, A. S., D. J. Sherrard, J. Jowsey, F. R. Singer, D. J. Baylink, N. Maloney, S. G. Massry, A. W. Norman, and J. W. Coburn. 1974b. 1,25-dihydroxycholecalciferol. Effect on skeletal lesions and plasma parathyroid hormone levels in uremic osteodystrophy. *Arch. Int. Med.*, **134:** 883.

10. Burton, B. T. 1977. Nutritional implications of renal disease. I. Current overview and general principles. *J. Am. Dietet. Assoc.*, **70:** 479.

11. Burton, B. T. 1974a. Current concepts of nutrition and diet in diseases of the kidney. I. General principles of dietary management. *J. Am. Dietet. Assoc.*, **65:** 623.

12. Burton, B. T. 1974b. Current concepts of nutrition and diet in diseases of the kidney. II. Dietary regimen in specific kidney disorders. *J. Am. Dietet. Assoc.*, **65:** 627.

13. Carmena, R. and F. L. Shapiro. 1972. Dietary management of chronic renal failure. Experience at Hennepin County General Hospital. *Geriatrics*, **27** (Mar.): 95.

14. Coburn, J. W., D. L. Hartenbower, and A. S. Brickman. 1976. Advances in vitamin D metabolism as they pertain to chronic renal disease. *Am. J. Clin. Nutr.*, **29:** 1283.

15. Comty, C. M. 1968. Long-term dietary management of dialysis patients. I. Pathologic problems and dietary requirements. *J. Am. Dietet. Assoc.*, **53:** 439.

16. de St. Jeor, S. T., B. J. Carlston, S. Christensen, R. K. Maddock, Jr., and F. H. Tyler. 1970. *Low Protein Diets for the Treatment of Chronic Renal Failure.* Salt Lake City, Utah: University of Utah Press.

17. de St. Jeor, S. T., B. J. Carlston, and F. H. Tyler. 1969. Planning low-protein diets for use in chronic renal failure. *J. Am. Dietet. Assoc.,* **54:** 32.

18. Department of Health, Education and Welfare. 1971. Hemodialysis manual. DHEW Publication No. (HSM) 72–7002.

19. Eastwood, J. B., T. C. B. Stamp, E. Harris, and H. E. de Wardener. 1976. Vitamin-D deficiency in the osteomalacia of chronic renal failure. *Lancet,* **2:** 1209.

20. Franklin, S. S., A. Gordon, C. R. Kleeman, and M. H. Maxwell. 1967. Use of a balanced low-protein diet in chronic renal failure. *J. Am. Med. Assoc.,* **202:** 477.

21. Giordano, C. 1963. Use of exogenous and endogenous urea for protein synthesis in normal and uremic subjects. *J. Lab. Clin. Med.,* **62:** 231.

22. Giovannetti, S. and Q. Maggiore. 1964. A low-nitrogen diet with proteins of high biological value for severe chronic uraemia. *Lancet,* **1:** 1000.

23. Goldsmith, R. S. and W. J. Johnson. 1973. Role of phosphate depletion and high dialysate calcium in controlling dialytic renal osteodystrophy. *Kidney Internat.,* **4:** 154.

24. Goodhart, R. S. and M. E. Shils, eds. 1973. *Modern Nutrition in Health and Disease,* 5th ed. Philadelphia: Lea and Febiger.

25. Hagler, L. and R. H. Herman. 1973. Oxalate metabolism. *Am. J. Clin. Nutr.,* **26:** 1242.

26. Halstead, S. B. and A. Valyasevi. 1967. Studies of bladder stone disease in Thailand. III. Epidemiologic studies in Ubol Province. *Am. J. Clin. Nutr.,* **20:** 1329.

27. Higgins, M. R., M. Grace, R. A. Ulan, D. S. Silverberg, K. B. Bettcher, and J. B. Dossetor. 1977. Anemia in hemodialysis patients. *Arch. Int. Med.,* **137:** 172.

28. Jamison, R. L. and R. H. Maffly. 1976. The urinary concentrating mechanism. *N. Eng. J. Med.,* **295:** 1059.

29. Jordan, W. L., J. E. Cimino, A. C. Grist, G. E. McMahon, and M. M. Doyle. 1967. Basic pattern for a controlled protein, sodium, and potassium diet. *J. Am. Dietet. Assoc.,* **50:** 137.

30. Kolff, W. J. 1972. Hemodialysis in the management of renal disease. *Ann. Rev. Med.,* **23:** 321.

31. Kopple, J. D. and M. E. Swendseid. 1974. Nitrogen balance and plasma amino acid levels in uremic patients fed an essential amino acid diet. *Am. J. Clin. Nutr.,* **27:** 806.

32. Lawson, V. K., M. N. Traylor, and M. R. Gram. 1976. An audio-tutorial aid for dietary instruction in renal dialysis. *J. Am. Dietet. Assoc.,* **69:** 390.

33. Lindner, A., B. Charra, D. J. Sherrard, and B. H. Scribner. 1974. Accelerated atherosclerosis in prolonged maintenance hemodialysis. *N. Eng. J. Med.,* **290:** 697.

34. Lonergan, E. T. and K. Lange. 1968. Use of a special protein-restricted diet in uremia. *Am. J. Clin. Nutr.,* **21:** 595.

35. Lowrie, E. G., J. M. Lazarus, C. L. Hampers, and J. P. Merrill. 1974. Cardiovascular disease in dialysis patients. *N. Eng. J. Med.,* **290:** 737.

36. Marshall, R. W., M. Cochran, and A. Hodgkinson. 1972. Relationships between calcium and oxalic acid intake in the diet and their excretion in the urine of normal and renal-stone-forming subjects. *Clin. Sci.,* **43:** 91.

37. Mayer, J. 1969. Nutrition and renal calculi. *Postgrad. Med.,* **46** (No. 2): 209.

38. McCosh, E. J., K. Solangi, J. M. Rivers, and A. Goodman. 1975. Hypertriglyceridemia in patients with chronic renal insufficiency. *Am. J. Clin. Nutr.,* **28:** 1036.

39. Niwa, T., T. Ito, E. Matsui, I. Ishiguro, and S. Kuwata. 1975. Plasma level and transfer

capacity of thiamin in patients undergoing long-term hemodialysis. *Am. J. Clin. Nutr.,* **28:** 1105.

40. Paine, C. J., M. D. Hargrove, Jr., and E. R. Eichner. 1976. Folic acid binding protein and folate balance in uremia. *Arch. Int. Med.,* **136:** 756.

41. Pennisi, A. J., E. T. Heuser, M. R. Mickey, A. Lipsey, M. H. Malekzadeh, and R. N. Fine. 1976. Hyperlipidemia in pediatric hemodialysis and renal transplant patients. *Am. J. Dis. Child.,* **130:** 957.

42. Piepmeyer, J. 1974. Planning diets controlled in oxalic acid content. *J. Am. Dietet. Assoc.,* **65:** 438.

43. Popovtzer, M. M., W. F. Pinggera, and J. B. Robinette. 1975. Secondary hyperparathyroidism. Conservative management in patients with renal insufficiency. *J. Am. Med. Assoc.,* **231:** 960.

44. Potter, D. E., C. J. Wilson, and M. B. Ozonoff. 1974. Hyperparathyroid bone disease in children undergoing long-term hemodialysis; treatment with vitamin D. *J. Ped.,* **85:** 60.

45. Rae, A. and M. Pendray. 1973. Advantages of peritoneal dialysis in chronic renal failure. *J. Am. Med. Assoc.,* **225:** 937.

46. Rae, A., P. Craig, and G. Miles. 1972. Home dialysis: its costs and problems. *C.M.A. Journal,* **106:** 1305.

47. Robinson, L. G. and A. H. Paulbitski. 1972. Diet therapy and educational program for patients with chronic renal failure. *J. Am. Dietet. Assoc.,* **61:** 531.

48. Rostand, S. G. 1976. Vitamin B_{12} levels and nerve conduction velocities in patients undergoing maintenance hemodialysis. *Am. J. Clin. Nutr.,* **29:** 691.

49. Schoolwerth, A. C. and J. E. Engle. 1975. Calcium and phosphorus in diet therapy of uremia. *J. Am. Dietet. Assoc.,* **66:** 460.

50. Spinozzi, N. S. and W. E. Grupe. 1977. Nutritional implications of renal disease. IV. Nutritional aspects of chronic renal insufficiency in childhood. *J. Am. Dietet. Assoc.,* **70:** 493.

51. Stein, P. G. and N. J. Winn. 1972. Diet controlled in sodium, potassium, protein, and fluid: use of points for dietary calculation. *J. Am. Dietet. Assoc.,* **61:** 538.

52. Stone, W. J., L. G. Warnock, and C. Wagner. 1975. Vitamin B_6 deficiency in uremia. *Am. J. Clin. Nutr.,* **28:** 950.

53. Sullivan, J. F. and A. B. Eisenstein. 1972. Ascorbic acid depletion during hemodialysis. *J. Am. Med. Assoc.,* **220:** 1697.

54. Swendseid, M. E. 1977. Nutritional implications of renal disease. III. Nutritional needs of patients with renal disease. *J. Am. Dietet. Assoc.,* **70:** 488.

55. Tsaltas, T. T. 1969. Dietetic management of uremic patients. I. Extraction of potassium from foods for uremic patients. *Am. J. Clin. Nutr.,* **22:** 490.

56. Valyasevi, A., S. Dhanamitta, and R. Van Reen. 1973. Studies of bladder stone disease in Thailand. XVI. Effect of 4-hydroxy-L-proline and orthophosphate supplementations on urinary composition and crystalluria. *Am. J. Clin. Nutr.,* **26:** 1207.

57. Williams, H. E. 1974. Nephrolithiasis. *N. Eng. J. Med.,* **290:** 33.

58. Wineman, R. J., J. A. Sargent, and L. Piercy. 1977. Nutritional implications of renal disease. II. The dietitian's key role in studies of dialysis therapy. *J. Am. Dietet. Assoc.,* **70:** 483.

59. Wintrobe, M. M., G. W. Thorn, R. D. Adams, E. Braunwald, K. J. Isselbacher, and R. G. Petersdorf (Eds.). 1974. *Harrison's Principles of Internal Medicine,* 7th ed. New York: McGraw-Hill.

60. Wright, P. L., P. J. Brereton, and D. E. M. Snell. 1970. Effectiveness of modified Giovannetti diet compared with mixed low-protein diet. *Metabolism,* **19:** 201.

CLIENT REFERENCES

1. Cost, J. S. 1975. Dietary Management of Renal Disease. Thorofare, N.J. 08086: Charles B. Slack, Publisher (6900 Grove Road).

2. de St. Jeor, S. T., B. J. Carlston, S. Christensen, R. K. Maddock, Jr., and F. H. Tyler. 1970. *Low Protein Diets for the Treatment of Chronic Renal Failure.* Salt Lake City, Utah: University of Utah Press.

3. Margie, J. D., C. F. Anderson, R. A. Nelson, and J. C. Hunt. *The Mayo Clinic Renal Diet Cookbook.* New York, N.Y. 10016: National Kidney Foundation (116 East 27th St.).

STUDY GUIDE

The kidneys function to maintain an appropriate interior milieu for all body cells.

1. Review the physiological functions of the normal kidney as it selectively filters blood and concentrates urine.

2. Describe several clinical tests for renal function.

Glomerulonephritis is characterized by inflammation of the glomeruli or immune glomerular injury.

3. Discuss possible relationships between infection and the development of acute glomerulonephritis.

4. Describe clinical signs and symptoms commonly associated with acute glomerulonephritis.

Nutritional care of a patient with glomerulonephritis is particularly important if edema, hypertension, persistent proteinuria, and/or oliguria are present.

5. Describe conditions under which a patient with glomerulonephritis might require a low-sodium diet and explain the rationale behind the use of the diet in each case.

6. Suggest appropriate levels of dietary protein for patients with acute glomerulonephritis and justify the suggestions.

The nephrotic syndrome may occur as a separate entity or as a stage in the progression of other kidney disorders.

7. List the three major characteristics of the nephrotic syndrome; also describe other characteristics often present.

8. Explain reasons for the development of hypoalbuminemia, proteinuria, and edema in patients with the nephrotic syndrome.

9. Outline dietary treatment that might be of benefit to a patient with the nephrotic syndrome and explain the rationale behind the suggestions. Also point out special problems that are likely to occur in implementing the desired dietary prescription.

Most progressive kidney disorders eventually reach a similar end-stage called the uremic syndrome or uremia.

10. Describe abnormal physiological conditions or symptoms commonly found in chronic renal failure and explain the possible underlying cause(s) of these manifestations.

11. Discuss the origin, characteristics, and rationale for G-G diets used in chronic renal failure.

12. Outline the basic principles of dietary treatment for chronic renal failure and suggest appropriate diet prescriptions based on these principles. Write diet patterns and menus.

13. Explain practical problems that a dietitian might encounter in striving for patient compliance with a 20-g protein diet and make suggestions for overcoming these problems.

14. Explain why adequate caloric intake is extremely important in the nutritional care of patients with chronic renal failure, either with or without dialysis.

Dialysis involves the diffusion of dissolved particles across a semipermeable membrane and has been successfully used in treating renal failure.

15. Explain the basic principles involved in hemodialysis and in peritoneal dialysis.

16. Describe several types of dialyzers and mechanisms for gaining access to the patient's circulation for repeated hemodialysis.

The dietary requirements of patients on hemodialysis vary individually with special attention to kilocalories, good quality protein, sodium, potassium, and fluid.

17. Suggest usual appropriate amounts of protein, sodium, potassium, and fluid for patients on maintenance dialysis and explain the rationale behind these suggestions. Write diet patterns.

18. Explain the importance of including a large proportion of the dietary protein from sources of high biological value.

19. Explain why vitamin supplements are commonly given to patients on maintenance hemodialysis as well as to nondialyzed patients with chronic renal failure.

20. Explain why patients on dialysis need to be carefully watched and treated on an individual basis for anemia and for bone problems.

21. Describe appropriate food groupings for use in developing basic diet patterns in the nutritional care of patients with chronic renal failure and explain the rationale behind these groupings.

Renal calculi may vary in chemical composition but knowledge of the composition is important in determining treatment.

22. Describe and discuss several theories that have been proposed to explain the pathogenesis of renal calculi.

23. Suggest and justify possible appropriate uses for the following diet prescriptions in the nutritional care of patients with renal calculi.
    (*a*) Low calcium, low vitamin D
    (*b*) Low calcium, low oxalate
    (*c*) High-dose pyridoxine therapy
    (*d*) Low oxalate
    (*e*) Acid-ash
    (*f*) Alkaline-ash

Appendix

Normal Laboratory Values*

Hematologic Values

Cell Counts

Erythrocytes: Males   4.6– 6.2 million/mm^3

           Females   4.2– 5.4 million/mm^3

           Children (varies with age)   4.5– 5.1 million/mm^3

Leukocytes

     Total   5000– 10,000/mm^3

     Differential

	Percentage	
Myelocytes	0	0/mm^3
Juvenile neutrophils	3– 5	150– 400/mm^3
Segmented neutrophils	54– 62	3000– 5,800/mm^3
Lymphocytes	25– 33	1500– 3,000/mm^3
Monocytes	3– 7	285– 500/mm^3
Eosinophils	1– 3	50– 250/mm^3
Basophils	0– 0.75	15– 50/mm^3

     (Infants and children have greater relative numbers of lymphocytes and monocytes)

Platelets   150,000– 350,000/mm^3

Reticulocytes: Adults   25,000– 75,000/mm^3

     0.5– 1.5% of erythrocytes

Corpuscular values of erythrocytes (adults)

     M.C.H. (mean corpuscular hemoglobin)   27– 31 pg

     M.C.V. (mean corpuscular volume)   80– 105 μ^3

     M.C.H.C. (mean corpuscular hemoglobin concentration)   32– 36%

Hematocrit

     Males   40– 54 ml/100 ml

     Females   37– 47 ml/100 ml

     Children (varies with age)   35– 49 ml/100 ml

Hemoglobin

     Males   14.0– 18.0 g/100 ml

     Females   12.0– 16.0 g/100 ml

     Children (varies with age)   11.2– 16.5 g/100 ml

Prothrombin time (one stage)   12.0– 14.0 s

[1] From P. B. Beeson and W. McDermott (Eds.). 1975. *Textbook of Medicine,* vol. II, 14th ed. Philadelphia: Saunders. M. M. Wintrobe, G. W. Thorn, R. D. Adams, E. Braunwald, K. J. Isselbacher, and R. G. Petersdorf (Eds.). 1974. *Harrison's Principles of Internal Medicine,* 7th ed. New York: McGraw-Hill.

Sedimentation rate	
Wintrobe: Males	0– 5 mm in 1 h
Females	0– 15 mm in 1 h
Westergren: Males	0– 15 in 1 hr
Females	0– 20 mm in 1 h

Blood, Plasma, and Serum Values

Ammonia, whole blood, venous	30– 70 μg/100 ml
Amylase, serum (Somogyi)	60– 180 units/100 ml
Arterial blood gases	
HCO_3^-	21– 18 meq/l
P_{CO_2}	35– 45 mmHg
pH	7.38– 7.44
P_{O_2}	80– 100 mmHg
Ascorbic acid, serum	0.4– 1.0 mg/100 ml
leukocytes	25– 40 mg/100 ml
Bilirubin, total, serum (Mallory-Evelyn)	0.3– 1.0 mg/100 ml
Direct, serum	0.1– 0.3 mg/100 ml
Indirect, serum	0.2– 0.7 mg/100 ml
Calcium, serum	4.5– 5.5 meq/l; 9– 11 mg/100 ml
Carbon dioxide-combining power, serum (sea level)	21– 28 meq/l; 50– 65 vol %
Carbon dioxide content, plasma (sea level)	21– 30 meq/l; 50– 70 vol %
Carotenoids, serum	50– 300 μg/100 ml
Ceruloplasmin, serum	27– 37 mg/100 ml
Cholesterol	
Total, serum (Man-Peters method)	180– 240 mg/100 ml
Esters, serum	100– 180 mg/100 ml
Creatinine, serum	1– 1.5 mg/100 ml
Fatty acids, serum	380– 465 mg/100 ml
Folic acid, serum	6– 15 ng/ml
Glucose (fasting)	
Blood (Nelson-Somogyi)	60– 90 mg/100 ml
Plasma	75– 105 mg/100 ml
Iron, serum	107 $\pm$ 31 μg/100 ml
Iron-binding capacity, serum	305 $\pm$ 32 μg/100 ml;
	20– 45% saturation
Ketones, total	0.5– 1.5 mg/100 ml
Lactic acid, blood	0,6– 1.8 meq/l
Lactic dehydrogenase, serum	
(Wrobleski)	200– 450 units/ml
(Wacker)	60– 100 units/ml
Lipids, total, serum	500– 600 mg/100 ml
Lipids, triglyceride, serum	50– 150 mg/100 ml
Magnesium, serum	1.5– 2.5 meq/l; 2– 3 mg/100 ml
Nitrogen, nonprotein, serum	15– 35 mg/100 ml
Osmolality, serum	280– 300 mOsm/kg water
Phospholipids, serum	150– 250 mg/100 ml
Phosphorus, inorganic, serum	1– 1.5 meq/l; 3– 4.5 mg/100 ml
Potassium, serum	3.5– 5.0 meq/l
Proteins, total, serum	5.5– 8.0 g/100 ml
Protein fractions, serum	
Albumin	3.5– 5.5 g/100 ml (50– 60%)
Globulin	2.0– 3.5 g/100 ml (40– 50%)
Pyruvic acid, serum	0– 0.11 meq/l
Riboflavin, erythrocyte	15– 19.9 μg/100 ml RBC

Sodium, serum	136– 145 meq/l
Thiamine (erythrocyte transketolase activity)	900– 1200 μg hexose/ml/h
Urea nitrogen, whole blood	10– 20 mg/100 ml
Uric acid, serum	3– 7 mg/100 ml
Vitamin A, serum	50– 100 μg/100 ml
Vitamin B$_{12}$, serum	200– 600 pg/ml
Vitamin E (tocopherols)	0.6– 1.5 mg/100 ml
Zinc, serum	120 $\pm$ 20 μg/100 ml

Urine

Ammonia	30– 50 meq/24 h
Calcium, usual diet	Less than 250 mg/24 h
Creatinine	15– 25 mg/kg body weight/24 h
Osmolality	38– 1400 mOsm/kg water
pH	4.6– 8.0; average 6.0
Solids, total	30– 70 g/l; average 50
Specific gravity	1.003– 1.030
Titratable acidity	20– 40 meq/24 h

Gastric Analysis

Basal gastric secretion (1 h)

	Concentration (Mean $\pm$ 1 SD)	Output (Mean $\pm$ 1 SD)
Male	25.8 $\pm$ 1.8 meq/l	2.57 $\pm$ 0.16 meq/h
Female	20.3 $\pm$ 3.0 meq/l	1.61 $\pm$ 0.18 meq/h

After histamine stimulation

Normal	Mean output = 11.8 meq/h
Duodenal ulcer	Mean output = 15.2 meq/h

After maximal histamine stimulation

Normal	Mean output = 22.6 meq/h
Duodenal ulcer	Mean output = 44.6 meq/h

Volume, fasting stomach content	50– 100 ml
Emptying time	3– 6 h
Specific gravity	1.006– 1.009
pH (adults)	0.9– 1.5

Index

80 81 82   10 9 8 7 6 5 4 3